Current Approach to Heart Failure

Maria Dorobanţu • Piotr Ponikowski
Frank Ruschitzka
Editors

Current Approach to Heart Failure

Second Edition

Springer

Editors
Maria Dorobanţu
Romanian Academy, Carol Davila
University of Medicine and Pharmacy
of Bucharest
Bucharest, Romania

Piotr Ponikowski
Institute of Heart Diseases
Wrocław Medical University
Wrocław, Poland

Frank Ruschitzka
Department of Cardiology
University Heart Center Department
of Cardiology
Zürich, Switzerland

ISBN 978-3-031-96561-6 ISBN 978-3-031-96562-3 (eBook)
https://doi.org/10.1007/978-3-031-96562-3

This Springer imprint is published by the registered company Springer Nature Switzerland AG
The registered company address is: Gewerbestrasse 11, 6330 Cham, Switzerland

Preface

It is with great pleasure that we present the second edition of *Current Approach to Heart Failure*. Since the publication of the first edition in 2017, the tremendous interest shown by readers and the significant number of downloads from the publisher's website have affirmed the value of this resource. This response has motivated us to update and expand the content, ensuring that it reflects the latest advancements in the rapidly evolving field of heart failure.

Heart failure continues to be a major global health challenge, with its incidence steadily increasing. In response, the medical community has made remarkable progress in understanding its pathophysiology, improving diagnostic tools, and refining treatment strategies. This second edition reflects these advancements, providing a comprehensive and practical guide for clinicians worldwide.

The book begins with foundational chapters on the epidemiology and pathophysiology of heart failure, incorporating new concepts that deepen our understanding of this complex syndrome. It then explores the critical role of imaging, with detailed chapters covering left ventricular systolic and diastolic dysfunction, right heart chambers, tricuspid valve, left atrial function, mitral regurgitation, aortic stenosis, cardiovascular magnetic resonance, and the increasingly valuable role of multimodality imaging.

On the therapeutic front, the book offers a detailed examination of contemporary pharmacological treatments, myocardial revascularization, ventricular arrhythmia management, mechanical circulatory support, cell and gene therapy, valvular surgery, and heart transplantation. It also addresses the challenges of managing heart failure in special populations, such as those with genetic cardiomyopathy, acute heart failure, preserved ejection fraction, frailty, oncologic conditions, and other unique patient groups.

This ambitious project would not have been possible without the exceptional contributions of our esteemed authors, each of whom is a renowned expert in their field. Their dedication, expertise, and hard work have made this book an authoritative and practical resource. We extend our heartfelt thanks to all contributors for their invaluable efforts.

We are also deeply grateful to Springer Publishing House for their partnership and support. We wish to thank Weston Grant and Ram Prasad Chandrasekar, whose guidance and encouragement were instrumental in bringing this project to fruition.

We are confident that this book will be an indispensable tool for doctors and healthcare professionals involved in the management of heart failure. Whether you are a seasoned cardiologist, a general practitioner, or a trainee, we hope this book will enhance your clinical practice and inspire further learning and collaboration.

Warm regards,

Bucharest, Romania — Maria Dorobanţu
Wrocław, Poland — Piotr Ponikowski
Zürich, Switzerland — Frank Ruschitzka

Contents

Part I
New Concepts on Mechanisms of Heart Failure

Chapter 1
New Concepts of Pathophysiology of Heart Failure

Tatiana Kuznetsova and Nicholas Cauwenberghs

Abstract It is of importance to better understand the pathophysiological mechanisms leading to heart maladaptation and the timely identification and management of patients at risk for developing symptomatic heart failure (HF). High blood pressure is the major modifiable risk factor for overt HF. In patients with hypertension the process of myocardial remodeling/dysfunction starts long before the onset of HF symptoms. The long-term increased afterload (high pressure) and, consequently, the chronically increased cardiac performance lead to left ventricular (LV) concentric remodeling, decreased longitudinal systolic deformation (strain), diastolic dysfunction and increased LV oxygen requirements. Atherosclerosis is another key pathological process leading to symptomatic HF. The buildup of plaque in the coronary arteries and therefore their narrowing lead to reduced oxygen supply to the heart muscle. The burdening of the heart resulting from the atherosclerotic process then accelerates the progression of cardiac remodeling and dysfunction. Recent studies revealed a high prevalence of asymptomatic LV systolic and diastolic dysfunction/remodeling in the community and their association with subclinical atherosclerotic lesions of coronary arteries. In this chapter we discussed the different aspects of cardiac maladaptive responses to a chronically increased hemodynamic load and atherosclerosis.

Keywords Hemodynamic load · Atherosclerosis · Concentric remodeling · Diastolic dysfunction · Deformation (strain) · Ventricular-arterial coupling

---

T. Kuznetsova (✉) · N. Cauwenberghs
Research Unit Hypertension and Cardiovascular Epidemiology, KU Leuven Department of Cardiovascular Sciences, University of Leuven, Leuven, Belgium
e-mail: tatiana.kouznetsova@kuleuven.be

M. Dorobanţu et al. (eds.), *Current Approach to Heart Failure*,
https://doi.org/10.1007/978-3-031-96562-3_1

Introduction

The normal heart is an efficient muscle that is designed to serve both as pump and integrator of two independent vascular systems, the pulmonary and systemic circulations. The capacity of the body to augment cardiac output, regulate systemic blood pressure (BP), and respond appropriately to elevations in heart rate and pre- and afterload depends on the properties of both the heart and the vasculature into which the left ventricle (LV) ejects blood [1]. Two components of systemic BP could be identified: the steady component, represented by mean arterial pressure (MAP), and the pulsatile component, represented by pulse pressure. MAP is determined by peripheral arterial resistance, which depends on the physical characteristics of the arterial tree and the volume of blood that the LV ejects. On the other hand, LV stroke volume and aortic compliance are major determinates of pulse pressure. In the absence of aortic stenosis, conventionally measured brachial BP provides a clinically useful estimate of LV afterload.

When a high afterload opposes LV ejection, reduction of the LV stroke volume could be observed in a short term. This reduction is further compensated by shifting the LV pump function to a higher energy level (the Frank-Starling mechanism) and by activating an autoregulatory mechanism (the Anrep response). However, the long-term increased afterload and, consequently, the chronically increased cardiac performance lead to adverse LV remodeling and dysfunction, increased LV oxygen requirements and eventually cause symptomatic heart failure (HF). On the other hand, the atherosclerotic process results in the build-up of plaque in the coronary arteries and therefore their narrowing leads to reduced oxygen supply to the heart muscle. Because the process of myocardial remodeling/dysfunction starts long before the onset of symptomatic HF, it is of importance to better understand the pathophysiological mechanisms leading to subclinical (asymptomatic) LV maladaptation and the timely identification of patients who are at risk for developing overt cardiac events. Hereby we discussed the different aspects of cardiac maladaptive responses to a chronically increased load as well as the burdening of the heart resulting from the atherosclerotic process.

LV Remodeling and Hypertrophy

For better understanding of cardiac mechanics, it is important to describe a relationship between pressure, volume, and wall stress of the LV. The law of Laplace is commonly used as a mathematical model to predict LV wall stress from given pressure and geometry [2]. According to this equation, LV wall stress is directly proportional to LV pressure and radius and is inversely proportional to the wall thickness of the LV (Fig. 1.1). Higher pressure can cause thickening of LV walls in order to accommodate an increased load and maintain normal wall tension. Indeed, hypertension induces a compensatory thickening of the LV wall in order to normalize

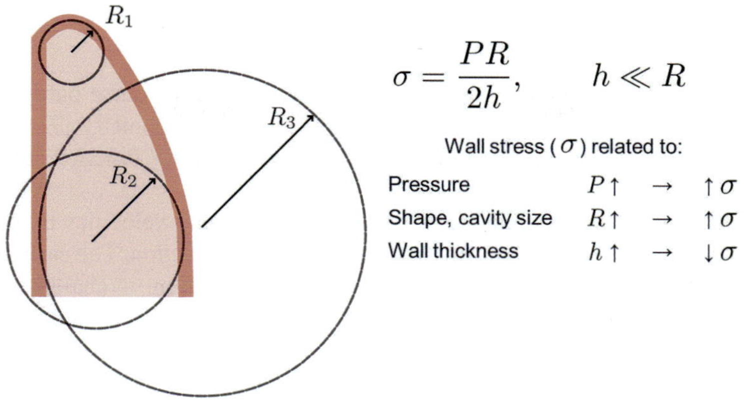

Fig. 1.1 Schematic representation of the law of Laplace, which states that wall tension is proportionate to the pressure (P) times radius (R). Therefore, wall stress (σ) is wall tension divided by wall thickness (h). At a given intraventricular pressure, wall stress increases with an increase in radius of the ventricular cavity

wall stress. Thus, patients with chronically increased afterload usually present with concentric remodeling or concentric LV hypertrophy, but have a normal-sized LV chamber and normal ejection fraction [3]. On the other hand, a hypertrophic LV is stiffer, so it requires elevated pressures to fill it, leading to a condition known as diastolic dysfunction.

Cardiac maladaptation such as LV remodeling or hypertrophy in response to chronically increased hemodynamic load is not a benign condition and is associated with increased risk of cardiovascular outcome, including HF [4, 5]. Several studies documented the relationship between LV hypertrophy detected by electrocardiography or echocardiography and an adverse prognosis. A meta-analysis including 48,545 subjects from 20 prospective studies showed that the adjusted risk of future cardiovascular morbidity associated with LV hypertrophy at baseline ranged from 1.5 to 3.5, with a weighted mean risk ratio of 2.3 for all studies together [6]. Several mechanisms may explain why adverse LV remodeling/hypertrophy is a harbinger of adverse cardiovascular outcomes. Firstly, LV hypertrophy or remodeling leads to increased LV stiffness and therefore diastolic filling abnormalities that predispose to symptomatic HF. Secondly, maladaptive LV remodeling leads to dysfunction of the autonomic nervous system, reduce coronary reserve, and increase LV oxygen requirements. Thirdly, it may predispose to ventricular arrhythmias and a greater risk of sudden death.

LV Diastolic Function

LV diastolic function tends to deteriorate over the adult life course particularly in patients with hypertension, paralleling changes in cardiac geometry [7]. Diastolic dysfunction refers to a condition in which abnormalities in LV function are present during diastole.

Assessment of intracardiac blood flows and myocardial velocities by echocardiography provide valuable information on LV diastolic function. The early stage of LV diastolic dysfunction, as impaired myocardial relaxation, is characterized by decreased transmitral early (E peak), and enhanced atrial (A peak) LV filling as well as less vigorous mitral annulus motion (e' peak) during early diastole. The more advanced stage of diastolic dysfunction is typically presented by increased LV end-diastolic filling pressure in response to increased LV stiffness. We might estimate LV filling pressure non-invasively by combining early transmitral blood flow velocity with early mitral annular velocity (E/e' ratio) [8]. Of notice, an accurate prediction of LV filling pressures for an individual patient requires further characterization of the intermediate E/e' group ("grey zone"), for instance by measurement of left atrial volume and deformation (strain), tricuspid regurgitation velocity and blood flow in the pulmonary vein [9].

Previous studies demonstrated that elderly women appear the most susceptible to the detrimental effects of increased pulsatile load on LV diastolic function [10–12]. This observation might be explained by the higher aortic pulsatile load and aortic stiffness, enhanced LV systolic performance, and lower LV compliance in women as compared to men [11, 13–15].

LV Deformation (Systolic Function)

LV deformation (strain) during systole is determined by the fiber structure and curvature of the myocardium and its interaction with local wall stress at the beginning of ejection, which decreases from the endocardium to epicardium and from the LV base to the apex [16]. During LV ejection, longitudinal deformation of the heart results from contraction of longitudinally oriented subendocardial and subepicardial fibers, whereas radial LV wall thickening mainly originates from contraction of circumferential fibers located in the mid-wall [17]. Gould et al. assessed the relation between the directional components of LV contraction and ejection fraction in 122 subjects with or without heart disease, by using angiocardiography [18]. The contribution of the longitudinal and radial components to total cardiac work was 14% and 40%, respectively [18]. It was suggested that separate analysis of the various components of LV systolic deformation might help us to understand the progression of LV systolic dysfunction at different stages of heart disease [19, 20].

Changes in LV Longitudinal Strain in Response to Increased MAP

Theoretical computer models of the heart predicted that LV systolic deformation in a longitudinal direction increases with higher cardiac output (preload) and decreases with increasing MAP (afterload) (Fig. 1.2) [21]. Because high systemic arterial pressure leads to increased LV wall stress, particularly deformation of the longitudinally oriented and less curved myofibers in the sub-endocardium is impaired. Thus, longitudinal systolic dysfunction could already be observed at early stages of progressive myocardial maladaptation related to chronically increased hemodynamic load [22].

Along similar lines, an experimental study involving an aortic banding model showed disparate changes in longitudinal and radial myocardial strain in response to acute alternation in LV afterload [23]. Longitudinal systolic function dramatically fell as afterload increased, whereas LV fractional shortening and radial strain were still preserved after mild banding [23]. Previous clinical studies reported depressed LV longitudinal function even in asymptomatic patients with hypertension as compared to normotensives controls [24–26]. In the presence of hypertension, subclinical impairment of LV longitudinal deformation appears worse if the high BP is longstanding and uncontrolled [27]. In another study in the general population, global longitudinal strain decreased significantly with increasing MAP (by 0.29% per 10 mmHg, $P < 0.01$) [6]. Moreover, LV longitudinal deformation declined stronger over time in individuals with higher MAP at baseline and stronger increase in MAP during follow-up [28].

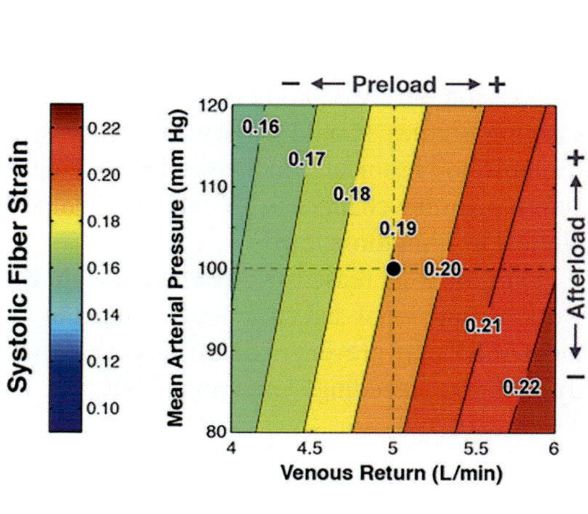

Fig. 1.2 Dependence of LV global LS (color gradient) to preload (venous return) and afterload (mean arterial pressure) in a normal heart. (Reproduced from Lumens et al. with permission [21])

Changes in LV Strain in Response to Increased Atrial Stiffness and Pulse Pressure

At systole, the heart ejects a volume of blood into the aorta and generates a forward pressure wave that is reflected at various sites in the arterial system. If the aorta is compliant, the aortic walls elastically expand to accommodate the ejected blood. An elastic aorta, therefore, dampens pulsatility and maintains a continuous blood flow from the heart to the periphery. Both hypertension and atherosclerosis accelerate the age-related stiffening of the large arteries including aorta, which plays a key role in the development of HF due to additional mechanical load on the heart [29]. Indeed, to expand stiffened arteries, the heart needs to produce greater pressure and therefore its energy expenditure increases [30–32]. In addition, increased pulse wave velocity (PWV) in stiffening arteries leads to an early return of the reflected wave which might, in turn, also augment late systolic LV load. On the other hand, as suggested recently, entrapment of reflected waves in the periphery might limit the influence of peripheral reflected waves on central hemodynamic and late systolic load [11].

Population studies showed that measures reflecting increased aortic stiffness such as a higher aortic PWV is associated with a higher risk of cardiovascular events including HF beyond traditional cardiovascular risk factors [33–36]. For instance, in an analysis including 7283 Framingham Study participants, greater aortic stiffness as reflected by increased aortic PWV was associated with multiple health outcomes [36]. In multivariable-adjusted analyses, a 1-SD increase in aortic PWV was associated with 20% and 21% higher risk for incidence of composite cardiovascular events and HF, respectively.

Along these lines, an age-dependent relationship between changes in LV radial systolic deformation and early and late systolic load was reported in a general population [14]. Radial strain increased significantly with higher central pulse pressure and PWV in middle-aged participants (50–60 years) only, whereas it decreased with these indexes in older subjects (above 70 years). These findings suggest that a chronic rise in pulse pressure increases LV load and enhances LV radial systolic performance, but eventually might lead to adverse LV remodeling and impaired radial deformation. This mechanism probably contributes to the development and progression of LV dysfunction in hypertensive patients. However, future serial imaging studies should clarify the progression of LV radial strain changes in response to chronically increased LV loading due to arterial stiffening. Figure 1.3 summarizes the changes in LV function components during the transition from subclinical to symptomatic HF.

Thus, both increased steady and pulsatile BP components evoke a complex network of functional and structural changes in the heart. As such, effective management of BP may prevent or delay the development of subclinical LV remodeling and dysfunction preceding symptomatic HF.

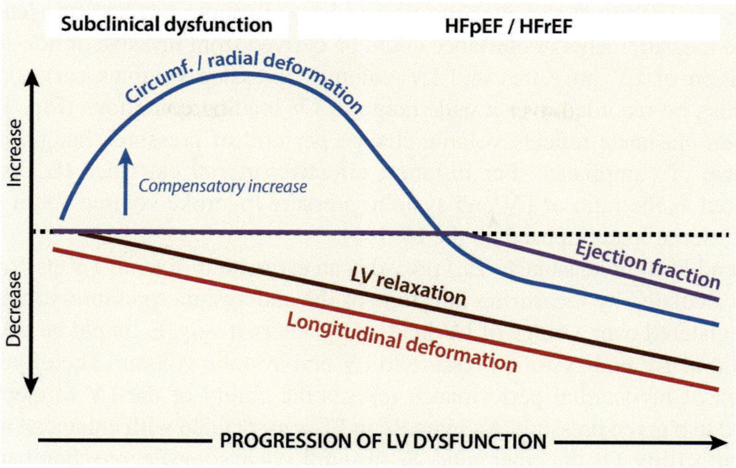

Fig. 1.3 The transition from subclinical to overt heart failure with preserved ejection fraction (HFpEF) or reduced ejection fraction (HFrEF) in arterial hypertension. Initially, hypertension-mediated changes in left ventricular (LV) function encompass reduced longitudinal shortening, and compensatory increased circumferential shortening to preserve LV ejection fraction. On the long run, circumferential/radial deformation progressively deteriorates, thereby gradually impairing the overall LV performance. (Modified from Ref. [37])

Atherosclerosis

Atherosclerosis, accelerated by hypertension, inflammation, and hypercholesterolemia is characterized by the buildup of plaques in the arterial walls. As highlighted in the previous section, the atherosclerotic process leads to an increase in arterial stiffness, which results to overload of the heart as it pumps against the increased pulsatile component. In addition, the accumulation of plaque in the coronary arteries and therefore their narrowing leads to reduced oxygen supply to the heart muscle. The burdening of the heart resulting from the atherosclerotic process then accelerates the progression to cardiac remodeling and dysfunction. Along these lines, several large-scale population studies have shown that subclinical coronary atherosclerotic disease burden, detected using coronary calcium scores, is independently associated with worse LV diastolic function and higher LV mass and volumes [38, 39].

Ventricular-Arterial Coupling

As highlighted in the previous section, the interaction of the heart with the systemic vasculature, or ventricular-arterial coupling, is a key determinant of cardiovascular performance. Therefore, simultaneous measurement of arterial and LV stiffness or elastance is important to better understand hemodynamic mechanisms leading to HF. The measurements of elastance could be derived from invasive or non-invasive registration of LV pressures and LV volumes (pressure-volumes curves), which might also be recorded over a wide range of LV loading conditions (Fig. 1.4). By definition elastance reflects volume change per unit of pressure change; it is the reciprocal of compliance. For instance, effective arterial elastance (E_a) could be calculated as the ratio of LV end-systolic pressure to stroke volume and it reflects the net arterial load imposed on the LV [40].

LV end-systolic elastance (E_{lv}) provides an estimate of overall LV performance and is calculated by measuring the slope of the end-systolic pressure-volume relations registered over a range of LV loads [40]. Alternatively, E_{lv} could be calculated as a ratio of LV end-systolic pressure to LV end-systolic volume. Therefore, E_{lv} as an index of myocardial performance reflects the ability of the LV to eject blood opposed to a given pressure. An increase in E_{lv} is associated with enhanced myocardial contractility. On the other hand, E_{lv} also reflects in some degree chamber geometry and passive myocardial stiffening, which could be altered in hypertensive patients. Indeed, numerous clinical studies [41–44] show that effective arterial and LV elastance based on invasive or non-invasive determination of LV volumes and end-systolic pressure are both increased in hypertensive patients. For instance, Cohen-Solal et al. [44] showed that E_a and E_{lv} as measured by angiography were significantly higher in 19 hypertensive patients as compared to 25 normotensive men. Later, Saba et al. [41] confirmed this finding using echocardiography for measurement of LV volumes and carotid pressure waveforms for assessment of ESP in 81 normotensive and 174 hypertensive patients. Furthermore, Chantler et al. [42] reported that the ventricular-arterial coupling ratio (E_a/E_{lv}) was about 25% lower in hypertensive compared with normotensive women. Along similar lines, we also

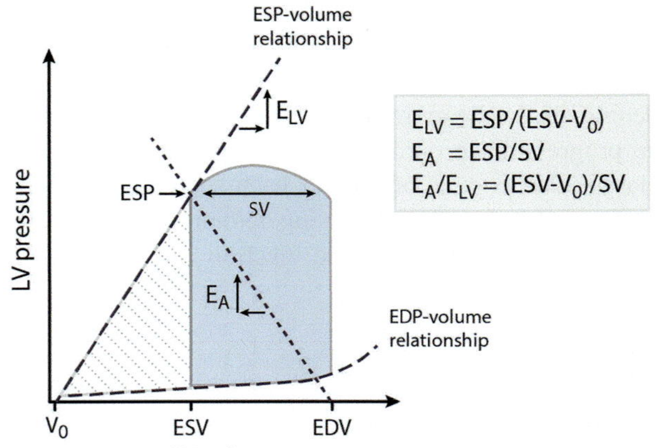

Fig. 1.4 Schematic representations of a pressure–volume loop and derived ventricular-arterial indexes. *EDV* indicates end-diastolic volume, *ESV* end-systolic volume, *ESP* end-systolic pressure, E_A arterial elastance, E_{LV} left ventricular end-systolic elastance, *LV* left ventricular, *SV* stroke volume

found that in hypertensive patients the ventricular-arterial coupling ratio at rest was 16.4% lower compared with normotensive subjects [43]. The lower ventricular-arterial coupling ratio in hypertensive patients was due to a disproportionate increase in E_{lv} compared with E_a (32% vs 10%) [43]. Therefore, in asymptomatic patients, a higher E_{lv} at rest might not only mean greater myocardial performance but also reflect geometrical and passive structural changes in hypertensive hearts.

Conclusion

As shown by epidemiological studies, hypertension and atherosclerosis are the most important modifiable risk factors for the development of symptomatic HF. Identifying patients at the early (asymptomatic) stages of HF would allow the institution of more aggressive risk management strategies and will likely decrease the progression to symptomatic disease.

In this regard, better understanding of pathophysiological mechanism of cardiac maladaptation in patients with hypertension is crucial for early detection of this condition. The chronically increased cardiac performance due to high afterload leads to LV concentric remodeling, impairment of LV systolic deformation and diastolic dysfunction. LV systolic and diastolic dysfunction coexists to varying degrees and appears very early in the course of hypertensive heart disease. Community-based studies revealed a higher than hitherto expected prevalence of LV systolic and diastolic dysfunction and their independent prognostic significance.

Hypertension and atherosclerosis also accelerate the age-related stiffening of the large arteries which plays an important role in the development of HF due to additional mechanical load on the heart. The heart typically adapts to confront higher systolic loads by both hypertrophy and LV stiffening. Increased vascular loading on the heart also contributes to LV dysfunction. Ventricular-arterial coupling disease has to be further explored in subjects with subclinical LV maladaptation.

References

1. De Tombe PP, Jones S, Burkhoff D, Hunter WC, Kass DA. Ventricular stroke work and efficiency both remain nearly optimal despite altered vascular loading. Am J Phys. 1993;264(6 Pt 2):H1817–24.
2. Moriarty TF. The law of Laplace. Its limitations as a relation for diastolic pressure, volume, or wall stress of the left ventricle. Circ Res. 1980;46(3):321–31.
3. Devereux RB, Roman MJ. Left ventricular hypertrophy in hypertension: stimuli, patterns, and consequences. Hypertens Res. 1999;22(1):1–9.
4. Zile MR, Gaasch WH, Patel K, Aban IB, Ahmed A. Adverse left ventricular remodeling in community-dwelling older adults predicts incident heart failure and mortality. JACC Heart Fail. 2014;2(5):512–22.

5. Velagaleti RS, Gona P, Pencina MJ, Aragam J, Wang TJ, Levy D, et al. Left ventricular hypertrophy patterns and incidence of heart failure with preserved versus reduced ejection fraction. Am J Cardiol. 2014;113(1):117–22.
6. Vakili BA, Okin PM, Devereux RB. Prognostic implications of left ventricular hypertrophy. Am Heart J. 2001;141(3):334–41.
7. Kuznetsova T, Thijs L, Knez J, Cauwenberghs N, Petit T, Gu YM, et al. Longitudinal changes in left ventricular diastolic function in a general population. Circ Cardiovasc Imaging. 2015;8(4):e002882.
8. Ommen SR, Nishimura RA, Appleton CP, Miller FA, Oh JK, Redfield MM, et al. Clinical utility of Doppler echocardiography and tissue Doppler imaging in the estimation of left ventricular filling pressures: a comparative simultaneous Doppler-catheterization study. Circulation. 2000;102(15):1788–94.
9. Kuznetsova T, Cauwenberghs N, Sabovčik F, Kobayashi Y, Haddad F. Evaluation of diastole by echocardiography for detecting early cardiac dysfunction: an outcome study. ESC Heart Fail. 2022;9(3):1775–83.
10. Shim CY, Park S, Choi D, Yang WI, Cho IJ, Choi EY, et al. Sex differences in central hemodynamics and their relationship to left ventricular diastolic function. J Am Coll Cardiol. 2011;57(10):1226–33.
11. Coutinho T, Borlaug BA, Pellikka PA, Turner ST, Kullo IJ. Sex differences in arterial stiffness and ventricular-arterial interactions. J Am Coll Cardiol. 2013;61(1):96–103.
12. Cauwenberghs N, Knez J, D'hooge J, Thijs L, Yang W-Y, Wei F-F, et al. Longitudinal changes in LV structure and diastolic function in relation to arterial properties in general population. JACC Cardiovasc Imaging. 2017;10(11):1307–16.
13. Borlaug BA. Sex, load, and relaxation: are women more susceptible to load-dependent diastolic dysfunction? J Am Coll Cardiol. 2011;57(10):1234–6.
14. Cauwenberghs N, Knez J, Tikhonoff V, D'hooge J, Kloch-Badelek M, Thijs L, et al. Doppler indexes of left ventricular systolic and diastolic function in relation to the arterial stiffness in a general population. J Hypertens. 2016;34(4):762–71.
15. Hayward CS, Kalnins WV, Kelly RP. Gender-related differences in left ventricular chamber function. Cardiovasc Res. 2001;49(2):340–50.
16. Choi HF, D'hooge J, Rademakers FE, Claus P. Distribution of active fiber stress at the beginning of ejection depends on left-ventricular shape. Conf Proc Annu Int Conf IEEE Eng Med Biol Soc IEEE Eng Med Biol Soc Annu Conf. 2010;2010:2638–41.
17. Spotnitz HM. Macro design, structure, and mechanics of the left ventricle. J Thorac Cardiovasc Surg. 2000;119(5):1053–77.
18. Gould KL, Kennedy JW, Frimer M, Pollack GH, Dodge HT. Analysis of wall dynamics and directional components of left ventricular contraction in man. Am J Cardiol. 1976;38(3):322–31.
19. Sengupta PP. Left ventricular transmural mechanics: tracking opportunities in-depth. J Am Soc Echocardiogr. 2009;22(9):1022–4.
20. Cheng S, Larson MG, McCabe EL, Osypiuk E, Lehman BT, Stanchev P, et al. Age- and sex-based reference limits and clinical correlates of myocardial strain and synchrony. Circ Cardiovasc Imaging. 2013;6(5):692–9.
21. Lumens J, Prinzen FW, Delhaas T. Longitudinal strain: "think globally, track locally". JACC Cardiovasc Imaging. 2015;8(12):1360–3.
22. Sengupta PP, Narula J. Reclassifying heart failure: predominantly subendocardial, subepicardial, and transmural. Heart Fail Clin. 2008;4(3):379–82.
23. Donal E, Bergerot C, Thibault H, Ernande L, Loufoua J, Augeul L, et al. Influence of afterload on left ventricular radial and longitudinal systolic functions: a two-dimensional strain imaging study. Eur J Echocardiogr. 2009;10(8):914–21.
24. Tadic M, Sala C, Carugo S, Mancia G, Grassi G, Cuspidi C. Myocardial strain in hypertension: a meta-analysis of two-dimensional speckle tracking echocardiographic studies. J Hypertens. 2021;39(10):2103–12.

25. Ballo P, Quatrini I, Giacomin E, Motto A, Mondillo S. Circumferential versus longitudinal systolic function in patients with hypertension: a nonlinear relation. J Am Soc Echocardiogr. 2007;20(3):298–306.
26. Baltabaeva A, Marciniak M, Bijnens B, Moggridge J, He FJ, Antonios TF, et al. Regional left ventricular deformation and geometry analysis provides insights in myocardial remodelling in mild to moderate hypertension. Eur J Echocardiogr. 2008;9(4):501–8.
27. Soufi Taleb Bendiab N, Meziane-Tani A, Ouabdesselam S, Methia N, Latreche S, Henaoui L, et al. Factors associated with global longitudinal strain decline in hypertensive patients with normal left ventricular ejection fraction. Eur J Prev Cardiol. 2017;24(14):1463–72.
28. Kuznetsova T, Nijs E, Cauwenberghs N, Knez J, Thijs L, Haddad F, et al. Temporal changes in left ventricular longitudinal strain in general population: clinical correlates and impact on cardiac remodeling. Echocardiography. 2019;36(3):458–68.
29. Kawaguchi M, Hay I, Fetics B, Kass DA. Combined ventricular systolic and arterial stiffening in patients with heart failure and preserved ejection fraction: implications for systolic and diastolic reserve limitations. Circulation. 2003;107(5):714–20.
30. Davies JE, Baksi J, Francis DP, Hadjiloizou N, Whinnett ZI, Manisty CH, et al. The arterial reservoir pressure increases with aging and is the major determinant of the aortic augmentation index. Am J Physiol Heart Circ Physiol. 2010;298(2):H580–6.
31. Wang JJ, O'Brien AB, Shrive NG, Parker KH, Tyberg JV. Time-domain representation of ventricular-arterial coupling as a windkessel and wave system. Am J Physiol Heart Circ Physiol. 2003;284(4):H1358–68.
32. Schultz MG, Davies JE, Hardikar A, Pitt S, Moraldo M, Dhutia N, et al. Aortic reservoir pressure corresponds to cyclic changes in aortic volume: physiological validation in humans. Arterioscler Thromb Vasc Biol. 2014;34(7):1597–603.
33. Vlachopoulos C, Aznaouridis K, Stefanadis C. Prediction of cardiovascular events and all-cause mortality with arterial stiffness. A systematic review and meta-analysis. J Am Coll Cardiol. 2010;55(13):1318–27.
34. Ben-Shlomo Y, Spears M, Boustred C, May M, Anderson SG, Benjamin EJ, et al. Aortic pulse wave velocity improves cardiovascular event prediction: an individual participant meta-analysis of prospective observational data from 17,635 subjects. J Am Coll Cardiol. 2014;63(7):636–46.
35. Tsao CW, Lyass A, Larson MG, Levy D, Hamburg NM, Vita JA, et al. Relation of central arterial stiffness to incident heart failure in the community. J Am Heart Assoc. 2015;4(11):e002189.
36. Vasan RS, Pan S, Xanthakis V, Beiser A, Larson MG, Seshadri S, et al. Arterial stiffness and long-term risk of health outcomes: the Framingham heart study. Hypertension. 2022;79(5):1045–56.
37. Cikes M, Solomon SD. Beyond ejection fraction: an integrative approach for assessment of cardiac structure and function in heart failure. Eur Heart J. 2016;37(21):1642–50.
38. Haddad F, Cauwenberghs N, Daubert MA, Kobayashi Y, Bloomfield GS, Fleischman D, et al. Association of left ventricular diastolic function with coronary artery calcium score: a project baseline health study. J Cardiovasc Comput Tomogr. 2022;16(6):498–508.
39. Yared GS, Moreira HT, Ambale-Venkatesh B, Vasconcellos HD, Nwabuo CC, Ostovaneh MR, et al. Coronary artery calcium from early adulthood to middle age and left ventricular structure and function. Circ Cardiovasc Imaging. 2019;12(6):e009228.
40. Sunagawa K, Sagawa K, Maughan WL. Ventricular interaction with the vascular system in terms of pressure-volume relationships. In: Ventriculo-vascular coupling: clinical, physiologic, and engineering aspects. New York: Springer; 1987. p. 210–39.
41. Saba PS, Ganau A, Devereux RB, Pini R, Pickering TG, Roman MJ. Impact of arterial elastance as a measure of vascular load on left ventricular geometry in hypertension. J Hypertens. 1999;17(7):1007–15.
42. Chantler PD, Melenovsky V, Schulman SP, Gerstenblith G, Becker LC, Ferrucci L, et al. The sex-specific impact of systolic hypertension and systolic blood pressure on arterial-ventricular coupling at rest and during exercise. Am J Physiol Heart Circ Physiol. 2008;295(1):H145–53.

43. Kuznetsova T, D'hooge J, Kloch-Badelek M, Sakiewicz W, Thijs L, Staessen JA. Impact of hypertension on ventricular-arterial coupling and regional myocardial work at rest and during isometric exercise. J Am Soc Echocardiogr. 2012;25(8):882–90.
44. Cohen-Solal A, Caviezel B, Himbert D, Gourgon R. Left ventricular-arterial coupling in systemic hypertension: analysis by means of arterial effective and left ventricular elastances. J Hypertens. 1994;12(5):591–600.

Chapter 2
Biomarkers for Heart Failure

Nicoleta-Monica Popa-Fotea and Maria Dorobanţu

Abstract Heart failure (HF) is the resultant consequence of various cardiovascular pathologies with different mechanisms and etiologies. These pathologies activate numerous pathophysiological pathways that drive to the initiation of neurohormonal system, oxidative stress, inflammation, myocardial stretch, and further on to fibrosis and apoptosis, resulting into a negative remodeling of the heart with impairment of the cardiac function. Despite the major advancement in the field of HF it is still characterized by high mortality and recurrent re-admissions with important burden on the health-care system. In this complex algorithm, an early diagnosis as well as prompt relapse of symptoms by specific biomarkers would contribute to a better prognosis and survival on long-term. This chapter discusses the most frequently used biomarkers in the clinical milieu, but also novel counterparts such as non-coding (microRNAs) or coding markers with their advantages and limitations.

Keywords Heart failure · Biomarkers · Inflammation · Fibrosis · Myocyte stretch · Myocyte injury · Neurohormonal activation · Oxidative stress

Introduction

Heart failure (HF) is a complex syndrome characterized by symptoms and/or signs induced by different cardiac conditions. The term HF is restricted to patients with clinical symptoms excluding the early phases with no clinical expression. The diagnosis of HF based solely on clinical data is challenging view the non-specific

N.-M. Popa-Fotea
Clinical Emergency Hospital, Bucharest, Romania

University of Medicine and Pharmacy "Carol Davila", Bucharest, Romania

M. Dorobanţu (✉)
University of Medicine and Pharmacy "Carol Davila", Bucharest, Romania

Romanian Academy, Bucharest, Romania

M. Dorobanţu et al. (eds.), *Current Approach to Heart Failure*,
https://doi.org/10.1007/978-3-031-96562-3_2

symptoms in the beginning of the disease, early diagnosis being paramount in reducing the mortality rate of the disease by the implementation of guideline-directed medical or interventional therapy whose efficiency in terms of reducing morbidity and mortality is proved in the most recent guidelines. Thus, biomarkers facilitating the early diagnosis are possible key elements as these could be able to establish the diagnosis and/or prognosis of cardiac dysfunction with high sensitivity and specificity at the very beginning of the heart dysfunction. A biomarker is defined by the International Program on Chemical Safety coordinated by the World Health Organization as "any substance, structure, or process that can be measured in the body or its products and influence or predict the incidence of outcome or disease" [1]. The ideal biomarker is capable of discriminating HF patients from healthy patients with an early expression in the progression of the disease, and easily and accurately detected by un-expensive methods. Few of the available biomarkers convey to the above mentioned characteristics, but each of them play a role in the continuum of HF diagnosis, risk stratification, prognosis and monitoring of treatment. Both the most recent European Society of Cardiology [2] and AHA/ACC/HFSA guidelines [3] provide solid evidence for natriuretic peptides in the diagnosis of HF with entire section dedicated to NPs role in heart failure management, being recommended as initial test in subjects with suspected HF to rule out the diagnosis. Unfortunately, the role of newer biomarkers is still not well established, thus not recommended for routine practice.

Biomarkers

Biomarkers are involved in numerous pathophysiological heart failure pathways with potential role in clinical diagnosis, prognosis or therapeutic monitoring. These can be divided into systemic or organ specific biomarkers and have been synthetized in Fig. 2.1. The systemic biomarkers play roles in neurohormonal activation (endothelin-1, anti-diuretic hormone (ADH), adrenomedullin (ADM) or mid-regional (MR)-pro-ADM, norepinephrine), oxidative stress (myeloperoxidase (MPO), uric acid, reactive oxygen species) and inflammation (C-reactive protein (CRP), procalcitonin, Il-1, Il-6, TNF-α). Among organ specific biomarkers are those with cardiac involvement promoting myocardial fibrosis and hypertrophy (galectin-3 or soluble source of tumorigenicity-2 (sST2)), myocyte injury (cardiac troponins (c-Tn) or high sensitivity c-Tn, heart-type fatty acid binding protein (h-FABP)), or myocardial stretch (brain natriuretic peptide (BNP) or N-terminal-pro-BNP (NT-pro-BNP), adrenomedullin, growth differentiation factor-15 (GDF-15), microRNAs) and markers depicting the cardio-renal syndrome (cystatin C and neutrophil gelatinase-associated lipocalin (NGAL)).

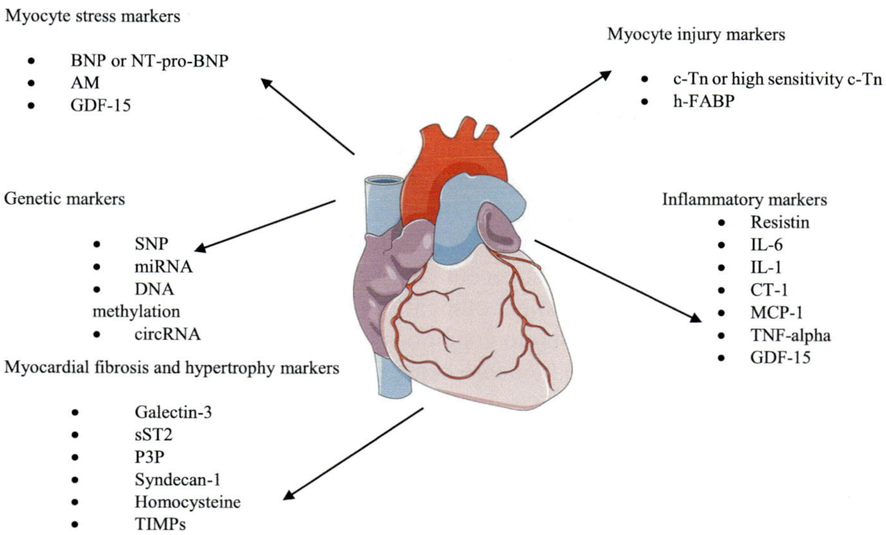

Fig. 2.1 Main biomarkers and their role in heart failure. *AM* adrenomedullin, *BNP* brain type natriuretic peptide, *circRNA* circular RNA, *CT-1* cardiotrophin-1, *c-Tn* cardiac troponin, *DNA* deoxyribonucleic acid, *Gal-3* galectine-3, *GDP-15* growth differentiation peptide-15, *h-FABP* heart-type fatty acid binding protein, *IL-1* interleukine-1, *IL-6* Interleukine-6, *MCP-1* monocyte chemoattractant protein-1, *miRNA* microRNAs, *MMPs* matrix metalloproteinases, *NT-pro-BNP* N-terminal-pro-brain type natriuretic peptide, *PIIINP* N-terminal pro-peptide of procollagen type III, *SNP* single nucleotide polymorphism, *sST2* soluble suppressor of tumorigenicity-2, *TIMPs* tissue inhibitor metalloproteinases, *TNF-alpha* tumor necrosis factor-alpha. (The Figure was partly generated using Servier Medical Art, provided by Servier, licensed under a Creative Commons Attribution 3.0 unported license)

Cardiac Specific Biomarkers

Myocyte Stress Markers

Natriuretic Peptides

The biomarkers with the highest level of recommendation according to the guidelines are natriuretic peptides (NP). In the most recent ESC HF guidelines, BNP/NT-pro-BNP have a class I level of recommendation, level of evidence B, to rule out a suspected chronic HF, and class IIa, level of evidence B to rule out acute HF. The thresholds to rule out the diagnosis of chronic HF are BNP < 35 pg/mL, NT-proBNP < 125 pg/mL or MR-proANP < 40 pmol/L and higher in the case of acute HF (BNP < 100 pg/mL, NT-proBNP < 300 pg/mL or MR-proANP < 120 pmol/L), values that are rather for excluding HF, than for confirming the diagnosis. Different from the ESC guidelines, the American counterparts, ACC/AHA/HFSA, recommend as class I, BNP/NT-proBNP to stratify the prognosis of patients admitted for HF, or as class IIa for estimating the prognosis after discharge for the long-term prognosis [3]. Notwithstanding, data about the association between changes in the plasmatic levels of natriuretic peptides and major adverse cardiovascular events are scarce. One study shows absolute risk increase in cardiovascular death or heart failure hospitalization for any two given concentrations of NPs in subjects with coronary artery disease and type 2 diabetes [4]. Although the same study pinpoints that a single NP measurement is predictive enough for the short-term outcomes without need for serial sampling, in accordance with ELIXA trial [5], this demonstrates that the most predictive NP is the most recent sample, the value on which clinicians should base to change their patient clinical course.

A special note is to be given to conditions associated with NP deficiency, the most frequently mentioned in literature being obesity and type 2 diabetes mellitus [6]; this state is associated with the development of cardiometabolic syndrome and could become a path for treatment. Furthermore, any other factors that interfere with the plasmatic values of BP, such as age, gender, race, in the direction of decreasing the values, can make HF diagnosis cumbersome mainly when BNP levels are under the clinically accepted cut-offs. The interpretation of BNP levels is to be considered in conjunction with all factors driving to increased levels, such renal dysfunction, sacubitril/valsartan, female gender, as all these may interfere with their interpretation. The notion of biomarker guided HF therapy is not new, but studies are not consistent in their results. The studies revealing favorable results by using NPs were small and the decrease in adverse events was driven mainly by a more careful monitoring of patients. The largest trial to date investigating a NT-proBNP guided management of reduced ejection HF (HFrEF) patients in the GUIDE-IT was terminated earlier as no superiority could be demonstrated [7]. Despite these unfavorable studies it is to mention that the patients with optimal adjusted guidelines directed medical therapy had better outcomes, supporting the idea derived from the guidelines that targeting the maximally tolerated dosages is more important than a biomarker guided treatment. The interception of the NP system proved to be essential for the treatment of HF, either through RAAS inhibitors or angiotensin receptor-neprilysin inhibition (ARNi), but this system can be targeted also at other levels with recombinant adeno-associated viral vectors encoding ANP, pro-BNP, but until now the methods used had a reduced rate of transduction and lack of effect [8]. Mutant ANP is a form of ANP that is resistant to the neprilysin degradation proving to be efficient in resistant arterial hypertension; a phase I clinical trial still recruiting patients of Afro American origin with resistant arterial hypertension analysis the properties of this drug although the long term effects are unknown (ClinicalTrials.gov identifier: NCT0454268). The stimulation of downstream signaling pathways such that of guanylate cyclase-A/cGMP/PKG could represent a new approach for the NP augmentation therapy; PDE9A is a phosphodiesterase that has a negative downregulation on the cGMP pathway and therefore inhibition of PDE9A proved to have positive influence on the neurohormonal activation and hemodynamic stress.

Adrenomedullin

Adrenomedullin (ADM) is a hormone with the role to decrease vascular resistance upregulated an increased volume overload inducing natriuresis and diuresis. ADM has a very short half-time making this an impractical biomarker, therefore MR-proADM is a better surrogate as it is release in equimolar ratio as ADM [9]. Congestion is the primary cause for re-admissions for most HF patients. Up-regulation of several pathways were demonstrated, among them ADM, one study showing this could be a potential biomarker in congestive HF [10], with others such as soluble ST2, GDF-15, FABP4, IL-6, FGF-23, FGF-21, CA-125 [11]. Furthermore, plasmatic ADM proved to be a marker for the severity of acute HF in subjects with acute coronary syndromes. Higher plasma MR-proADM levels in subjects with chronic HF correlates with increased risk of death and HF hospitalizations, and in combination with an increased use of loop diuretics are associated with a more higher likelihood of severe disease progression [12]. In contrast with NP decreasing irrespective of the residual congestion status, one study proved that MR-proADM was the best predictor for congestion [13], guiding physicians to more aggressively treat their patients. Adrecizumab, a monoclonal antibody against the N-terminal ADM, with a single intravenous infusion administration used in systemic inflammation and septic shock in AdrenOSS-2 trial, increases the levels of ADM by translocation of pre-existing ADM, maintaining this in circulation, with restoration of vascular integrity and less vasodilation, making this a potential target for HF therapy. A safety trial using a single infusion of adrecizumab in patients hospitalized with AHF (NCT04252937) is still recruiting patients and will produce more data about this new heart failure drug.

Growth Differentiation Factor-15 (GDF-15)

GDF-15 emerged as a relatively novel biomarker predicting cardiovascular events in some of the studies, while in others failed to show any correlation. A recent study, PARADIGM-HF is one of the studies showing discordance in GDF-15. Despite being a predictor of overall and cardiac mortality as well as a prognostic indicator of chronic HF in a meta-analysis [14], its plasmatic levels were not modified by sacubitril-valsartan, a drug that significantly decreases all these events compared with control. It is a marker that can predict the adverse outcomes during 1-year follow-up after an hospitalization of AHF in a multi-parametric predictor model [15] and furthermore a marker of sudden cardiac death due to incident myocardial infarction [16]. GDF-15 holds various roles in very different domains, such as estimating the bleeding risk in atrial fibrillation, or all-cause mortality, suggesting that it is rather an integrated systemic biomarker rather than a specific cardiac biomarker similar to others (Il-1, Il-6, hs-CRP).

MicroRNAs

MicroRNAs are non-coding RNAs that regulate at a post-translational level the expression of the mRNA. The aberrant activation of pathways in heart failure is associated with abnormal expression of miRNAs, that can be promising biomarkers. In a metanalysis that analyzed the profiling of miRNAs in HF in 55 studies revealed that mir-21, miR-30c, miR-210-3p, let-7i-5p, miR-129, let-7e-5p, and miR-622. The precise role of the mentioned above miRNAs is diverse covering all neurohormonal and cellular mechanism of HF. For example, miR-21 is involved in collagen expression in the heart, promoting fibrosis and hypertrophy, but its inhibition did not show favorable remodeling of the heart. miR-210 improves the heart function on a murine model of myocardial infarction by improving angiogenesis, this being the main miRNA involved in the stimulation of angiogenesis. miR-622 is increased in HF with reduced ejection function with good discrimination of HF as well as correlation with LVEF. miR-129-5p has a protective role by reduction inflammatory answer and hemodynamic parameters in a rat model of HF [17]. MicroRNA let-7i [18] suppresses cardiac inflammation and fibrosis by reducing the expression of IL-6 and other collagenases, its levels being reduced in dilated cardiomyopathy, coronary artery disease, while let-7e is increased in hypertensive individuals and heart development [19]. Thum and collaborators proved through the inhibition of miR-132 improves cardiac function and cardiomyocyte metabolism in a phase 1b, double-blind, place-controlled study [20]. Although this is only the start of the human use of antisense oligonucleotides in the treatment of HF, is a tremendous step forward for the field, with this new drug-proof of a concept. miR-1 is downregulated in patients with LVEF dysfunction and even lower in those with dilated left ventricle [21], the same being valid with miR-150-5p [22]. miRNA play also an important role in the assessment of the prognostic in HF. miR-22-3p correlated in a prospective study with the primary endpoint that included HF hospitalization, cardiovascular mortality, cardiac transplantation and left ventricle assistance device implantation [23]. miR-192 expression was associated with survival in ischemic cardiomyopathy compared with the non-ischemic cardiomyopathy and represents a prognostic marker in heart failure with ischemic etiology [24].

Myocyte Injury

Cardiac Troponins

Cardiac troponin I and T are isoforms unique for the cardiomyocyte being sensitive and specific for detecting for the cardiac injury. The increase of troponins is a frequent association in subjects presenting with acute HF even in the absence of myocardial ischemia. Although useful in risk stratification of both acute and chronic HF individuals, in the absence of acute coronary syndromes extremely cautious interpretation is required for clinicians, see that the actual troponin assays are extremely sensitive detecting increased levels even in healthy subjects seen the magnificent improvement in the immunoassays available on the market, with the limit of detection as low as 0.5 ng/ml. In a cohort of subjects with HFrEF admitted for decompensation, troponin I at 1 month independently predicted all-cause mortality, cardiovascular mortality and re-hospitalizations for HF at 1 year [25]. Similarly, in another study investigating this time HF with preserved ejection fraction elevated hs-TnT at discharge predicted adverse events [26]. Despite the role of hs-cTn in the diagnosis of myocardial infarction as cause of AHF, its informative role in chronic HF is still speculative. Troponin levels proved to predict prognosis expressed as cardiovascular death and HF hospitalization in subjects with stable ambulatory HF in a sub-analysis of subjects from TOPCAT [27]. Although it is not recommended to guide the drug therapy upon the hs-cTn levels, therapy with sacubitril/valsartan proved to with associated with lower hs-cTn at 1 and 2 months compared with those treated with enalapril [28], suggesting a possible role of this biomarker in the escalation of HF.

Heart-Type Fatty Acid Binding Protein (h-FABP)

Heart-type fatty acid binding protein (h-FABP) is protein found in the cytosol that transports long-chain fatty acids in the cardiomyocyte, its release in circulations being a consequence of the myocyte injury. Recognized as a marker of myocardial infarction, it has also roles in HF and pulmonary embolism. The dynamics of h-FABP predicted similarly with NP cardiac mortality and HF readmissions in a population of subjects with acute decompensated chronic HF. Other studies have found h-FABP to be a good predictor of outcomes in chronic stable HF, either with LV dysfunction of preserved LVEF [29]. In a small study it was shown that h-FABP is a very subtle biomarker of myocardial injury along with cardiac troponins with elevation in subjects with diastolic disfunction [30], but still asymptomatic.

Myocardial Fibrosis and Hypertrophy

In the cardiac specific category of biomarkers related to fibrosis and hypertrophy the most studied biomarkers are: soluble suppressor of tumorigenicity 2 (sST2), galectin-3 (Gal-3), N-terminal pro-peptide of procollagen type III (P3P), syndecan-1, homocysteine and tissue inhibitor metalloproteinases (TIMPs).

Soluble Suppressor of Tumorigenicity 2

ST2 is an IL-1 receptor family member that exists in two isoforms, soluble and transmembranar, its biological effects being through IL-33. The attachment of IL-33 to the transmembranar receptor-ST2 is cardioprotective by inhibition of myocardial fibrosis and cardiomyocyte hypertrophy. The other isoform, soluble ST2 exerts its effects by mediating the interaction of transmembrane ST2 with IL-33. Suppressor of tumorigenicity 2 secretion is activated by the mechanical strain of cardiac myocytes proportionally with diastolic overload [31]. The prognostic value of ST2 in acute HF and chronic HFrEF [32] is well established, many studies showing a good correlation with mortality at 1 year as well as with HF severity. Compared with other parameters, sST2 seems to be less depend on age, sex, renal function or body mass index, making this a better good marker for HF diagnosis in subjects with renal dysfunction compared with natriuretic peptides. A cut-off of 35 ng/ml predicted the risk of cardiovascular events making this a marker of monitoring chronic HF subjects [33]. In one study that enrolled both HFpEF and HFrEF proving prognostic correlations, the best was seen in hypertensive patients with HFpEF in direct correlation with high pulmonary wedge pressures and collagen dependent stiffness [34]. This supports the idea that ST2 is involved in HFpEF development at least by the pro-fibrotic effect in hypertensive subjects. A meta-analysis showed by pooling the data a difference of 1.56 ng/ml between those with severe and less severe disease [35]. Although not endorsed by guidelines for diagnosis and risk stratification of HF, sST2 has additional prognostic value. A combination with NPs, hs-cTn in a multi-parametric kit might increase the prognostic ability of each of the included biomarkers.

Galactin-3

Gal-3 is a member of the beta-galactosidase lectin family, released by activated macrophages in the cardiomyocytes as shown on heart biopsies, being colocalized with activated macrophages, inducing myocardial fibrosis and promoting ventricular remodeling. Studies proved that expression of Gal-3 in hypertrophic ventricles correlates with the development of HF [36]. Gal-3 is an independent marker of incident HF and all-cause mortality in Framingham Offspring Cohort [37]. As showed above Gal-3 is increased in chronic HF, but interestingly it has good discrimination value also for acute HF to identify individuals that need closed follow-up after discharge [37]. Gal-3 could be measured in asymptomatic individuals to identify fibrosis in early stages, and thus allowing the prompt initiation of specific treatment. In one study, Gal-3 serum levels proved to be superior to NT-proBNP in estimating short-term 60 days-prognosis with an area under the curve of 0.74 compared with 0.67. Additionally, Gal-3 in conjunction with NT-proBNP enhances the predictive value.

This biomarker has more prognostic than diagnostic value, a continuously increasing level translating greater risk for adverse cardiovascular outcomes [38].

Gal-3 has the ability to predict mortality up to 4 years after a single measurement at admission independently of other echocardiographic measurements [39].

N-Terminal Pro-peptide of Procollagen Type III (P3P)

N-terminal pro-peptide of procollagen III is a well-known marker of fibrosis in patients with hepatic disorders. One study showed an increase in P3P in a cohort of subjects with acute HF consequently to liver and renal dysfunction [40]. P3P is also a marker of target organ damage in hypertensive individuals which have significantly greater serum levels of P3P when exertional symptoms develop and in patients with advanced HF compared to asymptomatic counterparts [41]. It can be also used as a marker of prognosis, as higher levels of P3P is associated with a higher probability of developing HFpEF after 3 years of follow-up, along with other markers Gal-3, C-terminal pro-peptide of procollagen type I and NT-proBNP. In the RALES trial the administration of aldosterone antagonist, spironolactone, was associated with a decreased P3P in those having an increase of the baseline procollagen [42]. P3P is also an independent marker of prognosis for all-cause mortality in acute decompensated HF, with an incremental value in combination with NT-pro-BNP for survival [43]. Its levels increase in the process of remodeling in adult and pediatric populations with dilated cardiomyopathy being a marker of cardiac remodeling [44].

Syndecan-1

Syndecan-1 is a part of the transmembrane proteoglycan family to which growth factor binding glycosaminoglycans attaches. It plays an important role in regulating inflammation responses. In acute myocardial infarction the levels of syndecan-1 are elevated due to the damage of the glycocalyx [45]. Elevated levels of syndecan-1 are associated with worse outcomes in subjects with cardiogenic shock. It also correlated with clinical outcomes in HFpEF, but not in HFrEF in Trump et al. study [46], while in another study negative outcomes associated also with high syndecan-1 in reduced EF subjects of non-ischemic etiology [47]. Syndecan-1 is also a marker of liver and kidney impairment in acute heart failure, similar with NT-pro-BNP and troponins. A level of syndecan-1 higher than 120 ng/ml associated with mortality at 6 months after ST-segment elevation myocardial infarction independently of the myocardial injury as marker of endothelial disruption [48]. Apart from its role in HF, syndencan-1 was overexpressed in thoracic aortic aneurysm compared with healthy aortas, while in other reports syndecan-1 protected from the development of abdominal aortic aneurysm, the exact mechanism driving to these disparities being unknown [49]. One study (CIPHER) still recruiting patients with acute decompensated heart failure complicated by cardiogenic shock will phenotype this category of subjects to have a better understanding of the mechanism involved in cardiogenic shock (NCT04323371) through interleukine-6, angiopoietin 2, metabolomics, but also through endothelial glycocalyx perturbation markers, syndecan-1 and heparan sulfate.

Homocysteine

Meta-analysis showed an increase in the risk of coronary heart disease with the increase in homocysteine levels [50], but the impact of hyper-homocysteine on the incidence and prognosis of HF is unclear. In a Mendelian randomization study there was no link between higher homocysteine levels predicted genetically and appearance congestive HF or cardiomyopathy [51], while in another meta-analysis the plasmatic levels were raise in HF subjects compared with controls related with NYHA class. The levels of homocysteine are significantly increased in subjects with chronic HF [52] being associated with more decompensations and death. A cohort study showed that plasmatic homocysteine is an independent marker for adverse clinical events in subjects with reduced left ventricular ejection fraction HF [53]. Despite that numerous randomized trials investigated if acid folic supplementation to reduce homocysteine levels decreases coronary heart disease and HF the results reported are controversial and at present there is no recommendation for such treatment.

Metalloproteinases and Tissue Inhibitor Metalloproteinases (TIMPs)

Metalloproteinases are enzymes actively involved in the degradation of the extracellular matrix involved directly in left ventricular remodeling. Tissue inhibitor metalloproteinases bind to metalloproteinases to form a complex that will further inhibit the activity of MMPs. Concerning MMPs and TIMPs, even if each individual marker has an important contribution, panels with multi-markers increase the sensitivity and specificity of diagnosis.

Increased TIMP-1 correlates with reduced recovery of left ventricular ejection fraction in acute HF subjects [54]. TIMP-2 correlates with left ventricular ejection fraction, quality of life and functional capacity, as well as with MMP2 [55]. In Framingham study, TIMP-1 in the absence of HF, the plasmatic levels correlated with diabetes mellitus, active smoking status, but also with echocardiographic parameters suggestive a negative correlation with left ventricular function [56]. Irrespective of the cause of the HF the rise in TIMP-1 suggests this is a good marker for HF and possibly, a treatment target. Increased MMP2 and TIMP-4 with decreased MMP-8 correlated with diastolic left ventricular disfunction [57]. Increased overload is associated with cardiac expression of TIMP-1 and TIMP-2 in relation with the degree of interstitial fibrosis [58]. TIMP-3 deficiency in animal models induced dilated cardiomyopathy due to an increase in the activity of MMP-9 [59]. In subjects with chronic HF, TIMP-1 and not MMP-9 associated with overall mortality [60].

The increase of the ratio between MMP/TIMPs is associated with collagen accumulation and arterial hypertension. In more advanced hypertension, when there is also cardiac remodeling with diastolic HF, high MMP9/TIMP1 ratios is a sign of myocardium disfunction.

Inflammatory Biomarkers

Numerous biomarkers associated with inflammation are increased in HF, such as resistin, IL-6, IL-1, cardiotrophin-1 (CT-1), monocyte chemoattractant protein-1 (MCP-1), TNF-alpha, growth differentiation factor 15 (GDF-15), etc.

Resistin

Resistin is a hormone secreted by adipocytes being primary associated by diabetes mellitus, insulin resistance, but less with HF. Resistin correlated with pressure and volume overload in animal models, thus being a marker of neurohormonal stress at the level of the heart [61]. In a resistin knock-out model cardiac dysfunction and hypertrophy were diminished, the amelioration of heart function being related with decrease in myocardial fibrosis [62]. Resistin proves also to be a predictor of left ventricular remodeling and major adverse cardiovascular event post-acute myocardial infarction. Resistin is also a biomarker predicting incident HF, more precisely reduced left ventricular ejection HF and not preserved left ventricular ejection fraction HF.

Cardiotrophin-1

Cardiotrophin-1 (CT-1) is a member of the IL-6 cytokine superfamily, which included IL-11, leukemia inhibitory factor and ciliary neurotrophic factor. It was discovered as a cytokine with hypertrophic and cardioprotective effect. Its expression is present both in the fetal an adult heart, but also in other organs such as colon, ovaries, fetal kidney and lungs where has different and various functions. Zolk et al. showed that in the left ventricle with chronic HF there was an increase of the CT-1 mRA and protein expression as an answer to the hemodynamic overload [63]. CT-1 promotes beneficial cardiac remodeling by reducing caspase activation via casein kinase 2, suggesting that exogenous CT1 protein delivery could be a new therapeutic option. Furthermore, the plasmatic levels of CT-1 are predictive for mortality and heart failure after acute myocardial infarction, being a reliable marker for atherosclerotic cardiovascular disease [64].

IL-6

IL-6 is an important initiator of inflammation cascade inducing the secretion of C-reactive protein by the liver as well as a driver for changing the acute to chronic inflammation [65]. Higher concentrations of IL-6 are associated with worse outcomes in HF predicting major adverse cardiac events in chronic HF subjects or post-acute myocardial infarction [66]. RESCUE trial (Reduction in Inflammation in Patients With Advanced Chronic Renal Disease Utilizing Antibody Mediated IL-6 Inhibition) proved that ziltivekimab, a monoclonal anti-IL-6 reduced the markers of inflammation without serious side effects, such as infections or thrombocytopenia [67]. Making use of these results, ZEUS trial (NCT05021835) will compare ziltivekimab to placebo in patients with chronic kidney disease and elevated C-reactive protein to determine if this anti-inflammatory drug reduces cardiovascular events. Other outcomes of ZEUS will be the role of ziltivekimab on the contractile function.

IL-1

IL-1 is a major inflammatory marker in HF. The activation of IL-1β from the pro-protein is dependent on NOD-like receptor family, pyrin domain containing 3 (NLRP3) inflammasome and casapase-1. In HF, IL-1 derives cardiac dysfunction by inducing fibrosis, apoptosis, arterial stiffness and microvascular disfunction. The anti-IL-1 treatment in the form of anakinra, an IL-1 receptor antagonist proved to be efficient in both reduced left ventricular ejection HF [68] as well as preserved left ventricular ejection fraction HF [69] decreasing the risk for re-hospitalizations and death. When added to statins, in CANTOS study, canakinumab, a monoclonal antibody anti-IL-1β, reduced major adverse cardiovascular events compared with placebo [70].

MCP-1

The chemokine monocyte chemoattractant protein 1 (MCP-1) is key in the development of the atherosclerotic plaque inducing the progression of atherosclerosis, but it is also up-regulated in other cardiac diseases such as dilated cardiomyopathy or congestive HF, its expression being associated with the progression of the disease [71]. Considering the extensive role of MCP-1 in cardiac dysfunction, the anti-chemokines treatment for HF is a promising new path, but still after decades of experiments it is now at early stages. In a phase II clinical trial an anti CCR2(the cognate MCP-1 receptor)/CCR5 inhibitor showed improved of inflammation in subjects with non-alcoholic steatohepatitis [72], but the effects in HF have not been tried due to concerns regarding the dual role of the MCP-1 both in the downregulation of inflammation, but also in the stimulation of angiogenesis.

TNF-Alpha

TNF-alpha is a key pro-inflammatory marker that have been studied on a large scale in HF. The biological effects of TNF-alpha are mediated into the cell by NF-κB, that have dual effects depending on the type of receptors TNF-alpha activates: TNFα activation of TNF receptor 1 is deleterious while activation of TNF receptor 2 is beneficial. TNFα inhibits beta-adrenergic receptor function resulting in the inability of these receptors to respond to the sympathetic stimuli. The reduction in the beta-adrenergic receptor response increases the sympathetic hormones that like in a feedback loop elevates TNFα. The ATTACH study, a randomized, double-blind, placebo-controlled, pilot trial with Infliximab, a chimeric Monoclonal antibody to TNF-α, in patients with moderate-to-severe HF did not improve the clinical condition, but actually caused a deterioration [73], emphasizing once again the gap between proof of principle and hypothesis testing.

Genetic Biomarkers

Heart failure is a polygenic complex disease and the identification of specific HF loci as well as single nucleotide polymorphisms (SNP) is not associated with modifications in diagnosis and treatment. A systematic review addressed biomarkers in HF and showed that there is some associations of polymorphisms in specific genes with HF. Compared with the other genetic markers, SNP were determined only in peripheral blood, excluding the expression in cardiac tissue as SNP of a gene may include many allelic variants and thus complicated markers for screening [74]. Single nucleotide polymorphisms in many genes were found to be increased in HF such as HDC, VDR, ADA, HRH3, IL-17A, MHRT, HSPB7, ErbB4, TNF-alpha, LEP, AGT. DNA hypomethylation of B9 protein domain 1 and doublecortin-like kinase 2, and hypermethylation of neurotrimin with good under the curve areas for predicting HF also confirmed in myocardial tissue [75]. Circular RNA is a single stranded-RNA that different from linear RNA form a continuous loop with 3′ and 5′ ends joined together. From circRNA, hsa_circ_0097435 [76], hsa_circ_0112085, hsa_circ_0062960, hsa_circ_0053919 and hsa_circ_0014010 [77] were found to be highly expressed in peripheral blood of HF subjects. The cardiac-specific miRs (myomiRs), mir-208b(1), mir-208a(1), and mir-499(1), and the muscle-specific mir-1-1(4) and mir-133b(2) were significantly higher in subjects with advanced HF compared with healthy controls with decrease of these miRs after left ventricular assist device [78]. MiR-26a-5p and miR-150-5p were downregulated in advanced HF compared with moderate HF and healthy subjects [22]. The modification of lcRNA heart-disease-associated transcript 2 (Heat2) was validated in various cohort as a HF biomarker mainly in those with reduced ejection fraction [79], while RNA taurine upregulated gene 1 (TUG1) has good correlation in subjects with hypertensive preserved ejection fraction and NT-pro BNP [80]. The role of the transcriptome presented briefly above is demonstrated but the future of these markers in HF diagnosis and prognosis is directly related to multi-marker testing panels.

Conclusions

The current desiderate of personalized medicine in HF bases its principle on the identification of specific biomarkers that offers insights into the pathophysiological pathways to be interfered in the HF treatment. The ideal biomarkers has not been yet identified and continuous research is conducted to support more advanced and tailored HF-management.

References

1. United Nations Environment Programme., International Labour Organisation., World Health Organization., International Program on Chemical Safety. Biomarkers in risk assessment: validity and validation. World Health Organization; 2001.
2. Halvorsen S, Mehilli J, Cassese S, Hall TS, Abdelhamid M, Barbato E, De Hert S, de Laval I, Zakirov N, et al. 2022 ESC Guidelines on cardiovascular assessment and management of patients undergoing non-cardiac surgery. Eur Heart J. 2022;43(39):3826–924. https://doi.org/10.1093/eurheartj/ehac270.
3. Heidenreich PA, Bozkurt B, Aguilar D, Allen LA, Byun JJ, Colvin MM, Deswal A, Drazner MH, Dunlay SM, Evers LR, Fang JC, Fedson SE, Fonarow GC, Hayek SS, Hernandez AF, Khazanie P, Kittleson MM, Lee CS, Link MS, Milano CA, Nnacheta LC, Sandhu AT, Stevenson LW, Vardeny O, Vest AR, Yancy CW. 2022 AHA/ACC/HFSA Guideline for the Management of Heart Failure: a report of the American College of Cardiology/American Heart Association Joint Committee on Clinical Practice Guidelines. Circulation. 2022;145(18):e895–e1032. https://doi.org/10.1161/CIR.0000000000001063.
4. Wolsk E, Claggett B, Diaz R, Dickstein K, Gerstein HC, Køber L, Lewis EF, Maggioni AP, McMurray JJV, Probstfield JL, Riddle MC, Solomon SD, Tardif J, Pfeffer MA. Risk estimates of imminent cardiovascular death and heart failure hospitalization are improved using serial natriuretic peptide measurements in patients with coronary artery disease and type 2 diabetes. J Am Heart Assoc. 2022;11(8):e021327. https://doi.org/10.1161/JAHA.121.021327.
5. Wolsk E, Claggett B, Pfeffer MA, Diaz R, Dickstein K, Gerstein HC, Lawson FC, Lewis EF, Maggioni AP, McMurray JJV, Probstfield JL, Riddle MC, Solomon SD, Tardif J-C, Køber L. Role of B-type natriuretic peptide and N-terminal prohormone BNP as predictors of cardiovascular morbidity and mortality in patients with a recent coronary event and type 2 diabetes mellitus. J Am Heart Assoc. 2017;6(6):e004743. https://doi.org/10.1161/JAHA.116.004743.
6. Nyberg M, Terzic D, Ludvigsen TP, Mark PD, Michaelsen NB, Abildstrøm SZ, Engelmann M, Richards AM, Goetze JP. A state of natriuretic peptide deficiency. Endocr Rev. 2022;44(3):379–92. https://doi.org/10.1210/endrev/bnac029.

7. Felker GM, Anstrom KJ, Adams KF, Ezekowitz JA, Fiuzat M, Houston-Miller N, Januzzi JL, Mark DB, Piña IL, Passmore G, Whellan DJ, Yang H, Cooper LS, Leifer ES, Desvigne-Nickens P, O'Connor CM. Effect of natriuretic peptide–guided therapy on hospitalization or cardiovascular mortality in high-risk patients with heart failure and reduced ejection fraction. JAMA. 2017;318(8):713. https://doi.org/10.1001/jama.2017.10565.
8. Greenberg B, Butler J, Felker GM, Ponikowski P, Voors AA, Desai AS, Barnard D, Bouchard A, Jaski B, Lyon AR, Pogoda JM, Rudy JJ, Zsebo KM. Calcium upregulation by percutaneous administration of gene therapy in patients with cardiac disease (CUPID 2): a randomised, multinational, double-blind, placebo-controlled, phase 2b trial. Lancet. 2016;387(10024):1178–86. https://doi.org/10.1016/S0140-6736(16)00082-9.
9. Xue Y, Taub P, Iqbal N, Nguyen H, Clopton P, Daniels L, Maisel A. Elevated mid-region pro-adrenomedullin is associated with increased mortality in stable outpatients with diastolic dysfunction. J Card Fail. 2011;17(8):S3. https://doi.org/10.1016/j.cardfail.2011.06.010.
10. Ertmer C, Van Aken H, Westphal M. Adrenomedullin in the treatment of cardiovascular dysfunction and sepsis. In: Intensive care medicine: annual update 2007. Springer; 2007.
11. Pandhi P, Ter Maaten JM, Anker SD, Ng LL, Metra M, Samani NJ, Lang CC, Dickstein K, de Boer RA, van Veldhuisen DJ, Voors AA, Sama IE. Pathophysiologic processes and novel biomarkers associated with congestion in heart failure. Heart Fail. 2022;10(9):623–32. https://doi.org/10.1016/J.JCHF.2022.05.013.
12. Špinarová M, Špinar J, Špinarová L, Krejčí J, Goldbergová-Pávková M, Pařenica J, Ludka O, Málek F, Ošťádal P, Benešová K, Jarkovský J, Lábr K. Relation between mid-regional pro-adrenomedullin in patients with chronic heart failure and the dose of diuretics in 2-year follow-up-data from FAR NHL registry. Medicina (Kaunas, Lithuania). 2022;58(10):1477. https://doi.org/10.3390/MEDICINA58101477.
13. Kremer D, Ter Maaten JM, Voors AA. Bio-adrenomedullin as a potential quick, reliable, and objective marker of congestion in heart failure. Eur J Heart Fail. 2018;20(9):1363–5. https://doi.org/10.1002/EJHF.1245.
14. Luo J-W, Duan W-H, Song L, Yu Y-Q, Shi D-Z. A meta-analysis of growth differentiation factor-15 and prognosis in chronic heart failure. Front Cardiovasc Med. 2021;8:1590. https://doi.org/10.3389/fcvm.2021.630818.
15. Gürgöze MT, van Vark LC, Baart SJ, Kardys I, Akkerhuis KM, Manintveld OC, Postmus D, Hillege HL, Lesman-Leegte I, Asselbergs FW, Brunner-la-Rocca H-P, van den Bos EJ, Orsel JG, de Ridder SPJ, Pinto YM, Boersma E. Multimarker analysis of serially measured GDF-15, NT-proBNP, ST2, GAL-3, cTnI, creatinine, and prognosis in acute heart failure. Circ Heart Fail. 2023;16(1):e009526. https://doi.org/10.1161/CIRCHEARTFAILURE.122.009526.
16. Andersson J, Fall T, Delicano R, Wennberg P, Jansson J-H. GDF-15 is associated with sudden cardiac death due to incident myocardial infarction. Resuscitation. 2020;152:165–9. https://doi.org/10.1016/j.resuscitation.2020.05.001.
17. Xiao N, Zhang J, Chen C, Wan Y, Wang N, Yang J. miR-129-5p improves cardiac function in rats with chronic heart failure through targeting HMGB1. Mamm Genome. 2019;30(9–10):276–88. https://doi.org/10.1007/s00335-019-09817-0.
18. Wang X, Wang H-X, Li Y-L, Zhang C-C, Zhou C-Y, Wang L, Xia Y-L, Du J, Li H-H. MicroRNA Let-7i negatively regulates cardiac inflammation and fibrosis. Hypertension. 2015;66(4):776–85. https://doi.org/10.1161/HYPERTENSIONAHA.115.05548.
19. Bao M-H, Feng X, Zhang Y-W, Lou X-Y, Cheng Y, Zhou H-H. Let-7 in cardiovascular diseases, heart development and cardiovascular differentiation from stem cells. Int J Mol Sci. 2013;14(11):23086–102. https://doi.org/10.3390/ijms141123086.
20. Täubel J, Hauke W, Rump S, Viereck J, Batkai S, Poetzsch J, Rode L, Weigt H, Genschel C, Lorch U, Theek C, Levin AA, Bauersachs J, Solomon SD, Thum T. Novel antisense therapy targeting microRNA-132 in patients with heart failure: results of a first-in-human Phase 1b randomized, double-blind, placebo-controlled study. Eur Heart J. 2021;42(2):178–88. https://doi.org/10.1093/eurheartj/ehaa898.

21. Tomaniak M, Sygitowicz G, Błaszczyk O, Kołtowski Ł, Puchta D, Malesa K, Kochanowski J, Sitkiewicz D, Filipiak KJ. miR-1, miR-21, and galectin-3 in hypertensive patients with symptomatic heart failure and left ventricular hypertrophy. Kardiol Pol. 2018;76(6):1009–11. https://doi.org/10.5603/KP.2018.0117.
22. Scrutinio D, Conserva F, Passantino A, Iacoviello M, Lagioia R, Gesualdo L. Circulating microRNA-150-5p as a novel biomarker for advanced heart failure: a genome-wide prospective study. J Heart Lung Transplant. 2017;36(6):616–24. https://doi.org/10.1016/J.HEALUN.2017.02.008.
23. van Boven N, Akkerhuis KM, Anroedh SS, Rizopoulos D, Pinto Y, Battes LC, Hillege HL, Caliskan KC, Germans T, Manintveld OC, Cornel J-H, Constantinescu AA, Boersma E, Umans VA, Kardys I. Serially measured circulating miR-22-3p is a biomarker for adverse clinical outcome in patients with chronic heart failure: the Bio-SHiFT study. Int J Cardiol. 2017;235:124–32. https://doi.org/10.1016/j.ijcard.2017.02.078.
24. Klenke S, Eul S, Peters J, Neumann T, Adamzik M, Frey UH. Circulating miR-192 is a prognostic marker in patients with ischemic cardiomyopathy. Futur Cardiol. 2018;14(4):283–9. https://doi.org/10.2217/fca-2017-0108.
25. Greene SJ, Butler J, Fonarow GC, Subacius HP, Ambrosy AP, Vaduganathan M, Triggiani M, Solomon SD, Lewis EF, Maggioni AP, Böhm M, Chioncel O, Nodari S, Senni M, Zannad F, Gheorghiade M. Pre-discharge and early post-discharge troponin elevation among patients hospitalized for heart failure with reduced ejection fraction: findings from the ASTRONAUT trial. Eur J Heart Fail. 2018;20(2):281–91. https://doi.org/10.1002/ejhf.1019.
26. Suzuki S, Motoki H, Masatoshi M, Okuma Y, Shoin W, Okano T, Kimura K, Ebisawa S, Okada A, Kuwahara K. Prognostic significance of high-sensitivity cardiac troponin in patients with heart failure with preserved ejection fraction. Heart Vessel. 2019;1:3. https://doi.org/10.1007/s00380-019-01393-2.
27. Myhre PL, O'Meara E, Claggett BL, de Denus S, Jarolim P, Anand IS, Beldhuis IE, Fleg JL, Lewis E, Pitt B, Rouleau JL, Solomon SD, Pfeffer MA, Desai AS. Cardiac troponin I and risk of cardiac events in patients with heart failure and preserved ejection fraction. Circ Heart Fail. 2018;11(11):e005312. https://doi.org/10.1161/CIRCHEARTFAILURE.118.005312.
28. Packer M, McMurray JJV, Desai AS, Gong J, Lefkowitz MP, Rizkala AR, Rouleau JL, Shi VC, PARADIGM-HF Investigators and Coordinators, et al. Angiotensin receptor neprilysin inhibition compared with enalapril on the risk of clinical progression in surviving patients with heart failure. Circulation. 2015;131(1):54–61. https://doi.org/10.1161/CIRCULATIONAHA.114.013748.
29. Kutsuzawa D, Arimoto T, Watanabe T, Shishido T, Miyamoto T, Miyashita T, Takahashi H, Niizeki T, Takeishi Y, Kubota I. Ongoing myocardial damage in patients with heart failure and preserved ejection fraction. J Cardiol. 2012;60(6):454–61. https://doi.org/10.1016/j.jjcc.2012.06.006.
30. Setsuta K, Seino Y, Kitahara Y, Arau M, Ohbayashi T, Takano T, Mizuno K. Elevated levels of both cardiomyocyte membrane and myofibril damage markers predict adverse outcomes in patients with chronic heart failure. Circulation. 2007;72(4):569–74.
31. Bartunek J, Delrue L, Van Durme F, Muller O, Casselman F, De Wiest B, Croes R, Verstreken S, Goethals M, de Raedt H, Sarma J, Joseph L, Vanderheyden M, Weinberg EO. Nonmyocardial production of ST2 protein in human hypertrophy and failure is related to diastolic load. J Am Coll Cardiol. 2008;52(25):2166–74. https://doi.org/10.1016/j.jacc.2008.09.027.
32. Bayes-Genis A, Zhang Y, Ky B. ST2 and patient prognosis in chronic heart failure. Am J Cardiol. 2015;115(7):64B–9B. https://doi.org/10.1016/j.amjcard.2015.01.043.
33. Januzzi JL, Pascual-Figal D, Daniels LB. ST2 testing for chronic heart failure therapy monitoring: the international ST2 consensus panel. Am J Cardiol. 2015;115(7 Suppl):70B–5B. https://doi.org/10.1016/j.amjcard.2015.01.044.
34. Zile MR, Baicu CF, Ikonomidis JS, Stroud RE, Nietert PJ, Bradshaw AD, Slater R, Palmer BM, Van Buren P, Meyer M, Redfield MM, Bull DA, Granzier HL, LeWinter MM. Myocardial stiffness in patients with heart failure and a preserved ejection fraction: contributions

of collagen and titin. Circulation. 2015;131(14):1247–59. https://doi.org/10.1161/CIRCULATIONAHA.114.013215.
35. Ip C, Luk KS, Yuen VLC, Chiang L, Chan CK, Ho K, Gong M, Lee TTL, Leung KSK, Roever L, Bazoukis G, Lampropoulos K, Li KHC, Tse G, Liu T, Network IHIS (IHIS). Soluble suppression of tumorigenicity 2 (sST2) for predicting disease severity or mortality outcomes in cardiovascular diseases: a systematic review and meta-analysis. Int J Cardiol Heart Vasc. 2021;37:100887. https://doi.org/10.1016/J.IJCHA.2021.100887.
36. Sharma UC, Pokharel S, van Brakel TJ, van Berlo JH, Cleutjens JPM, Schroen B, André S, Crijns HJGM, Gabius H-J, Maessen J, Pinto YM. Galectin-3 marks activated macrophages in failure-prone hypertrophied hearts and contributes to cardiac dysfunction. Circulation. 2004;110(19):3121–8. https://doi.org/10.1161/01.CIR.0000147181.65298.4D.
37. Ho JE, Liu C, Lyass A, Courchesne P, Pencina MJ, Vasan RS, Larson MG, Levy D. Galectin-3, a marker of cardiac fibrosis, predicts incident heart failure in the community. J Am Coll Cardiol. 2012;60(14):1249–56. https://doi.org/10.1016/J.JACC.2012.04.053.
38. Daniels LB, Clopton P, Laughlin GA, Maisel AS, Barrett-Connor E. Galectin-3 is independently associated with cardiovascular mortality in community-dwelling older adults without known cardiovascular disease: the rancho Bernardo study. Am Heart J. 2014;167(5):674–682.e1. https://doi.org/10.1016/J.AHJ.2013.12.031.
39. Shah RV, Chen-Tournoux AA, Picard MH, van Kimmenade RRJ, Januzzi JL. Galectin-3, cardiac structure and function, and long-term mortality in patients with acutely decompensated heart failure. Eur J Heart Fail. 2010;12(8):826–32. https://doi.org/10.1093/eurjhf/hfq091.
40. Shirakabe A, Okazaki H, Matsushita M, Shibata Y, Shigihara S, Nishigoori S, Sawatani T, Sasamoto N, Kiuchi K, Atsukawa M, Itokawa N, Arai T, Kobayashi N, Asai K. Type III procollagen peptide level can indicate liver dysfunction associated with volume overload in acute heart failure. ESC Heart Fail. 2022;9(3):1832–43. https://doi.org/10.1002/ehf2.13878.
41. Bielecka-Dabrowa A, Michalska-Kasiczak M, Gluba A, Ahmed A, Gerdts E, von Haehling S, Rysz J, Banach M. Biomarkers and echocardiographic predictors of myocardial dysfunction in patients with hypertension. Sci Rep. 2015;5:8916. https://doi.org/10.1038/srep08916.
42. Zannad F, Alla F, Dousset B, Perez A, Pitt B. Limitation of excessive extracellular matrix turnover may contribute to survival benefit of spironolactone therapy in patients with congestive heart failure. Circulation. 2000;102(22):2700–6. https://doi.org/10.1161/01.CIR.102.22.2700.
43. Yao Y, Feng L, Sun Y, Wang S, Sun J, Hu B. Myocardial fibrosis combined with NT-proBNP improves the accuracy of survival prediction in ADHF patients. BMC Cardiovasc Disord. 2021;21(1):264. https://doi.org/10.1186/s12872-021-02083-6.
44. Kaufman BD, Videon N, Zhang X, Harris MA, Shaddy RE, Goldmuntz E. Procollagen type III amino-terminal propeptide: a serum biomarker of left ventricular remodelling in paediatric dilated cardiomyopathy. Cardiol Young. 2015;25(2):228–36. https://doi.org/10.1017/S1047951113001820.
45. Reitsma S, Slaaf DW, Vink H, Van Zandvoort MAMJ, Oude Egbrink MGA. The endothelial glycocalyx: composition, functions, and visualization. Pflugers Arch. 2007;454(3):345–59.
46. Tromp J, van der Pol A, Klip IT, de Boer RA, Jaarsma T, van Gilst WH, Voors AA, van Veldhuisen DJ, van der Meer P. Fibrosis marker syndecan-1 and outcome in patients with heart failure with reduced and preserved ejection fraction. Circ Heart Fail. 2014;7(3):457–62. https://doi.org/10.1161/CIRCHEARTFAILURE.113.000846.
47. Liu W, Wang Y, Zheng J, Song D, Zheng S, Ren L, Wang Y, Yao Y, Wang Y, Liu Y, Bai R, Dong J, Liu T. Syndecan-1 as an independent risk factor for the incidence of adverse cardiovascular events in patients having stage C and D heart failure with non-ischemic dilated cardiomyopathy. Clin Chim Acta. 2019;490:63–8. https://doi.org/10.1016/J.CCA.2018.12.022.
48. Wernly B, Fuernau G, Masyuk M, Muessig JM, Pfeiler S, Bruno RR, Desch S, Muench P, Lichtenauer M, Kelm M, Adams V, Thiele H, Eitel I, Jung C. Syndecan-1 predicts outcome in patients with ST-segment elevation infarction independent from infarct-related myocardial injury. Sci Rep. 2019;9(1):18367. https://doi.org/10.1038/s41598-019-54937-x.

49. Zalghout S, Vo S, Arocas V, Jadoui S, Hamade E, Badran B, Oudar O, Charnaux N, Longrois D, Boulaftali Y, Bouton M-C, Richard B. Syndecan-1 is overexpressed in human thoracic aneurysm but is dispensable for the disease progression in a mouse model. Front Cardiovasc Med. 2022;9:720. https://doi.org/10.3389/fcvm.2022.839743.
50. Humphrey LL, Fu R, Rogers K, Freeman M, Helfand M. Homocysteine level and coronary heart disease incidence: a systematic review and meta-analysis. Mayo Clin Proc. 2008;83(11):1203–12. https://doi.org/10.4065/83.11.1203.
51. Wang X, Chen Z, Tian W, Zhang J, Li Q, Ju J, Xu H, Chen K. Plasma homocysteine levels and risk of congestive heart failure or cardiomyopathy: a mendelian randomization study. Front Cardiovasc Med. 2023;10:47. https://doi.org/10.3389/fcvm.2023.1030257.
52. Maurer M, Burri S, de Marchi S, Hullin R, Martinelli M, Mohacsi P, Hess OM. Plasma homocysteine and cardiovascular risk in heart failure with and without cardiorenal syndrome. Int J Cardiol. 2010;141(1):32–8. https://doi.org/10.1016/j.ijcard.2008.11.131.
53. Iqbal NS, Wu Y, Hazen S, Tang WHW. Elevated plasma homocysteine identifies patients with chronic heart failure at increased cardiovascular risk. J Card Fail. 2012;18(8):S87. https://doi.org/10.1016/j.cardfail.2012.06.521.
54. Tseng CH, Huang WM, Sung SH. Tissue inhibitor of metalloproteinase (TIMP)-1 predicts negative remodeling and recovery of ejection fraction in acute heart failure with reduced ejection fraction. Eur Heart J. 2022;43(Suppl_2):ehac544.1086. https://doi.org/10.1093/eurheartj/ehac544.1086.
55. Bhalla V, Georgiopoulou VV, Azeem AA, Marti CN, Cole RT, Laskar SR, De Staercke C, Hooper WC, Smith AL, Kalogeropoulos AP, Butler J. Matrix metalloproteinases, tissue inhibitors of metalloproteinases, and heart failure outcomes. Int J Cardiol. 2011;151(2):237–9. https://doi.org/10.1016/j.ijcard.2011.06.048.
56. González A, López B, Querejeta R, Zubillaga E, Echeverría T, Díez J. Filling pressures and collagen metabolism in hypertensive patients with heart failure and normal ejection fraction. Hypertension (Dallas, Tex: 1979). 2010;55(6):1418–24. https://doi.org/10.1161/HYPERTENSIONAHA.109.149112.
57. Zile MR, Desantis SM, Baicu CF, Stroud RE, Thompson SB, McClure CD, Mehurg SM, Spinale FG. Plasma biomarkers that reflect determinants of matrix composition identify the presence of left ventricular hypertrophy and diastolic heart failure. Circ Heart Fail. 2011;4(3):246–56. https://doi.org/10.1161/CIRCHEARTFAILURE.110.958199.
58. Heymans S, Schroen B, Vermeersch P, Milting H, Gao F, Kassner A, Gillijns H, Herijgers P, Flameng W, Carmeliet P, Van de Werf F, Pinto YM, Janssens S. Increased cardiac expression of tissue inhibitor of metalloproteinase-1 and tissue inhibitor of metalloproteinase-2 is related to cardiac fibrosis and dysfunction in the chronic pressure-overloaded human heart. Circulation. 2005;112(8):1136–44. https://doi.org/10.1161/CIRCULATIONAHA.104.516963.
59. Kassiri Z, Oudit GY, Sanchez O, Dawood F, Mohammed FF, Nuttall RK, Edwards DR, Liu PP, Backx PH, Khokha R. Combination of tumor necrosis factor-α ablation and matrix metalloproteinase inhibition prevents heart failure after pressure overload in tissue inhibitor of metalloproteinase-3 knock-out mice. Circ Res. 2005;97(4):380–90. https://doi.org/10.1161/01.RES.0000178789.16929.cf.
60. Frantz S, Störk S, Michels K, Eigenthaler M, Ertl G, Bauersachs J, Angermann CE. Tissue inhibitor of metalloproteinases levels in patients with chronic heart failure: an independent predictor of mortality. Eur J Heart Fail. 2008;10(4):388–95. https://doi.org/10.1016/j.ejheart.2008.02.015.
61. Chemaly ER, Kang S, Zhang S, McCollum L, Chen J, Bénard L, Purushothaman K-R, Hajjar RJ, Lebeche D. Differential patterns of replacement and reactive fibrosis in pressure and volume overload are related to the propensity for ischaemia and involve resistin. J Physiol. 2013;591(21):5337–55. https://doi.org/10.1113/jphysiol.2013.258731.
62. Zhao B, Lebeche D. Abstract 313: inhibition of resistin protects against heart failure injury by targeting Gadd45α. Circ Res. 2019;125(Suppl_1) https://doi.org/10.1161/res.125.suppl_1.313.

63. Zolk O, Ng LL, O'Brien RJ, Weyand M, Eschenhagen T. Augmented expression of cardiotrophin-1 in failing human hearts is accompanied by diminished glycoprotein 130 receptor protein abundance. Circulation. 2002;106(12):1442–6. https://doi.org/10.1161/01.CIR.0000033117.39335.DF.
64. Khan SQ, Kelly D, Quinn P, Davies JE, Ng LL. Cardiotrophin-1 predicts death or heart failure following acute myocardial infarction. J Card Fail. 2006;12(8):635–40. https://doi.org/10.1016/j.cardfail.2006.06.470.
65. Hanna A, Frangogiannis NG. Inflammatory cytokines and chemokines as therapeutic targets in heart failure. Cardiovasc Drugs Ther. 2020;34(6):849–63. https://doi.org/10.1007/s10557-020-07071-0.
66. Maeda K, Tsutamoto T, Wada A, Mabuchi N, Hayashi M, Tsutsui T, Ohnishi M, Sawaki M, Fujii M, Matsumoto T, Kinoshita M. High levels of plasma brain natriuretic peptide and interleukin-6 after optimized treatment for heart failure are independent risk factors for morbidity and mortality in patients with congestive heart failure. J Am Coll Cardiol. 2000;36(5):1587–93. https://doi.org/10.1016/S0735-1097(00)00912-8.
67. Ridker PM, Devalaraja M, Baeres FMM, Engelmann MDM, Hovingh GK, Ivkovic M, Lo L, Kling D, Pergola P, Raj D, Libby P, Davidson M, RESCUE Investigators. IL-6 inhibition with ziltivekimab in patients at high atherosclerotic risk (RESCUE): a double-blind, randomised, placebo-controlled, phase 2 trial. Lancet (London, England). 2021;397(10289):2060–9. https://doi.org/10.1016/S0140-6736(21)00520-1.
68. Abbate A, Van Tassell BW, Biondi-Zoccai G, Kontos MC, Grizzard JD, Spillman DW, Oddi C, Roberts CS, Melchior RD, Mueller GH, Abouzaki NA, Rengel LR, Varma A, Gambill ML, Falcao RA, Voelkel NF, Dinarello CA, Vetrovec GW. Effects of interleukin-1 blockade with anakinra on adverse cardiac remodeling and heart failure after acute myocardial infarction [from the Virginia Commonwealth University-Anakinra Remodeling Trial (2) (VCU-ART2) pilot study]. Am J Cardiol. 2013;111(10):1394–400. https://doi.org/10.1016/j.amjcard.2013.01.287.
69. Van Tassell BW, Arena R, Biondi-Zoccai G, Canada JM, Oddi C, Abouzaki NA, Jahangiri A, Falcao RA, Kontos MC, Shah KB, Voelkel NF, Dinarello CA, Abbate A. Effects of interleukin-1 blockade with anakinra on aerobic exercise capacity in patients with heart failure and preserved ejection fraction (from the D-HART pilot study). Am J Cardiol. 2014;113(2):321–7. https://doi.org/10.1016/j.amjcard.2013.08.047.
70. Ridker PM, Everett BM, Thuren T, MacFadyen JG, Chang WH, Ballantyne C, Fonseca F, Nicolau J, Koenig W, Anker SD, Kastelein JJP, Cornel JH, Pais P, Pella D, Genest J, Cifkova R, Lorenzatti A, Forster T, Kobalava Z, Vida-Simiti L, Flather M, Shimokawa H, Ogawa H, Dellborg M, Rossi PRF, Troquay RPT, Libby P, Glynn RJ. Antiinflammatory therapy with canakinumab for atherosclerotic disease. N Engl J Med. 2017;377(12):1119–31. https://doi.org/10.1056/NEJMoa1707914.
71. Behr TM, Wang X, Aiyar N, Coatney RW, Li X, Koster P, Angermann CE, Ohlstein E, Feuerstein GZ, Winaver J. Monocyte chemoattractant protein-1 is upregulated in rats with volume-overload congestive heart failure. Circulation. 2000;102(11):1315–22. https://doi.org/10.1161/01.CIR.102.11.1315.
72. Ratziu V, Sanyal A, Harrison SA, Wong VW-S, Francque S, Goodman Z, Aithal GP, Kowdley KV, Seyedkazemi S, Fischer L, Loomba R, Abdelmalek MF, Tacke F. Cenicriviroc treatment for adults with nonalcoholic steatohepatitis and fibrosis: final analysis of the phase 2b CENTAUR study. Hepatology (Baltimore, Md). 2020;72(3):892–905. https://doi.org/10.1002/hep.31108.
73. Chung ES, Packer M, Lo KH, Fasanmade AA, Willerson JT. Randomized, double-blind, placebo-controlled, pilot trial of infliximab, a chimeric monoclonal antibody to tumor necrosis factor-α, in patients with moderate-to-severe heart failure. Circulation. 2003;107(25):3133–40. https://doi.org/10.1161/01.CIR.0000077913.60364.D2.

74. Chair S-Y, Chan J-Y-W, Waye M-M-Y, Liu T, Law B-M-H, Chien W-T. Exploration of potential genetic biomarkers for heart failure: a systematic review. Int J Environ Res Public Health. 2021;18(11):5904. https://doi.org/10.3390/ijerph18115904.
75. Meder B, Haas J, Sedaghat-Hamedani F, Kayvanpour E, Frese K, Lai A, Nietsch R, Scheiner C, Mester S, Bordalo DM, Amr A, Dietrich C, Pils D, Siede D, Hund H, Bauer A, Holzer DB, Ruhparwar A, Mueller-Hennessen M, Weichenhan D, Plass C, Weis T, Backs J, Wuerstle M, Keller A, Katus HA, Posch AE. Epigenome-wide association study identifies cardiac gene patterning and a novel class of biomarkers for heart failure. Circulation. 2017;136(16):1528–44. https://doi.org/10.1161/CIRCULATIONAHA.117.027355.
76. Han J, Zhang L, Hu L, Yu H, Xu F, Yang B, Zhang R, Zhang Y, An Y. Circular RNA-expression profiling reveals a potential role of Hsa_circ_0097435 in heart failure via sponging multiple microRNAs. Front Genet. 2020;11:212. https://doi.org/10.3389/fgene.2020.00212.
77. Sun Y, Jiang X, Lv Y, Liang X, Zhao B, Bian W, Zhang D, Jiang J, Zhang C. Circular RNA expression profiles in plasma from patients with heart failure related to platelet activity. Biomol Ther. 2020;10(2):187. https://doi.org/10.3390/biom10020187.
78. Akat KM, Moore-McGriff D, Morozov P, Brown M, Gogakos T, Correa Da Rosa J, Mihailovic A, Sauer M, Ji R, Ramarathnam A, Totary-Jain H, Williams Z, Tuschl T, Schulze PC. Comparative RNA-sequencing analysis of myocardial and circulating small RNAs in human heart failure and their utility as biomarkers. Proc Natl Acad Sci. 2014;111(30):11151–6. https://doi.org/10.1073/pnas.1401724111.
79. Boeckel J-N, Perret MF, Glaser SF, Seeger T, Heumüller AW, Chen W, John D, Kokot KE, Katus HA, Haas J, Lackner MK, Kayvanpour E, Grabe N, Dieterich C, von Haehling S, Ebner N, Hünecke S, Leuschner F, Fichtlscherer S, Meder B, Zeiher AM, Dimmeler S, Keller T. Identification and regulation of the long non-coding RNA Heat2 in heart failure. J Mol Cell Cardiol. 2019;126:13–22. https://doi.org/10.1016/j.yjmcc.2018.11.004.
80. Zhang S, Jin R, Li B. Serum NT-proBNP and TUG1 as novel biomarkers for elderly hypertensive patients with heart failure with preserved ejection fraction. Exp Ther Med. 2021;21(5):446. https://doi.org/10.3892/etm.2021.9874.

Chapter 3
The Kidney and Electrolyte Imbalances in Heart Failure

Mugurel Apetrii and Adrian Covic

Abstract Electrolyte imbalances are prevalent and dangerous complications in heart failure (HF) patients, arising from both the physiological changes of HF and the side effects of medications like diuretics and RAAS inhibitors. Key imbalances include hyponatremia, hypokalemia, hyperkalemia, and hypomagnesemia, each contributing to increased arrhythmia risk and mortality. Effective management of these electrolyte imbalances is crucial for optimizing patient outcomes in HF. Understanding their underlying mechanisms and early detection are essential for appropriate intervention. Future research should focus on developing targeted strategies and guidelines for managing electrolyte imbalances in HF to improve prognosis and reduce mortality.

Keywords Heart failure · Kidney disease · Electrolytes · Arrythmia · Mortality
Electrolyte imbalances are common and potentially dangerous complication among patients with heart failure (HF). These complications can arise from two main sources: firstly, the physiological changes inherent to HF, which trigger neurohumoral responses such as activation of the renin-angiotensin-aldosterone system (RAAS) and sympathetic stimulation; secondly, they can result from the side effects of medications like diuretics or RAAS inhibitors. Patients with HF often exhibit deficiencies in sodium, magnesium, and potassium, the latter two being particularly involved in the onset of cardiac arrhythmias. Hyperkalemia, which can arise from angiotensin-converting-enzyme (ACE) inhibitors, angiotensin II receptor blockers (ARBs) or aldosterone receptor blockers usage, can lead to myocardial conduction slowing, potentially predisposing individuals to arrhythmias. Early detection of these abnormalities and understanding their underlying physiological mechanisms are crucial for effectively managing these patients.

M. Apetrii · A. Covic (✉)
University of Medicine and Pharmacy "Grigore T Popa", Iasi, Romania

Dr CI Parhon University Hospital, Iasi, Romania

M. Dorobanţu et al. (eds.), *Current Approach to Heart Failure*,
https://doi.org/10.1007/978-3-031-96562-3_3

Hyponatremia

Hyponatremia is the most prevalent electrolyte abnormality in hospitalized patients. Mild to moderate hyponatremia is typically found in 10% of individuals with HF, although various reports suggest a higher prevalence. For instance, in the OPTIME-CHF trial, 27% of participants exhibited mild hyponatremia ranging from 132 to 135 mEq/L [1], while in the ESCAPE trial, 25.3% had hyponatremia at admission and 18% of subjects experienced persistent hyponatremia during hospitalization [2]. These patients experienced higher in-hospital and post-discharge mortality rates and longer hospital stays compared to those with normal sodium levels. Despite its significance, there are currently no established guidelines for managing hyponatremia in HF patients.

Pathogenesis

HF impairs the body's ability to excrete ingested water by elevating levels of antidiuretic hormone (ADH), regardless of ejection fraction status. Although overhydrated patients with HF exhibit increased extracellular fluid volumes, the body perceives a volume depletion due to decreased effective arterial blood volume as a result of reduced cardiac output, which reduces pressure on the baroreceptors in the carotid sinus and renal afferent arteriole. This condition triggers an activation of RAAS, increase of ADH and norepinephrine [3] therefore limiting the sodium and water excretion in an effort to restore perfusion pressure to normal levels. The extent of neurohumoral activation typically correlates with the severity of cardiac dysfunction, measured by left ventricular ejection fraction or functional class [3].

Hyponatremia serves both as a long-term predictor of adverse prognosis in HF but it also predicts poor short-term outcomes in hospitalized HF patients. Moreover, the severity of hyponatremia, paralleled by ADH release, holds prognostic significance, with patient survival significantly reduced once serum sodium falls below 135 mEq/L while a sodium that is persistently below 125 mEq/L indicates a near end-stage heart disease [4].

Clinical Manifestations

Hyponatremia in HF patients typically progresses slowly, with symptoms emerging only below 120 mEq/L, indicating severe heart disease and a poor prognosis. Some patients with moderate chronic hyponatremia (120–129 mEq/L) may exhibit subtle neurological manifestations, potentially improved by gradual serum sodium correction; these include reduced mental, social, and physical functioning scores, and in older adults, loss of balance and falls [5].

Therapeutic Considerations

Correction of hyponatremia hasn't shown to improve hemodynamic abnormalities or clinical outcomes in severe chronic HF. Specific therapy is advised for severe hyponatremia, symptomatic cases, or when there's concern about increased fall/fracture risk from asymptomatic hyponatremia.

Fluid restriction is the cornerstone of therapy for symptomatic or worsening severe hyponatremia. However, fluid restriction is often poorly tolerated in HF patients due to increased thirst stimulated by reduced tissue perfusion and enhanced antidiuretic hormone release. Several days of restriction are required to see any results from this treatment. Currently, no studies have examined the safety or tolerability of this approach in hyponatremia in chronic HF.

ACE inhibitors, ARBs, and loop diuretics are commonly used in HF with reduced ejection fraction and may raise serum sodium concentrations through various mechanisms, including improving cardiac function and decreasing water reabsorption.

In recent years, sodium-glucose cotransporter 2 (SGLT2) inhibitors have demonstrated improvements in HF outcomes for patients with and without diabetes mellitus, in addition to their beneficial effects on type 2 diabetes mellitus and chronic kidney disease (CKD). Beyond their well-established cardioprotective effects, recent clinical studies have shown that SGLT2 inhibitors significantly increase serum sodium levels by inducing osmotic diuresis [6, 7]. Additionally, there is evidence suggesting that SGLT2 inhibitors can modulate non-osmotic sodium storage, leading to reduced skin sodium content and interstitial fluid volume [8]. Consequently, the oral administration of SGLT2 inhibitors is emerging as a promising treatment option for hyponatremia in heart failure patients.

Vasopressin receptor antagonists, such as tolvaptan and conivaptan, selectively induce water diuresis and may help correct hyponatremia, particularly in patients with chronic HF who haven't responded to other treatments. Tolvaptan, a selective V2 receptor inhibitor, has shown efficacy in raising serum sodium levels and improving symptoms in HF patients, but concerns about its safety (i.e., hepatotoxicity) and potential for overly rapid correction of hyponatremia exist. Conivaptan, which blocks both the V2 and V1a receptors, also induces water diuresis and increases serum sodium levels among HF patients. By blocking V1a receptors, it reduces afterload, potentially enhancing systemic hemodynamics in those with reduced ejection fraction. This medication could be beneficial for HF patients with symptomatic hyponatremia and as an adjunct to diuretic therapy for those with fluid overload. However, its use may be limited by hypotension.

Combining loop diuretics with hypertonic saline infusion has been effective for treating hyponatremia in HF patients by promoting electrolyte-free water losses and preventing volume depletion in some studies. Even if this approach may improve hyponatremia and preserve kidney function compared to diuretics alone, this approach remains controversial.

For patients unresponsive to aggressive diuretic treatment, hemodialysis can be considered for both removing the excess intravascular fluid and the correction of hyponatremia. However, studies have not shown clinical benefits of ultrafiltration over diuretic therapy, nor does it preserve renal function. Prior to opting for a mechanical fluid removal strategy, consultation with a kidney specialist is advisable.

Hypokalemia

Hypokalemia is frequently observed in individuals with HF and serves as a significant independent predictor of mortality [9]. Hypokalemia tends to be more pronounced in advanced HF patients undergoing intensive diuretic therapy and experiencing an increased activity of the renin-angiotensin system.

Pathogenesis

Several mechanisms contribute to hypokalemia in chronic heart failure. Firstly, reduced renal perfusion activates the RAAS, leading to aldosterone release, which promotes sodium retention and potassium excretion. Secondly, stimulation of the β2 adrenergic receptor by elevated circulating catecholamines enhances sodium reabsorption and potassium excretion, and shifts potassium into the intracellular compartment. Thirdly, the use of loop diuretics or a combination of loop and thiazide diuretics causes further renal potassium loss and contraction alkalosis further aggravating hypokalemia. Additionally, low intracellular magnesium exacerbates renal potassium wasting by releasing the inhibition of the renal outer medullary potassium (ROMK) channel, necessitating combined magnesium and potassium supplementation to increase tissue potassium levels. As heart failure progresses, the increasing severity of neurohormonal and pharmacological imbalances can further elevate the risk of hypokalemia.

Clinical Manifestations

Potassium depletion poses a risk for increased ventricular arrhythmias, and hypokalemia can exacerbate arrhythmias induced by HF therapies such as digitalis, while also compromising the efficacy of antiarrhythmic drugs by altering myocardial electrophysiological properties. Approximately 50% of deaths from heart failure are sudden, often due to arrhythmias. In cases of sudden cardiac death, myocardial potassium levels are frequently lower compared to controls, and survivors may exhibit hypokalemia, possibly resulting from a potassium shift from the intravascular compartment. Whether hypokalemia precedes and triggers the episode or occurs as a consequence of resuscitation remains uncertain; however, a correlation has been found between decreased serum potassium (<4.4 mEq/L) and sudden cardiac death.

Potassium depletion can lead to diastolic dysfunction, while high potassium levels protect against hypertensive endothelial dysfunction and mediates vasodilation via rectifying potassium channels and the sodium-potassium-ATPase in vascular smooth muscle cells and therefore restoring the nitric oxide bioavailability [10]. Furthermore, targeting a higher plasma K to high-normal levels mitigates the systolic and diastolic left ventricular function in patients with low-normal to moderately reduced left ventricular ejection fraction [11]. These positive effects could be explained by an increase in intracellular K which improves contractility as well as impulse generation coupled with a lowering of intracellular sodium which is a hallmark of heart failure.

Therapeutic Considerations

While diuretics and adrenergic stimulation can induce hypokalemia, neurohormonal blockade using ACE inhibitors, angiotensin receptor blockers, beta-blockers, and aldosterone antagonists may cause hyperkalemia. Thus, serum potassium levels should be regularly monitored in these patients.

The treatment of hypokalemia depends on its severity and etiology. Unlike hyponatremia, in which the total body sodium deficit can be readily estimated, serum potassium may not accurately reflect total body stores. Mild hypokalemia of heart failure patients can be managed with aldosterone receptor antagonists like spironolactone or eplerenone, while severe cases may require potassium supplementation. Symptomatic or severe hypokalemia should be corrected with a solution of intravenous potassium: 10–40 mEq infused over 2–3 h (infusion rate should not to exceed 10 mEq/h). In less urgent situations, oral supplementation is preferred and safer: 50–100 mEq/d divided two-four times per day. Long-term treatment should be based on the recognition of the hypokalemia cause. Therefore, hypokalemia in HF warrants close monitoring and management to mitigate adverse outcomes and optimize cardiovascular health. Routine potassium replacement should be considered in HF patients, even if initial potassium levels appear normal.

Hyperkalemia

Hyperkalemia is a significant concern in HF patients since it could exacerbate the symptoms of heart failure and complicate its management. It can cause electrical issues ranging from conduction system abnormalities to life-threatening rhythm disorders and interfere with defibrillator function. Additionally, hyperkalemia can lead to the reduction or discontinuation of RAAS inhibitors and angiotensin-neprilysin inhibitors, which are essential for HF therapy. Furthermore, hyperkalemia is associated with increased hospital length of stay and mortality [12].

The prevalence of hyperkalemia in heart failure varies widely, depending on the population and criteria used for diagnosis, ranging from 1% to 16% in different studies [13–15] due to differences in how hyperkalemia is defined. Trials consistently demonstrate a link between potassium levels and mortality in chronic HF. Incident hyperkalemia, though not directly associated with increased mortality, often leads to RAAS inhibitors downtitration or discontinuation, which independently increases mortality.

Pathogenesis

In the setting of hyperkalemia, it's important to verify the accuracy of the measurement since pseudo hyperkalemia, a falsely elevated serum potassium, could occur favorized by factors such as hemolysis, phlebotomy technique or errors in the laboratory. Pseudo hyperkalemia should be suspected when there is no apparent cause for the hyperkalemia in an asymptomatic patient who has no clinical or electrocardiographic manifestations of hyperkalemia "True" hyperkalemia in HF patients is due to decreased potassium excretion or increased intake (see Table 3.1).

Medication like RAAS inhibitors frequently cause hyperkalemia in HF patients by inhibiting angiotensin-II-mediated aldosterone secretion by the adrenal gland. Additionally, they cause efferent arteriolar vasodilation, which reduces the glomerular filtration rate by altering renal blood flow. Mineralocorticoid receptor antagonists directly block aldosterone secretion, leading to hyperkalemia by decreasing the renal excretion of potassium.

Other comorbidities such as chronic kidney disease or diabetes play a significant role in the development of hyperkalemia. Kidney injury, which may occur in the context of cardiorenal syndrome (types I and II), leads to hyperkalemia due to reduced renal potassium excretion. Under normal conditions, the kidneys excrete 90% of all potassium, with only 10% reaching the distal tubule. Here, excess potassium is excreted into the urine by the principal cells in the renal collecting duct, a process facilitated by the Na+/K+ ATPase and luminal sodium channels. This

Table 3.1 Common causes of hyperkalemia in heart failure patients

Increased dietary potassium intake
Metabolic acidosis
Hyperglycemia
Medication: RAAS inhibitors, K sparing diuretics, Angiotensin–neprilysin inhibitors, Beta-blockers, calcineurin inhibitors, heparin
Chronic kidney disease
Acute kidney injury
Type IV renal tubular acidosis

regulation is influenced by both sodium concentration and serum aldosterone levels at the distal tubule. In heart failure, decreased renal blood flow and perfusion pressure trigger renin secretion by the juxtaglomerular cells, initiating the RAAS cascade. In healthy individuals, elevated aldosterone levels promote potassium excretion. However, in heart failure patients, increased aldosterone levels enhance sodium reabsorption, reducing the amount of sodium delivered to the distal nephron and impairing potassium excretion [16].

CKD can also lead to impaired renin release, resulting in hyporeninemic hypoaldosteronism, which is a cause of hyperkalemia. Additionally, aldosterone resistance can occur in CKD, further contributing to hyperkalemia. Type IV renal tubular acidosis, characterized by a hypoaldosteronism state, also leads to hyperkalemia. This condition can be inherited or acquired, often seen in individuals with diabetes or those taking certain medications such as ACE inhibitors, MRAs, NSAIDs, heparin, beta blockers, digitalis, trimethoprim, and cyclosporine.

Dietary potassium intake must also be considered in patients with hyperkalemia. Potassium supplements and sodium substitutes that are high in potassium need to be accounted for. Other potential causes of hyperkalemia in the general population include adrenal insufficiency, metabolic acidosis, and trauma leading to rhabdomyolysis.

Clinical Manifestations

The most severe effects of hyperkalemia include muscle weakness or paralysis, cardiac conduction abnormalities, and arrhythmias, often occurring at potassium levels of ≥7.0 mEq/L in chronic hyperkalemia or potentially even at lower levels during acute rises in serum potassium. Patients experiencing skeletal muscle or cardiac manifestations typically display one or more characteristic ECG abnormalities associated with hyperkalemia. These changes can include high peaked T waves with a shortened QT interval as initial findings, followed by progressive lengthening of the PR interval and QRS duration, disappearance of the P wave, and eventually widening of the QRS complex to a sine wave pattern.

Hyperkalemia can also cause various conduction abnormalities and arrhythmias, including right bundle branch block, left bundle branch block, bifascicular block, advanced atrioventricular block, sinus bradycardia, sinus arrest, slow idioventricular rhythms, ventricular tachycardia, ventricular fibrillation, and asystole.

Furthermore, hyperkalemia significantly increases the risk of mortality in various patient populations, including those with and without preexisting cardiovascular disease, different severities of chronic kidney disease, and critically ill hospitalized patients. Rapid-onset hyperkalemia may pose a greater mortality risk than slowly developing hyperkalemia, with arrhythmia playing a pivotal role in the increased mortality.

Early correction of serum potassium levels is associated with reduced mortality in hyperkalemic patients presenting to the emergency department or intensive care unit.

Hyperkalemia interferes with renal ammonium excretion, limiting acid excretion and potentially leading to the development of metabolic acidosis. Several mechanisms contribute to this effect, including intracellular alkalosis, reduced NH4+ reabsorption in the thick ascending limb of the loop of Henle, and diminished proximal tubular ammoniagenesis.

Therapeutic Considerations

Effective management of hyperkalemia in heart failure involves a proactive strategi including regular monitoring and medication adjustment. Frequent monitoring of serum potassium levels is crucial, especially after initiating or adjusting medications that affect potassium. The American Heart Association recommends monitoring potassium levels every 1–2 weeks during medication titration and periodically thereafter. Adjusting doses or discontinuing RAAS inhibitors may be necessary in the presence of hyperkalemia. Balancing the benefits of these medications against the risk of hyperkalemia requires careful clinical judgment. Studies suggest that careful down-titration can mitigate hyperkalemia without significantly compromising heart failure outcomes.

Acute Management of Hyperkalemia in HF

Given the cardiotoxic effects of hyperkalemia, stabilizing the membrane with calcium is essential, especially if ECG changes related to hyperkalemia are present. To acutely lower the potassium levels, agents that shift potassium from the extracellular to the intracellular space are used, such as insulin, salbutamol, and sodium bicarbonate. Loop diuretics, which inhibit the Na+/K+/2Cl− cotransporter in the loop of Henle, increase sodium delivery to the distal nephron, stimulating potassium excretion. They are typically reserved for hyperkalemic patients who are volume overloaded. In severe cases of hyperkalemia associated with cardiac electrical abnormalities or in cases of hyperkaliemia refractory to medical management, hemodialysis may be necessary.

Chronic Management of Hyperkaliemia in HF

Limiting dietary potassium intake can help manage mild hyperkalemia. Dietitian-guided interventions have shown to reduce serum potassium levels effectively.

Sodium polystyrene sulfate (SPS), the oldest potassium-binding resin, has been used for the past 60 years. SPS binds potassium ions in the intestine in exchange for sodium ions, but this binding is nonspecific and can also involve calcium and magnesium. The use of SPS is mainly limited by its side effects, which can include nausea, vomiting, constipation, or diarrhea, as well as severe adverse events such as ulcers and perforations. Additionally, SPS increases the sodium load (1500 mg of sodium in 15 g) which may lead to worsening hypertension or heart failure symptoms.

Newer binder, such as patiromer and sodium zirconium were designed to address the limitations of the early generation binding resins. Clinical trials have demonstrated their efficacy and safety in heart failure patients. Patients with hyperkalemia and concomitant HF and/or CKD have higher rates of hospital visits and longer stays. Those with both HF and hyperkalemia incur significantly higher healthcare costs, averaging over four times more than normokalaemia patients. Even if these newer agents remain expensive, they may overall save costs to the healthcare system.

Sodium-glucose cotransporter 2 (SGLT2) inhibitors reduce the risk of cardiorenal events in people with HF with or without chronic kidney disease. Recent findings from a metanalysis of more than 50,000 patients, revealed that SGLT2 inhibitors effectively lowered the risk of serious hyperkalemia (defined as serum potassium ≥6.0 mmol/L) without increasing the risk of hypokalemia.

This risk reduction was observed consistently across various participant characteristics, including different levels of kidney function, albuminuria, history of heart failure, and concurrent use of diuretics. The study suggests that the decreased risk of serious hyperkalemia associated with SGLT2 inhibitors may enable greater use of renin angiotensin-aldosterone system inhibitors in individuals with type 2 diabetes and either chronic kidney disease or heart failure [17].

Hypomagnesemia

Magnesium is an essential mineral involved in various physiological processes, has gained increased attention for its potential role in the pathophysiology and management of HF. Magnesium plays pivotal roles in cardiovascular health, influencing cardiac rhythm, vascular tone, and myocardial contractility.

Hypomagnesemia is a commonly encountered condition in individuals with HF, and may be due in part to diuretic therapy [18], but its effect on mortality is still a matter of debate. For instance, a study of over 1000 patients with class III or IV heart failure found no correlation between initial hypomagnesemia and 6-month survival [19] while another study found that serum magnesium levels ≤2 mEq/L were linked to higher all-cause and cardiovascular mortality risks (hazard ratios 1.23 and 1.38, respectively) [20].

Emerging evidence suggests hypomagnesemia is not only a risk amplifier in HF patients but is also a risk factor for the development of HF. Thus, in the ARIC cohort of 14,709 patients, those in the lowest quintile of serum magnesium had a 2.6-fold higher risk of heart failure over a median of 20.6 years compared to those in the highest quintile [21].

Pathogenesis

Magnesium participates in numerous enzymatic processes and serves as a crucial component in mitochondrial structure and function. Additionally, it regulates cellular potassium permeability and influences calcium uptake and distribution [22].

Magnesium plays pivotal roles in cardiovascular health, influencing cardiac rhythm, vascular tone, and myocardial contractility. Within the myocardium, magnesium facilitates ATP-dependent ion pumps, regulating intracellular calcium levels and modulating myocardial contractility. Additionally, magnesium acts as a physiological calcium antagonist, counteracting the effects of calcium on vascular smooth muscle and promoting vasodilation. Furthermore, magnesium modulates cardiac electrical activity by influencing ion channel function, thereby regulating cardiac excitability and maintaining normal sinus rhythm.

Clinical Manifestations

Hypomagnesemia is associated with increased arrhythmic risks, including atrial and ventricular arrhythmias. Moreover, magnesium deficiency exacerbates myocardial dysfunction, impairs endothelial function, and promotes inflammation, thereby predisposing patients to cardiovascular events and worsening heart failure symptoms. Conversely, magnesium supplementation has shown promising effects in improving myocardial function, reducing arrhythmic events, and alleviating heart failure symptoms in select patient populations.

Therapeutic Considerations

The therapeutic utility of magnesium in heart failure management remains an area of active investigation. Magnesium supplementation, either orally or intravenously, holds potential as an adjunctive therapy in heart failure patients with concomitant magnesium deficiency or recurrent arrhythmias. However, optimal dosing regimens, patient selection criteria, and long-term efficacy warrant further research. Moreover, the safety profile of magnesium supplementation, particularly in patients with renal impairment or electrolyte disturbances, necessitates cautious monitoring and individualized therapy.

Conclusion

Electrolyte imbalances in HF patients are common and can lead to serious complications, including arrhythmias and increased mortality. These imbalances often result from HF-related physiological changes and medications like diuretics and RAAS inhibitors. Hyponatremia is the most prevalent and is linked to higher mortality and longer hospital stays. Managing it involves fluid restriction and, in some cases, vasopressin receptor antagonists. Hypokalemia, frequently due to intensive diuretic therapy, increases arrhythmia risk and requires careful potassium level monitoring and supplementation. Hyperkalemia, often caused by RAAS inhibitors, poses significant risks, including life-threatening arrhythmias and management challenges, requiring both acute and chronic management strategies. Hypomagnesemia, commonly due to diuretics, increases arrhythmia risk and impairs myocardial function. Magnesium supplementation shows promise but requires careful patient selection and monitoring.

Understanding the intricate interplay between electrolytes and heart failure pathophysiology is essential for guiding targeted interventions aimed at optimizing patient outcomes. Future research should focus on the optimal role, dosing strategies, and clinical impact of electrolytes for heart failure management with the purpose of improving prognosis for affected individuals.

References

1. Gheorghiade M, et al. Relationship between admission serum sodium concentration and clinical outcomes in patients hospitalized for heart failure: an analysis from the OPTIMIZE-HF registry. Eur Heart J. 2007;28:980–8. https://doi.org/10.1093/eurheartj/ehl542.
2. Gheorghiade M, et al. Characterization and prognostic value of persistent hyponatremia in patients with severe heart failure in the ESCAPE Trial. Arch Intern Med. 2007;167:1998–2005. https://doi.org/10.1001/archinte.167.18.1998.
3. Benedict CR, et al. Relation of neurohumoral activation to clinical variables and degree of ventricular dysfunction: a report from the Registry of Studies of Left Ventricular Dysfunction. SOLVD Investigators. J Am Coll Cardiol. 1994;23:1410–20. https://doi.org/10.1016/0735-1097(94)90385-9.
4. Goldberg A, et al. Hyponatremia and long-term mortality in survivors of acute ST-elevation myocardial infarction. Arch Intern Med. 2006;166:781–6. https://doi.org/10.1001/archinte.166.7.781.
5. Renneboog B, Musch W, Vandemergel X, Manto MU, Decaux G. Mild chronic hyponatremia is associated with falls, unsteadiness, and attention deficits. Am J Med. 2006;119(71):e71–8. https://doi.org/10.1016/j.amjmed.2005.09.026.
6. Refardt J, et al. A randomized trial of empagliflozin to increase plasma sodium levels in patients with the syndrome of inappropriate antidiuresis. J Am Soc Nephrol. 2020;31:615–24. https://doi.org/10.1681/asn.2019090944.
7. Yeoh SE, et al. Relationship of dapagliflozin with serum sodium: findings from the DAPA-HF trial. JACC Heart Fail. 2022;10:306–18. https://doi.org/10.1016/j.jchf.2022.01.019.

8. Bjornstad P, et al. The potential roles of osmotic and nonosmotic sodium handling in mediating the effects of sodium-glucose cotransporter 2 inhibitors on heart failure. J Card Fail. 2021;27:1447–55. https://doi.org/10.1016/j.cardfail.2021.07.003.
9. Cleland JG, Dargie HJ, Robertson I, Robertson JI, East BW. Total body electrolyte composition in patients with heart failure: a comparison with normal subjects and patients with untreated hypertension. Br Heart J. 1987;58:230–8. https://doi.org/10.1136/hrt.58.3.230.
10. Zhou MS, Kosaka H, Yoneyama H. Potassium augments vascular relaxation mediated by nitric oxide in the carotid arteries of hypertensive Dahl rats. Am J Hypertens. 2000;13:666–72. https://doi.org/10.1016/s0895-7061(99)00269-1.
11. Winsløw U, et al. The effect of increased plasma potassium on myocardial function; a randomized POTCAST substudy. Int J Card Imaging. 2023;39:2097–106. https://doi.org/10.1007/s10554-023-02914-x.
12. Núñez J, et al. Long-term potassium monitoring and dynamics in heart failure and risk of mortality. Circulation. 2018;137:1320–30. https://doi.org/10.1161/circulationaha.117.030576.
13. Desai AS, et al. Incidence and predictors of hyperkalemia in patients with heart failure: an analysis of the CHARM Program. J Am Coll Cardiol. 2007;50:1959–66. https://doi.org/10.1016/j.jacc.2007.07.067.
14. Pitt B, et al. The effect of spironolactone on morbidity and mortality in patients with severe heart failure. Randomized Aldactone Evaluation Study Investigators. N Engl J Med. 1999;341:709–17. https://doi.org/10.1056/nejm199909023411001.
15. Rossignol P, et al. Unravelling the interplay between hyperkalaemia, renin-angiotensin-aldosterone inhibitor use and clinical outcomes. Data from 9222 chronic heart failure patients of the ESC-HFA-EORP Heart Failure Long-Term Registry. Eur J Heart Fail. 2020;22:1378–89. https://doi.org/10.1002/ejhf.1793.
16. Sarwar CM, et al. Hyperkalemia in heart failure. J Am Coll Cardiol. 2016;68:1575–89. https://doi.org/10.1016/j.jacc.2016.06.060.
17. Neuen BL, et al. Sodium-glucose cotransporter 2 inhibitors and risk of hyperkalemia in people with type 2 diabetes: a meta-analysis of individual participant data from randomized. Controll Trials Circ. 2022;145:1460–70. https://doi.org/10.1161/circulationaha.121.057736.
18. Cooper HA, Dries DL, Davis CE, Shen YL, Domanski MJ. Diuretics and risk of arrhythmic death in patients with left ventricular dysfunction. Circulation. 1999;100:1311–5. https://doi.org/10.1161/01.cir.100.12.1311.
19. Eichhorn EJ, et al. Clinical and prognostic significance of serum magnesium concentration in patients with severe chronic congestive heart failure: the PROMISE Study. J Am Coll Cardiol. 1993;21:634–40. https://doi.org/10.1016/0735-1097(93)90095-i.
20. Adamopoulos C, et al. Low serum magnesium and cardiovascular mortality in chronic heart failure: a propensity-matched study. Int J Cardiol. 2009;136:270–7. https://doi.org/10.1016/j.ijcard.2008.05.006.
21. Lutsey PL, et al. Serum magnesium, phosphorus, and calcium are associated with risk of incident heart failure: the Atherosclerosis Risk in Communities (ARIC) Study. Am J Clin Nutr. 2014;100:756–64. https://doi.org/10.3945/ajcn.114.085167.
22. Touyz RM, de Baaij JHF, Hoenderop JGJ. Magnesium Disorders. N Engl J Med. 2024 6;390(21):1998-2009. https://doi.org/10.1056/NEJMra1510603. PMID: 38838313.

Part II
Role of Cardiac Imaging in the Evaluation of Heart Failure

Chapter 4
Assessment of Left Ventricular Systolic and Diastolic Dysfunction

Bogdan A. Popescu, Carmen C. Beladan, and Anca D. Mateescu

Abstract Echocardiography is the imaging method of choice in the evaluation of patients with heart failure (HF) due to its accuracy, availability, low cost and safety profile. It provides a wealth of information about left and right ventricular size, geometry and function, left atrium size, valve function, pulmonary pressures, and the pericardium. It provides evidence about the cause of HF, which is critical for the selection of the best treatment. The assessment of left ventricular (LV) ejection fraction (EF) is essential to differentiate HF with reduced ejection fraction from HF with preserved EF and HF with mid-range EF, and therefore to guide proper therapies based on LVEF cut-off values. Abnormalities in diastolic function are extremely common in patients with HF and either reduced or preserved LVEF and may have prognostic implications. Since LV diastolic dysfunction is thought to be the main pathophysiological abnormality in patients with HFpEF, evaluation of LV diastolic function and filling pressure is of utmost importance for both diagnostic and prognostic purposes. Thus, the information provided by a comprehensive echo exam aids greatly in the better management of HF patients.

Keywords Echocardiography · Left ventricular systolic function · Left ventricular diastolic function

Introduction

The diagnosis of heart failure (HF) can be sometimes difficult because symptoms are not specific, especially in the elderly, and signs can be absent, particularly in patients receiving treatment, or may have a low reproducibility. Thus, the key to the diagnosis of HF is the evidence of an underlying cardiac cause. Cardiovascular imaging has a central role in the diagnosis and identification of the HF etiology.

B. A. Popescu (✉) · C. C. Beladan · A. D. Mateescu
University of Medicine and Pharmacy "Carol Davila", Euroecolab, Emergency Institute for Cardiovascular Diseases "Prof. Dr. C. C. Iliescu", Bucharest, Romania

M. Dorobanţu et al. (eds.), *Current Approach to Heart Failure*,
https://doi.org/10.1007/978-3-031-96562-3_4

Echocardiography is a diagnostic test that accurately and noninvasively provides information about structural and functional abnormalities and can assess the underlying cause so that an optimal management strategy can be implemented. Due to its accuracy, availability, low cost and safety profile, echocardiography is the imaging method of choice in the evaluation of patients with HF [1].

Transthoracic echocardiography (TTE) is the imaging method that usually underlines the first diagnosis of HF in urgent, elective, or screening settings [2]. TTE can provide a wealth of information about left and right ventricular size, geometry and function, left atrium size, valve function, pulmonary pressures, and the pericardium.

The left ventricular (LV) ejection fraction (EF) is useful to differentiate HF with reduced ejection fraction (HFrEF, when EF $< 40\%$) from HF with preserved EF (HFpEF, EF $\geq 50\%$), and HF with mid-range EF (HFmrEF, EF between 40% and 50%) [3]. Abnormalities in diastolic function are very common in patients with heart failure and either reduced or preserved LVEF and may have prognostic implications. Around half of all patients with HF have a normal LV EF [4, 5] and the frequency of this syndrome continues to increase as the prevalence of risk factors involved (e.g. older age, female sex, hypertension) is growing.

Assessment of Left Ventricular Systolic Function

The most common indication for echocardiography is the evaluation of LV function. Echocardiography offers several methods for assessment of systolic function, most of them being indirect estimates of LV systolic performance. Thus, echocardiography may evaluate the percentage change in LV dimension (e.g. LV fractional shortening, LVFS; or LV ejection fraction, LVEF), parameters of LV myocardial deformation (e.g. LV strain and strain rate), the rate of change in intracavitary pressure (i.e. LV dp/dt), or parameters related to the LV output (e.g. stroke volume, cardiac output).

Left Ventricular Fractional Shortening

Fractional shortening (FS) is a percentage change in LV dimensions that is usually obtained by 2D-guided M-mode imaging. It is calculated as the difference between LV end-diastolic and end-systolic diameters divided by LV end-diastolic diameter:

$$\mathrm{FS}(\%) = (\mathrm{LVEDD} - \mathrm{LVESD}) / \mathrm{LVEDD} \times 100.$$

Although easy to measure and widely used, this method has several limitations: it is load dependent, it does not evaluate LV longitudinal function, it may not be representative for the whole ventricle, particularly in the presence of regional wall motion abnormalities (e.g. in patients with coronary artery disease or conduction abnormalities). This parameter is now rarely used for diagnosis or clinical decision making.

Left Ventricular Ejection Fraction

2D Echocardiography

The LVEF is the most commonly used method for assessing LV systolic function [6]. It has proved useful in diagnosis and risk stratification in a variety of cardiovascular diseases and is the basis for recommendations of several important therapies, allocated to patients based on their LVEF [3].

It represents the percentage of LV end-diastolic volume ejected in the following systole. It is therefore calculated as stroke volume divided by LV end-diastolic volume: LVEF = (LVEDV − LVESV)/LVEDV × 100.

Left ventricular volumes may be estimated from 2D echocardiography in different moments of the cardiac cycle. End-diastole is defined as the first frame after mitral valve closure or the frame in which LV volume is the largest [6]. End-systole is defined as the frame after aortic valve closure or the frame in which the LV volume is the smallest. Currently, the recommended 2D method to assess LV EF is the biplane method of disks (modified Simpson's rule). This technique requires two orthogonal apical views. Reliable visualization of the LV endocardial border is essential for reliable LV volume measurements. When the acoustic window is suboptimal, the use of a trans-pulmonary contrast agent to better delineate the endocardial border is recommended [6]. Also, harmonic imaging may improve the definition of the endocardial border.

The normal values for LVFS and LVEF are included in recommendations documents and may be slightly different between TTE and cardiac magnetic resonance (CMR) imaging [6].

Although LVEF carries important prognostic information and is the basis for many therapeutic decisions, it is not an index of contractility, and it simply reflects the volume changes during the cardiac cycle. Thus, it depends on volumes, preload, afterload, heart rate, and valvular function and it does not describe intrinsic myocardial function [3].

For example, LVEF may be preserved in patients with significant mitral regurgitation, despite a reduced forward stroke volume. Moreover, the stroke volume may be normal in patients with HFrEF because of LV dilation, whereas it may be reduced in patients with HFpEF and severe concentric LV hypertrophy. Therefore, LVEF must always be interpreted in clinical context.

Another limitation of LVEF as a measure of LV systolic function is its late impairment in conditions affecting LV function. Thus, LVEF decreases only late in the course of many diseases being unable to detect early LV dysfunction and to trigger initiation of proper treatment. Thus, it has to be combined with more sensitive measures of LV dysfunction.

From a technical standpoint, the accuracy of LVEF estimation by 2DE is affected by image quality, endocardial border definition, ventricular geometry, and representative orthogonal imaging planes.

2D echocardiography is less accurate compared with the gold imaging standard for quantification of LV volumes and LVEF, cardiac magnetic resonance (CMR) [7]. The reasons for the underestimation of LV volumes and EF by echocardiography involve reliance on geometric assumptions and commonly encountered foreshortening of the LV. This underestimation may be overcome using three-dimensional echocardiography (3DE) [8].

3D Echocardiography

3DE may provide measurements of LV volumes and ejection fraction independent of geometric assumptions about LV shape [9–11]. Experience indicates that LV volume measurements are more reliable and accurate with real-time 3DE than with 2DE and also avoid LV foreshortening and geometric assumptions about LV shape [8, 12]. Comparisons of 3DE LV volume determinations with 2DE and CMR imaging measurements showed that LV volume was significantly underestimated by 2DE, and much less by 3DE [12]. Mor-Avi et al. showed in their study that the accuracy of 3DE in volumetric assessments is similar to that of the gold standard CMR [13].

Also, 3DE has proved accurate in assessing LV volumes in remodeled ventricles after myocardial infarction and in evaluating the global LV dyssynchrony [14]. The LV cavity shape allows the extraction of quantitative information in patients with LV dysfunction (e.g. the 3D sphericity index) [9, 15].

Data Acquisition

There are two different methods for data acquisition using 3DE imaging: real-time and multiple-beat. Real-time refers to the acquisition of multiple pyramidal data sets per second in a single heartbeat. This method is limited by poor temporal and spatial resolution although it overcomes the limitations imposed by rhythm disturbances or respiratory motion. Multiple-beat 3DE refers to multiple acquisitions of narrow volumes of data over several heart beats that are subsequently stitched together to form a single volumetric data set. Therefore, this method provides images of higher temporal resolution, although imaging artifacts due to respiratory motion or irregular cardiac rhythms may limit it [9]. In atrial fibrillation, however, the single-beat acquisition is superior because the absence of stitching artifacts is more important than the image quality.

In clinical practice, to quantify LV volumes, LVEF, and LV shape in patients with heart failure, a gated 3DE full volume data set from the apical window must be acquired. It is best to use a wide-angle acquisition in the apical window so as to include the entire ventricle. The acquisition is obtained during breath hold to minimize the risk of artifacts. In multi-beat acquisitions, stitching artifacts can easily be detected in the transversal plane. The transducer frequency and overall gain should be adjusted accordingly to improve image quality. If the acoustic window is limited, then acquisition may be combined with the infusion of contrast to improve delineation of the endocardial border [9].

Images may be displayed with either orthogonal long-axis views or multiple short-axis views. The examiner may obtain multiple slices from the same volumetric data set and different orientations. An advantage of a 3D data set over 2D is the ability to avoid foreshortening [16, 17].

Analysis

Image analysis may be performed offline, using a dedicated 3D software, or online, with a software intrinsic to the ultrasound machine. Following manual identification of the mitral annulus and LV apex, the program automatically identifies the endocardial surface using a deformable shell model [9]. For the calculation of LV volumes, the LV trabeculae and papillary muscles should be included within the LV cavity. The end-diastolic LV volume will be automatically computed directly from voxel counts. After that, end-systole will be selected by identifying the frame in which the LV volume is smallest. Endocardial border detection, including initialization, will then be repeated on this frame to obtain end-systolic volume. The 3DE LV EF will be calculated from these LV volumes (Fig. 4.1).

Also, the LV volumes can be segmented, which allows for regional LV function assessment. Regional LV volumes are divided into 17 segments, and the relative contribution of each volume segment to the global LV systolic function can be established. Time-volume curves can be generated to evaluate each LV volume segment changes over time and also the presence of dyssynchrony. This may be of particular interest in guiding optimal LV lead placement for cardiac resynchronization therapy (CRT). The accuracy of LVEF measurements may guide a more appropriate selection of patients who are suitable for CRT.

The real-time 3D imaging of the LV may also be used during stress echocardiography. Preliminary clinical studies have confirmed the feasibility of this technique and reported sensitivity and specificity comparable to 2D stress imaging. An advantage of real-time 3D stress echo would be the reduced acquisition time [18, 19].

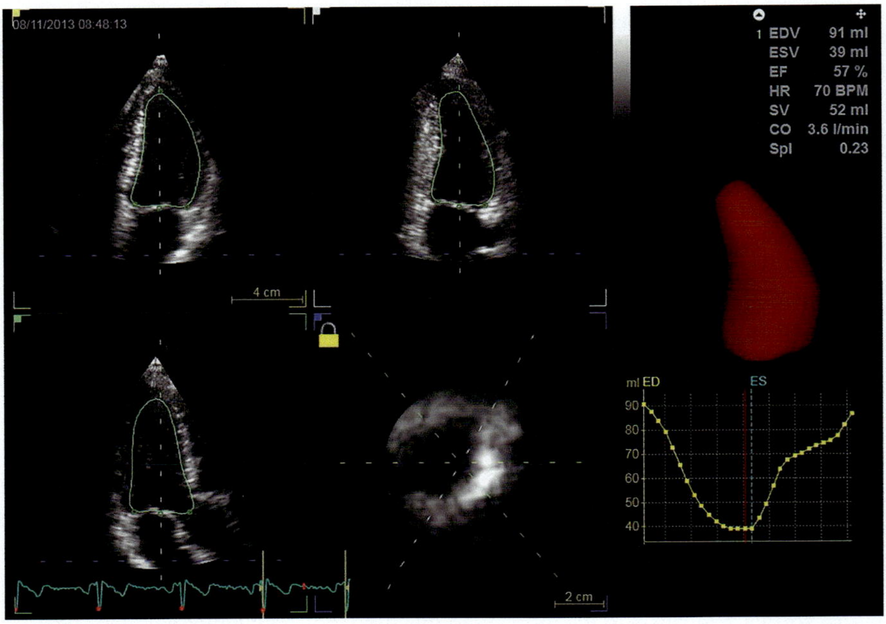

Fig. 4.1 The assessment of left ventricular ejection fraction by 3D echocardiography

Stroke Volume and Cardiac Output

Other approaches commonly used to assess LV systolic function are stroke volume (SV) and cardiac output (CO) estimates.

Stroke volume can be determined through volumetric or Doppler methods.

Volumetric Method SV can be measured by subtracting LV end-systolic volume from LV end-diastolic volume, obtained by the Simpson method or by 3D echocardiography, as previously described. The difference should be equal to the SV across the LVOT if there is no valvular regurgitation.

Doppler Method Stroke volume can be measured by multiplying the velocity time integral (VTI) in the LV outflow tract (LVOT) by the LVOT area. The VTI in the LVOT can be measured by PW Doppler from the apical five-chamber/long-axis view, while LVOT diameter (D_{LVOT}) is usually measured in the parasternal long-axis view (Fig. 4.2) and it is used to calculate the LVOT area assuming it has a circular shape.

$$\text{The formula used is}: \mathrm{SV} = \pi \times \left(\mathrm{D_{LVOT}}^2/4\right) \times \mathrm{LVOT\,VTI}\left(\mathrm{ml}\right).$$

Although this is a useful method to estimate cardiac output, it has some limitations. Small errors in the measurement of LVOT diameter lead to significant errors

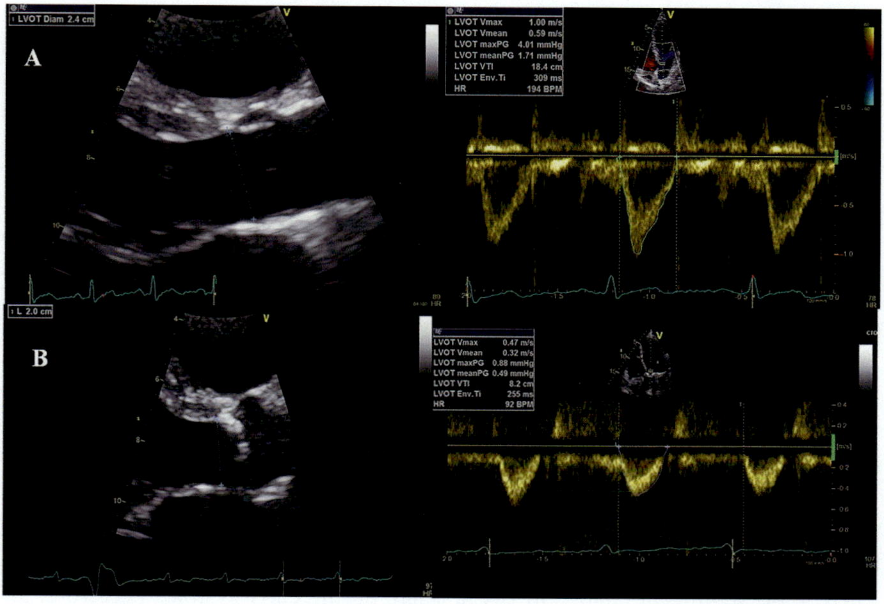

Fig. 4.2 Determination of stroke volume by Doppler method. The first patient (**a**) has a normal SV: LVOT 2.4 cm, LVOT VTI 18.4 cm, SV 83 ml. The second patient (**b**) has a reduced SV due to severe LV systolic dysfunction: LVOT 2 cm, LVOT VTI 8.2 cm, SV 25 ml. *LVOT* left ventricular outflow tract, *VTI* velocity time integral, *SV* stroke volume

in the calculation of LVOT area (because the radius of the outflow tract is squared). Moreover, the LVOT is often oval, not circular so using the assumption of a circular area implies an inherent error in many cases.

The presence of significant valve regurgitation may affect the use of SV as a measure of LV systolic function. For example, the presence of significant aortic regurgitation would increase the SV, overestimating the LV systolic performance. Cardiac output can be calculated multiplying the SV by the heart rate, while the cardiac index can then be obtained dividing the cardiac output by the body surface area [6].

LV Regional Function

Even though measures of global LV function provide quantification of overall cardiac performance, the regional function can vary substantially, such as in ischemic heart disease. Acute myocardial infarction (MI) can cause regional wall motion abnormalities in a specific coronary distribution. Currently, regional wall motion is assessed qualitatively using a scoring system based on a 17-segment model. In this system, each segment is scored as normal or hyperkinetic (1 point), hypokinetic (2 points), akinetic (3 points), or dyskinetic (4 points) [6]. The wall motion score index (WMSI) is the average value of all analyzed segments. Therefore, a normokinetic LV has a WMSI score of 1.0, and the index increases as wall motion abnormalities become more severe. This score also has prognostic value and a higher score is an independent predictor of morbidity and mortality, including increased hospitalizations for heart failure following MI [20]. Although MI is the most likely reason for regional wall motion abnormalities, other conditions (such as myocarditis or sarcoidosis) can affect myocardial function regionally, but usually not in a definite coronary distribution.

Doppler Methods of LV Systolic Function Evaluation

Rate of LV Pressure Increase

The rate of LV pressure increase during isovolumic contraction, LV dP/dt, reflects force development and thus represents a parameter of myocardial contractility. There is no significant change in LA pressure during early systole. Therefore, the mitral regurgitation (MR) jet velocity is the instantaneous systolic pressure in the LV and reflects LVdP/dt. According to the simplified Bernoulli equation ($G = 4 \times v^2$), pressure gradients may be estimated from measured velocities. Thus, the pressure change calculated from the slope of the CW Doppler spectrum of MR between 1 m/sec (G = 4 mm Hg) and 3 m/sec (G = 36 mm Hg) is 32 mm Hg, while the time interval between these two moments is directly measured. Thus, the dP/dt is calculated from the following formula: LV dP/dt = 32 mm Hg/time.

While normal values are usually ≥12,000 mm Hg/sec, values less than 1000 mm Hg/sec indicate LV systolic dysfunction, and values less than 600 mm Hg/sec imply severely impaired LV systolic function and are associated with poor outcome [21] (Fig. 4.3).

This parameter is complementary to LVEF and is useful mainly when decreased or increased afterload (e.g. significant MR, significant aortic stenosis, respectively) coexist, and the LVEF over/underestimates the LV contractile function. In these settings, dP/dt may be a useful index of LV contractile reserve.

Although the method is very appealing, it has several limitations: the MR signal is needed; small differences in measuring the time interval will lead to large differences in calculated dP/dt; this parameter cannot be used in the presence of acute MR (due to the very high LA pressure).

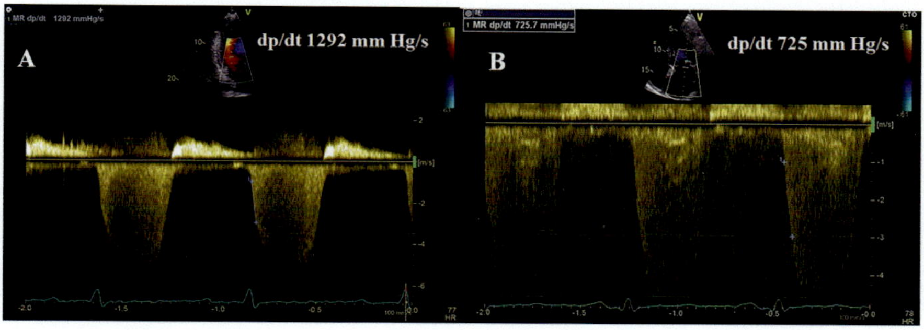

Fig. 4.3 Determination of Doppler-derived LV dP/dt from the continuous-wave Doppler spectrum of the mitral regurgitation jet. The time interval between the moments corresponding to velocities of 1 m/sec and 3 m/sec, respectively, is directly measured. (**a**) Dp/dt in a patient with normal left ventricular systolic function = 1292 mm Hg/s. (**b**) Dp/dt in a patient with reduced left ventricular ejection fraction of 30%: dp/dt of 725 mm Hg/s

Myocardial Deformation Imaging

Novel advanced echocardiographic techniques to image the myocardial mechanics have been developed in the past years. Myocardial deformation imaging is a method for the assessment of intrinsic myocardial function.

The efficient systolic pumping of the LV is a complex process requiring a coordinated contraction of the myocardial fibers. The LV has a complex anatomy with the endocardial and the epicardial fibers orientated in a double helical pattern. The subendocardial fibers have a right-handed orientation, while the subepicardial fibers have a left-handed orientation, forming a helical structure [22]. When it contracts, the LV changes shape and deforms in different directions: it shortens in the longitudinal direction, it thickens in the radial direction, and it shortens circumferentially [22]. Moreover, as the oppositely oriented double helical fibers contract, this leads to a twisting of the LV as the apex rotates in the opposite direction compared to the base. The twisting motion of the LV helps squeezing the blood into the aorta, contributing to a more efficient ejection [23].

During LV ejection, elastic potential energy is stored due to the deformation of the subendocardial fiber matrix. Its subsequent elastic recoil causes rapid untwisting which is associated with the release of restoring forces, creating suction gradients that contribute to early LV diastolic filling by active suction of blood from the atria [22–24].

This complex deformation of the LV in three directions is, therefore, essential for both LV systolic and diastolic function and its impairment contributes to the occurrence of LV dysfunction as the precursor of HF.

It is known that the impairment of longitudinal function is an early marker of LV dysfunction that precedes the drop in LVEF. The use of advanced echocardiography techniques allows measurements of different parameters describing myocardial mechanics, such as myocardial displacement, velocity, strain, and strain rate, in different directions (e.g. longitudinal, radial, and circumferential). Such measurements can be performed either with tissue Doppler or speckle tracking echocardiography.

Tissue Doppler imaging (TDI) allows the preferential sampling of myocardial motion which has lower velocities and larger amplitudes compared to that of the blood flow. TDI is most often recorded using pulsed-wave (PW) or color Doppler. The recorded waves are then analyzed and used to offer information about the myocardial function. The peak systolic myocardial velocity S recorded at the LV base, reflects longitudinal myocardial fiber shortening and has been used to assess LV systolic function in patients with HF. While S values are uniformly reduced in HFrEF, reduced S-wave values as determined by PW-TDI have been reported in a large proportion (around 50%) of patients with HFpEF [25, 26]. These findings suggest that TDI may detect impairment of longitudinal function as an early marker of LV dysfunction, that precedes the drop in LVEF.

One major limitation of assessing LV function by measuring myocardial velocities by TDI is that the translational motion of the heart or tethering by adjacent segments may influence the measured velocities. Assessing LV deformation may overcome this limitation.

Strain (deformation) refers to the actual change in length of the myocardium during the cardiac cycle as compared to its initial value and is expressed as a percentage. Therefore, shortening is expressed as negative values, while lengthening/thickening as positive values.

Strain rate is the rate of instantaneous change in deformation, and is calculated as the difference between two velocities (V) normalized to the distance (d) between them: Strain rate = (V1 − V2)/d. This parameter is expressed as "s^{-1}" [27].

The measurement of LV strain and strain rate by TDI is limited by the requirement of parallel alignment of the Doppler cursor with the direction of myocardial motion. This limits its application to the segments which can be properly insonated and cannot be applied to the whole ventricle and for all types of myocardial deformation.

In clinical practice, measuring strain and strain rate has proved useful to detect abnormalities of both LV systolic and diastolic function in patients with infiltrative cardiomyopathies [28]. Moreover, it can help to differentiate restrictive cardiomyopathy (reduced early diastolic strain rate) from constrictive pericarditis (increased early diastolic strain rate) [29].

One of the most studied applications of TDI is the evaluation of LV dyssynchrony. Intersegmental delay in peak systolic longitudinal contraction between different segments (abnormal > 65 ms), and the standard deviation of time to peak velocity of 12 basal- and mid-LV segments (abnormal >30 ms) are parameters of LV dyssynchrony [30, 31].

Several studies have reported good sensitivity and specificity of TDI techniques in predicting echocardiographic and clinical response after cardiac resynchronization therapy (CRT) [32–34]. However, the negative and/or controversial results of some trials [35] lead to the lack of inclusion of such methods in the recommendations for CRT in HF guidelines [3]. Nonetheless, there may be circumstances where the echocardiographic assessment of LV synchrony may be beneficial. The colocation of the LV lead at the site of maximal delay has been shown to be beneficial in randomized clinical trials [36]. Evidence of mechanical delay may help predict the CRT response when the QRS complex is of intermediate duration or the morphology is not typical of left bundle branch block.

In conclusion, it may be useful in selected cases, in a comprehensive approach, to select borderline candidates, to guide device optimization and to assess response during follow-up.

Doppler-based methods to assess myocardial strain and particularly strain rate are relatively noisy and require dedicated acquisition during scanning, thus limiting their usefulness. The angle-dependent nature inherent to a Doppler technique represents another limitation.

Speckle tracking echocardiography (STE) is a method based on 'speckles' formed by reflection, scattering and interference of the ultrasound beam in the myocardial tissue [37]. The 'speckles' can be tracked frame to frame throughout the entire cardiac cycle and information about tissue motion and its derivatives, including strain and strain rate can be obtained. Strain imaging based on STE has proved to be more reliable and easier to use, although it has poorer temporal resolution than Doppler-based techniques do. Due to its relative angle-independence, STE can be applied to all LV segments, irrespective of the insonation angle. Thus, STE-derived myocardial strain can be measured for all LV segments in the longitudinal, circumferential, and radial directions by using the appropriate imaging plane [28] (Fig. 4.4).

The most robust parameter of LV systolic function assessed by STE is LV global longitudinal strain (GLS), calculated by averaging the different segmental values measured (Fig. 4.5). GLS has proved to be highly feasible and reproducible in the clinical setting [38, 39]. Moreover, LV GLS is an accurate and widely available method for the early detection of subclinical LV longitudinal dysfunction, which occurs before LVEF impairment [27, 40]. It has also been shown that GLS provides incremental prognostic data over LVEF in unselected patients undergoing echocardiography for evaluation of the LV function at rest [38, 39]. Therefore, whenever possible, STE-derived GLS shall be obtained and reported to provide a quantitative analysis of LV longitudinal function [41].

Because of the vendor variability of STE analysis, there is no clear cut-off value of GLS, however, a range from −18% to −22% can be reasonable in a healthy person. The lower the absolute value of GLS is below 18%, the more likely it is to be abnormal [27].

In the early phases of the STE-derived strain measurements, the main limitation was the significant inter-vendor variability, and vendor-independent software was used to circumvent this problem [42]. Since the publication of the consensus paper from the European Association of Cardiovascular Imaging/American Society of Echocardiography/ Industry standardization task force [37], inter-vendor differences in GLS measurements have been markedly reduced to levels similar to those of standard parameters, including LVEF [43–45].

GLS has proved useful both for diagnostic purposes in identifying early LV dysfunction in patients with HFpEF [3] and for prognostic purposes in patients with

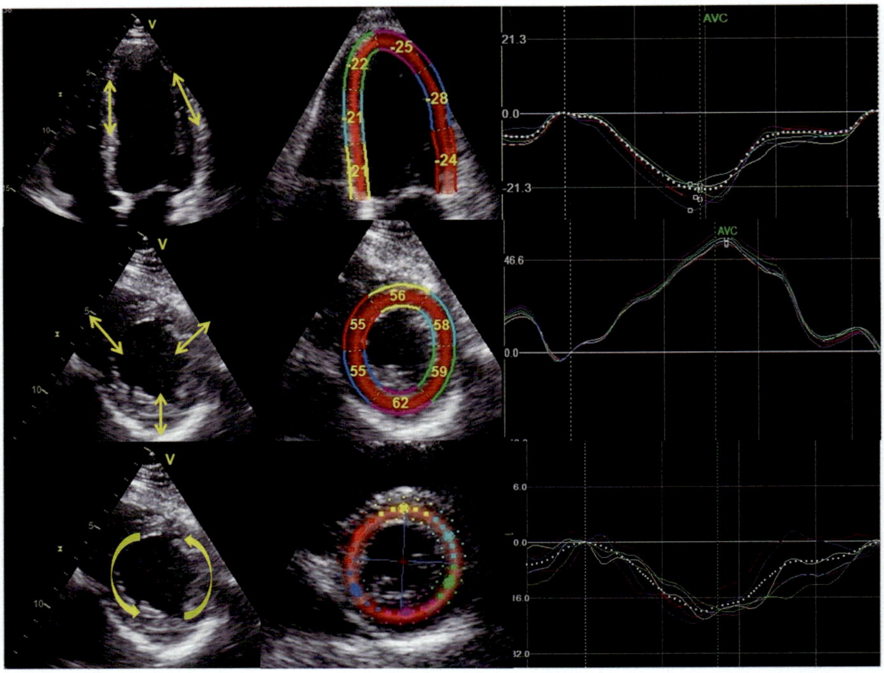

Fig. 4.4 Strain imaging based on 2D speckle tracking echocardiography. On the left column: the directions of myocardial deformation which are assessed (arrows): longitudinal deformation (upper row), radial deformation (middle row), and circumferential deformation (lower row). On the middle column: the peak systolic strain values are displayed for each LV segment. On the right column: the color-coded segmental deformation curves for all LV segments in the longitudinal (upper row), radial (middle row), and circumferential (lower row)

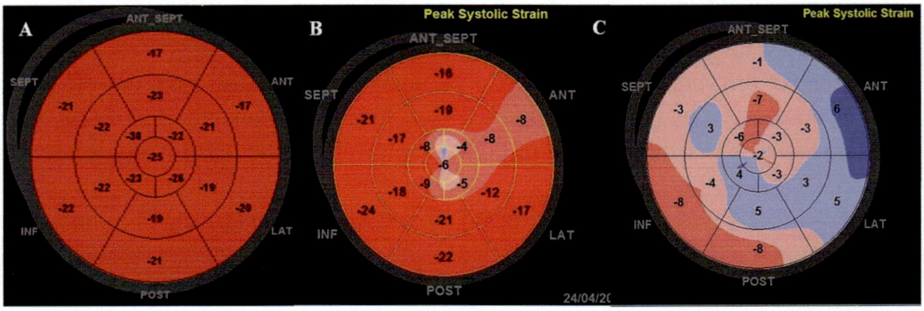

Fig. 4.5 Left ventricular global longitudinal strain (GLS) displayed in the bull's eye format. (**a**) Normal global and regional longitudinal strain in a healthy individual. (**b**) Segmental myocardial dysfunction with a specific coronary distribution (the left anterior descending territory), in a patient with an old anterior myocardial infarction. (**c**) Diffusely reduced global longitudinal strain (not following a specific coronary distribution) in a patient with dilated cardiomyopathy and normal coronary arteries

HfrEF [46]. Moreover, the bulls' eye display of individual segmental values allows rapid identification of LV dysfunction patterns: diffuse in dilated cardiomyopathy, following a specific coronary distribution in patients with coronary disease, or following a specific regional pattern in other disease settings (Fig. 4.5). The latter may be particularly useful in identifying the etiology of LV dysfunction in patients with HFpEF. Thus, apical sparing of longitudinal myocardial deformation has been described in amyloidosis (Fig. 4.6) while regional reductions in LV longitudinal strain in the most hypertrophied areas of the LV has been shown in patients with hypertrophic cardiomyopathy [47] (Fig. 4.7).

The apical sparing in amyloidosis may assume considerable importance in the context of the emerging recognition of transthyretin amyloidosis in low-flow low-gradient aortic stenosis and in HFpEF. While apical sparing probably does not differentiate among the different types of amyloidosis, this pattern distinguishes cardiac amyloidosis from other diagnoses, including Fabry disease and Friedreich ataxia [48].

A recently published clinical validation of an elliptical LV model explains the inconsistency of the association of GLS and global circumferential strain with EF, through the roles of wall thickness and short-axis diameter [49]. Global circumferential strain is much more closely associated with EF than GLS. More importantly, increased LV wall thickness or reduced LV diameter contribute to preserved LV EF contrary to LV longitudinal reduction, but also LV circumferential shortening. Thus, patients with myocardial dysfunction, but a small and hypertrophied LV have a preserved EF despite an impaired GLS. This important observation indicates a benefit of GLS, irrespective of the technique of EF estimation. Accordingly, GLS has been incorporated into guidelines for multimodality cardiovascular imaging of patients with hypertrophic cardiomyopathy as it adds important prognostic information [50].

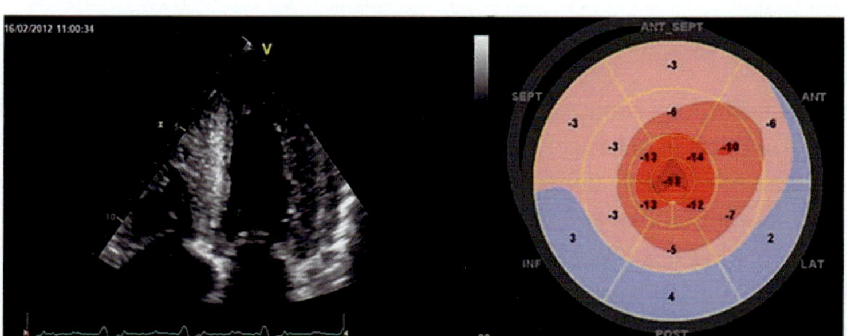

Fig. 4.6 Left ventricular global longitudinal strain (GLS) displayed in the bull's eye format (right panel) reveals apical sparing of longitudinal myocardial deformation in a patient with cardiac amyloidosis (left panel)

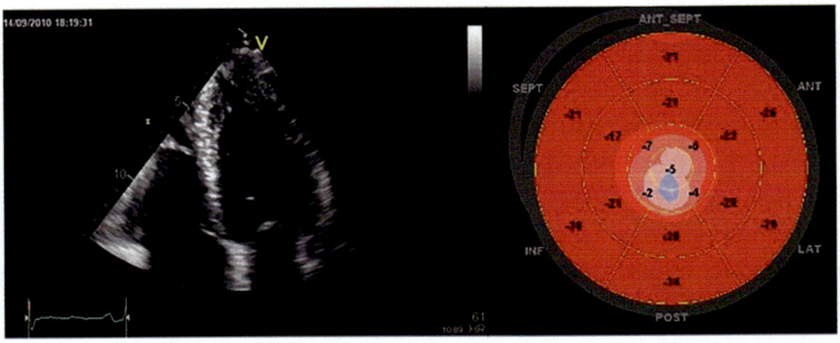

Fig. 4.7 Left ventricular global longitudinal strain (GLS) displayed in the bull's eye format (right panel) shows regional reduction in LV longitudinal strain in the LV apical hypertrophied area in a patient with apical hypertrophic cardiomyopathy (left panel)

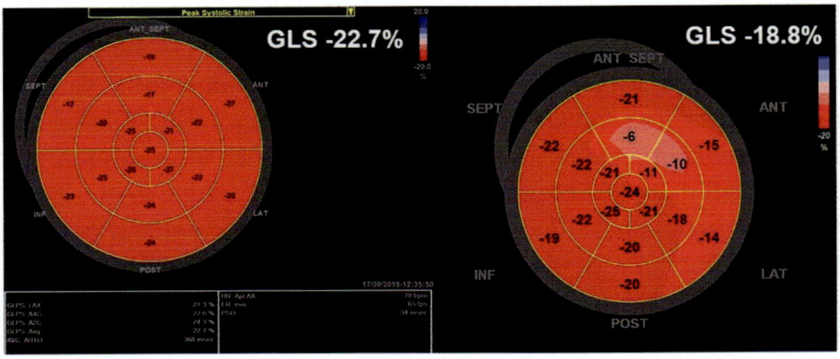

Fig. 4.8 ΔGLS reduction of 17% in a 46 y/o patient with cancer and without cardiovascular risk factors after 4 cycles of trastuzumab therapy (approximately 4 months) while baseline LV EF of 62% did not significantly change during follow-up

Asymptomatic LV Dysfunction

As mentioned above, GLS may identify subclinical LV systolic dysfunction, which has been associated with a greater risk of developing HF or recurrent HF hospitalizations [51].

The most common scenario in which GLS is currently used to assess asymptomatic LV dysfunction is in cancer therapeutics-related cardiac dysfunction (CTRCD). The incidence of CTRCD depends on risk profiles, cumulative anthracycline dose, and therapy combinations [52, 53].

Impairments in GLS precede reductions in LV EF and a 10–15% early reduction in GLS by STE during therapy appears to be the most useful parameter for the prediction of cardiotoxicity [54] (Fig. 4.8). Accordingly, GLS measurement is incorporated into consensus guidelines for an abnormal cardiotoxic response as a >15% relative reduction in GLS from baseline [55]. The use of GLS for routine surveillance provides a potentially early window for the initiation of cardio-protective therapy (CPT). Studies have shown that a GLS-based approach to cardiac surveillance followed by initiation of CPT reduced the degree of reduction in LVEF and the incidence of CTRCD at 1-year follow-up [56, 57].

Heart Failure

Reduced LV strain values were reported in patients with HFrEF, however, studies have also described reductions in myocardial deformation in both longitudinal and circumferential directions in patients with HFpEF [58]. Thus, systolic function abnormalities are quite prevalent in HFpEF, can be detected by echocardiography, and may contribute to the pathophysiology of this syndrome.

The prognostic utility of longitudinal deformation has been robustly demonstrated in patients with reduced and preserved LV EF. GLS is also a predictor of outcome in preclinical HF [59, 60]. Accordingly, GLS has been incorporated into the most recent version of the ACC/AHA guidelines on HF as a useful echocardiographic parameter for the definition of asymptomatic stage B HF (pre-HF), as LV EF is often not reduced in the preclinical phase, and there is a benefit for a comprehensive assessment of myocardial dysfunction by other contractile markers, such as GLS [51].

In patients with HFpEF, reduced longitudinal systolic function can identify patients with more advanced myocardial disease and at a higher risk for adverse events [61].

GLS has been associated with outcomes in symptomatic HFpEF [62] as well as in HFrEF, where strain adds value for outcome stratification of patients with an LV EF <22% [45].

Moreover, GLS independently predicted mortality in acute HF while LV EF did not, a change that reflects the evolution to a predominance of the HFpEF phenotype, which was less common when the classical prognostic data about LV EF were assembled [63].

Strain imaging has also shown prognostic value over traditional imaging markers of LV function after acute myocardial infarction [64].

Valvular Heart Disease

LVEF has prognostic value in patients presenting with aortic stenosis (AS), and this has been used as a criterion for valve replacement in asymptomatic AS [65]. However, in most asymptomatic patients, an LVEF <50% is uncommon, and patients with an LVEF of 50–59% fare almost as badly. Moreover, LVEF is an insensitive marker of LV systolic function, especially in the setting of LV hypertrophy. The phenotype of paradoxical low-flow low-gradient AS is characterized by a small, often hypertrophied LV, typically associated with HFpEF, and alternative parameters for LV function may be needed. GLS detects subclinical dysfunction and has incremental prognostic value over traditional risk markers including haemodynamic severity, symptom class, and LVEF in patients with AS [66]. Moreover, impaired LV GLS is associated with reduced survival in asymptomatic patients with significant AS and normal LVEF [67]. Incorporation of GLS into risk models may improve the identification of the optimal timing for AV replacement.

Impaired LV longitudinal function correlates with LV fibrosis and is associated with poor symptomatic recovery and even deterioration following surgery for symptomatic severe AS [68].

Speckle tracking methods can also be used to assess ventricular rotation and to derive LV twist and torsion. Twist and untwist are important contributors to systole and diastole respectively [24].

Changes in LV volumes between end-diastole to end-systole also do not account for the complexity of myocardial mechanics related to systole.

Impaired LV twist has been described in patients with dilated cardiomyopathy, and reversed apical rotation correlated to the severity of LV systolic and diastolic dysfunction [69].

However, the clinical applications of measuring LV rotation and twist are limited because of technical challenges in obtaining images at sufficient temporal resolution, as well as being able to measure the distance over which torsion develops, and both of these barriers may be scaled by technical developments, such as faster single-beat 3-dimensional (3D) capabilities. In addition, there is high interobserver variability as well as a lack of properly validated normal values.

The assessment of GLS has become a clinically useful alternative to LVEF for the measurement of LV systolic function, while the clinical applications are numerous and expanding. However, experience and proper training are very important.

Assessment of Left Ventricular Diastolic Function

Echocardiographic assessment of LV diastolic function is an essential component of the comprehensive assessment of patients with suspected or confirmed HF diagnosis.

LV diastolic dysfunction (LVDD) is usually the consequence of abnormal LV relaxation, reduced restoring forces and increased LV chamber stiffness, leading to increased cardiac filling pressures [70]. With impaired relaxation, LV filling progressively shifts from early to late diastole and left atrial (LA) contraction becomes responsible for a substantial proportion of LV diastolic filling and cardiac output. In the early stages, as long as LA function is preserved and with an adequate filling period, LV filling pressures (LVFP) remain normal and LVDD is asymptomatic. With further deterioration of LV diastolic function and loss of diastolic reserve, LVFP increase leading to upstream congestion and symptomatic LVDD initially with exercise and eventually at rest [71, 72].

In HFrEF patients, LV diastolic function is virtually always impaired. Thus, when evaluating diastolic function in this setting, the focus is mainly on estimating

LVFP, since it can guide therapy, monitor the disease course and improve outcomes. In patients with suspected HFpEF, on the other hand, the focus is on detecting the presence of LVDD which is the likely cause of HF and fundamental to the diagnosis [70].

A broad spectrum of echocardiographic techniques and parameters may be used to reveal impaired LV relaxation, reduced restoring forces, increased diastolic stiffness, increased LA pressure and LV end-diastolic pressure (LVEDP) in patients presenting with symptoms or signs of HF.

Echocardiographic Diagnosis of Left Ventricular Diastolic Dysfunction in Patients with HFpEF

By demonstrating relevant structural heart disease and LVDD in patients with clinical features of HF and preserved LVEF, echocardiography can provide key diagnostic criteria for HFpEF [3].

Relevant cardiac structural alterations are represented by *pathological LV hypertrophy* (LVH) and *LA dilation*, whereas functional abnormalities (e.g. changes in LV relaxation, compliance or stiffness, indices of increased LVFP) are best reflected by mitral inflow velocities, mitral annular e' velocities, E/e' ratio and tricuspid regurgitation velocity (TRV). Furthermore, since systole and diastole are tightly coupled, echocardiographic markers of LV systolic longitudinal dysfunction can be used as an indication of myocardial disease, supporting the diagnosis of LVDD in patients with inconclusive data. In these cases of uncertainty, pathological "L" velocity in mitral inflow, increased amplitude or duration of atrial reversal velocity in pulmonary vein flow, a shift to an impaired relaxation pattern in mitral inflow with Valsalva maneuver may provide additional information to confirm the diagnosis of LVDD [70].

It should be noted that, according to current guidelines, the term "preserved" LVEF refers to LVEF >50%. LVEF between 40% and 50% in patients with signs and symptoms of HF, along with relevant structural alterations and LVDD supports the diagnosis of HF with mid-range LVEF (HFmrEF). Since LVDD is thought to be the main pathophysiological abnormality in patients with HFpEF and perhaps HFmrEF, LV diastolic function evaluation is of utmost importance in both clinical situations and follows the same diagnostic pathway [3].

2D and 3D echocardiography may reveal structural abnormalities of the heart representing either the cause or the consequence of LVDD and expressing its severity and duration.

Pathological LVH, defined as abnormally increased LV mass in untrained subjects, is a marker of impaired myocardial relaxation and increased stiffness, which strongly suggest the presence of LVDD. It is the most prevalent structural cardiac abnormality reported in patients with HFpEF, and it was independently associated with an increased risk of morbidity and mortality in this setting [6, 73, 74].

The currently recommended method for LV mass estimation in patients without significant cardiac geometry distortions relies on M-mode or 2D echocardiographic linear measurements of LV diastolic diameter and wall thickness as most studies relating LV mass to prognosis are based on this method. However, the linear dimension method using the cubed formula (with LV modeled as a prolate ellipse) may be inaccurate in many HF patients exhibiting asymmetric ventricular hypertrophy. Two-dimensional methods based on either the area-length or truncated ellipsoid technique are less dependent on geometrical assumptions and more suited for LV mass estimation in patients with regional variations in wall thickness. The main limitations of 2D methods are related to methodology, low reproducibility, and limited prognostic data [6].

Three-dimensional echocardiography provides a more accurate estimation of LV mass in patients with remodeled ventricles since it is free of geometric assumptions. However, prognostic data with 3D methods are still scarce [6, 9].

Uniform reference values for LV mass are difficult to define since LV mass may vary with gender, age, body size, obesity and geographic area. Moreover, there is still a controversy related to the term of LV mass indexing (height, weight or body surface area) [6].

The upper limits for normal LV mass currently recommended with 2D measurements, indexed to BSA, are 88 g/m^2 in women and 102 g/m^2 in men. Left ventricular DD should be suspected when LV mass by linear measurements is >95 g/m^2 in women and >115 g/m^2 in men [3, 6]. There is insufficient available data in healthy subjects to recommend reference values for LV mass with 3D echocardiography.

Different patterns of LV remodeling were reported in patients with HFpEF. While concentric LV remodeling/hypertrophy is common, some patients present with normal LV geometry or even with an eccentric pattern. Thus, further assessment of ventricular geometry and function in broader HFpEF populations will be needed to establish the prevalence, correlates, and prognostic significance of these measures [75].

Left atrial (LA) dilation is an important feature for the diagnosis of HFpEF, suggesting the presence of LVDD with long standing increased LVFP. Moreover, LA size emerged as an independent outcome predictor in patients with HFpEF [74].

Bradycardia, atrial arrhythmias, significant mitral valve disease, high-output states may lead to LA dilation on their own, altering the relationship between LA size and LVFP [70, 76]. Thus, LA size value as a supportive finding for the diagnosis of HFpEF is limited in these settings.

2D echocardiography is currently recommended to assess LA size. The anteroposterior diameter, widely used for LA assessment, often underestimates the real LA size in patients with asymmetric LA remodeling [77]. Thus, LA volume, which provides a more accurate assessment of LA size and has superior prognostic value when compared to area or diameter, should be used to estimate LA dilation [6, 78].

3D echocardiography allows a better assessment of LA size due to lack of geometric assumptions, higher accuracy than 2D echo in determining LA volume when compared to CMR, and better prognostic value. However, its use for LA size assessment is still limited by the lack of a standardized methodology, variability, and the limited normative data [6].

Scaling LA volume to body size by dividing it to body surface area is recommended. The cut-off value for normal LA volume is 34 ml/m^2 which is also the reference value for the diagnosis of LVDD and for LVFP assessment [3, 6, 70]. However, LA volume index <34 ml/m^2 does not rule out the LVDD when other relevant parameters are strongly suggesting it. A normal LA volume has been reported in patients with early stages of diastolic dysfunction or with acute elevations of LVFP [6].

In a study comparing echocardiographic features of patients with HFpEF vs non-failing hypertensive subjects with LVH, the product of LV mass index and LA volume emerged as the best predictor of HF-pEF [79]. Thus, the association of LVH and LA dilation in patients experiencing exercise dyspnea increases the likelihood of HFpEF.

Increased LA volume without associated increase of LVFP may be found in athletes, in patients with atrial rhythm disturbances, mitral valve disease, high output states, heart transplants with biatrial technique or in patients with chronic, compensated HF [6].

Conventional Doppler echocardiography is critical to reaching meaningful conclusions regarding LV diastolic function.

Mitral inflow parameters (peak early filling velocity E, peak atrial contraction velocity A, the E/A ratio, E velocity deceleration time, and isovolumic relaxation time IVRT), continue to play a significant role in the workup of HFpEF patients [70]. However, the age and load dependency of these parameters limit their use as first-line tools in this process [80].

Slowing of LV relaxation and of LV pressure decay, in the absence of elevated LA pressure, leading to "impaired LV relaxation" pattern, may be encountered in the early stages of LVDD, but also with increasing age, higher heart rate, right ventricular overload, and other conditions [81]. On the other hand, several studies reported cases of patients presenting with acute or chronic HFpEF showing "impaired relaxation pattern" and increased LVFP probably due to markedly delayed LV relaxation (Fig. 4.9) [82–84].

Moreover, a "pseudonormal" filling pattern in patients with progressive LV diastolic dysfunction and increased LA pressure which restores the early diastolic gradient between the LA and the LV (E/A ratio > 1) may be difficult to differentiate from normal transmitral filling. Further information supporting the presence of LVDD in this setting may be obtained from response to *Valsalva maneuver and pulmonary venous flow analysis*. Thus, a decrease in E/A ratio with Valsalva Maneuver of more than 0.5 in patients with baseline E/A > 1 is highly accurate for "pseudonormal filling" due to increased LVFP and supports the presence of LVDD. Likewise, an increase in pulmonary vein atrial reversal wave Ar, with a difference between Ar duration and mitral A in duration >30 msec has a good accuracy in predicting elevated LVEDP in patients with abnormal LV relaxation [70].

Echocardiographic assessment of *pulmonary artery systolic pressure* (PASP) based on Doppler assessment of tricuspid regurgitation jet peak velocity and inferior vena cava evaluation by 2D echocardiography, should not be overlooked when assessing LV diastolic function in patients with suspected HFpEF. In previous

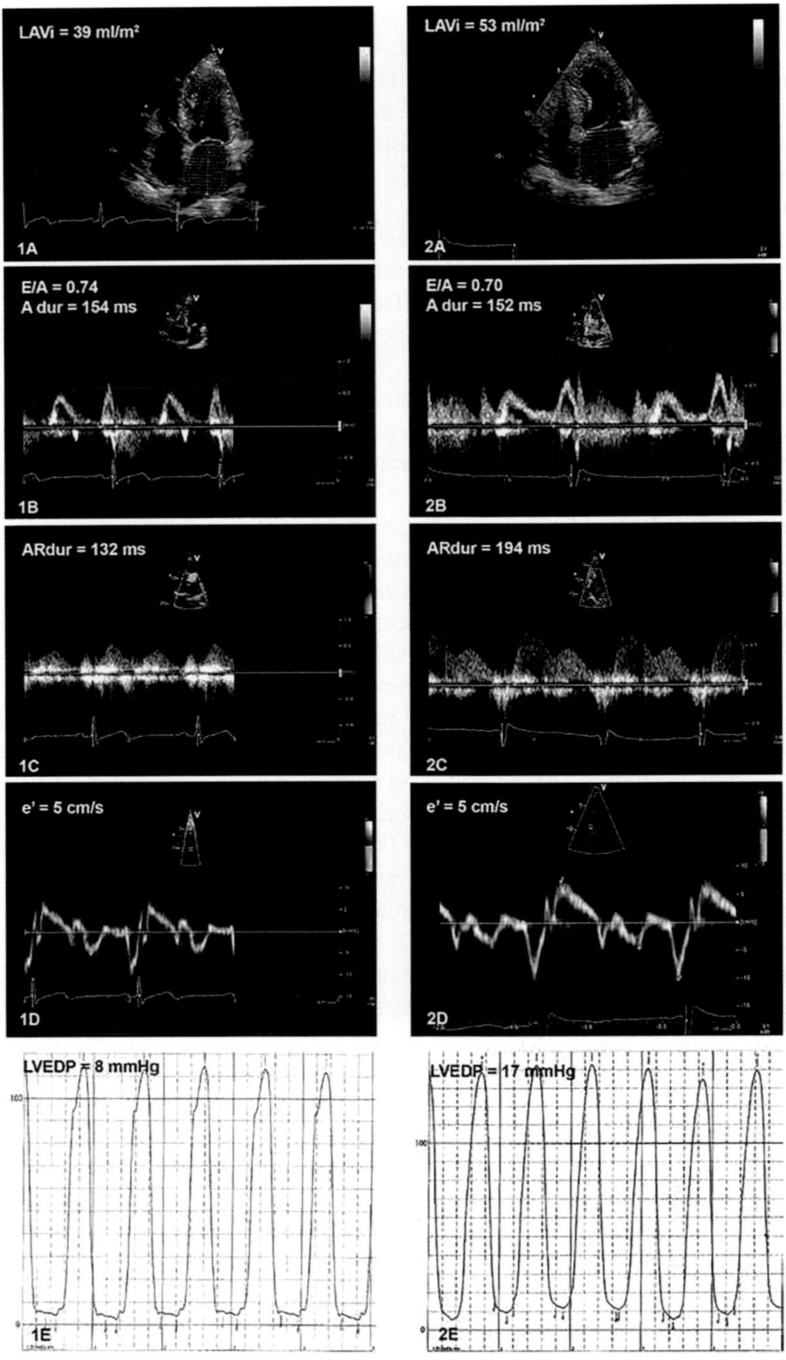
LAVi = 39 ml/m²
1A
LAVi = 53 ml/m²
2A
E/A = 0.74
A dur = 154 ms
1B
E/A = 0.70
A dur = 152 ms
2B
ARdur = 132 ms
1C
ARdur = 194 ms
2C
e' = 5 cm/s
1D
e' = 5 cm/s
2D
LVEDP = 8 mmHg
1E
LVEDP = 17 mmHg
2E

studies, PASP estimated by echocardiography emerged as a better predictor of HFpEF when compared to other echocardiographic parameters associated with LVDD (E/e' ratio, LA volume, and LV wall thickness). Elevated PASP values can identify patients with increased LVFP due to LVDD, provided pulmonary vascular disease or other potential causes of PH such as valvular heart disease, lung disease, chronic thromboembolic disease, and obstructive sleep apnea have been excluded [70, 85, 86]. **Tissue Doppler** derived *mitral annular velocities* are currently considered key echocardiographic measurements in assessing LV diastolic function. The mitral annulus early diastolic velocities (septal and lateral e') are of primary interest as they decrease with impaired LV relaxation and are less preload dependent compared to mitral inflow early diastolic velocity (E wave) in patients with myocardial disease [70, 81, 87, 88]. Whereas the E/A ratio of the mitral inflow exhibits a U-shaped relationship with progressive LVDD, the e' velocities decrease in a continuous manner being less affected by the gradual increase in LVFP. It was suggested that the decrease in e' velocities precedes the reduction in E/A ratio with 10–15 years [87, 89]. Therefore, normal e' velocity is unusual in patients with LVDD related to a myocardial abnormality or disease, which is the main reason why evaluation of diastolic function should begin with e' in patients with normal LVEF [1]. The E/e' ratio is thought to be a reflection of LVFP and can be used as a marker of LVDD. The correlation between E/e' and LVFP has been confirmed in patients with both HFrEF and HFpEF [89, 90]. To date, reduced e' and elevated E/e' are incorporated in guidelines as evidence of LVDD [70].

Although mitral annular velocities are less load dependent than conventional parameters of diastolic function, slowing of myocardial relaxation with increasing age can account for the decrease in both mitral E/A ratio and e' velocities. Moreover, several studies suggested that E/e' is not sensitive enough to detect HFpEF in an

Fig. 4.9 Echocardiographic findings in two patients with normal LVEF and impaired relaxation pattern, yet significantly different left ventricular end-diastolic pressure (LVEDP) at cardiac catheterization. The figure presents: measurements of left atrial volume from the apical four-chamber view—first row **a**; pulsed wave Doppler tracings of mitral inflow—second row **b**; pulsed wave Doppler tracings of pulmonary venous flow—third row **c**; mitral annulus velocities at the septal site—fourth row **d**; left ventricular pressure curves recorded at cardiac catheterization: fifth row **e**. Patient 1 (left column) had a normal LVEDP of 8 mm Hg (**1e**) while patient 2 (right column), who had LV hypertrophy, had a significantly increased LVEDP of 17 mm Hg (**2e**). Both patients had a very similar impaired relaxation filling pattern (**1b**, **2b**). The impaired LV relaxation was confirmed by the reduced early diastolic velocity e': 5 cm/s in both (**1d**, **2d**). Both patients had a dilated left atrium, but the severity of LA dilation was higher in patient 2 (53 ml/m^2, **2a**) compared to patient 1 (39 ml/m^2, **1a**). Although both patients had an E/e' ratio of 8 and a very similar S/D ratio at pulmonary venous flow (**1c**, **2c**), the time difference between pulmonary vein AR duration and mitral A-wave duration was increased only in patient 2 (42 ms). In patient 1 AR duration was actually shorter than mitral A-wave duration (132 ms vs 154 ms), indicating normal LVEDP. In these patients the careful assessment of AR duration and mitral A-wave duration and the size of the LA suggested a higher LVEDP in patient 2 despite the similarity in all the other echo parameters. This example underlines the importance of a comprehensive multi-parameter approach for the evaluation of LV diastolic function. (Reprinted with permission from Ref. [72])

early stage of the disease, when alterations in diastolic processes are very subtle [91–93].

The recently updated recommendations for the evaluation of LV diastolic function by echocardiography proposed four variables to be evaluated when searching for the presence of LV DD in patients with normal LVEF. Three out of the four recommended variables are Doppler-derived indices: *annular e' velocity* (septal e' < 7 cm/sec, lateral e' < 10 cm/sec), *average E/e' ratio* > 14 (E/e' lat > 13 or E/e' sep > 15), and *peak TR velocity* > 2.8 m/sec. Left atrial maximum volume index > 34 mL/m^2 is the fourth parameter required for the diagnosis of LVDD [70].

More than half of the available parameters should meet these cutoff values to make the diagnosis of LVDD [1]. If more than two (or 50%) of the available parameters do not satisfy these cutoff values, LV diastolic function will be considered normal. Between these two situations the study is considered inconclusive [70] (Fig. 4.10).

In patients with suspected HFpEF and inconclusive diastolic function parameters, evaluation of LV longitudinal systolic function may aid the diagnosis, providing evidence of myocardial dysfunction. Parameters such as mitral annular plane systolic excursion using M-mode (MAPSE), tissue Doppler–derived mitral annulus systolic velocity (S), and LV global longitudinal strain (GLS) by speckle-tracking may provide further insight when assessing LV diastolic function, since previous studies have demonstrated a close relationship between systole and diastole and a high prevalence of systolic longitudinal dysfunction in HFpEF population [94, 95].

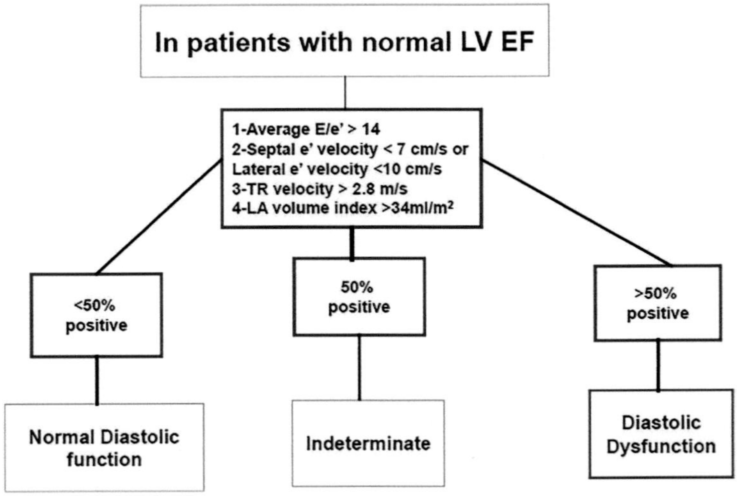

Fig. 4.10 Algorithm for diagnosis of LV diastolic dysfunction in subjects with normal LVEF. (Reprinted with permission from Ref. [70])

Echocardiographic Assessment of Left Ventricular Filling Pressures and Diastolic Dysfunction Grade

Evaluation of LVFP and grading LVDD with echocardiography are two essential components of LV diastolic function assessment in patients with HF irrespective of LVEF. The clinical purpose of LVDD grading is mainly the prognostic stratification of patients whereas the evaluation of LVFP offers an estimate of invasively measured capillary wedge pressure, mean LA pressure, and LV end-diastolic pressure which is clinically relevant for diagnosis (particularly in HFpEF patients), monitoring and guiding therapy [70].

Different evidence emerged from validation studies in patients with preserved or reduced LVEF, and thus, two algorithms were used for several years for grading LVDD and estimating LVFP according to LVEF. Recently, the previously published decision trees merged into one single algorithm (Fig. 4.11). The principal variables recommended for the assessment of LV diastolic function grade include mitral flow velocities, mitral annular e' velocity, E/e' ratio, peak velocity of TR jet, and LA maximum volume index [70].

Of note, the algorithm was based on expert consensus and has not been validated at the time of its publication. Its use has been recommended in the absence of: atrial fibrillation, left bundle branch block, ventricular paced rhythm, at least moderate

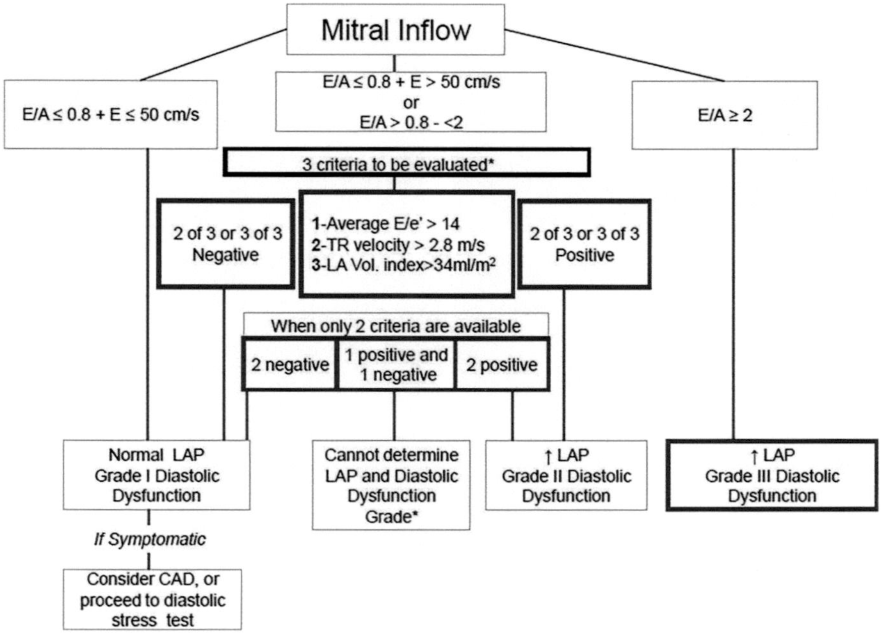

Fig. 4.11 Algorithm for estimation of LV filling pressures and grading LV diastolic function in patients with depressed LVEFs and patients with myocardial disease and normal LVEF after consideration of clinical and other 2D data. (Reprinted with permission from Ref. [70])

mitral annular calcification, more than moderate mitral regurgitation/stenosis, mitral valve repair or prosthetic mitral valve, LV assist devices [70].

Based on this new approach, in patients with preserved LVEF and structural and/or functional heart abnormalities as well as in patients with LV systolic dysfunction (reduced LVEF), LVDD is assumed to be present and the echocardiographic examination should focus on the assessment of LVFP.

In patients with HFrEF, the transmitral inflow pattern is usually sufficient to predict LAP (Fig. 4.12). In this population the restrictive filling pattern (RFP, E/A > 2) indicates grade III LVDD, and it was associated with higher rates of adverse events than non-RFP patients. Moreover, the response of RFP to loading manipulation represents an even stronger predictive marker, since a significant rate of major events was reported in patients with irreversible RFP. The "pseudonormal" filling pattern has also been shown to predict poor outcomes in patients with HF, which was similar to that seen with RFP in some studies. In patients with chronic HF, changes in transmitral flow patterns after chronic optimized therapy are correlated with changes in pulmonary wedge pressure, are accompanied by changes in functional capacity, and provide relevant independent prognostic information [96–99]. Deceleration time of mitral E velocity is usually short with RFP (<160 ms)

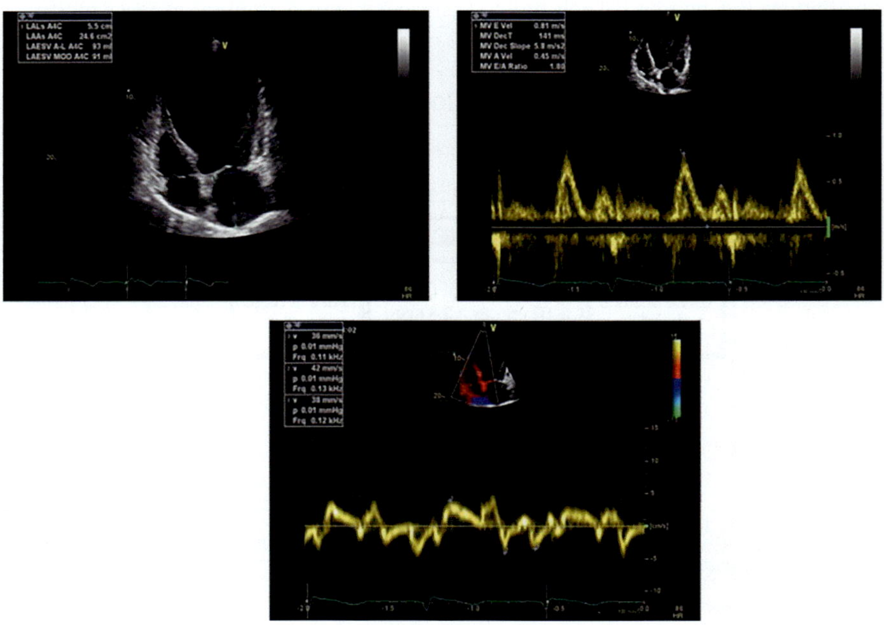

Fig. 4.12 Echocardiographic evaluation of LV diastolic function in a patient with HFrEF: E 81 cm/s, E/A ratio 1.8, EDT 140 ms, LVEF = 20%. The combination of LVEF<35% and restrictive filling pattern with EDT < 150 ms is highly suggestive of increased LVFP. LAVi was 51 ml/m^2 and E/e's ep = 20, also suggestive of high LVFP. At left heart catheterization the measured LVEDP was 20 mm Hg, confirming the echo estimates

and an important predictor of outcome in patients with reduced LVEF, symptomatic or asymptomatic [100].

With a "pseudonormal pattern" or when E/A ratio < 0.8 with a peak E velocity of >50 cm/sec, additional parameters are required to estimate LAP and conclude the grade of LVDD. Among these, average E/e' ratio > 14 supports the presence of elevated LVFP [70]. Several studies reported a high power of e' velocity and E/e' ratio to predict adverse events in patients after acute myocardial infarction, with and without HF [101, 102]. Increased LA volume index (<34 ml/m^2) and peak TR velocity (>2.8 m/s) are the other two recommended parameters supporting the presence of increased LVFP in this setting, both shown to be robust predictors of outcome in HFrEF patients [103–105]. If one of the three main parameters is not available, pulmonary venous flow S/D ratio < 1 may is consistent with elevated LVFP [70].

In patients with myocardial disease and preserved LVEF the recommended approach for LVFP assessment starts with a careful screening for cardiac structural and functional changes relevant in this setting: LA dilation, pathological LV hypertrophy, elevated PASP, provided that alternative explanations for these alterations have been excluded. The proposed algorithm is similar to that for patients with depressed LVEF.

It should be noted that in patients with dyspnea on exertion and preserved LVEF, the echocardiographic diagnosis of grade I LVDD with normal resting LAP should not exclude the presence of cardiac dyspnea, and stress echocardiography is recommended in this setting.

Echocardiographic exercise testing has recently been added to the set of criteria that should be fulfilled for the diagnosis of HFpEF [3, 106]. The recommendation is based on previous studies reporting a lack of diastolic reserve leading to increased LVFP with exercise in patients with LVDD compared to healthy subjects [107–110]. The test may improve de specificity of diagnosing HFpEF in patients with no apparent signs of central fluid overload, grade 1 diastolic dysfunction, which indicates delayed myocardial relaxation and normal filling pressures at rest [70, 101]. On the contrary, no valuable diagnostic input will be gained by extending the recommendation of a diastolic stress test to patients with normal heart and diastolic function at rest (it is unlikely that they will experience dyspnea due to diastolic dysfunction and elevated filling pressures with exercise), or to patients with abnormal findings at baseline consistent with elevated LV filling pressures (LVFP will further increase with exercise) [70].

A diastolic echocardiographic stress test can be performed using a semi-supine bicycle ergometer exercise protocol with the assessment of mitral inflow velocities, mitral annulus tissue Doppler velocities, and peak TR velocity by CW Doppler at baseline, during each stage including peak exercise, and in recovery (Table 4.1).

When the only abnormal finding of a diastolic stress test is an isolated increase in exercise peak TR velocity, available data should be analyzed with caution. Peak TR velocity may increase in healthy subjects due to increased pulmonary blood flow with exercise [70].

Table 4.1 The interpretation of the diastolic stress test [70]

	Resting septal e′	Resting lateral e′	Exercise average e/e′	Exercise septal e/e′	Exercise peak TR velocity
Normal test	<7 cm/s	<10 cm/s	<10	<10	<2.8 m/s
Definitely abnormal test	<7 cm/s	<10 cm/s	>14	>15	>2.8 m/s

When resting echocardiography and diastolic stress test are inconclusive an invasive hemodynamic investigation may be performed in selected patients in order to explain their symptoms of heart failure or dyspnea, especially with exertion [70].

Recently, **LA deformation analysis using 2D-speckle tracking echocardiography (STE)** emerged as a promising non-invasive technique that can help to estimate LVFP and diagnose HFpEF when the assessment of LVFP remains inconclusive.

In the 2022 European Association of Cardiovascular Imaging (EACVI) consensus for the multimodality imaging in patients with HFpEF, LA reservoir strain was included as an additive, third parameter, to estimate LVFP in the group of indeterminate readings, where one of the three criteria is missing and the remaining two are conflicting [106]. The optimal cut-off value proposed for LA strain to differentiate between normal and elevated LVFP in this document are 18% for LA reservoir strain and 8% for pump strain when defining PCWP >12 mmHg as elevated. These values are based on the results of a multicenter study that enrolled 322 patients with different cardiovascular disease and a median LVEF of 55%, aiming to compare LA strain and other echocardiographic parameters with invasively measured LVFP. The authors concluded that LA reservoir and pump strain are determined predominantly by LV GLS and LVFP. Accuracy of LA strains to identify elevated LVFP was best in patients with reduced LV systolic function. High values of LA pump strain, however, identified normal LVFP with good accuracy in patients with normal systolic function [111].

Current and Future Perspective on Diastolic Function Evaluation

The 2016 algorithm for the echocardiographic assessment of LVFP has been tested and validated in subsequent studies against invasively measured LVFP. Most of these studies have shown the superiority of the integrated multiparametric approach over each single parameter used alone but they have also shown significant differences in the correlations of the recommended echocardiographic parameters with invasively measured LVFP [112–115]. These results show that the 2016 recommendations are clinically useful and superior to the previous ones, and practical recommendations about the echo assessment of LVFP have been proposed [116]. However, there is still need for further validation and refinements. At the same time, the limitations of these classification schemes built by experts and based on the same conventional parameters with their well-known drawbacks, call for different approaches to be tested.

The evaluation of diastolic function by echocardiography continues to evolve, and future directions in this field are likely to include advancements in technology, standardization of techniques, and a deeper understanding of the mechanisms involved.

Recent studies have demonstrated that artificial intelligence (AI) and machine learning algorithms have the potential to enhance the accuracy and efficiency of diastolic function assessment from different perspectives. AI algorithms can automate the measurement process, accurately identifying key parameters such as mitral inflow velocities (E and A waves), tissue Doppler velocities, and deceleration time, reducing the risk of human error and ensuring consistent measurements [117]. AI models can recognize patterns within echocardiographic data, allowing it to identify subtle abnormalities indicative of diastolic dysfunction and can analyze vast amounts of echocardiographic data, clinical variables, and outcomes to predict the risk of developing diastolic dysfunction or related cardiovascular events [118, 119]. Predictive analytics can help clinicians identify high-risk patients for early intervention. Moreover, AI algorithms can integrate echocardiographic data with other clinical information, such as patient demographics, medical history, and laboratory results. This holistic approach enables a more comprehensive assessment of diastolic function in the context of the patient's overall health. However, the development and validation of AI models require large and diverse datasets as well as close collaboration between clinicians, data scientists, and researchers to ensure the accurate interpretation and clinical relevance of AI-driven diastolic function assessments.

In summary, echocardiography is an essential tool in the comprehensive assessment of LV function in HF. It provides valuable information that helps guide diagnosis, treatment decisions, and general management of patients with HF. Ongoing research focuses on refining and developing advanced imaging techniques, such as 3D echocardiography, strain imaging, and contrast-enhanced imaging, to provide more detailed and accurate assessments of LV function. Researchers are exploring the integration of artificial intelligence and machine learning algorithms to assist in the automated analysis of echocardiographic images and how echocardiography can be integrated with other imaging modalities, such as magnetic resonance imaging or computed tomography, to provide a more comprehensive understanding of LV structure and function. At the other end of the spectrum the increasing use of handheld ultrasound devices may greatly help for rapid assessment of LV function, particularly in point-of-care or resource-limited settings.

References

1. Kirkpatrick JN, Vannan MA, Narula J, Lang RM. Echocardiography in heart failure: applications, utility, and new horizons. J Am Coll Cardiol. 2007;50:381–96.
2. Garbi M, Edvardsen T, Bax J, Petersen SE, McDonagh T, Filippatos G, et al. Reviewer panel: EACVI appropriateness criteria for the use of cardiovascular imaging in heart failure derived from European National Imaging Societies voting. Eur Heart J Cardiovasc Imaging. 2016;17:711–21.

3. Ponikowski P, Voors AA, Anker SD, Bueno H, Cleland JG, Coats AJ, et al. 2016 ESC Guidelines for the diagnosis and treatment of acute and chronic heart failure. Eur Heart J. 2016;37(27):ehw128. [Epub ahead of print].
4. Owan TE, Hodge DO, Herges RM, Jacobsen SJ, Roger VL, Redfield MM. Trends in prevalence and outcome of heart failure with preserved ejection fraction. N Engl J Med. 2006;355:251–9.
5. Mann DL, Zipes DP, Libby P, Bonow RO. Braunwald's heart disease: a textbook of cardiovascular medicine. 10th ed. ISBN-13, 9781455751341. Elsevier; 2001.
6. Lang RM, Badano LP, Mor-Avi V, Afilalo J, Armstrong A, Ernande L, et al. Recommendations for cardiac chamber quantification by echocardiography in adults: an update from the American Society of Echocardiography and the European Association of Cardiovascular Imaging. Eur Heart J Cardiovasc Imaging. 2015;16:233–70.
7. Bellenger NG, Burgess MI, Ray SG, Lahiri A, Coats AJ, Cleland JG, et al. Comparison of left ventricular ejection fraction and volumes in heart failure by echocardiography, radionuclide ventriculography, and cardiovascular magnetic resonance. Are they interchangeable? Eur Heart J. 2000;21:1387–96.
8. Jacobs LD, Salgo IS, Goonewardena S, Weinert L, Coon P, Bardo D, et al. Rapid online quantification of left ventricular volume from real-time three-dimensional echocardiographic data. Eur Heart J. 2006;27:460–8.
9. Lang RM, Badano LP, Tsang W, Adams DH, Agricola E, Buck T, et al. EAE/ASE recommendations for image acquisition and display using three-dimensional echocardiography. Eur Heart J Cardiovasc Imaging. 2012;13:1–46.
10. Dorosz JL, Lezotte DC, Weitzenkamp DA, Allen LA, Salcedo EE. Performance of 3-dimensional echocardiography in measuring left ventricular volumes and ejection fraction: a systematic review and meta-analysis. J Am Coll Cardiol. 2012;59:1799–808.
11. Muraru D, Badano LP, Peluso D, Dal Bianco L, Casablanca S, Kocabay G, et al. Comprehensive analysis of left ventricular geometry and function by three-dimensional echocardiography in healthy adults. J Am Soc Echocardiogr. 2013;26:618–28.
12. Caiani EG, Corsi C, Zamorano J, Sugeng L, MacEneaney P, Weinert L, et al. Improved semiautomated quantification of left ventricular volumes and ejection fraction using 3-dimensional echocardiography with a full matrix-array transducer: comparison with magnetic resonance imaging. J Am Soc Echocardiogr. 2005;18:779–88.
13. Mor-Avi V, Jenkins C, Kuhl HP, Nesser HJ, Marwick TH, Franke A, et al. Real-time 3-dimensional echocardiographic quantification of left ventricular volumes: multicenter study for validation with magnetic resonance imaging and investigation of sources of error. JACC Cardiovasc Imaging. 2008;1:413–23.
14. Arai K, Hozumi T, Matsumura Y, Sugioka K, Takemoto Y, Yamagishi H, et al. Accuracy of measurement of left ventricular volume and ejection fraction by new real-time three-dimensional echocardiography in patients with wall motion abnormalities secondary to myocardial infarction. Am J Cardiol. 2004;94:552–8.
15. Mannaerts HF, van der Heide JA, Kamp O, Stoel MG, Twisk J, Visser CA. Early identification of left ventricular remodelling after myocardial infarction, assessed by transthoracic 3D echocardiography. Eur Heart J. 2004;25:680–7.
16. Hung J, Lang R, Flachskampf F, Shernan SK, McCulloch ML, Adams DB, et al. 3D echocardiography: a review of the current status and future directions. J Am Soc Echocardiogr. 2007;20:213–33.
17. Van der Heide JA, Kleijn SA, Aly MF, Slikkerveer J, Kamp O. Three-dimensional echocardiography for left ventricular quantification: fundamental validation and clinical applications. Neth Heart J. 2011;19(10):423–31.
18. Matsumura Y, Hozumi T, Arai K, Sugioka K, Ujino K, Takemoto Y, et al. Non-invasive assessment of myocardial ischaemia using new real-time three-dimensional dobutamine stress echocardiography: comparison with conventional two-dimensional methods. Eur Heart J. 2005;26:1625–32.

19. Ahmad M, Xie T, McCulloch M, Abreo G, Runge M. Realtime three-dimensional dobutamine stress echocardiography in assessment stress echocardiography in assessment of ischemia: comparison with two-dimensional dobutamine stress echocardiography. J Am Coll Cardiol. 2001;37:1303–9.
20. Kan G, Visser CA, Koolen JJ, Dunning AJ. Short and long term predictive value of admission wall motion score in acute myocardial infarction. A cross sectional echocardiographic study of 345 patients. Br Heart J. 1986;56:422–7.
21. Kolias TJ, Aaronson KD, Armstrong WF. Doppler-derived dP/dt and -dP/dt predict survival in congestive heart failure. J Am Coll Cardiol. 2000;36(5):1594–9.
22. Beladan CC, Călin A, Roşca M, Ginghină C, Popescu BA. Left ventricular twist dynamics: principles and applications. Heart. 2014;100:731–40.
23. Sengupta PP, Tajik AJ, Chandrasekaran K, Khandheria BK. Twist mechanics of the left ventricle: principles and application. JACC Cardiovasc Imaging. 2008;1:366–76.
24. Nakatani S. Left ventricular rotation and twist: why should we learn? J Cardiovasc Ultrasound. 2011;19:1–6.
25. Yip G, Wang M, Zhang Y, Fung JW, Ho PY, Sanderson JE. Left ventricular long axis function in diastolic heart failure is reduced in both diastole and systole: time for a redefinition? Heart. 2002;87:121–5.
26. Yu CM, Lin H, Yang H, Kong SL, Zhang Q, Lee SW. Progression of systolic abnormalities in patients with "isolated" diastolic heart failure and diastolic dysfunction. Circulation. 2002;105:1195–201.
27. Mor-Avi V, Lang RM, Badano LP, Belohlavek M, Cardim NM, Derumeaux G, et al. Current and evolving echocardiographic techniques for the quantitative evaluation of cardiac mechanics: ASE/EAE consensus statement on methodology and indications endorsed by the Japanese Society of Echocardiography. J Am Soc Echocardiogr. 2011;24:277–313.
28. Koyama J, Ray-Sequin PA, Falk RH. Longitudinal myocardial function assessed by tissue velocity, strain, and strain rate tissue Doppler echocardiography in patients with AL (primary) cardiac amyloidosis. Circulation. 2003;107:2446–52.
29. Palka P, Lange A, Donnelly JE, Nihoyannopoulos P. Differentiation between restrictive cardiomyopathy and constrictive pericarditis by early diastolic Doppler myocardial velocity gradient at the posterior wall. Circulation. 2000;102:655–62.
30. Bax JJ, Bleeker GB, Marwick TH, Molhoek SG, Boersma E, Steendijk P, et al. Left ventricular dyssynchrony predicts response and prognosis after cardiac resynchronization therapy. J Am Coll Cardiol. 2004;44:1834–40.
31. Bax JJ, Abraham T, Barold SS, Breithardt OA, Fung JW, Garrigue S, et al. Cardiac resynchronization therapy: part 1—issues before device implantation. J Am Coll Cardiol. 2005;46:2153–67.
32. Pitzalis MV, Iacoviello M, Romito R, Massari F, Rizzon B, Luzzi G, et al. Cardiac resynchronization therapy tailored by echocardiographic evaluation of ventricular asynchrony. J Am Coll Cardiol. 2002;40:1615–22.
33. Yu CM, Bleeker GB, Fung JW, Schalij MJ, Zhang Q, van der Wall EE, et al. Left ventricular reverse remodeling but not clinical improvement predicts long-term survival after cardiac resynchronization therapy. Circulation. 2005;112:1580–6.
34. Stellbrink C, Breithardt OA, Franke A, Sack S, Bakker P, Auricchio A, et al. Impact of cardiac resynchronization therapy using hemodynamically optimized pacing on left ventricular remodeling in patients with congestive heart failure and ventricular conduction disturbances. J Am Coll Cardiol. 2001;38:1957–65.
35. Yu CM, Abraham WT, Bax J, Chung E, Fedewa M, Ghio S, et al. Predictors of response to cardiac resynchronization therapy (PROSPECT)-study design. Am Heart J. 2005;149:600–5.
36. Khan FZ, Virdee MS, Palmer CR, Pugh PJ, O'Halloran D, Elsik M, et al. Targeted left ventricular lead placement to guide cardiac resynchronization therapy: the TARGET study: a randomized, controlled trial. J Am Coll Cardiol. 2012;59:1509–18.

37. Voigt JU, Pedrizzetti G, Lysyansky P, Marwick TH, Houle H, Baumann R, et al. Definitions for a common standard for 2D speckle tracking echocardiography: consensus document of the EACVI/ASE/Industry Task Force to standardize deformation imaging. Eur Heart J Cardiovasc Imaging. 2015;16:1–11.
38. Yingchoncharoen T, Agarwal S, Popovic ZB, Marwick TH. Normal ranges of left ventricular strain: a meta-analysis. J Am Soc Echocardiogr. 2013;26:185–91.
39. Stanton T, Leano R, Marwick TH. Prediction of all-cause mortality from global longitudinal speckle strain: comparison with ejection fraction and wall motion scoring. Circ Cardiovasc Imaging. 2009;2:356–64.
40. Thomas JD, Badano LP. EACVI-ASE-industry initiative to standardize deformation imaging: a brief update from the co-chairs. Eur Heart J Cardiovasc Imaging. 2013;14:1039–40.
41. Galderisi M, Cosyns B, Edvardsen T, Cardim N, Delgado V, Di Salvo G, et al. Standardization of adult transthoracic echocardiography reporting in agreement with recent chamber quantification, diastolic function, and heart valve disease recommendations: an expert consensus document of the European Association of Cardiovascular Imaging. Eur Heart J Cardiovasc Imaging. 2017;18:1301–10.
42. Negishi K, Lucas S, Negishi T, Hamilton J, Marwick TH. What is the primary source of discordance in strain measurement between vendors: imaging or analysis? Ultrasound Med Biol. 2013;39:714–20.
43. Farsalinos KE, Daraban AM, Ünlü S, Thomas JD, Badano LP, Voigt JU. Head-to-head comparison of global longitudinal strain measurements among nine different vendors. J Am Soc Echocardiogr. 2015;28:1171–81.
44. Yang H, Marwick TH, Fukuda N, Oe H, Saito M, Thomas JD, et al. Improvement in strain concordance between two major vendors after the strain standardization initiative. J Am Soc Echocardiogr. 2015;28:642–8.
45. Potter E, Marwick TH. Assessment of left ventricular function by echocardiography: the case for routinely adding global longitudinal strain to ejection fraction. JACC Cardiovasc Imaging. 2018;11:260–74.
46. Sengeløv M, Jørgensen PG, Jensen JS, Bruun NE, Olsen FJ, Fritz-Hansen T, et al. Global longitudinal strain is a superior predictor of all-cause mortality in heart failure with reduced ejection fraction. JACC Cardiovasc Imaging. 2015;8:1351–9.
47. Phelan D, Collier P, Thavendiranathan P, Popović PB, Hanna M, Plana JC, et al. Relative apical sparing of longitudinal strain using two-dimensional speckle-tracking echocardiography is both sensitive and specific for the diagnosis of cardiac amyloidosis. Heart. 2012;98:1442–8.
48. Tribouilloy C, Rusinaru D, Mahjoub H, Goissen T, Levy F, Peltier M. Impact of echocardiography in patients hospitalized for heart failure: a prospective observational study. Arch Cardiovasc Dis. 2008;101:465–73.
49. Stokke TM, Hasselberg NE, Smedsrud MK, Sarvari SI, Haugaa KH, Smiseth OA, et al. Geometry as a confounder when assessing ventricular systolic function: comparison between ejection fraction and strain. J Am Coll Cardiol. 2017;70:942–54.
50. Nagueh SF, Phelan D, Abraham T, Armour A, Desai MY, Dragulescu A, et al. Recommendations for multimodality cardiovascular imaging of patients with hypertrophic cardiomyopathy: an update from the American Society of Echocardiography, in Collaboration with the American Society of Nuclear Cardiology, the Society for Cardiovascular Magnetic Resonance, and the Society of Cardiovascular Computed Tomography. J Am Soc Echocardiogr. 2022;35(6):533–69.
51. Heidenreich PA, Bozkurt B, Aguilar D, Allen LA, Byun JJ, Colvin MM, et al. 2022 AHA/ACC/HFSA Guideline for the management of heart failure: executive summary: a report of the American College of Cardiology/American Heart Association Joint Committee on Clinical Practice Guidelines. Circulation. 2022;145:876–94.
52. Plana JC, Galderisi M, Barac A, Ewer MS, Ky B, Scherrer-Crosbie M, et al. Expert consensus for multimodality imaging evaluation of adult patients during and after cancer therapy:

a report from the American Society of Echocardiography and the European Association of Cardiovascular Imaging. J Am Soc Echocardiogr. 2014;27:911–39.
53. Chen J, Long JB, Hurria A, Owusu C, Steingart RM, Gross CP. Incidence of heart failure or cardiomyopathy after adjuvant trastuzumab therapy for breast cancer. J Am Coll Cardiol. 2012;60:2504–12.
54. Thavendiranathan P, Poulin F, Lim KD, Plana JC, Woo A, Marwick TH. Use of myocardial strain imaging by echocardiography for the early detection of cardiotoxicity in patients during and after cancer chemotherapy: a systematic review. J Am Coll Cardiol. 2014;63:2751–68.
55. Lyon AR, López-Fernández T, Couch LS, Asteggiano R, Aznar MC, Bergler-Klein J, et al. 2022 ESC Guidelines on cardio-oncology developed in collaboration with the European Hematology Association (EHA), the European Society for Therapeutic Radiology and Oncology (ESTRO) and the International Cardio-Oncology Society (IC-OS): developed by the Task Force on Cardio-Oncology of the European Society of Cardiology (ESC). Eur Heart J. 2022;43:4229–361.
56. Negishi T, Thavendiranathan P, Negishi K, Marwick TH. Rationale and design of the strain surveillance of chemotherapy for improving cardiovascular outcomes: the SUCCOUR trial. J Am Coll Cardiol Img. 2018;11:1098–105.
57. Thavendiranathan P, Negishi T, Somerset E, Negishi K, Penicka M, Lemieux J, et al. Strain-guided management of potentially cardiotoxic cancer therapy. J Am Coll Cardiol. 2021;77:392–401.
58. Kraigher-Krainer E, Shah AM, Gupta DK, Santos A, Claggett B, Pieske B, et al. PARAMOUNT Investigators. Impaired systolic function by strain imaging in heart failure with preserved ejection fraction. J Am Coll Cardiol. 2014;63:447–56.
59. Biering-Sørensen T, Biering-Sørensen SR, Olsen FJ, Sengeløv M, Godsk Jørgensen P, Mogelvang R, et al. Global longitudinal strain by echocardiography predicts long-term risk of cardiovascular morbidity and mortality in a low-risk general population: the Copenhagen City Heart Study. Circ Cardiovasc Imaging. 2017;10:e005521.
60. Kuznetsova T, Cauwenberghs N, Knez J, Yang WI, Herbots L, D'hooge J, et al. Additive prognostic value of left ventricular systolic dysfunction in a population-based cohort. Circ Cardiovasc Imaging. 2016;9:9.
61. Argulian E, Narula J. Advanced cardiovascular imaging in clinical heart failure. JACC Heart Fail. 2021;9:699–709.
62. Huang W, Chai SC, Lee SGS, MacDonald MR, Leong KTG. Prognostic factors after index hospitalization for heart failure with preserved ejection fraction. Am J Cardiol. 2017;119:2017–20.
63. Park JJ, Park JB, Park JH, Cho GY. Global longitudinal strain to predict mortality in patients with acute heart failure. J Am Coll Cardiol. 2018;71:1947–57.
64. Hung CL, Verma A, Uno H, Shin SH, Bourgoun M, Hassanein MH, et al. Longitudinal and circumferential strain rate, left ventricular remodeling, and prognosis after myocardial infarction. J Am Coll Cardiol. 2010;56:1812–22.
65. Vahaniana A, Beyersdorf F, Praz F, Milojevic M, Baldus S, Bauersachs J, et al. 2021 ESC/EACTS Guidelines for the management of valvular heart disease: developed by the Task Force for the management of valvular heart disease of the European Society of Cardiology (ESC) and the European Association for Cardio-Thoracic Surgery (EACTS). ESC/EACTS Scientific Document Group. Eur Heart J. 2022;43:561–632.
66. Kearney LG, Lu K, Ord M, Patel SK, Profitis K, Matalanis G, et al. Global longitudinal strain is a strong independent predictor of all-cause mortality in patients with aortic stenosis. Eur Heart J Cardiovasc Imaging. 2012;13:827–33.
67. Magne J, Cosyns B, Popescu BA, Carstensen HG, Dahl J, Desai MY, et al. Distribution and prognostic significance of left ventricular global longitudinal strain in asymptomatic significant aortic stenosis: an individual participant data meta-analysis. JACC Cardiovasc Imaging. 2019;12:84–92.

68. Weidemann F, Herrmann S, Störk S, Niemann M, Frantz S, Lange V, et al. Impact of myocardial fibrosis in patients with symptomatic severe aortic stenosis. Circulation. 2009;120:577–84.
69. Popescu BA, Beladan CC, Calin A, Muraru D, Deleanu D, Rosca M, et al. Left ventricular remodelling and torsional dynamics in dilated cardiomyopathy: reversed apical rotation as a marker of disease severity. Eur J Heart Fail. 2009;11:945–51.
70. Nagueh SF, Smiseth OA, Appleton CP, Byrd BF 3rd, Dokainish H, Edvardsen T, et al. Recommendations for the evaluation of left ventricular diastolic function by echocardiography: an update from the American Society of Echocardiography and the European Association of Cardiovascular Imaging. J Am Soc Echocardiogr. 2016;29:277–314.
71. Oh JK, Park SJ, Nagueh SF. Established and novel clinical applications of diastolic function assessment by echocardiography. Circ Cardiovasc Imaging. 2011;4:444–55.
72. Beladan CC, Iliesiu AM, Popescu AC, Coman IM, Ginghina C, Popescu BA. Imaging assessment of left ventricular diastolic function: current and emerging methods. Acta Cardiol. 2016;71:379–88.
73. Zile MR, Baicu CF, Gaasch WH. Diastolic heart failure abnormalities in active relaxation and passive stiffness of the left ventricle. N Engl J Med. 2004;350:1953–9.
74. Zile MR, Gottdiener JS, Hetzel SJ, McMurray JJ, Komajda M, McKelvie R, et al. Prevalence and significance of alterations in cardiac structure and function in patients with heart failure and a preserved ejection fraction. Circulation. 2011;124:2491–501.
75. Shah AM. Ventricular remodeling in heart failure with preserved ejection fraction. Curr Heart Fail Rep. 2013;10:341–9.
76. Asrar U, Haq M, Mutha V, Rudd N, Hare DL, Wong C. Heart failure with preserved ejection fraction—unwinding the diagnosis mystique. Am J Cardiovasc Dis. 2014;4:100.
77. Lester SJ, Ryan EW, Schiller NB, Foster E. Best method in clinical practice and in research studies to determine left atrial size. Am J Cardiol. 1999;84:829–32.
78. Pritchett AM, Jacobsen SJ, Mahoney DW, Rodeheffer RJ, Bailey KR, Redfield MM. Left atrial volume as an index of left atrial size: a population-based study. J Am Coll Cardiol. 2003;41:1036–43.
79. Melenovsky V, Borlaug BA, Rosen B, Hay I, Ferruci L, Morell CH, et al. Cardiovascular features of heart failure with preserved ejection fraction versus nonfailing hypertensive LVH in the urban Baltimore community: the role of atrial remodeling/dysfunction. J Am Coll Cardiol. 2007;49:198–207.
80. Ogunyankin KO. Assessment of left ventricular diastolic function: the power, possibilities, and pitfalls of echocardiographic imaging techniques. Can J Cardiol. 2011;27:311–8.
81. Kavianipour M, Farkhooy A, Flachskampf FA. Role of echocardiography in the diagnosis of heart failure with preserved left ventricular systolic function: update 2013. Curr Cardiovasc Imaging Rep. 2013;6:523–33.
82. Dalsgaard M, Kjaergaard J, Pecini R, Iversen KK, Kober L, Moller JE, et al. Left ventricular filling pressure estimation at rest and during exercise in patients with severe aortic valve stenosis: comparison of echocardiographic and invasive measurements. J Am Soc Echocardiogr. 2009;22:343–9.
83. Bogaty P, Mure P, Dumesnil JG. New insights into diastolic dysfunction as the cause of acute left-sided heart failure associated with systemic hypertension and/or coronary artery disease. Am J Cardiol. 2002;89:341–5.
84. Dumesnil JG, Pibarot P. Doppler assessment of diastolic function at rest and during exercise: distinguishing myth from reality. J Am Soc Echocardiogr. 2009;22:343–9.
85. Lam CSP, Roger VL, Rodeheffer RJ, Borlaug BA, Enders FT, Redfield MM. Pulmonary hypertension in heart failure with preserved ejection fraction. J Am Coll Cardiol. 2009;53:1119–26.
86. Oktay AA, Shah SJ. Diagnosis and management of heart failure with preserved ejection fraction: 10 key lessons. Curr Cardiol Rev. 2015;11:42–52.
87. Sohn DW, Chai IH, Lee DJ, Kim HC, Kim HS, Oh BH, et al. Assessment of mitral annulus velocity by Doppler tissue imaging in the evaluation of left ventricular diastolic function. J Am Coll Cardiol. 1997;30:474–80.

88. Nagueh SF, Middleton KJ, Kopelen HA, Zoghbi WA, Quinones MA. Doppler tissue imaging: a noninvasive technique for evaluation of left ventricular relaxation and estimation of filling pressures. J Am Coll Cardiol. 1997;30:1527–33.
89. Garcia MJ, Thomas JD, Klein AL. New Doppler echocardiographic applications for the study of diastolic function. J Am Coll Cardiol. 1998;32:865–75.
90. Ommen SR, Nishimura RA, Appleton CP, Miller FA, Oh JK, Redfield MM, et al. Clinical utility of Doppler echocardiography and tissue Doppler imaging in the estimation of left ventricular filling pressures: a comparative simultaneous Doppler-catheterization study. Circulation. 2000;102:1788–94.
91. Huis in't Veld AE, de Man FS, van Rossum AC, Handoko ML. How to diagnose heart failure with preserved ejection fraction: the value of invasive stress testing. Neth Heart J. 2016;24:244–51.
92. Penicka M, Bartunek J, Trakalova H, Hrabakova H, Maruskova M, Karasek J, et al. Heart failure with preserved ejection fraction in outpatients with unexplained dyspnea: a pressure-volume loop analysis. J Am Coll Cardiol. 2010;55:1701–10.
93. Santos M, Rivero J, McCullough SD, West E, Opotowsky AR, Waxman AB, et al. E/e' ratio in patients with unexplained dyspnea: lack of accuracy in estimating left ventricular filling pressure. Circ Heart Fail. 2015;8:749–56.
94. Wang J, Khoury DS, Yue Y, Torre-Amione G, Nagueh SF. Preserved left ventricular twist and circumferential deformation, but depressed longitudinal and radial deformation in patients with diastolic heart failure. Eur Heart J. 2008;29:1283–9.
95. Wenzelburger FW, Tan YT, Choudhary FJ, Lee ES, Leyva F, Sanderson JE. Mitral annular plane systolic excursion on exercise: a simple diagnostic tool for heart failure with preserved ejection fraction. Eur J Heart Fail. 2011;13:953–60.
96. Whalley GA, Doughty RN, Gamble GD, Wright SP, Walsh HJ, Muncaster SA, et al. Pseudonormal mitral filling pattern predicts hospital re-admission in patients with congestive heart failure. J Am Coll Cardiol. 2002;39:1787–95.
97. Pozzoli M, Traversi E, Cioffi G, Stenner R, Sanarico M, Tavazzi L. Loading manipulations improve the prognostic value of Doppler evaluation of mitral flow in patients with chronic heart failure. Circulation. 1997;95:1222–30.
98. Somaratne JB, Whalley GA, Gamble GD, Doughty RN. Restrictive filling pattern is a powerful predictor of heart failure events post acute myocardial infarction and in established heart failure: a literature-based metaanalysis. J Card Fail. 2007;13:346–5.
99. Traversi E, Pozzoli M, Cioffi G, Capomolla S, Forni G, Sanarico M, et al. Mitral flow velocity changes after 6 months of optimized therapy provide important hemodynamic and prognostic information in patients with chronic heart failure. Am Heart J. 1996;132(4):809–19.
100. Giannuzzi P, Temporelli PL, Bosmini E, Silva P, Imparato A, Corra U, et al. Independent and incremental prognostic value of Doppler-derived mitral deceleration time of early filling in both symptomatic and asymptomatic patients with left ventricular dysfunction. J Am Coll Cardiol. 1996;28:383–90.
101. Bruch C, Klem I, Breithardt G, Wichter T, Gradaus R. Diagnostic usefulness and prognostic implications of the mitral E/E' ratio in patients with heart failure and severe secondary mitral regurgitation. Am J Cardiol. 2007;100:860–5.
102. Dini FL, Conti U, Fontanive P, Andreini D, Panicucci E, De Tommasi SM. Prognostic value of N-terminal pro-type-B natriuretic peptide and Doppler left ventricular diastolic variables in patients with chronic systolic heart failure stabilized by therapy. Am J Cardiol. 2008;102:463–8.
103. Damy T, Goode KM, Kallvikbacka-Bennett A, Lewinter C, Hobkirk J, Nikitin NP, et al. Determinants and prognostic value of pulmonary arterial pressure in patients with chronic heart failure. Eur Heart J. 2010;31:2280–90.
104. Miller WL, Grill DE, Borlaug BA. Clinical features, hemodynamics, and outcomes of pulmonary hypertension due to chronic heart failure with reduced ejection fraction: pulmonary hypertension and heart failure. JACC Heart Fail. 2013;1:290–9.

105. Meris A, Amigoni M, Uno H, Thune JJ, Verma A, Køber L, et al. Left atrial remodelling in patients with myocardial infarction complicated by heart failure, left ventricular dysfunction, or both: the VALIANT Echo study. Eur Heart J. 2009;30:56–65.
106. Smiseth OA, Morris DA, Cardim N, Cikes M, Delgado V, Donal E, et al. Multimodality imaging in patients with heart failure and preserved ejection fraction: an expert consensus document of the European Association of Cardiovascular Imaging. Eur Heart J Cardiovasc Imaging. 2022;23:e34–61.
107. Kraigher-Krainer E, Shah AM, Gupta DK, Santos A, Claggett B, Pieske B, et al. Impaired systolic function by strain imaging in heart failure with preserved ejection fraction. J Am Coll Cardiol. 2014;63:447–56.
108. Borlaug BA, Nishimura RA, Sorajja P, Lam CSP, Redfield MM. Exercise hemodynamics enhance diagnosis of early heart failure with preserved ejection fraction. Circ Heart Fail. 2010;3:588–95.
109. Westermann D, Kasner M, Steendijk P, Spillmann F, Riad A, Weitmann K, et al. Role of left ventricular stiffness in heart failure with normal ejection fraction. Circulation. 2008;117:2051–60.
110. Borlaug BA, Olson TP, Lam CSP, Flood KS, Lerman A, Johnson BD, et al. Global cardiovascular reserve dysfunction in heart failure with preserved ejection fraction. J Am Coll Cardiol. 2010;56:845–54.
111. Inoue K, Khan FH, Remme EW, Ohte N, García-Izquierdo E, Chetrit M, et al. Determinants of left atrial reservoir and pump strain and use of atrial strain for evaluation of left ventricular filling pressure. Eur Heart J Cardiovasc Imaging. 2021;23:61–70.
112. Andersen OS, Smiseth OA, Dokainish H, Abudiab MM, Schutt RC, Kumar A, et al. Estimating left ventricular filling pressure by echocardiography. J Am Coll Cardiol. 2017;69:1937–48.
113. Lancellotti P, Galderisi M, Edvardsen T, Donal E, Goliasch G, Cardim N, et al. Echo-Doppler estimation of left ventricular filling pressure: results of the multicentre EACVI Euro-Filling study. Eur Heart J Cardiovasc Imaging. 2017;18:961–8.
114. Balaney B, Medvedofsky D, Mediratta A, Singh A, Ciszek B, Kruse E, et al. Invasive validation of the echocardiographic assessment of left ventricular filling pressures using the 2016 diastolic guidelines: head-to-head comparison with the 2009 guidelines. J Am Soc Echocardiogr. 2018;31:79–88.
115. Sato K, Grant ADM, Negishi K, Cremer PC, Negishi T, Kumar A, et al. Reliability of updated left ventricular diastolic function recommendations in predicting elevated left ventricular filling pressure and prognosis. Am Heart J. 2017;189:28–39.
116. Popescu BA, Beladan CC, Nagueh SF, Smiseth OA. How to assess left ventricular filling pressures by echocardiography in clinical practice. Eur Heart J Cardiovasc Imaging. 2022;23:1127–9.
117. Elwazir MY, Akkus Z, Oguz D, Ye Z, Oh JK. Fully automated mitral inflow doppler analysis using deep learning. In: 2020 IEEE 20th international conference on bioinformatics and bioengineering (BIBE); 2020. p. 691–6.
118. Valsaraj A, Kalmady SV, Sharma V, Frost M, Sun W, Sepehrvand N, et al. Development and validation of echocardiography-based machine-learning models to predict mortality. EBioMedicine. 2023;90:104479.
119. Kaptein YE, Karagodin I, Zuo H, Lu Y, Zhang J, Kaptein JS, et al. Identifying Phenogroups in patients with subclinical diastolic dysfunction using unsupervised statistical learning. BMC Cardiovasc Disord. 2020;20:367.

Chapter 5
The Role of Atrial Functional Assessment in Heart Failure

Matteo Cameli and Federico Landra

Abbreviations

AF	Atrial fibrillation
AFL	Atrial flutter
LAA	Left atrial appendage
CT	Computed tomography
CMR	Cardiac magnetic resonance
HF	Heart failure
HFpEF	Heart failure with preserved ejection fraction
HFrEF	Heart failure with reduced ejection fraction LA Left atrium/left atrial
EmF	Emptying fraction
LV	Left ventricle/left ventricular
RV	Right ventricle/right ventricular
LVEF	Left ventricular ejection fraction
LA	Left atrium/left atrial
RA	Right atrium/right atrial
PALS	Peak atrial longitudinal strain
STE	Speckle tracking echocardiography
TDI	Tissue Doppler imaging
PH	Pulmonary hypertension

The Role of Atria

The atria are thin-walled chambers whose electromechanical and endocrine role is of critical relevance for the overall heart functioning. First of all, the atria act as a reservoir during ventricular systole, a conduit for blood transiting from veins to the ventricles, an active contractile chamber that augments left ventricular (LV) and

M. Cameli (✉) · F. Landra
Department of Medical Biotechnologies, Division of Cardiology, University of Siena, Siena, Italy

M. Dorobanţu et al. (eds.), *Current Approach to Heart Failure*,
https://doi.org/10.1007/978-3-031-96562-3_5

right ventricular (RV) filling in late diastole and a suction source that refills itself in early systole. Through these various mechanical functions, the atria modulate ventricular filling [1, 2]. Particularly, atria reservoir function is mainly determined by atrial compliance/stiffness and is influenced by the base descent during systole and breathing phases; also, RV generates a driving pressure transmitted through the pulmonary circulation to help left atrium (LA) filling, while the systemic venous return is determined by a peripheral-to-central pressure gradient. Atria conduit function is inversely related to reservoir function and is strongly modulated by ventricular lusitropy. Atrial pump function, as for each cardiac chamber, is dependent on contractility, preload (venous return) and afterload (LV and RV end-diastolic pressure). Of note, the Frank–Starling law applies to atrial mechanics as well, with atrial emptying fraction increasing as atrial filling volume increases, in a non-linear fashion because of a drop in contractility after a certain degree of dilation [3].

Aside from their hemodynamic role in global cardiac performance, the atria are typically responsible for the rhythm of the heart. The rhythm profoundly influences both atrial and ventricular function. Sinus rhythm represents the ideal rhythm, allowing a regular, adequately timed depolarization of both the atria and the ventricles. Also, the atrio-ventricular node, located at the apex of the triangle of Koch in the right atrium (RA), regulates the atrio-ventricular synchrony, a key determinant in ventricular filling. Despite sinus rhythm, intra-atrial, inter-atrial (mainly via the Bachmann's bundle) and atrio-ventricular conduction abnormalities may alter atrial function and reduce atrio-ventricular synchrony, with consequent risk of heart failure (HF), stroke and death. Abnormal rhythms, such as atrial fibrillation (AF), atrial flutter (AFL), atrial tachycardia or paced rhythms, all lead to atrial dysfunction and, on the long run, to structural and electrophysiological abnormalities known under the term 'remodelling' [4]. Contributing up to 30% of total LV stroke volume in normal individuals, the loss of atrial contribution to LV filling and stroke volume with AF leads to hemodynamic deterioration [5]. Also, AF and AFL may promote the formation of clots into left atrial appendage (LAA) with potentially fatal consequences such as stroke. LAA itself is still a mysterious entity but it seems that it significantly contributes to the hemodynamic, hemostatic, electrical and also neuroendocrine function of LA [6]. Indeed, LA also acts as volume sensor with the atrial wall releasing natriuretic peptides in response to stretch, generating natriuresis, vasodilatation and inhibition of the sympathetic nervous system and renin-angiotensin-aldosterone system.

Atrial Functional Assessment

In light of the abovementioned reasons, both right and left atria are relevant for the overall cardiac performance. However, as for the RV in contrast to the LV, the RA has long been overshadowed by the LA. Nowadays much more importance is being attributed to the whole right heart, as a result of a wider comprehension of its pathophysiological processes and advances in interventional cardiology. The functioning of the right heart is mostly influenced by left-sided diseases, even though it may be altered also in other conditions such as non-type 2 pulmonary hypertension (PH), valvular diseases, AF and so on, and, importantly, carries prognostic value [7–10]. As the 'other atrium in heart failure', few studies have investigated the RA in the context of HF in contrast to the LA so far, even though the remodelling process is not limited to the LA only [11]. Nonetheless, it has already been reported that RA functional assessment may be useful for risk stratification both in patients with and without HF and in those with pulmonary hypertension [12–15]. Recently, a comprehensive review of multimodality anatomical and functional assessment of the RA has been published [16]. Echocardiography is recognized as the most useful mean of investigation when it comes to atrial assessment, because of its accessibility, portability, and its real time assessment with high temporal resolution. Aside from anatomical aspects which are not the purpose of the present issue, for RA functional assessment the most useful projection is the RV-focused apical view optimized for RA visualization [17]. Three-dimensional total emptying fraction (EmF), composed of passive and active EmF, and two-dimensional reservoir RA strain, composed of RA conduit strain and RA contractile strain, both reflects the different mechanical phases of atrial function, namely the reservoir, conduit and contraction phases and are the two most widely recognized functional parameters [18]. Distinction of active and passive EmF requires additional calculation of pre-A RA volume (pre-atrial systole volume), from which active and passive emptying RA volumes are derived. For this purpose, identifying the frame corresponding to the peak of the P wave on ECG tracing is essential. Standardized definitions and techniques for using 2D speckle tracking echocardiography (STE) of both RA and LA strain have been recently synthetized in a consensus document [17]. Also, a recent publication has reported the echocardiographic reference ranges of global longitudinal strain for all cardiac chambers, therefore including RA and LA, using guideline-directed dedicated views [19]. Cardiac magnetic resonance (CMR) and computed tomography (CT) are far less employed even though they both have higher spatial resolution. Similar functional variables have been translated from echocardiography to such examination modalities for atrial assessment.

On the counterpart, the LA has been widely studied in the last years and it is now a well-established marker of LV dysfunction, particularly in the field of HF with preserved ejection fraction (HFpEF) and LV diastolic dysfunction. Indeed, LA primary function is LV filling modulation, therefore functional LA abnormalities appear at the initial stages of the disease. Recent studies have shown that LA dysfunction may be much more than a surrogate disease marker, but may contribute to the pathogenesis of HFpEF and it is expected to become a real therapeutic target [20]. Moreover, LA function has been shown to be a strong predictor of poor outcomes such as HF, AF, stroke and mortality. For these purposes, doppler analysis of transmitral and pulmonary vein flows, tissue doppler assessment of mitral annulus velocities, LA volumes, estimated pulmonary artery systolic pressure and, recently, by LA strain by speckle tracking echocardiography (STE) are all call into action [21]. The E wave of the transmitral flow reflects LA conduit function, while the A wave provides information about the booster pump function [22]. Moreover, in the presence of reduced LV compliance and elevated filling pressures, atrial contraction may result in flow reversal into the pulmonary veins [1, 23, 24]. Regarding tissue doppler imaging (TDI), an excellent correlation between mitral annulus a′ and atrial function has been demonstrated in a large number of studies [1]. Both LV systolic and diastolic function affect LA contractile function. As such, a higher LV ejection fraction is associated with a higher a′, while a restrictive LV diastolic filling is associated with a lower a′ [25]. TDI has been used to calculate LA strain as well, but insonation angle dependency, which is the main technical challenge of doppler echocardiography, has limited its spreading [26]. Also, TDI-based LA strain has been used to calculate an index of LA stiffness using LA pressure estimate with E/e′. This index was able to differentiate between HFrEF and HFpEF, and between HFpEF and left ventricular diastolic dysfunction without HF [27]. Recently, the limitations coming from angle dependency have been overcome with atrial longitudinal strain measurement obtained from the analysis of myocardial deformation of the LA using STE (Fig. 5.1). First described in 2009 [28], increasing evidence has emerged suggesting that this imaging modality is highly promising for LA function assessment, providing a comprehensive functional assessment of the LA [29]. As shown by recent studies, LA strain brings considerable feasibility and reproducibility [29–32]. As already mentioned for RA strain, standardized definitions and

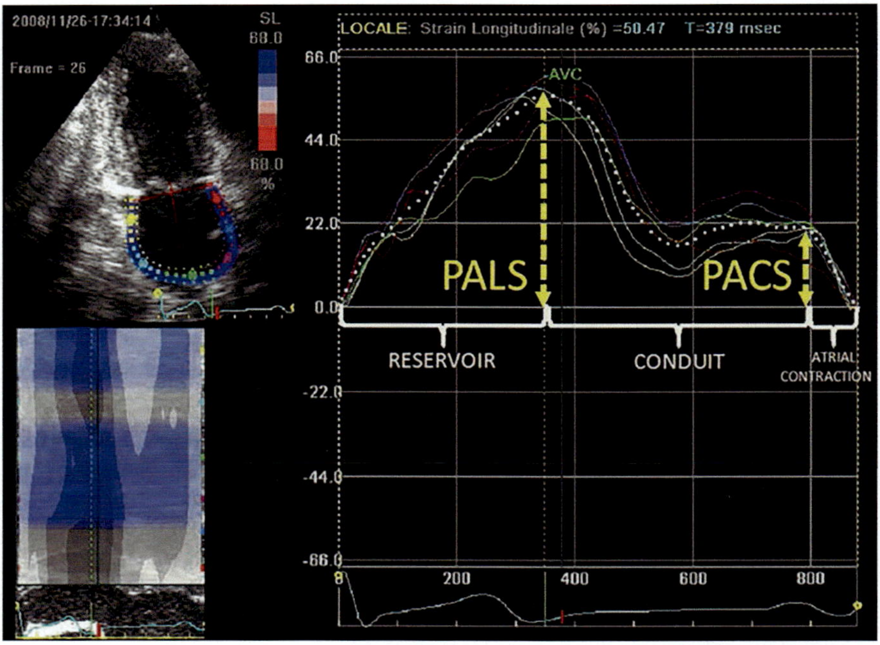

Fig. 5.1 Composite figure showing the measurement of Peak Atrial Longitudinal Strain (PALS) using the speckle tracking echocardiography (STE) from an apical two-chamber view, in a representative subject. The dashed curve represents the average atrial longitudinal strain along the cardiac cycle (AVC aortic valve closure)

techniques for using 2D STE of LA strain as well as echocardiographic reference ranges have been recently reported [17, 19]. Apical views, both four chamber and two chamber views (to obtain a biplane calculation of LA strain), should be optimized in terms of orientation, depth and gain to obtain a complete visualization of the LA throughout the whole cardiac cycle and avoid foreshortening of the LA. As for the RA, the LA function can be assessed with real-time three-dimensional echocardiography, which allows to measure volumetric changes of the LA during cardiac cycle and to quantify the contribution of LA contraction to LV filling, through the measurement of LA EmF [33]. Finally, LA function can be assessed also by CMR and CT. Again, echocardiography is most often used in clinical practice, since the cost/effectiveness and the added clinical value of using either CMR or CT, instead of echocardiography, remains to be demonstrated.

Atrial Function in Heart Failure

The understanding of HF hemodynamics has traditionally focused on LV structure and function, with the LA being considered simply as a passive transport chamber that empties into the LV. Regarding the right heart, it has been similarly neglected in the first instance. However, over the last decades, there has been increasing recognition of the importance of LA and right sided structures in the pathophysiology of HF. LA volume has been the first recognized parameter reflecting the goodness of LV diastolic function, and subsequently considered a predictor of adverse cardiovascular outcomes in HF. More recently, LA function has emerged as a novel determinant of clinical status and outcomes in HF, and perhaps an even more robust prognostic marker than LA volume [3].

HF is now recognized as a progressive disorder in which asymptomatic risk factors (Stage A) lead to a pre-clinical stage of LV dysfunction (Stage B) and finally to the clinically manifest stage of symptomatic HF (Stages C and D). While the role of LV functional changes in the staged progression of HF has been well described, the role of LA dysfunction has received relatively little attention. Increases in LA volume initially enhance LA contractility according to the Frank–Starling mechanism. Thus, the relative contribution of LA pump function increases, whereas conduit function decreases, in the presence of abnormal LV relaxation such as in Stage B patients. As LV filling pressures further increase in Stage C HF, LA enlargement reaches the limits of LA preload reserve, and LA conduit function becomes predominant [34]. Similar adaptive mechanisms occur in the right heart as well, such for example as a consequence of RV disfunction caused by PH. As such, increased RA pressure determines RA remodelling, dilatation and dysfunction, with worsening of RV filling, pulmonary perfusion, and systemic congestion [35]. Therefore, pathological LA enlargement can be viewed as an adaptive response with an initial increase of LA volume and serves to maintain LV stroke volume and cardiac output. However, continued LA enlargement eventually results in decreased LA compliance, reduced reservoir and contractile pump functions, and consequent increased incidence of atrial arrhythmias [36]. Indeed, one manifestation of the LA disease, defined as a complex of subclinical structural, electrophysiological, and functional changes with the potential to produce clinical consequences, is AF. When AF occurs the atrial pump function is lost, which means significant reduction in LV stroke volume, and a pro-thrombotic state is established. Impaired atrial contractile reserve and LA enlargement independently predict morbidity and mortality, AF onset or recurrence, and severity of functional impairment in HF patients [37, 38]. Moreover, AF begets AF and AF contributes to progressive LA dysfunction in a vicious cycle. A fibro-inflammatory process seems to be at the base of this relationship. For these reasons, some have defined rhythm control strategies the fifth pillar of HF care, confirming the trend towards considering LA dysfunction a real therapeutic target [39, 40]. An inverse process, called reverse remodelling, may occur especially in the earliest phases of LA disease, resulting from the reduction of LA volume and restoration of specific functional parameters. AF ablation favors not only LA but also RA reverse remodelling and pre-procedural LA strain may predict ablation outcome [41–44]. Most studies have used a 15% change in LA volume to define LA reverse remodelling. LA strain has also been used for the purpose, but there is inconsistency with regards to the change of LA strain which may be clinically significant. However, LA function restoration may be more sensitive than changes in LA volume to detect therapeutic effects. The possibility of reverse remodelling and its clinical significance at more advanced stages of LA dysfunction has not been proven yet. On the other hand, not only is LA function probably more sensitive to detect the effects of therapeutic interventions, but also several studies have shown that LA dysfunction may precede LA structural changes in different clinical settings [45, 46]. Indeed, the decrease of LA reservoir and the increase of LA pump functions are the first manifestations of the burden of diastolic dysfunction [47]. Therefore, assessment of LA remodelling may be critical even in the pre-clinical stages of HF, namely patients in stages A and B, and LA reverse remodelling to evaluate the effect of preventive measures (Fig. 5.2). For instance, physical activity and weight loss in obese patients have shown positive results in terms of LA reverse remodelling and incidence of arrhythmias [48].

Growing evidence suggests that LA dysfunction is an active contributor to symptoms [49–52] and disease progression [29, 53]. However, even though LA remodelling is becoming increasingly recognized as a key determinant of HF pathophysiology, its mechanisms are still poorly understood. Prior studies suggest greater adverse effects from loss of LA function in HFpEF compared with HF with reduced ejection fraction (HFrEF) [54]. LA reverse remodelling in the context of HFrEF has been observed in patients treated with HF disease modifier drugs. Also, it has been shown that LA reverse remodelling in patients receiving a CRT predicted better outcomes independently from concomitant LV reverse remodelling (the so called 'complete left-side reverse remodelling'). Therefore, LA function once again could be an independent therapeutic target in HF care. Regarding HFpEF, LA functional assessment is crucial for its diagnosis [55]. Doppler evaluation of transmitral flow pattern, TDI of the mitral annulus velocity and, recently, LA reservoir strain are used to define LV filling pressures. In fact, in cases in which conflicting findings are documented,

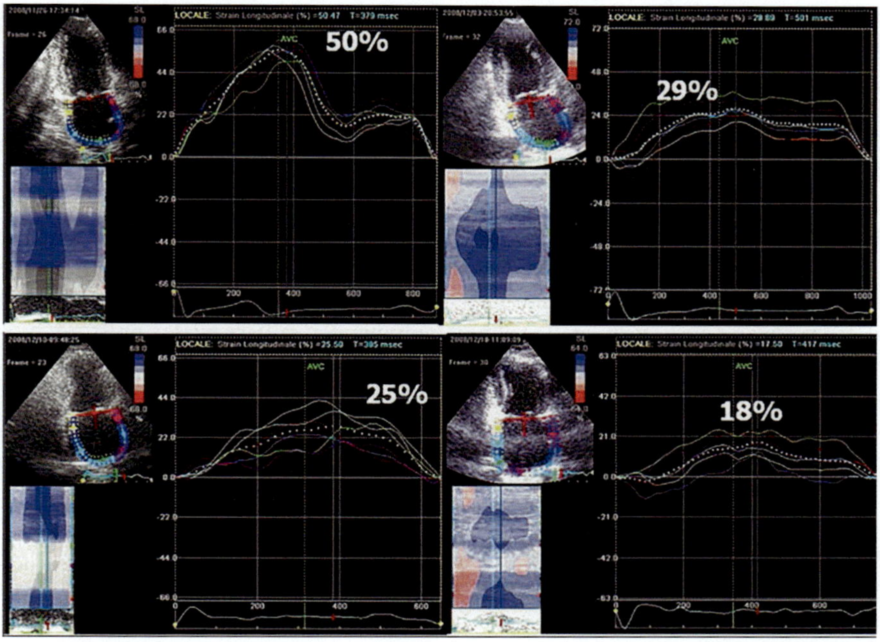

Fig. 5.2 Peak atrial longitudinal strain measurements in a healthy subject (**a**) and in a hypertensive (**b**), diabetic (**c**) and hypertensive-diabetic (**d**) patients. Atrial strain appeared reduced in hypertensive and in diabetics. In the case of association of the two diseases the reduction is even more evident

LA reservoir strain (cut-off 18%) has recently gained relevance in determining whether LV filling pressure is normal or elevated. LA function is dependent not only on LA intrinsic contractile properties but it is also strongly influenced by LV function in terms of LV end-diastolic pressure, which represents the afterload that the LA has to face. Previous studies have investigated the effect of LV end-diastolic pressure on LA wall tension, demonstrating that elevated LV end-diastolic pressure is associated with a decrease in LA reservoir values. In other words, higher LV filling pressures are associated to reduced LA deformation. In fact, atrial longitudinal strain has demonstrated a good correlation with pulmonary capillary wedge pressure [56–59]. When LV filling pressures are high and there are signs and symptoms of HF, HFpEF diagnosis is reasonable. However, there are cases in which the echocardiographic examination may be inconclusive, therefore additional investigation or use of multiparametric scores are recommended [60]. Aside from diagnostic purposes, LA functional assessment in the context of HFpEF is reasonably useful for the evaluation of treatment effects and again could be eligible for treatment target as well. For instance, drug treatment with ARNI in the PARAMOUNT trial showed a significant reduction in LA size and volume at follow-up, even without apparent effects on LV size and diastolic function [61]. Regarding the RA, its involvement in HF has still to be thoroughly elucidated. Chirinos et al. reported that HFrEF patients have a reduced RA function in terms of reservoir, conduit and pump properties [62].

Differently, in HFpEF only RA conduit function was altered, while reservoir and pump function were normal.

Finally, LA function assessment resulted particularly useful also in the clinical settings of end-stage HF. Treatment in these patients are difficultly capable of initiating a LA reverse remodelling process because of the advanced stage of atrial disease. However, in this subset of patients an accurate estimation of left ventricular filling pressure may be useful to assure proper management because of a precarious hemodynamic balance. The E/e′ ratio, the most widely employed echocardiographic parameter for the estimation of ventricular filling pressure, proved inadequate for this purpose [59]. In a population of patients with advanced HF, LA longitudinal deformation analysis correlated well with pulmonary capillary wedge pressure, providing a better estimation of LV filling pressures [63].

Conclusion

Our understanding of atrial function is rapidly evolving, and data are accumulating to suggest that this is a powerful biomarker for HF and potentially a therapeutic target.

There have been tremendous advances in terms of our ability to characterize and quantify atrial function using non-invasive imaging. STE provides detailed information regarding atrial mechanics.

Future Directions

Despite considerable data demonstrating the utility of LA function in predicting cardiovascular events, risk stratification strategies incorporating these parameters are not currently exploited in clinical practice.

Secondly, LA reverse remodelling is a favorable process that has been observed as a consequence of various HF treatments. Whether this could be eligible to a real therapeutic target remains to be determined.

References

1. Blume GG, Mcleod CJ, Barnes ME, Seward JB, Pellikka PA, Bastiansen PM, Tsang TRM. Left atrial function: physiology, assessment, and clinical implications. Eur J Echocardiogr. 2011;12:421–30.
2. Cameli M, Lisi M, Righini FM, Mondillo S. Novel echocardiographic techniques to assess left atrial size, anatomy and function. Cardiovasc Ultrasound. 2012;10:4.
3. Shah AM, Lam CSP. Function over form? Assessing the left atrium in heart failure. Eur Heart J. 2015;36:711–4.

4. Cronin EM, Vedage N, Israel CW. Alternative atrial pacing site to improve cardiac function: focus on Bachmann's bundle pacing. Eur Heart J Suppl. 2023;25(Suppl G):G44–55. https://doi.org/10.1093/eurheartjsupp/suad118. PMID: 37970517; PMCID: PMC10637835.
5. Leung DY, Boyd A, Ng AA, Chi C, Thomas L. Echocardiographic evaluation of left atrial size and function: current understanding, pathophysiologic correlates, and prognostic implications. Am Heart J. 2008;156(6):1056–64.
6. Alkhouli M, Di Biase L, Natale A, et al. Nonthrombogenic roles of the left atrial appendage: JACC review topic of the week. J Am Coll Cardiol. 2023;81(11):1063–75. https://doi.org/10.1016/j.jacc.2023.01.017.
7. Carluccio E, Biagioli P, Alunni G, Murrone A, Zuchi C, Coiro S, Riccini C, Mengoni A, D'Antonio A, Ambrosio G. Prognostic value of right ventricular dysfunction in heart failure with reduced ejection fraction: superiority of longitudinal strain over tricuspid annular plane systolic excursion. Circ Cardiovasc Imaging. 2018;11(1):e006894. https://doi.org/10.1161/CIRCIMAGING.117.006894. PMID: 29321212.
8. Landra F, Sciaccaluga C, Pastore MC, Gallone G, Barilli M, Fusi C, Focardi M, Cavigli L, D'Ascenzi F, Natali BM, Bernazzali S, Maccherini M, Valente S, Cameli M, Mandoli GE. Right ventricular myocardial work for the prediction of early right heart failure and long-term mortality after left ventricular assist device implant. Eur Heart J Cardiovasc Imaging. 2023;25(1):jead193. https://doi.org/10.1093/ehjci/jead193. Epub ahead of print. PMID: 37542478.
9. Papanastasiou CA, Bazmpani MA, Kokkinidis DG, Zegkos T, Efthimiadis G, Tsapas A, Karvounis H, Ziakas A, Kalogeropoulos AP, Kramer CM, Karamitsos TD. The prognostic value of right ventricular ejection fraction by cardiovascular magnetic resonance in heart failure: a systematic review and meta-analysis. Int J Cardiol. 2022;368:94–103. https://doi.org/10.1016/j.ijcard.2022.08.008. Epub 2022 Aug 10. PMID: 35961612.
10. Anastasiou V, Papazoglou AS, Moysidis DV, Daios S, Tsalikakis D, Giannakoulas G, Karamitsos T, Delgado V, Ziakas A, Kamperidis V. The prognostic value of right ventricular longitudinal strain in heart failure: a systematic review and meta-analysis. Heart Fail Rev. 2023;28(6):1383–94. https://doi.org/10.1007/s10741-023-10329-y. Epub 2023 Jun 13. PMID: 37308615; PMCID: PMC10575809.
11. Borlaug BA, Obokata M. The other atrium in heart failure. JACC Cardiovasc Imaging. 2019;12(8 Pt 1):1471–3. https://doi.org/10.1016/j.jcmg.2018.08.019. Epub 2018 Oct 17. PMID: 30343068.
12. Jain S, Kuriakose D, Edelstein I, Ansari B, Oldland G, Gaddam S, Javaid K, Manaktala P, Lee J, Miller R, Akers SR, Chirinos JA. Right atrial phasic function in heart failure with preserved and reduced ejection fraction. JACC Cardiovasc Imaging. 2019;12(8 Pt 1):1460–70. https://doi.org/10.1016/j.jcmg.2018.08.020. Epub 2018 Oct 17. PMID: 30343071; PMCID: PMC6461533.
13. Querejeta Roca G, Campbell P, Claggett B, Solomon SD, Shah AM. Right atrial function in pulmonary arterial hypertension. Circ Cardiovasc Imaging. 2015;8(11):e003521; discussion e003521. https://doi.org/10.1161/CIRCIMAGING.115.003521. PMID: 26514759; PMCID: PMC4629509.
14. D'Alto M, D'Andrea A, Di Salvo G, Scognamiglio G, Argiento P, Romeo E, Di Marco GM, Mattera Iacono A, Bossone E, Sarubbi B, Russo MG. Right atrial function and prognosis in idiopathic pulmonary arterial hypertension. Int J Cardiol. 2017;248:320–5. https://doi.org/10.1016/j.ijcard.2017.08.047. Epub 2017 Aug 24. PMID: 28844500.
15. Bhave NM, Visovatti SH, Kulick B, Kolias TJ, McLaughlin VV. Right atrial strain is predictive of clinical outcomes and invasive hemodynamic data in group 1 pulmonary arterial hypertension. Int J Cardiovasc Imaging. 2017;33(6):847–55. https://doi.org/10.1007/s10554-017-1081-7. Epub 2017 Feb 6. PMID: 28168563; PMCID: PMC5645792.
16. Lang RM, Cameli M, Sade LE, Faletra FF, Fortuni F, Rossi A, Soulat-Dufour L. Imaging assessment of the right atrium: anatomy and function. Eur Heart J Cardiovasc Imaging.

2022;23(7):867–84. https://doi.org/10.1093/ehjci/jeac011. Erratum in: Eur Heart J Cardiovasc Imaging. 2022 May 03. PMID: 35079782.
17. Badano LP, Kolias TJ, Muraru D, Abraham TP, Aurigemma G, Edvardsen T, D'Hooge J, Donal E, Fraser AG, Marwick T, Mertens L, Popescu BA, Sengupta PP, Lancellotti P, Thomas JD, Voigt JU, Industry representatives; Reviewers: This document was reviewed by members of the 2016–2018 EACVI Scientific Documents Committee. Standardization of left atrial, right ventricular, and right atrial deformation imaging using two-dimensional speckle tracking echocardiography: a consensus document of the EACVI/ASE/Industry Task Force to standardize deformation imaging. Eur Heart J Cardiovasc Imaging. 2018;19(6):591–600. https://doi.org/10.1093/ehjci/jey042. Erratum in: Eur Heart J Cardiovasc Imaging. 2018 Jul 1;19(7):830-833. PMID: 29596561.
18. Peluso D, Badano LP, Muraru D, Dal Bianco L, Cucchini U, Kocabay G, Kovàcs A, Casablanca S, Iliceto S. Right atrial size and function assessed with three-dimensional and speckle-tracking echocardiography in 200 healthy volunteers. Eur Heart J Cardiovasc Imaging. 2013;14(11):1106–14. https://doi.org/10.1093/ehjci/jet024. Epub 2013 Feb 19. PMID: 23423966.
19. Nyberg J, Jakobsen EO, Østvik A, Holte E, Stølen S, Lovstakken L, Grenne B, Dalen H. Echocardiographic reference ranges of global longitudinal strain for all cardiac chambers using guideline-directed dedicated views. JACC Cardiovasc Imaging. 2023;16(12):1516–31. https://doi.org/10.1016/j.jcmg.2023.08.011. Epub 2023 Nov 1. PMID: 37921718.
20. Inciardi RM, Bonelli A, Biering-Sorensen T, Cameli M, Pagnesi M, Lombardi CM, Solomon SD, Metra M. Left atrial disease and left atrial reverse remodelling across different stages of heart failure development and progression: a new target for prevention and treatment. Eur J Heart Fail. 2022;24(6):959–75. https://doi.org/10.1002/ejhf.2562. Epub 2022 Jun 6. PMID: 35598167; PMCID: PMC9542359.
21. Mandoli GE, Sisti N, Mondillo S, Cameli M. Left atrial strain in left ventricular diastolic dysfunction: have we finally found the missing piece of the puzzle? Heart Fail Rev. 2020;25(3):409–17. https://doi.org/10.1007/s10741-019-09889-9. PMID: 31773504.
22. Lupu S, Mitre A, Dobreanu D. Left atrium function assessment by echocardiography—physiological and clinical implications. Med Ultrason. 2014;16(2):152–9.
23. Iuchi A, Oki T, Tabata T, Manabe K, Kageji Y, Sasaki M, et al. Changes in pulmonary venous and transmitral flow velocity patterns after cardioversion of atrial fibrillation. J Cardiol. 1995;25:317–24.
24. Basnight MA, Gonzalez MS, Kershenovich SC, Appleton CP. Pulmonary venous flow velocity: relation to hemodynamics, mitral flow velocity and left atrial volume, and ejection fraction. J Am Soc Echocardiogr. 1991;4:547–58.
25. Yu CM, Fung JW, Zhang Q, Kum LC, Lin H, Yip GW, et al. Tissue Doppler echocardiographic evidence of atrial mechanical dysfunction in coronary artery disease. Int J Cardiol. 2005;105:178–85.
26. Zhang Q, Yip GW, Yu CM. Approaching regional left atrial function by tissue Doppler velocity and strain imaging. Europace. 2008;10(Suppl 3):iii62–9. https://doi.org/10.1093/europace/eun237. PMID: 18955401.
27. Kurt M, Wang J, Torre-Amione G, Nagueh SF. Left atrial function in diastolic heart failure. Circ Cardiovasc Imaging. 2009;2(1):10–5. https://doi.org/10.1161/CIRCIMAGING.108.813071. PMID: 19808559.
28. Cameli M, Caputo M, Mondillo S, Ballo P, Palmerini E, Lisi M, Marino E, Galderisi M. Feasibility and reference values of left atrial longitudinal strain imaging by two-dimensional speckle tracking. Cardiovasc Ultrasound. 2009;7:6. https://doi.org/10.1186/1476-7120-7-6.
29. Hoit BD. Left atrial size and function: role in prognosis. J Am Coll Cardiol. 2014;63:493–505.
30. Kim DG, Lee KJ, Lee S, Jeong SY, Lee YS, Choi YJ, Yoon HS, Kim JH, Jeong KT, Park SC, Park M. Feasibility of two-dimensional global longitudinal strain and strain rate imaging for the assessment of left atrial function: a study in subjects with a low probability of cardiovascular disease and normal exercise capacity. Echocardiography. 2009;26:1179–87.

31. Saraiva RM, Demirkol S, Buakhamsri A, Greenberg N, Popović ZB, Thomas JD, Klein AL. Left atrial strain measured by two-dimensional speckle tracking represents a new tool to evaluate left atrial function. J Am Soc Echocardiogr. 2010;23:172–80.
32. Okamatsu K, Takeuchi M, Nakai H, Nishikage T, Salgo IS, Husson S, Otsuji Y, Lang RM. Effects of aging on left atrial function assessed by two-dimensional speckle tracking echocardiography. J Am Soc Echocardiogr. 2009;22:70–5.
33. Murata M, Iwanaga S, Tamura Y, Kondo M, Kouyama K, Murata M, Ogawa S. Real-time three-dimensional echocardiographic quantitative analysis of left ventricular diastolic dysfunction. Am J Cardiol. 2008;8:1097–102.
34. Pellicori P, Zhang J, Lukaschuk E, Joseph AC, Bourantas CV, Loh H, Bragadeesh T, Clark AL, Cleland JGF. Left atrial function measured by cardiac magnetic resonance imaging in patients with heart failure: clinical associations and prognostic value. Eur Heart J. 2015;36:733–42.
35. Vonk Noordegraaf A, Galiè N. The role of the right ventricle in pulmonary arterial hypertension. Eur Respir Rev. 2011;20(122):243–53. https://doi.org/10.1183/09059180.00006511. PMID: 22130817; PMCID: PMC9487747.
36. Pagel PS, Kehl F, Gare M, et al. Mechanical function of the left atrium: new insights based on analysis of pressure-volume relations and Doppler echocardiography. Anesthesiology. 2003;98:975–94.
37. Cameli M, Sciaccaluga C, Loiacono F, Simova I, Miglioranza MH, Nistor D, Bandera F, Emdin M, Giannoni A, Ciccone MM, Devito F, Guaricci AI, Favale S, Lisi M, Mandoli GE, Henein M, Mondillo S. The analysis of left atrial function predicts the severity of functional impairment in chronic heart failure: the FLASH multicenter study. Int J Cardiol. 2019;286:87–91. https://doi.org/10.1016/j.ijcard.2019.03.063. Epub 2019 Mar 29. PMID: 30955880.
38. Cameli M, Pastore MC, Mandoli GE, Nistor D, Lisi E, Tok ÖÖ, Cavigli L, Romano A, Mondillo S. Prognosis and risk stratification of patients with advanced heart failure (from PROBE). Am J Cardiol. 2019;124(1):55–62. https://doi.org/10.1016/j.amjcard.2019.03.041. Epub 2019 Apr 9. PMID: 31047653.
39. Marrouche NF, Brachmann J, Andresen D, Siebels J, Boersma L, Jordaens L, Merkely B, Pokushalov E, Sanders P, Proff J, Schunkert H, Christ H, Vogt J, Bänsch D, CASTLE-AF Investigators. Catheter ablation for atrial fibrillation with heart failure. N Engl J Med. 2018;378(5):417–27. https://doi.org/10.1056/NEJMoa1707855. PMID: 29385358.
40. Sohns C, Fox H, Marrouche NF, Crijns HJGM, Costard-Jaeckle A, Bergau L, Hindricks G, Dagres N, Sossalla S, Schramm R, Fink T, El Hamriti M, Moersdorf M, Sciacca V, Konietschke F, Rudolph V, Gummert J, Tijssen JGP, Sommer P, CASTLE HTx Investigators. Catheter ablation in end-stage heart failure with atrial fibrillation. N Engl J Med. 2023;389(15):1380–9. https://doi.org/10.1056/NEJMoa2306037. Epub 2023 Aug 27. PMID: 37634135.
41. Motoki H, Negishi K, Kusunose K, Popović ZB, Bhargava M, Wazni OM, Saliba WI, Chung MK, Marwick TH, Klein AL. Global left atrial strain in the prediction of sinus rhythm maintenance after catheter ablation for atrial fibrillation. J Am Soc Echocardiogr. 2014;27(11):1184–92. https://doi.org/10.1016/j.echo.2014.08.017. Epub 2014 Sep 23. PMID: 25260436; PMCID: PMC4425733.
42. Tsao HM, Hu WC, Wu MH, Tai CT, Chang SL, Lin YJ, Lo LW, Huang CC, Hu YF, Sheu MH, Chang CY, Chen SA. The impact of catheter ablation on the dynamic function of the left atrium in patients with atrial fibrillation: insights from four-dimensional computed tomographic images. J Cardiovasc Electrophysiol. 2010;21(3):270–7. https://doi.org/10.1111/j.1540-8167.2009.01618.x. Epub 2009 Oct 5. PMID: 19804542.
43. Wylie JV Jr, Peters DC, Essebag V, Manning WJ, Josephson ME, Hauser TH. Left atrial function and scar after catheter ablation of atrial fibrillation. Heart Rhythm. 2008;5(5):656–62. https://doi.org/10.1016/j.hrthm.2008.02.008. Epub 2008 Feb 8. PMID: 18452866.
44. Müller H, Noble S, Keller PF, Sigaud P, Gentil P, Lerch R, Shah D, Burri H. Biatrial anatomical reverse remodelling after radiofrequency catheter ablation for atrial fibrillation: evidence from real-time three-dimensional echocardiography. Europace. 2008;10(9):1073–8. https://doi.org/10.1093/europace/eun187. Epub 2008 Jul 14. PMID: 18628258.

45. Inciardi RM, Claggett B, Minamisawa M, Shin SH, Selvaraj S, Gonçalves A, Wang W, Kitzman D, Matsushita K, Prasad NG, Su J, Skali H, Shah AM, Chen LY, Solomon SD. Association of left atrial structure and function with heart failure in older adults. J Am Coll Cardiol. 2022;79(16):1549–61. https://doi.org/10.1016/j.jacc.2022.01.053. PMID: 35450571.
46. Morris DA, Takeuchi M, Krisper M, Köhncke C, Bekfani T, Carstensen T, Hassfeld S, Dorenkamp M, Otani K, Takigiku K, Izumi C, Yuda S, Sakata K, Ohte N, Tanabe K, Osmanoglou E, Kühnle Y, Düngen HD, Nakatani S, Otsuji Y, Haverkamp W, Boldt LH. Normal values and clinical relevance of left atrial myocardial function analysed by speckle-tracking echocardiography: multicentre study. Eur Heart J Cardiovasc Imaging. 2015;16(4):364–72. https://doi.org/10.1093/ehjci/jeu219. Epub 2014 Nov 3. PMID: 25368210.
47. Kokubu N, Yuda S, Tsuchihashi K, Hashimoto A, Nakata T, Miura T, Ura N, Nagao K, Tsuzuki M, Wakabayashi C, Shimamoto K. Noninvasive assessment of left atrial function by strain rate imaging in patients with hypertension: a possible beneficial effect of renin-angiotensin system inhibition on left atrial function. Hypertens Res. 2007;30:13–21.
48. Thomas L, Abhayaratna WP. Left atrial reverse remodeling: mechanisms, evaluation, and clinical significance. JACC Cardiovasc Imaging. 2017;10(1):65–77. https://doi.org/10.1016/j.jcmg.2016.11.003. PMID: 28057220.
49. Donal E, Raud-Raynier P, DePlace C, Gervais R, Rosier A, Roulaud M, Ingels A, Carre F, Daubert JC, Denjean A. Resting echocardiographic assessments of left atrial function and filling pressure interest in the understanding of exercise capacity in patients with chronic congestive heart failure. J Am Soc Echocardiogr. 2008;21:703–10.
50. Welles CC, Ia K, Kwan DM, Whooley MA, Schiller NB, Turakhia MP. Left atrial function predicts heart failure hospitalization in subjects with preserved ejection fraction and coronary heart disease: longitudinal data from the Heart and Soul Study. J Am Coll Cardiol. 2012;59:673–80.
51. Tan YT, Wenzelburger F, Lee E, Nightingale P, Heatlie G, Leyva F, Sanderson JE. Reduced left atrial function on exercise in patients with heart failure and normal ejection fraction. Heart. 2010;96:1017–23.
52. Melenovsky V, Borlaug BA, Rosen B, Hay I, Ferruci L, Morell CH, Lakatta EG, Najjar SS, Kass DA. Cardiovascular features of heart failure with preserved ejection fraction versus nonfailing hypertensive left ventricular hypertrophy in the urban Baltimore community: the role of atrial remodelling/dysfunction. J Am Coll Cardiol. 2007;49:198–207.
53. Gottdiener JS, Kitzman DW, Aurigemma GP, Arnold AM, Manolio TA. Left atrial volume, geometry, and function in systolic and diastolic heart failure of persons > or =65 years of age (the cardiovascular health study). Am J Cardiol. 2006;97:83–9.
54. Olsson LG, Swedberg K, Ducharme A, Granger CB, Michelson EL, McMurray JJ, Puu M, Yusuf S, Pfeffer MA, Investigators CHARM. Atrial fibrillation and risk of clinical events in chronic heart failure with and without left ventricular systolic dysfunction: results from the Candesartan in Heart failure-Assessment of Reduction in Mortality and morbidity (CHARM) program. J Am Coll Cardiol. 2006;47:1997–2004.
55. Smiseth OA, Morris DA, Cardim N, Cikes M, Delgado V, Donal E, Flachskampf FA, Galderisi M, Gerber BL, Gimelli A, Klein AL, Knuuti J, Lancellotti P, Mascherbauer J, Milicic D, Seferovic P, Solomon S, Edvardsen T, Popescu BA. Reviewers: this document was reviewed by members of the 2018–2020 EACVI Scientific Documents Committee. Multimodality imaging in patients with heart failure and preserved ejection fraction: an expert consensus document of the European Association of Cardiovascular Imaging. Eur Heart J Cardiovasc Imaging. 2022;23(2):e34–61. https://doi.org/10.1093/ehjci/jeab154. PMID: 34729586.
56. Wakami K, Ohte N, Asada K, Fukuta H, Goto T, Mukai S, Narita H, Kimura G. Correlation between left ventricular end-diastolic pressure and peak left atrial wall strain during left ventricular systole. J Am Soc Echocardiogr. 2009;22:847–51.
57. Cameli M, Lisi M, Mondillo S, Padeletti M, Ballo P, Tsioulpas C, Bernazzali S, Maccherini M. Left atrial longitudinal strain by speckle tracking echocardiography correlates well with left ventricular filling pressures in patients with heart failure. Cardiovasc Ultrasound. 2010;8:14.

58. Cameli M, Sparla S, Losito M, Righini FM, Menci D, Lisi M, D'Ascenzi F, Focardi M, Favilli R, Pierli C, Fineschi M, Mondillo S. Correlation of left atrial strain and Doppler measurements with invasive measurement of left ventricular end-diastolic pressure in patients stratified for different values of ejection fraction. Echocardiography. 2016;33(3):398–405.
59. Mullens W, Borowski A, Curtin R, Thomas J, Tang W. Tissue Doppler imaging in the estimation of intracrdiac filling pressure in decompensated patients with advanced systolic heart failure. Circulation. 2009;119:62–70.
60. Pieske B, Tschöpe C, de Boer RA, Fraser AG, Anker SD, Donal E, Edelmann F, Fu M, Guazzi M, Lam CSP, Lancellotti P, Melenovsky V, Morris DA, Nagel E, Pieske-Kraigher E, Ponikowski P, Solomon SD, Vasan RS, Rutten FH, Voors AA, Ruschitzka F, Paulus WJ, Seferovic P, Filippatos G. How to diagnose heart failure with preserved ejection fraction: the HFA-PEFF diagnostic algorithm: a consensus recommendation from the Heart Failure Association (HFA) of the European Society of Cardiology (ESC). Eur Heart J. 2019;40(40):3297–317. https://doi.org/10.1093/eurheartj/ehz641. Erratum in: Eur Heart J. 2021 Mar 31;42(13):1274. PMID: 31504452.
61. Zile MR, Jhund PS, Baicu CF, Claggett BL, Pieske B, Voors AA, Prescott MF, Shi V, Lefkowitz M, McMurray JJ, Solomon SD, Prospective Comparison of ARNI With ARB on Management of Heart Failure With Preserved Ejection Fraction (PARAMOUNT) Investigators. Plasma biomarkers reflecting profibrotic processes in heart failure with a preserved ejection fraction: data from the prospective comparison of ARNI with ARB on management of heart failure with preserved ejection fraction study. Circ Heart Fail. 2016;9(1):e002551. https://doi.org/10.1161/CIRCHEARTFAILURE.115.002551. PMID: 26754625; PMCID: PMC5485256.
62. Chirinos J, Satija V, Gaddam S, et al. Right atrial function in heart failure with preserved and reduced ejection fraction. J Am Coll Cardiol. 2018;71(11_Suppl):A1604. https://doi.org/10.1016/S0735-1097(18)32145-4.
63. Cameli M, Mandoli GE, Loiacono F, Dini FL, Henein M, Mondillo S. Left atrial strain: a new parameter for assessment of left ventricular filling pressure. Heart Fail Rev. 2016;21(1):65–76.

Chapter 6
Heart Failure and Mitral Regurgitation—What We Need to Know?

Maria Dorobanţu and Maria Florescu

Abstract Mitral regurgitation is a growing cardiac issue and is associated with increase morbidity and mortality. This condition represents a very heterogenous disease, which can by *a primary defect* of mitral valve apparatus that through volume overload can lead to left ventricular dysfunction and heart failure, or can be *secondary* to left ventricular remodeling and dysfunction due to an ischemic or non-ischemic cause. Definition of mechanism and etiology of MR and correct grading are essential for management strategy and timing. Extended Heart Team and multimodality imagistic techniques and multi-parametric approach of patients with mitral regurgitation and heart failure are, therefore, mandatory. When indicated, mitral surgery is the treatment of choice in primary mitral regurgitation and with heart failure patients, with repair whenever is possible, meanwhile, the initial cornerstone of management is optimized guideline-directed medical treatment, with surgical or percutaneous trans-catheter intervention as second line of therapy in patients with secondary mitral regurgitation. Our review will discuss aspects regarding the anatomy and function of the complex mitral apparatus, mechanisms, etiologies and pathophysiology of mitral regurgitation and heart failure, different diagnostic tools and management strategies and timing in both primary and secondary mitral regurgitation.

Keywords Heart failure · Primary mitral regurgitation · Secondary mitral regurgitation · Extended heart team · Multimodality imaging techniques · Surgical mitral valve repair · Percutaneous trans-catheter edge-to edge repair

M. Dorobanţu
University of Medicine and Pharmacy "Carol Davila", Bucharest, Romania

Romanian Academy, Bucharest, Romania

M. Florescu (✉)
Emerald Medical Center, Bucharest, Romania

M. Dorobanţu et al. (eds.), *Current Approach to Heart Failure*,
https://doi.org/10.1007/978-3-031-96562-3_6

Abbreviations

ACE	angiotensin converting enzyme
AI	artificial intelligence
AF	atrial fibrillation
ARBs	angiotensin receptor blockers
ASE	American Society of Echocardiography
CRT	cardiac resynchronization therapy
CABG	coronary artery by-pass grafting
CAD	coronary artery disease
cMR	cardiac magnetic resonance
CWD	continuous wave Doppler
CT	computed tomography
CPET	cardiopulmonary exercise testing
DCMP	dilated cardiomyopathy
EACVI	European Association of Cardiovascular Imaging
ECG	electrocardiogram
EF	ejection fraction
EROA	effective regurgitant orifice area
FED	fibroelastic deficiency
GLS	global longitudinal strain
GDMT	guideline directed medical therapy
HF	heart failure
HFrEF	heart failure with reduced ejection fraction
IHD	ischemic heart disease
LA	left atrium
LV	left ventricle
LAD artery	left anterior descending artery
LBBB	left bundle branch block
LVESD	left ventricular end systolic diameter
LVEDD	left ventricular end diastolic diameter
LVESV	left ventricular end systolic volume
LVEDV	left ventricular end diastolic volume
LVOT	left ventricular outflow tract
LVTSV	left ventricular total stroke volume
LGE	late gadolinium enhancement
MD	myxomatous disease
MI	myocardial infarction
MR	mitral regurgitation
MV	mitral valve
MVP	mitral valve prolapse
NYHA	New York Heart Association
PCI	percutaneous coronary interventions
PISA	proximal isovelocity surface area

PsH	pulmonary systolic hypertension
PM	papillary muscles
PSLA	parasternal long axis
PVSFR	pulmonary vein systolic flow reversal
PWD	pulsed wave Doppler
QoL	quality of life
RCTs	randomized clinical trials
RV	right ventricle
RegVol	regurgitant volume
RegFrac	regurgitant fraction
SMR	secondary mitral regurgitation
SGLT2 inhibitors	sodium-glucoze co-transporter 2 inhibitors
sPAP	systolic pulmonary arterial pressure
TEER	transcatheter edge-to edge repair
TVI	time velocity integral
TTE	transthoracic echocardiography
TEER	trans-catheter edge to edge repair
TEE	transesophageal echocardiography
Va	aliasing velocity
VHD	valvular heart disease

Introduction

Mitral regurgitation (MR) affects 3–5% of general population and is associated with increased morbidity and mortality [1]. In EURO Heart Survey II, this defect encountered 21% of all valvular diseases and, through significant ventricular volume overload, can be the primary cause of ventricular dysfunction and heart failure (HF)—primary MR, or can develop secondary to preexisting ventricular remodeling and dysfunction– secondary MR [2]. The mitral valve (MV) is a very complex anatomical and functional structure and identification of the MR etiology and mechanism and correct grading of the severity are essential for the appropriate management timing and strategy [3]. If primary MR necessitates immediately surgery when criteria are indicated, in secondary MR optimized guideline-directed medical treatment for HF is the initial management step, with surgical or percutaneous transcatheter intervention as second line of treatment. However, in real life, patients with native valvular heart disease (VHD) are still referred to medical evaluation at a late stage of the disease, more than 40% of them being in New York Heart Association (NYHA) class III to IV and 10–30% of them being hospitalized in the last year [2]. Left untreated, severe primary MR will initiate a cascade of events leading to HF and death with 1—year mortality up to 57%, as seen in Fig. 6.1 [4, 5]. On the other hand, 1 out of 5 patients with established HF had moderate to severe secondary MR associated with a poor short- and long-term prognosis [6]. Even if the multimodality imaging is now more frequently used and the recommendations for interventions in

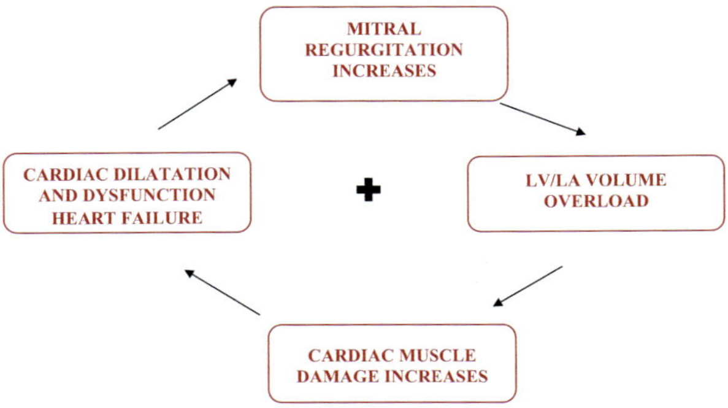

Fig. 6.1 Mitral regurgitation cascade leading to heart failure. *LA* left atrium, *LV* left ventricle

symptomatic patients with severe MR are better applied, stress testing remains underused in asymptomatic patients and late referral for surgical or percutaneous interventions indicates the urgent need for more prompt MR diagnostic [2]. Moreover, population aging and the high burden of comorbidities underline the need for an expanded multidisciplinary Heart Team approach to evaluate the risk-benefit ratio of the different modalities of interventions [1, 7]. The main intervention in primary MR remains surgery, meanwhile technological advances within the last years made percutaneous trans-catheter mitral valve procedures safe and feasible in clinical practice in certain categories of patients with both primary and secondary MR with heart failure. Therefore, in our review we will discuss: ***(I) the anatomy of the mitral valve; (II) the etiology, classification, and natural history of primary and secondary MR; (III) the diagnostic techniques for primary and secondary MR; (IV) the different management strategies based on etiology for primary and secondary MR,*** emphasizing the role of the newest percutaneous trans-catheter MV interventions in patients with severe MR and heart failure. We also will outline the current evidence and limitations and the importance of the appropriate selection of patients according to the new guideline recommended medical and device strategy [8–10].

Mitral Valve Anatomy

MV apparatus is a complex and dynamic structure that includes synchronous involvement of the following elements: mitral annulus, valvular leaflets, chordae tendinae, papillary muscles and left ventricular (LV) wall to allow blood flow in diastole from the left atrium (LA) to the LV, and to prevent regurgitation during systole [3]. Alterations at any level can lead to leaflets closure abnormality and a degree of blood regurgitation. Understanding of the mitral valve anatomy is essential for correct diagnosis and optimal timing and planning for interventions in significant MR patients [3, 8–10].

Mitral Valve Leaflets

Mitral valve has two leaflets—anterior leaflet, located in the posterior part of the aortic root forming the fibrous mitro-aortic continuity and posterior leaflet. Tissue of the mitral leaflets are attached to the mitral annulus with a length between 0.5 and 1 cm and is very important for the coaptation and leaflets closure [11]. On contrary to the atrial surface, which is smooth, the rough zone starting at 1 cm from the distal leaflets tips ensures the perfect closure of the leaflets in LV and is called the coaptation zone, as seen in Fig. 6.2 [11]. The anterior leaflet has a semicircular shape or sail shape, is bigger and thicker than the posterior one, with fibrosa layer more representative, covering one-third of the annular ring and two-third of the valve orifice [11]. This leaflet has no indentations, however, for medical purposes it is divided into lateral (A1), central (A2), and medial scallops (A3) [11]. The posterior leaflet represents two-third of the annular circumference and only one—third of the valve orifice and is divided into three scallops by true slits—lateral (P1), central

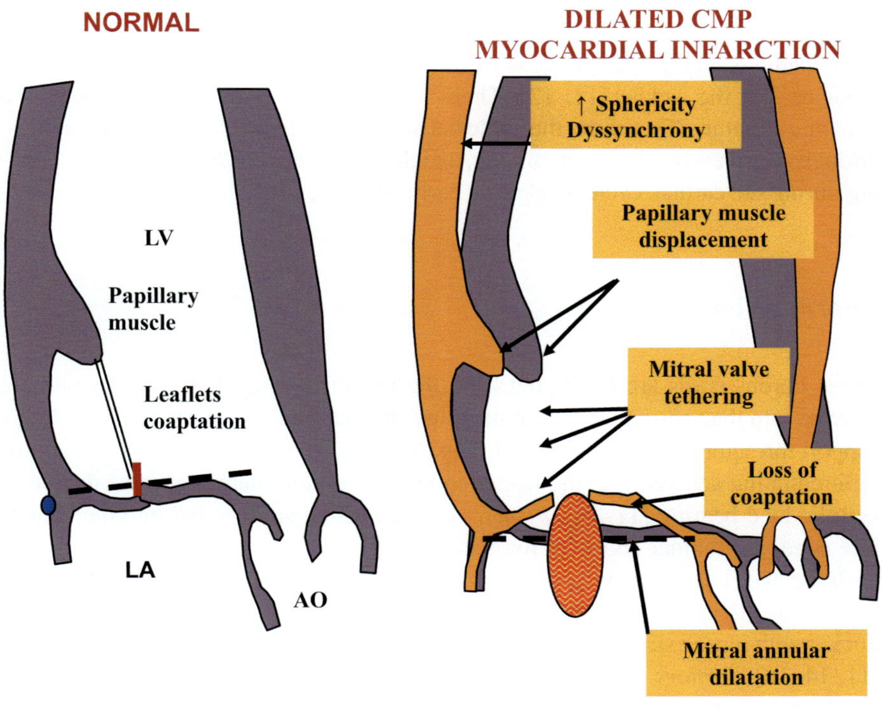

Fig. 6.2 The pathophysiology of secondary MR in dilated cardiomyopathy and myocardial infarction. There are present: papillary muscles displacement and increased sphericity and dyssnchrony, mitral annular dilatation, leaflets tethering with loss of coaptation (right side of the diagram) versus normal mitral valve apparatus in systole—there is no tethering forces, with normal length of leaflets coaptation in the mitral valve annular plane [11]. *DCMP* dilated cardiomyopathy, *MI* myocardial infarction, *MR* mitral regurgitation, *LA* left atrium, *LV* left ventricle

(P2), and medial scallops (P3) [11]. Commissures—anterolateral and posteromedial—are made from additional leaflets tissue found at the anterolateral—A1-P1—and posteromedial—A3-P3 parts [11]. Cardiac muscle cells are present in both leaflets near the mitral annulus and this tissue is excitable from the atrial side, before the LV, being responsible for early closure of the mitral valve in the isovolumic phase of the LV contraction and preventing early MR [11, 12]. Even if the interstitial cells present in the leaflets are inactive, pathological or physiological volume overload stress or annular dilatation can lead to the interstitial cells proliferation, suggesting that there is an adaptation mechanism with leaflets increasing in these conditions [11–13].

Mitral Valve Annulus

This structure represents the intersections of the mitral leaflets, LA and LV—in so called atrioventricular junction [14]. It has a saddle shape and represents a muscular structure in the posterior part, what makes it more susceptible to dilatation than the anterior part [14]. On contrary, the anterior annulus is fibrous, continuing with the aortic annulus and fibrous skeleton of the heart and represents the most important atrial part of the saddle [11, 12]. There are several studies showing that it is a dynamic structure. Therefore, the angle between the aortic valve and mitral annulus, through mitral aortic fibrous continuity, and the size of the mitral annulus are changing during the cardiac cycle preventing early MR [11, 12, 15].

Chordae Tendineae

These fibrous cords are originated from the tips of the papillary muscles and are inserted into the ventricular face of the mitral leaflets and commissures, providing a support throughout systole, as seen in Fig. 6.3 [14]. There are three types of chords differentiating according to the leaflet point of insertion, therefore to the degree of systolic load-bearing [11, 14]. *Primary chords*, which are inserted into the leaflets free edge, are thinner and with limited extensibility, therefore they prevent leaflet prolapse and flail and they do not bear significant loads [11, 14]. *Secondary chords* insert into the anterior leaflet rough zone and into the posterior leaflet body, are thicker with more extensibility, therefore they are bearing an important systolic bear [11, 14, 16]. *Tertiary chords* are attached to the basal LV wall and the base of the posterior leaflet, connecting the posterior annulus and leaflet to the papillary muscle, maintaining the valve-ventricular continuity [14, 16].

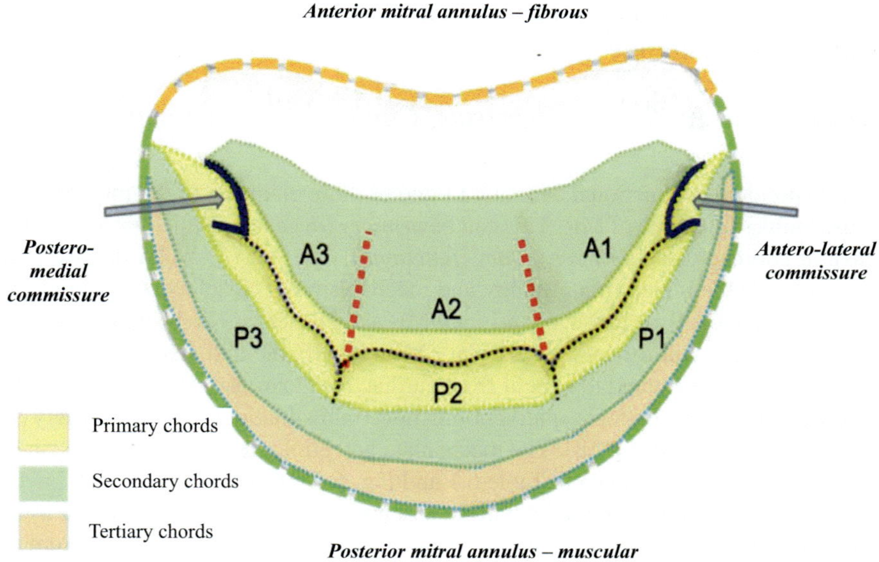

Fig. 6.3 Ventricular face of the mitral valve—mitral valve annulus, leaflets and tendinae chords. (Reproduced from [14], no permission required)

Papillary Muscles and Left Ventricular Walls

There are two groups of papillary muscles (PM): antero-lateral, which is the largest and having two heads arising from a mid to apical border between the lateral and inferolateral wall, and postero-medial arising from the mid to apical inferior wall, comprising three heads—anterior, intermediate and posterior [14]. The PM give chords to both leaflets: the antero-lateral to P1, A1 and medial part of P2 and A2, while the postero-medial supplies P3, A3 and lateral part of P2 and A2 [14]. The posterior descending artery is typically the only source of perfusion for the postero-medial PM, which extend from the right coronary artery in 70–80% of the patients, from left circumflex artery in 5–10% and from both left and right systems in 10–20% of patients [14]. On contrary, the antero-lateral PM has two sources of perfusion—from the left anterior descending (LAD) and from the circumflex artery [11, 14]. During the mid and late systolic phase, through PM contraction, the leaflets are kept under direct tension, avoiding the anterior motion of the leaflets and, therefore, the LV outflow tract obstruction [11, 14].

Mitral Regurgitation Mechanisms, Etiologies, Classification and Pathophisiology

Mitral Regurgitation Mechanisms, Etiologies, and Classification

Any anatomical or functional anomaly of one or more elements of the mitral apparatus results in a degree of MR. This can be *primary* (*degenerative*)—due to a mitral valve or chordae disease or *secondary* (*functional*) due to a LV or LA disease [14, 17]. Defining the underlying etiology and mechanism of the defect is essential for further management, as for severe primary MR and HF surgery is the first choice, in particular repair, and for severe secondary MR and HF, the first step is to optimize the medical treatment and to benefit from cardiac resynchronization therapy (CRT) or mitral valve trans-catheter interventions in certain situations, leaving surgery as the last options [8–10, 14, 18]. The mechanism and etiologies of MR are described by Carpantier and are shown in Table 6.1 and Fig. 6.4 [14, 19, 20].

Type I MR with normal leaflet motion and poor coaptation and apposition as in isolated annular dilation or in mitral valve perforation [11]. The most common mechanism is annular dilatation resulting in secondary MR due to LV or LA dilatation. However, the pure annular dilatation from severe LA enlargement caused by atrial fibrillation (AF)—so called secondary *atrial MR is* still poorly understood [11, 14, 19]. This can appear in the late course of AF with severe annular dilatation, when the protective mechanisms against MR—chords that are providing from papillary muscles to both MV leaflets holding them together and the strong fibrous skeleton of the mitral annulus—are overwhelmed [21, 22]. On the other hand, loss of normal LA function—contraction and relaxation, leads to loss of mechanism of leaflets closure [11]. Patients with significant secondary atrial MR tends to be older (majority more than 80 years old), female, with chronic history of AF, with non-dilated LV and usually LV ejection fraction (EF) > 50% [11, 14, 23]. The outcome of atrial secondary MR is poor, partly due to the advanced age and co-morbidities of patients, with HF hospitalization significantly higher when compared to primary MR or other etiology [11, 14, 23]. The optimal treatment is different and may consists of diuretics, rate or rhythm control of AF, including ablation and possible mitral annuloplasty [23]. Other causes of type 1 MR associated with leaflets perforation can be infective endocarditis, iatrogenic trauma in cardiac surgery, specific drugs or congenital [3, 11, 14].

Type II MR is characterized by excessive leaflets motion due to MV prolapse or fail, which can affect one or both leaflets, one or more scallops or commissures [3, 11]. A rare ischemic cause with papillary muscle ruptured can occur following acute myocardial infarction (MI) [3, 14]. The most frequent types are myxomatous disease (MD) or Barlow disease or fibroelastic deficiency (FED) [3, 11, 14]. In MD, there is a generalized thickening and redundancy of both leaflets, usually with involvement of multiple scallops and MR appears in mid-systole [3, 11, 19]. On contrary, in FED, there is a thickening of a single segment, usually P2, with redundancy and possible ruptured chordae, while the rest of the valve is thin and the MR

Table 6.1 Mitral valve apparatus morphology, cardiac response and remodeling, and mitral regurgitation jet description in primary and secondary ischemic vs non-ischemic MR

	Primary MR	Secondary MR Ischemic	Secondary MR Non-ischemic
Etiology	Fibrotic, myxomatuous, calcifications	Inferior MI	Idiopathic CMP, non-ischemic CMP
LV remodeling	Global if severe MR	Mostly inferior wall	Global dilatation with increased sphericity
LA remodeling	Present to severe	Variable	Mostly severe
MV annulus	Dilated, dynamic function present	Less dynamic, mild to moderate dilatation	Usually severe dilatation, flattening, non-dynamic
Morphology			
Thickening	Moderate to severe	No/mild	No/mild
Prolapse or flail	Variable	No/mild	No/mild
Calcificatio	Variable	No/mild	No/mild
Papillary muscles distance	Normal	Increased posterior papillary inter-valvular fibrosa distance	Increased interpapillary muscles distance
Tethering pattern	None	Asymmetric	Symmetric
Systolic tenting	None	Increased	Significant increased
MR jet direction	Eccentric or central	Eccentric-posterior	Usually, central
CWD	Late systolic (MVP), holo-systolic (flail or calcification)	Uniform through systole	Biphasic pattern—proto- and tele-systolic, mid-systolic dropout
PISA	Usual hemispheric	Not hemispheric	Not hemispheric/biphasic

Adapted from Ref. [14, 19]
CMP cardiomyopathy, *CWD* continuous wave Doppler, *LA* left atrium, *LV* left ventricle, *MI* myocardial infarction, *MR* mitral regurgitation, *MV* mitral valve, *MVP* mitral valve prolapse, *PISA* proximal isovelocity surface area. Sometimes, the mechanism of MR is mixt, primary and secondary

is holo-systolic [11, 14, 19]. Specific leaflet prolapse or flail cause override of the leaflet directing the regurgitant jet in the opposite direction as seen in Fig. 6.4 [14]. Moreover, mitral annulus dynamics are abnormal as an intrinsic part of the MD and has an essential role in aggravating the MR, meanwhile in FED the annular dilatation and dysfunction is only secondary to MR [11], these findings being important in further surgical plan [11, 24].

Type III MR is associated with limited leaflets motion, leading to a coaptation in the LV, as also seen in Fig. 6.4. This can be primary—as in rheumatic disease, post inflammatory condition such as collagen valvular disease, radiation injury, carcinoid syndrome or drug-induced inflammatory changes, with the most restriction in diastole—*Type IIIa*, or can be secondary to LV remodeling and dysfunction with a restriction of leaflet mainly in systole—*Type IIIb* [14]. It can appear due to an

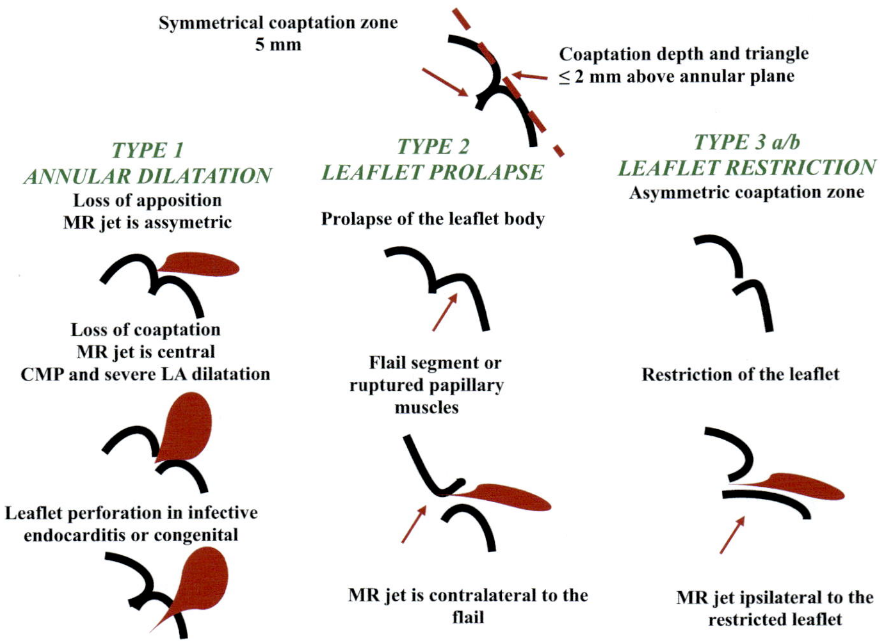

Fig. 6.4 Mitral regurgitation mechanisms and etiologies according to the leaflet motion and Carpantier classification. Competent mitral valve function and motions of the leaflets in systole are shown in the top diagram. (Adapted from [14], no permission required). Carpantier Type 1 MR describes normal valve leaflets motion in case of annular dilation as seen in DCMP of severe LA dilatation with loss of leaflets coaptation and apposition or as seen in perforation of the mitral valve as seen in infective endocarditis; Carpantier Type II describes excessive valve leaflets in case of redundant valve tissue and annulus into the LA or in case of leaflet flail when the primary chordae support is loss and the leaflet tip everts and points into the LA; Carpantier Type III refers to the reduced leaflets motion—Type IIIa where there is a diastolic restriction of leaflet motion due to a primary leaflet disease as in rheumatic disease and shortening of the valve or Type IIIb where there is a systolic restriction of the leaflet due to a LAV or LA disease and the leaflets are normal, but they are tethered. There is a wall motion anomaly that can affect papillary muscle function in ischemic cause or a LV dilation or dissynchrony that can lead to increased tension in subvalvular apparatus and prevents leaflet return to annular plane to meet the opposite leaflet in systole. *DCMP* dilated cardiomyopathy, *LA* left atrium, *LV* left ventricle, *MR* mitral regurgitation

ischemic or non-ischemic cause. Type IIIb occurs with global LV dilatation and mitral annulus enlargement or segmental LV remodeling with posterior and apical displacement of papillary muscles leading to excessive valvular tenting, as seen in Fig. 6.2 [11, 14, 25].

Mitral Regurgitation Pathophysiology

In most cases, *primary MR* worsens over time and have a chronic course, with development of HF in late stages of the disease. In time, due to a volume overload, both LA and LV will be transformed in compliant chambers, with addition of sarcomeres and rearrangement of myocardial fibers resulting in eccentric LV hypertrophy to maintain normal wall stress and adequate cardiac output in the compensated phase of MR [3, 14]. Also, in this phase, LA will enlarge to improve compliance and decrease pulmonary venous pressures [3, 26]. However, during the progression of the disease, afterload increases and LV contractility could eventually decrease with the development of subclinical LV dysfunction and thereafter, overt HF with poor prognosis [3, 27].

On the other hand, *secondary MR* has a very complex pathophysiology due to the imbalance between valve closing forces—which are decreased (by reduced LV contractility and mitral annulus contraction, LV dyssynchrony and increased LA pressure), and leaflets tethering forces—which are increased (by LV dilatation and sphericity, papillary muscles displacement and asymmetry, annular dilation and flattening, along with mitral valve mal-function and fibrotic mal-adaptative leaflet thickening and fibrosis) as shown in Fig. 6.2 [7]. More specifically, in inferior/posterior myocardial infarction (MI), there is a restricted motion of posterior leaflet mostly in systole, and ischemia determines that myocardial segments underlying the papillary muscle to bulge outward and posteriorly, pulling the leaflet away from their normal coaptation resulting in *ischemic MR*, as seen in Fig. 6.4 [28]. Secondary MR may also occur as a consequence of a LV muscle disease and its dilatation in the absence of coronary artery disease (CAD), so called *non—ischemic MR*. It is important to remember that secondary MR is a dynamic defect and any factor that affects LV afterload (high blood pressure, physical activity, or medication) or LV preload (medication or hydration status), as well as heart rhythm or conduction system disturbances may impact the severity of MR. On the other hand, in ischemic MR, could reflect the combination of viable and no-viable myocardial ratio [7, 29, 30]. All over, in patients with HF, significant secondary MR is an indicator of poor prognosis and the change from a LV disease "marker" to a HF "determinant" is essential in determining the optimal management, more specific the need for valve interventions [7, 31].

As already mentioned, in the last years has been described other form of secondary MR, due to LA enlargement and mitral annular dilatation and flattening, in patients with long history with AF, where LV is less dilated and has a normal LVEF—*atrial MR*. Identification of this mechanism is very important since the treatment is completely different [7, 32].

Diagnostic Techniques of Mitral Regurgitation and Heart Failure

Diagnosis, correct description of the mechanism and etiology, and accurate grading of the defect severity are crucial for the optimal management of patients with MR and HF, since primary MR and secondary MR have different type of treatment approach and the timing of intervention is essential for prognosis.

The initial diagnosis of MR is based on the patient history and physical examination, in order to define functional capacity, haemodynamic and volume status, and HF symptoms and severity [7]. Electrocardiogram (ECG) is also an important tool to demonstrate cardiac rhythm (sinus rhythm or not) and to define intraventricular conduction delay as left bundle branch block (LBBB) and to measure QRS duration, essential data for cardiac resynchronization therapy indication where feasible [7]. Laboratory measurements, more specific level of hemoglobin and iron, renal and hepatic function, natriuretic peptides and troponins help in global understanding of the HF status associated with MR. Coronary invasive or non-invasive angiography diagnosed potentially associated CAD in these patients. Moreover, ventriculography in selected cases can provide information over LV function and grading the MR severity [7]. However, the most important diagnostic tool are *imagistic techniques*, emphasizing the role of *integrated multi-modality imagistic and multi-parameters approach* for the diagnosis of MR, description of the mechanism and cause and grading the severity, also for the evaluation of the consequences of the MR on the cardiac dimensions and function and on pulmonary pressure. Therefore, (1) T*ransthoracic echocardiography—standard 2D echocardiography or novel methods—3D echocardiography or speckle tracking echocardiography*—is the key and first tool to describe integrated structural and functional assessment of the MV, grading the severity of the defect, LV and LA, associated valve disease, RV function, and estimated pulmonary pressure; (2) *Transesophageal echocardiography* may provide more accurate images of the mitral valve anatomy and function and is essential for surgical plan in mitral valve repair or percutaneous trans-catheter interventions; (3) *Stress echocardiography—with exercise* in primary MR can help in surgical management decision and in the assessment of ischemic MR, to evaluate haemodynamic interaction between MR severity and LV function, or *with dobutamine* for the evaluation of induced myocardial ischemia, but its precise role remains unclear; (4) *Cardiac magnetic resonance (cMR)* allows precise measurement of LV volumes and ejection fraction, identification of fibrosis or scar and myocardial viability and accurate quantification of MR severity [7, 29].

Primary Mitral Regurgitation

Morphology *"First, look at the valve!"* All echocardiographic evaluation should begin with full anatomical MV apparatus description, in the presence of MVP mixomatous changes—prolapse, flail, ruptured or elongated chordae, MV degeneration—thickening, calcifications, MV infection—endocarditis—vegetations, perforation, aneurysm, inflammatory—rheumatic, irradiation, collagen systemic disease, drugs, congenital—mitral cleft, parachute MV [33]. MVP is defined as a systolic displacement of the mitral leaflets into LA of at least 2 mm from the annular plane from parasternal long axis view (PSLA) [19]. As a part of the MVP disease, a flail occurs commonly from rupture of the marginal primary chordae and the leaflet edge, and not just the leaflet body is in the LA with free motion [19]. The presence of the flail almost always defines a severe MR and is associated with poor prognosis; an extreme form of prolapse represents papillary muscle rupture [19, 34]. The presence of a mitral annulus disjunction in MVP should be checked due to its ventricular arrhythmic risk [33, 35]. Other echocardiographic feature that should be described in MVP disease is clef-like indentations, which are deep separation exceeding 50% of the mitral valve leaflet depth and is best characterized by 3D echocardiography [33, 36]. Sometime, it is difficult to clearly differentiate between primary or secondary MR in the presence of retraction of a single or both leaflets, associated with MV annulus dilatation and, moreover, an initially secondary MR can worsen with valve degeneration and lead to a "tertiary" or "mixed" MR [37]. As seen in Fig. 6.4, analysis of jets using the color Doppler helps in understanding the MR mechanism—for example, isolated posterior MVP resulting in an eccentric anterior MR jet towards the interatrial septum or associated cleft-like indentations may lead to atypical MR jet or multiple jets [33, 38].

Data regarding *echocardiographic* assessment of morphology and MR severity are shown in Table 6.2.

Haemodynamic Consequences and Consideration in Echocardiographic Assessment of MR

In the early phase of chronic MR, there is a LA volume overload, and in the later stages a pressure overload, however, the increased LV stroke volume will compensate the MR flow to maintain LV forward stroke volume. In time, this will progress to LV dilatation according to the Frank Starling law, therefore LV volumes and diameters should be carefully measured in patients with MR [19, 33]. Patients with severe MR may have spherical mid-to-apical LV end-systolic remodeling resulting in higher LV end-systolic volume (ESV) and almost normal LV end systolic diameter (ESD) [19, 33]. However, LVESD is an important parameter of LV impairment in severe MR, and it must be integrated with systolic function and afterload

Table 6.2 Severe mitral regurgitation criteria according to 2D echocardiography in primary vs secondary mitral regurgitation [8–10]

	Primary MR	Secondary MR
Qualitative		
MV morphology	Flail, ruptured papillary muscles, severe retraction, perforation, severe MVP	Normal leaflets, loss of coaptation, severe leaflet tethering and tenting
Color flow jet area	Large central jet >50% of LA, eccentric jet with Coanda effect	Large central jet >50% of LA or eccentric impinging jet
Flow convergence	Large, holo-systolic	Large, holo-systolic
CWD jet	Holo-systolic, dense, triangular	Holo-systolic, dense, triangular
Semiquantitative		
Vena contracta width (mm)	≥7 mm (≥8 mm for biplane)	≥7 mm (≥8 mm for biplane)
Pulmonary vein flow	Systolic flow reversal	Systolic flow reversal
Mitral inflow	Dominant E wave > 1.2 m/s	Dominant E wave > 1.2 m/s
TVI mitral/TVI aortic	>1.4	>1.4
Quantitative		
EROA (2D PISA/mm^2)	≥40 mm^2	≥40 mm^2 (may be ≥30 mm^2 if elliptical regurgitant orifice area)
Regurgitant volume (ml/beat) Volumetric method	≥60 ml	≥60 ml (may be ≥45 ml if low flow condition)
Regurgitant fraction (%) Volumetric method	≥50%	≥50%
Structural		
Left ventricle	Dilated ESD ≥ 40 mm	Dilated
Left atrium	Dilated (diameter ≥ 55 mm, volume ≥ 60 ml/m^2)	Dilated

2D echocardiography two-dimensional echocardiography, *ESD* end systolic diameter, *EROA* effective regurgitant orifice area, *LA* left atrium, *LV* left ventricle, *MR* mitral regurgitation, *MV* mitral valve, *PISA* proximal isovelocity surface area, *TVI* time velocity integral

condition. LA volume measurement is a strong predictor of prognosis in primary MR and should be always assessed. In advanced stage of MR, the symptoms of heart failure will occur, along with LV dysfunction and signs of pulmonary hypertension (PH) [33, 39, 40].

However, due to a reduced afterload, severe MR is associated long time with normal or even supranormal LVEF or LV global longitudinal strain (GLS), therefore these parameters may overestimate LV contractility [33, 41]. A low aortic VTI despite of a LVEF > 60% is suggestive for significant MR. Prompt surgery is necessary in a severe primary MR with LVEF < 60% [8–10]. There have been proposed a new classification for cardiac damage, both LV and right ventricle (RV) damage in asymptomatic patients with moderate to severe MR, including also LV GLS and RV dysfunction with significant prognostic role [42–44]. Recent study from MIDA—Quantitative registry suggested that parameters such as LA dilatation, AF, high pulmonary pressure and/or at least moderate tricuspid regurgitation could have a prognostic role for survival after MR surgery [45]. To notice, even if LV ESD dilatation > 40 mm is an important parameter used for indication of surgery in severe MR, in several cases of severe MR this could be relatively normal, due to the fact that normal LV volumes decrease with age and are lower in women [46].

Quantitative assessment of mitral regurgitation severity includes: (1) calculation of EROA, area of the loss of leaflets coaptation; (2) measurements of mitral regurgitant volume (RegVol) and (3) mitral regurgitant fraction (RegFrac) [8, 9, 33]. These parameters with certain prognostic value could be obtain using the proximal isovelocity surface area (PISA) method, or indirectly, based on the mass conservation using volumetric method [33, 47]. The PISA method relies on the assumption that the regurgitant flow is constant over time and orthogonal to well-defined isovelocity hemisphere, however this condition is very rarely encountered in real life in patients with primary MR [48, 49]. Therefore, in wall-constrained eccentric MR jet, as in commissural MR or posterior valve prolapse, multiple jets, extensive Barlow's disease with bi-leaflets prolapse and diffuse inter-commissural regurgitation, the calculation of the RegVol using PISA method is not reliable [50].

Volumetric method assesses MR severity using the principle according to that the amount of blood volume across the MV (trans-mitral volume) is equal to that ejected into the aorta across the aortic valve (trans-aortic volume), therefore in isolated MR, LV total stroke volume (LV TSV) equals the aortic forward stroke volume (anterograde flow) plus the mitral RegVol (retrograde flow). Moreover, the RegFrac can be calculated dividing RegVol by the LVTSV. This method could be applicable for grading the severity of MR in patients with sinus rhythm when PISA method is not reliable. In real life, 2D and 3D transthoracic echocardiography (TTE) volumetric method for calculation of RegVol and RegFrac should be done routinely in patients with MR when 3D echo is feasible, and the biggest LV volumes between those obtained by 2D vs 3D-TTE should be selected for measurement of LVTSV [33]. In conclusion, to avoid the mistaking the quantitative methods, studies recommend reporting PISA assessing EROA and volumetric method for RegVol and RegFrac [33].

3D-transthoracic echocardiography for measuring vena contracta area and proximal flow convergence can be used to better describe the complex geometry of the MV apparatus and the loss of coaptation and apposition between leaflets, considering that EROA is a three-dimensional structure [51]. Although recent improvements in 3D echo increase spatial and temporal resolution, in clinical practice use of 3D VCA and PISA remained limited to a few specialized echo laboratories, but we expected that the limitations may be overcome by artificial intelligence (AI) based tools [33].

In conclusion, the final echocardiographic report should classify the MR as severe or significant, moderate, mild or "indeterminate". According to the ESC guideline, the severe primary MR is define using the criteria listed in Table 6.2 [8]. If there is a certain diagnosis of severe MR, and at least one indication for MV surgery, as we will further discuss, the intervention should be planned after Heart Team discussion, in relation to MV repair probability and patient's preference and risk

[33]. Moreover, in case of significant, MR but no heart failure symptoms or equivocal symptoms, *cardiopulmonary exercise testing (CPET)* or *exercise stress echocardiography* could be indicated to estimate the functional capacity and hemodynamic tolerance of MR, to unmask the PH or to reveal the low peak oxygen consumption, associated with poor prognosis [33, 52].

Figure 6.5 shows an integrated echocardiographic approach of a severe primary MR due to an extreme anterior MV prolapse and flail, using conventional 2D echocardiography, 3D echocardiography and speckle tracking imaging.

In several situation, such an AF, eccentric or multiple jets, extensive bi-commissural leak, wall constrained jet, late systolic MR jet or in women or old persons with complex MV morphology, a second line examination methods—*cardiac magnetic resonance—cMR or transesophageal echocardiography—TEE*—should be applied. In the last years, there are several studies that demonstrated the advantages of cMR in staging MR, description of morphology and arrhythmic risk stratification, however this method should be performed in patients able to hold breath and when the main remaining question is to quantify the severity of MR [53]. However, in a recent paper, Vermes et al. showed that cMR has become an excellent tool in assessment of mitral valve prolapse, providing accurate data of both LV and RV dimension and function, mitral annulus motion and MR severity, along to the ability to assess focal or diffuse myocardial fibrosis [54]. Finally, using the late

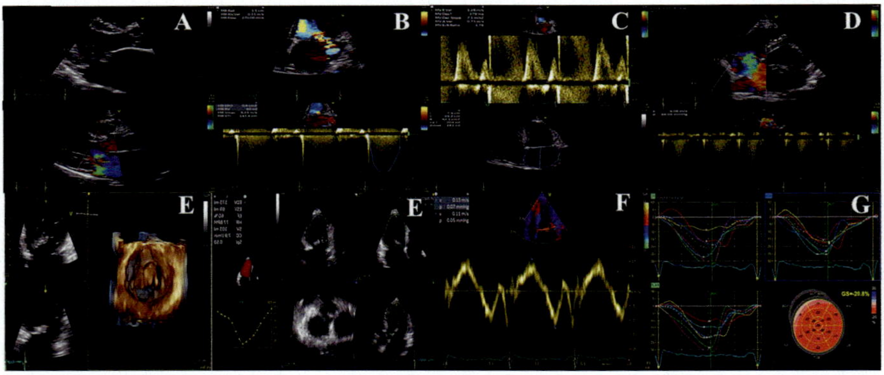

Fig. 6.5 Integrated echocardiographic assessment of a severe primary mitral regurgitation in a patient with symptoms of heart failure NYHA III (with courtesy of Dr. Oana Ionita). (**a**) 2D echocardiography shows a severe anterior MV prolapse/flail, with relatively eccentric jet; (**b**) a quantitative assessment of the defect using PISA method shows a regurgitant volume 60 ml, the patient has a dilated LV, with LVESD 42 mm; (**c**) predominant E wave on PWD and severely dilated LA; (**d**) RV is slightly dilated with moderate secondary TR and there is elevated PH; (**e**) 3D echocardiographic reconstruction of the MV prolapse/ flail and LVEF measurement; (**f**) TVI mitral annulus systolic velocities measurements; (**g**) LV GLS is −20%. This echocardiographic evaluation indicates mitral valve surgery as a management. *EF* ejection fraction, *ESD* end systolic diameter, *GLS* global longitudinal strain, *LV* left ventricle, *LA* left atrium, *MV* mitral valve, *PISA* proximal isovelocity surface area, *PH* pulmonary hypertension, *PWD* pulsed wave Doppler, *RV* right ventricle, *TR* tricuspid regurgitation, *TVI* tissue velocity imaging, *STE* speckle tracking echocardiography

gadolinium enhancement (LGE) and T1 mapping, focal and diffuse fibrosis and calculation of the extracellular volume can be measured, identifying patients with high risk of ventricular arrhythmias [54].

Transesophageal echocardiography, with 3D high resolution imaging is the second-line imagistic technique when there is a need for comprehensive mitral apparatus description along with grading the MR. It could be useful in cases of MR due to infective endocarditis, giving information about the structures around the MV [9]. Also, this is a method of choice to assess the probability of MV repair, with 3D imaging offering a surgical view of the valve. TEE before surgery will help to predict the surgical plan, although the final decision about repair versus replacement of the valve will be made in the operating room. To remember, MR is load dependent, therefore the grading of severity could be influenced by the TEE conditions—under general anesthesia or light sedation [19, 33]. Moreover, intraoperative TEE verify the results of the MV repair and, since even mild residual MR after repair may lead in time to repair failure, surgeons strive for near perfect interventions. The results of the valve repair should be evaluated after physiological filling pressure and blood pressure have been completely established [9, 55].

Secondary Mitral Regurgitation

Current guidelines recommend using transthoracic echocardiography as the first line of imaging technique for diagnosis of secondary MR, description of etiology, LV dimensions and function, grading the severity of MR and estimation of pulmonary arterial pressure [8, 9].

Morphology As seen in Table 6.1, in secondary MR the leaflets are relatively normal, although minor thickening and calcification may be present [19]. LV adverse remodelling from ischemic cause—most frequently inferior MI or multiple MI or non-ischemic cause, such as dilated cardiomyopathy, leads to apical tethering of one or both leaflets and papillary muscle displacement with incomplete mitral closure (Fig. 6.2). The leaflets are apically displaced, with restricted posterior motion in ischemic pattern and the P3 segment tethered more apically than P1 in dilated cardiomyopathy leading to an irregular regurgitant orifice or even double orifice [56].

Using echocardiography, a "hockey stick" sign or "seagull" sign, a bend in the body of the anterior leaflet from tethering of the basal or strut chordae, and a posterior regurgitant jet can be seen. It is important to note that that a severely restricted posterior leaflet due to ischemic wall motion abnormality may result in anterior leaflet override, however this leaflet is not prolapsing and not representing a mixed etiology [19].

The degree of leaflets tethering is a very important parameter that can be used in planning an eventual surgery. This can be assessed by: **tenting area** at mid-systole—the area measurement from the leaflet tips to the annular plane; **coaptation height/**

depth—the maximal distance from leaflets tips to the annular plane, which is correlated with the severity of secondary/ischemic MR, **interpapillary muscles distance**, **the tenting volume**—measured by 3D echocardiography. However, even there is a correlation between these parameters and the severity of the secondary MR, these are not able to differentiate mild, moderate, or severe MR [19, 57].

In secondary MR, there is a significant annular dilatation mostly along with leaflets tethering and in very few cases of severe LA dilatation from long history of atrial fibrillation, single annular dilatation can cause significant MR [19, 33]. Furthermore, echocardiography should describe posterior leaflet length, valve area or associated valvular anomalies, and the parameters of LV anatomy and functions: end diastolic and end-systolic diameters and volumes, LVEF, sphericity index, interpapillary muscles distance, regional or global LV contractility anomalies/dysfunction. Although several etiologies may coexist in an individual patient, the predominant mechanism should be identified to distinguish between those with primary MR and reduced LV function and those with true secondary MR. In several cases there are mixed MR etiologies and has to be described, for example a long standing moderate primary MR due to MV prolapse can be complicated with ischemic MR due to a myocardial infarction.

Grading the severity in secondary MR is more challenging than in primary MR due to several factors, such as: the LV TSV (total stroke volume) may be decreased in case of LV dysfunction and, therefore, RegVol may be lower than in primary MR (less than 60 ml for severe MR if LVTSV is reduced); the regurgitant orifice is no longer circular, may be semilunar or elliptical, affecting VC width measurement (which is usually not seen) and possible leading to underestimated EROA by 2D PISA method [8, 14, 19]. Moreover, EROA measurement may be influenced by the LV dimensions and function. As seen in Table 6.2, an EROA of at least 0.4 cm^2 define a severe MR, however a lower 0.3 cm^2 cut off calculated by PISA method is more likely to be severe due to the above considerations. Added to this, parameters of cardiac chambers remodeling are not so useful, because they are already abnormal due to the underlying cardiomyopathy, such as blunted systolic pulmonary venous flow pattern due to elevated LA pressure [9, 14, 19]. Because of elevated LA pressure, a compliant and dilated LA and reduced LVEF, an inverted systolic flow is not commonly seen in severe secondary MR [9, 14, 19]. Finally, the dynamic pattern of secondary MR makes the grading of severity jet more difficult, being very important to report blood pressure, volume status and cardiac rhythm. Several studies demonstrated that an EROA of secondary MR based on PISA method of 0.2 cm^2, the previous cut off used in guidelines to define significant secondary MR, is associated with poor prognosis, however is still not known if the severe prognostic value is primarily due to the MR or to the degree of irreversible myocardial damage, fibrosis and LV dysfunction [8, 9, 14]. Moreover, current studies did not demonstrate that surgical correction of significant secondary MR improves outcomes [8, 9, 14, 19], and define lesser degree of MR as significant could lead to unnecessary interventions [8, 9]. On the other hand, reduction of MR severity in selected patients using MitraClip can lead to a decreasing of LV and LA remodeling and improving NYHA functional class, despite of moderate residual MR [17].

In fact, the present guidelines define secondary MR as a severe defect with the same cut off as primary MR using EROA based on 2D PISA ≥ 0.4 cm^2, and may be considered severe if EROA is 0.3–0.39 cm^2 if the orifice is elliptical; RegVol ≥ 60 ml, and may be considered severe if RegVol is 45–59 ml and RegFrac is ≥50%, and may be considered if it is 40–49% [8, 9]. However, further research is needed to better grade the severity of secondary MR using multi-imaging methods approach—2D and 3D echocardiography or transesophageal echocardiography, along with cMR to assess the LA and LV remodeling, keeping in mind that the principal goal of this severity grading is to identify the patients who will benefit from mitral valve intervention which can change the clinical course of the disease. The ***proportionality of secondary MR***, a recent concept that describes the fact that secondary MR is a consequence of LV disease and treatment should target this LV dysfunction will be detailed in the management section [58]. When the LV function is severely depressed and LV severely dilated, a large EROA and RegFrac of MR is ***proportionate*** with the degree of LV dilatation (is noticed that in case of LVEF around 30% and a LVEDV of 220–260 ml, an EROA will be 0.3 cm^2) and this group of patients with HF would benefit from optimized medical treatment or device for LV dilatation and dysfunction [58]. On contrary, less severe LV remodeling with similar EROA and RegFrac defines a ***disproportionate MR*** to the degree of LV dilatation (an EROA of 0.3–0.4 cm^2 with a LVEDV of 160–200 ml) and this group of patients could benefit from percutaneous interventions [58].

Finally, we have to pay attention to several general echocardiographic considerations: (1) Secondary MR is a very dynamic phenomenon and severity may vary significantly according to loading conditions, therefore grading should be done in stable patients with controlled blood pressure, under optimal medical treatment, and interpreted cautiously in decompensated patients under inotropic support or fluid overload; (2) Quantitative assessment of secondary MR has low reproducibility, being highly operator-dependent and is inaccurate if the regurgitant orifice is elliptical (as in multiple cases) or in case of multiple jets, therefore multiple parameters should be measured; (3) Intraventricular conduction abnormalities, such as LBBB and RV pacing increase the severity of secondary MR, grade 1 AV block can lead to diastolic secondary MR and the secondary MR is very difficult to assess in atrial fibrillation [14, 19].

Exercise echocardiography can be useful in evaluating patients with secondary MR, unmask the symptoms and define the functional capacity, a poor contractility reserve during exercise having a worse prognosis [8, 9]. Increase of EROA with 0.13 cm^2 during exercise is associated with adverse outcome in secondary MR [8, 9]. *Transesophageal echocardiography (TEE)* can be used in secondary MR to correctly identify the underlying causes, localize the valve pathology and to plan the percutaneous valve procedures or surgery [8, 9]. However, the jet may appear larger on TEE and, due to the sedative use, secondary MR may appear less severe if the blood pressure is very low. Moreover, recent guidelines recommend ***cMR*** as a diagnostic tool for secondary MR and myocardial viability, offering an accurate assessment of both ventricles and atrium remodelling and function, in addition to identification of myocardial scar (ischemic or not) [8, 9, 14].

General Echocardiographic Consideration for Mitral Valve Surgery

Severe primary MR, as soon as the symptoms or signs of LV dysfunction, LA remodeling, increase the PH or AF occur represents a class I indication for surgery, mitral valve repair being preferred when possible. It has been demonstrated that if repair is performed before onset of LV impairment it has the potential to restore normal life expectancy [8–10, 14]. In cases where the likelihood of reparability is high and surgical risk is low, early surgery should be performed, therefore several echocardiographic parameters should be report. Classical, the indexes that indicates surgery are: LVESD $\geq$ 40 mm, LV dilatation by Simpson's biplane volume, a LVEF $\leq$ 60%, an increased systolic pulmonary arterial pressure (sPAP), a severe LA dilatation $\geq$ 60 ml/m^2 and mitral flail [8, 9]. Other important parameter is the valve morphology, since the likelihood of repair decreases with complexity of valve defects and, although surgery in isolated P2 prolapse has demonstrated good long-term durability, bi-leaflet defects, isolated anterior valve prolapse or associated of P1 and P3 or commissural involvement, annulus or leaflet calcifications require greater surgical expertise and could be less durable [14, 19]. All these unfavorable morphological parameters should be described in a complete echocardiographic report. Regarding ***secondary MR***, there have been described several unfavorable echocardiographic parameters for the MV repair: leaflet coaptation high > 10 mm; tenting area > 2.5–3 cm^2; inter-papillary muscle distance > 20 mm; global LV remodeling with LVEDD > 65 mm/LVESD > 51 mm, ESV > 140 ml; systolic sphericity index > 0.7, as seen in Fig. 6.6 [14].

For the prediction of MV repair durability with ***MV clip using trans-catheter interventions in primary MR***, the unfavorable parameters are: large flail gap > 10 mm; LVEDD > 70 mm; flail width or size of prolapsing segment > 15 mm; LVEDV > 200 mL; small MV orifice < 4 cm^2 and in ***secondary MR*** are:

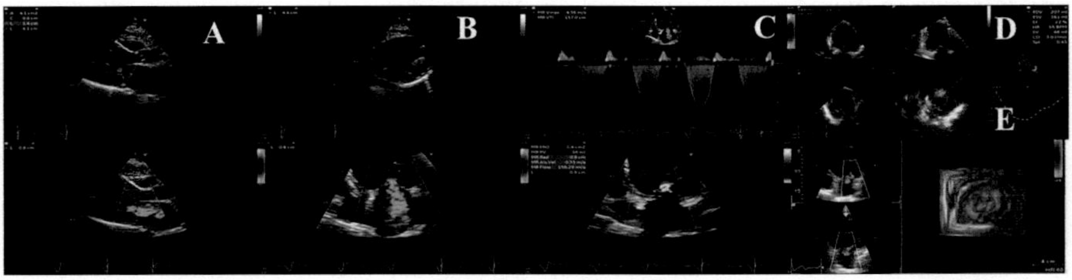

Fig. 6.6 Integrated 2D and 3D echocardiographic approach in a patient with ischemic dilated cardiomyopathy. (With courtesy of Dr. Oana Ionita). (**a**) 2D echocardiography shows a very dilated LV, with thin, necrotic walls in parasternal long axis view and apical 4C view, with measurement of leaflet coaptation high and tenting area; (**b**) in short axis view measurement of inter-papillary muscle distance; (**c**) severe secondary MR calculated using PISA method (**d**) 3D echocardiography shows global LV remodeling with dilated LVEDV and very depressed LVEF; (**e**) 3D echocardiography measurement of vena contracta. *EF* ejection fraction, *EDV* end diastolic volume, *LV* left ventricle, *MR* mitral regurgitation, *PISA* proximal isovelocity surface area

LVEDD > 70 mm; LVEDV > 200 ml; LVEDV index > 96 ml/m^2; posterior leaflet length < 6/10 mm [14].

Management Strategies in Mitral Regurgitation and Heart Failure

Severe untreated MR is associated with poor prognosis, increasing the burden of HF and AF and risk of death irrespective of etiology [3]. Factors such as high functional class NYHA III or IV, RV dysfunction, new onset AF, association of tricuspid regurgitation, secondary etiology and echocardiographic parameters (EROA $\geq$ 0.4 cm^2 or 0.3–0.39 cm^2 in secondary MR) are predictive for worse outcome in patients with significant MR [3].

Chronic MR has a very long compensated stage, and decompensated phase occurs late in the course of the disease depending on MR severity and associated cardiac changes. The latest stage, decompensated, is defined by the presence of HF symptoms and suboptimal LV structural and functional parameters due to the failure of compensatory mechanisms-LVESD > 40 mm and LVEF < 60% [8, 9]. The transition time between compensated stages and decompensated phase with heart failure is less well-defined, but the correct identification of this point is essential for ideal timing of MV intervention to stop the progression of MR and heart failure.

The regular follow-up should be done for the asymptomatic patients with significant MR with periodic clinical exam and TTE to prevent the irreversible evolution toward the LV dysfunction and PH [8, 9]. However, patients with severe MR should be evaluated by the extended, multi-disciplinary Heart Team when the valve intervention is considered and an individual risks should be calculated for specific surgical and/or trans-catheter procedures, using online tools when available, and discussed before the procedure as a part of a shared decision-making process together with the patient [8, 9]. Risk assessment for surgical mitral procedure comprises calculation of ***STS—score for the death index event*** (http://riskcalc.sts.org/stswebriskcalc/#/) or ***EUROSCORE II risk*** calculator can be used (http://www.euroscore.org/calc.html); the assessment of different frailty score indexes, evaluation of specific comorbidities and procedures specific risk [8].

Management in Primary Mitral Regurgitation and Heart Failure

Recent guidelines showed that the development of symptoms in severe MR is an indication for mitral intervention, even if the LV is preserved, indicating changes in LA or LV compliance, decrease in RV function or development of PH [8, 9]. New onset of AF, significant PH and severe dilatation of LA (>60 ml/m^2) are other indicators for valve interventions. Cardiac biomarkers and global LV longitudinal strain may be helpful to orient the timing of interventions in asymptomatic patients with severe MR [8, 9, 59, 60].

Guideline Directed Medical Treatment (GDMT)

Diuretics or other vasodilator therapy that may decrease symptoms do not change the poor prognosis of severe MR left unoperated, MV surgery being the only intervention that improve the natural history of the disease [8, 9]. However, GDMT for LV systolic dysfunction or systemic arterial hypertension should be indicated as in any patient with these conditions [8, 9, 61].

Mitral Valve Interventions for Severe Primary MR

- Recent guidelines recommend *surgical intervention* as a class I of indication for symptomatic patients with degenerative severe MR irrespective of LV function or asymptomatic patients with LVEF $\leq$ 60%, LVESD $\leq$ 40 mm or new onset of AF and sPAP > 50 mm hg or high likelihood of durable repair, low surgical risk, significant LA dilatation (>60 ml/m^2) or LV dilatation and decrease in LV function at $\geq$3 repeated echocardiographic exams [8–10]. The appearance of symptoms is an indication for prompt mitral valve surgery, even if they are mildly and LV function is normal, since the symptoms are associated with worse prognosis [62]. MV repair is the surgical intervention of chose whenever the successful and durable repair is possible [8, 9, 63]. Accurate evaluation of the valve anatomy, especially with intraoperative TEE is essential for surgical repair success, mostly demonstrated in single posterior scallop MV involvement. In cases of repair of the posterior leaflet and annuloplasty, the mortality rate is <1% and the freedom from reoperation at 15–20 years is 95% [64]. Anterior and bileaflets defects require more complicated repair and studies demonstrated that, at 15–20 years, 60% of these cases are free from moderate to severe residual MR and 80% free from reoperation, when the surgery is done in an experience center [65].
- The MV replacement should be performed only when MV repair is not feasible even after the first attempt, however is preferable to a poor repair. In an experienced center, mini—invasive surgical approach has similar results as full median sternotomy [8, 9]. In rheumatic severe MR, MV repair may be considered (class IIb) when is indicated if durability is expected in an experienced Comprehensive Valve Center when the disease is not so advanced or in patients in whom a mechanical prosthesis cannot be used due to the anticoagulant concern [8, 9, 66]. However, one third of patients who underwent to repair had significant stenosis or regurgitation at 10 years [66].
- In severely symptomatic HF (functional class NYHA III or IV) or when the surgical risk is prohibitive, interventional therapy should be considered, either

trans-catheter edge-to edge repair (TEER) or trans-catheter MV replacement (MVR). TEER with the anterior and posterior leaflets clip together is an option when the valve anatomy is favorable and patient's life expectancy is at least 1 year [67]. Several studies have demonstrated a reduction in the MR severity and LV remodeling and improvement of symptoms in selected patients only, since the general date showed a better outcome with surgery in comparison with TEER [68]. Therefore, when STS score is >6 and Frailty index is 2–4, echocardiographic parameters are essential to decide between the 2 procedures, TEER or trans-catheter MVR [69].

- An EROA > 0.4 cm^2, MV medium diastolic gradient < 5 mm hg, A2/P2 scallops involvement, normal leaflet motion, no calcification, posterior leaflet length > 10 mm, coaptation > 2 mm, flail gap < 10 mm, flail width < 15 mm, LVEF > 25% and LVEDD > 70 mm are indexes that favor TEER. When there are significant calcification, leaflets restriction, P1/P3 segments involvement or multiple TEER devices, posterior leaflet length < 10 mm, flail gap > 10 mm, flail width > 15 mm, MV cleft or perforation, trans-catheter MVR is preferred [69]. This intervention is a domain of interest of the future and several trials are studying the results since this procedure is much more challenging than this of the aortic valve because the MV is a very complex structure [70, 71].

Management for Secondary MR and Heart Failure

Symptoms of HF in secondary MR are first attributable to the myocardial ischemia or primary myocardial diseases and, in first stages, respond to the myocardial revascularization or optimized GDMT. Pharmacological treatment, cardiac devices, surgery and trans-catheter methods and criteria for their ideal use are evolving [7, 72]. Even more than in primary MR, extended Heart Team has an essential role in management decisions and must include at least an HF specialist, a cardiovascular imaging specialist, a cardiac electrophysiologist, a cardiac surgeon and an interventional cardiologist with expertise in trans-catheter interventions, who supposed to meet regularly and discuss the complexity of the MV anatomy based on the clinical particular setting of the patient [7, 73].

Guideline Directed Medical Treatment (GDMT)

ACC/AHA and ESC HF guideline recommend as class I of indication in patients with severe secondary MR and HF with reduced EF (HFrEF) optimization of GDMT addressed to LV dysfunction before any MV intervention, including changing of ACE inhibitors/ARBs with sacubitril –valsartan, beta blockers, aldosterone antagonists, SGLT2 inhibitors and/or ivabradine, and diuretics with a guideline recommended or tolerated doses (maximum doses) and biventricular pacing or coronary revascularization when indicated [8–10, 74]. Several studies suggested a reduction in secondary MR severity along with the improvement in LV geometry and function with drugs [74, 75].

Diuretics, nitrates or hydralazine may also improve the HF symptoms in patients with severe secondary MR by decreasing the LV preload and afterload. Furthermore, oral anticoagulants are mandatory in patients with AF and significant secondary MR and rhythm or rate control therapy, such as catheter ablation for atrial fibrillation can be used to reduce the severity of atrial secondary MR [32].

Usually, secondary MR is responsive to optimization of GDMT, including cardiac resynchronization therapy—CRT- and coronary revascularization, which should be done by an expert in HF treatment [8, 9]. When HF symptoms are truly refractory to these, the decision of surgical or trans-catheter treatment should be evaluated immediately [8–10].

Cardiac Resynchronization Therapy (CRT)

Intraventricular conduction delay and dyssynchrony, such as bundle branch block, may aggravate the secondary MR through different mechanisms [7, 76]. CRT procedure may decrease LV remodeling, reduce the papillary muscles dyssynchrony, ameliorate LV systolic function in cases with significant QRS prolongation. Therefore, due to decreasing of MV tethering and increasing MV closing forces, the effect could be also to reduce the secondary MR severity at rest and during exercise [7, 77]. CRT may ameliorate the overall survival in patients with secondary MR and in those who fulfill the recommended criteria for CRT, short term reduction of MR severity being associated with favorable prognosis, meanwhile persistent MR predicts worse survival [8, 78]. However, it is very important to pay attention to the selection of candidates at CRT, regarding the fact that the extensive post ischemic myocardial scar may not respond to this therapy.

The ACC guideline for HF recommend CRT for patients with LVEF $\leq$ 35% in sinus rhythm, with left bundle branch block (LBBB) and QRS duration $\geq$ 150 ms on electrocardiogram (ECG), in functional class NYHA II, III or ambulatory IV on optimized GDMT in order to reduce mortality, symptoms of HF and improve the quality of life, with implicit economic benefits as a class I of indication, and as a class IIa—in patients with LVEF $\leq$ 35% in sinus rhythm, in functional class NYHA II, III or ambulatory IV with non-LBBB and QRS duration $\geq$ 150 ms on electrocardiogram (ECG) or with LBBB and QRS duration 120–149 ms. Also, in patients with atrial fibrillation and LVEF $\leq$ 35%, CRT will have the same benefits if the patient requires ventricular pacing or is meeting the CRT criteria or in case of atrioventricular node ablation and 100% ventricular pacing with CRT [10].

Figure 6.7 shows a beneficial effect of the CRT on a MR severity and LVEF, with improvement of symptoms in a patient with LBBB on ECG with tri-coronary arteries disease and HF symptoms of NYHA III despite maximal GDMT.

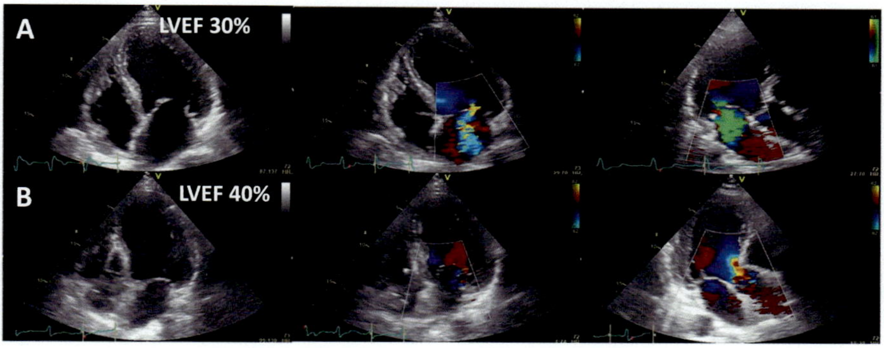

Fig. 6.7 shows a beneficial effect of the CRT on a MR severity and LVEF, with improvement of symptoms in a patient with LBBB on ECG (a QRS duration of 156 ms), with tri-coronary arteries disease and HF symptoms of NYHA III despite maximal GDMT. (**a**) Severe LVEF reduction and severe MR evaluated by 2D echocardiography before CRT; and (**b**) After CRT there is a significant MR reduction, improvement in LVEF and patient's symptoms. *CRT* cardiac resynchronization therapy, *ECG* electrocardiogram, *LBBB* left ventricular bundle branch block, *LVEF* Left ventricular ejection fraction, *GDMT* guided directed medical treatment, *MR* mitral regurgitation

Coronary Revascularization

Conditions such as coronary artery disease (CAD) must be addressed in patients with significant secondary MR, especially in the presence of LV dysfunction, by percutaneous coronary interventions (PCI) or surgical revascularization—coronary artery by-pass grafting (CABG) [3]. There are limited data investigating the effects of CABG alone on the severity secondary MR in selected cases, although the beneficial results of surgical revascularization were demonstrated in patients with HF [7, 79]. Several studies demonstrated that secondary MR is improved in almost 50% of patients after isolated CABG, however data on the beneficial effects of PCI on severity of secondary MR are scares, being observed in one third of patients in one small study and associated with improved survival, and could be in relation to the extension of myocardial perfusion defects [7, 80].

Mitral Valve Surgery for Significant Secondary MR

The role of surgical MV repair or replacement to interrupt the progressive cycle of LV volume overload, LV dilation, and moreover increasing LV volume and progressive secondary MR is less well established, although some patients may symptomatically benefit. Moreover, choosing between the two types of MV surgery—*repair or replacement*—is still debatable. Finally, in patients with severe HF and secondary MR refractory to standard therapies, consideration should be given to mechanical LV assist devices and heart transplantation [10].

Current guidelines recommend *MV surgery as a class IIa of indication* in patients with severe secondary MR when CABG or other valve surgery is undertaken for the treatment of myocardial ischemia [8–10], and as *a class IIb of indication* in patients with severe secondary atrial MR due to atrial annular dilation with preserved LV systolic function (LVEF > 50%) who have persistent symptoms (NYHA class III or IV) despite therapy for HF and therapy for associated AF or other comorbidities, in patients with LVEF < 50% with persistent severe symptoms (NYHA III or IV) despite optimized GDMT [8–10]. Also, ESC and ACC guidelines recommend that in patients with CAD and severe secondary MR related to systolic dysfunction (LVEF < 50%), who are undergoing to MV surgery, ***chordal sparing mitral valve replacement*** may be reasonable against downsized annuloplasty repair [8–10]. However, these recommendations were made before the data supporting the benefits of trans-catheter valve repair were available, and the evidence for supporting surgical intervention for secondary MR remains poor and the type of intervention must be tailored for individual patients [7].

In 2016, the CTSN trial data showed that, for severe ischemic mitral regurgitation, there were no significant difference between MV replacement with total chordae preservation and MV repair in left ventricular reverse remodeling or survival at 2 years, however, recurrent MR appeared more frequently in the repair group, resulting in more heart-failure–related adverse events and cardiovascular admissions [81]. In 2019, a study demonstrated that in selected patients with severe secondary MR and no significant LV remodeling, MV repair with undersized complete rigid ring, reduces the severity of MR and LV dilatation and improves the symptoms of HF [8, 82]. This may be indicated (class IIb) in patients who do not have important basal aneurysm or dyskinesia or significant valve tethering or LV dilatation (LVEDD < 65 mm). Additional valvular or subvavlular techniques repair or MV replacement should be recommended in patients with echocardiographic predictors of repair failure: leaflet coaptation height > 10 mm; leaflet coaptation area > 2.5–3 cm^2; interpapillary muscle distance > 20 mm; global LV remodeling LVEDD > 65 mm, LVESD > 51 mm, ESV > 140 mL; systolic sphericity index > 0.7 [14, 83]. However, it is important to remind that recommendations for isolated MV surgery in secondary MR are very limited due to a high surgical risk, high rates of recurrence and the lack of beneficial effects evidence [84].

On the other hand, in patients with secondary atrial MR, in the first stages when LV is not so dilated and LVEF is usually normal, mitral ring annuloplasty and surgical ablation for AF may be an option [85]. Rhythm restoration, trans catheter intervention and surgical procedures may address significant atrial secondary MR, but only surgery can treat at least four mechanisms of disease: LA dilatation with atrial plication, mitral annulus dilatation and pseudo-prolapse of the anterior leaflet with annuloplasty with or without neo-chords, insufficient leaflet remodeling and atriogenic leaflet tethering with patch augmentation, and rhythm control with Cox-Maze procedure [86].

In summary, it is reasonable for patients with severe secondary MR with indication for surgery and with high predicted risk for MR recurrence after potential MV repair, to have a MV replacement. If a patient has a symptomatic secondary MR, but no predictive factors for MR recurrence, then MV repair may be considered. Both recommendations advocate for optimization of medical and cardiac device therapy prior to surgery [8–10]. Patients with advanced HF and severe SMR may better benefit by cardiac transplantation or LV assist device implantation (either as destination therapy or a bridge to transplantation) [7].

Trans-Catheter Edge-to Edge Repair

MitraClip for the management of significant secondary MR has become the first line option for trans-catheter intervention in Europe, having the largest clinical experience and safety [7]. Two randomized clinical trials (RCTs)—COAPT and MITA-FR have assessed the results and safety in patients with symptoms of HF and significant MR despite optimizing GDMT, who were ineligible for surgery by the expanded Heart Team [8–10, 87–90].

In the MITRA—FR trial, a French Multicenter Percutaneous Repair Trial, 304 patients with severe MR defined as EROA > 20 mm^2 or regurgitant volume > 30 mL, LEVEF between 15% and 40%, no limit of end-systolic dimeter of LV, NYHA class II–II and history of at least one HF hospitalization within 1 year and, unsuitable for surgery were randomized to undergo MitraClip implantation and optimized GDMT or GDMT alone [88, 89]. The results showed no difference between groups regarding the all-cause mortality or HF hospitalization at 12 months (HR 1.16, 95% CI 0.73–1.84). Furthermore, the study showed no beneficial effects on functional status, 6-min walking distance, quality of life, or LV end-diastolic volumes [87, 88]. At 24 month follow up no changes were reported in these findings, with no impact of MitraClip implantation on all-cause mortality or HF hospitalization [91].

On contrary, in the COAPT study, with recently 5 years follow-up results published, 614 patients with moderate-to severe or severe MR who remained asymptomatic despite the medical treatment were assigned either to receive MitraClip along with optimized GDMT or to receive GDMT only [90]. The rate of HF hospitalization, all-cause mortality, the risk of death for HF, and safety were analyzed for 5 years. Hospitalization for HF (HR 0.53; 95% CI 0.41–0.68), all-cause mortality (HR 0.72; 95% CI, 0.58–0.89), death or hospitalization for HF within 5 years (HR 0.53; 95% CI, 0.44–0.64) were lower in the device group than in the GDMT group. They reported at 5 years of follow-up an incidence of 1.4% device safety events, respectively 4 of 293 treated patients, with all the events occurring within 30 days after the procedure [90]. These results sustained those published in 2018 [89]. Moreover, improvements were also observed in LV remodeling, renal outcomes, hospitalizations (primarily related to HF, both fatal and nonfatal), and patient symptoms, with significant improvements in quality of life (QoL) starting at 1 month and sustained out to 5 years. Benefits were seen among elderly patients, although benefit in HF hospitalization was greater among younger patients. In the overall population, changes in LV dimensions at 6 months on echocardiogram were seen in both arms. However, favorable remodeling appeared to have a positive impact on outcomes between 6 months and 2 years in both arms, but only the association between CV death and change in LVED volume index was statistically significant. The beneficial impact of TEER + GDMT over GDMT alone at 2 years did not appear to be driven by more favorable remodeling with TEER. At 4 years, stroke/TIA rates were similar between MitraClip + GDMT vs. GDMT alone [92].

Several papers tried to explain these conflicting results of the two trials: the different design and size of study populations, use of concomitant therapy, comorbidities, several technical factors and selection of patients, from which most important was echocardiographic assessment of secondary MR severity and LV remodeling [8, 93]. As we already noticed, Graybourn et al. proposed a concept of disproportionate secondary MR reflecting greater severity in relation to LV dimensions, majority patients from COAPT study having these echocardiographic findings EROA > 0.3 cm^2, LVEDD < 70 mm, EDVix < 96 ml/m^2 and were more likely to respond to TEER [58]. Moreover, the more frequent use of multiple clips in COAPT population as a technical difference between the two studies may be other reason for the better long-term reduction of SMR and better outcome in these patients, highlighting the importance of best possible results achieving immediately after MitraClip implantation [7]. Figure 6.8 shows a MitraClip percutaneous implantation in a patient with severe secondary MR and depressed systolic function and prohibitive surgical risk, with optimal result.

Robinson et al. proposed an echocardiographic algorithm to orient the optimal management in such heterogeneous population with significant secondary MR, shown in Fig. 6.9 [14]. An EROA/LVEDV ratio of 0.14 mm^2/ml is an index proposed for differentiate between those patients in whom medical therapy should be optimized and those in whom percutaneous intervention could have significant benefit, although not implemented in routine clinical practice [14]. Moreover, they propose to consider futility in patients with heart failure and severe MR in very severe LV and LA remodeling and dysfunction (LVEF < 15%), severe RV dysfunction and pulmonary hypertension (PH) or lung disease and severe elevated NT–proBNP (>5000–10,000) [14].

Therefore, current guideline recommend that TEER should be consider in patients with severe secondary MR who fulfill the COAPT inclusion criteria along with optimized GDMT by a specialist in HF after a careful discussion in expanded Heart Team [8]. Adammo et al. demonstrated that in real life MitraClip is beneficial for the right selected patients, defining a COAPT-like profile, including specific echocardiographic and clinical criteria [94]. Therefore, all of the next 3 criteria should be fulfilled to define a COAPT criteria: (1) absence of LV severe impairment (LVEF ≥ 20% and LVEDD ≤ 70 mm), (2) absence of LV severe impairment and/or severe PH (TAPSE ≥ 15 mm and systolic velocity on tissue Doppler imaging ≥ 8 cm/s; less than severe tricuspid regurgitation; systolic arterial pulmonary pressure ≤ 70 mm hg), and (3) absence of hemodynamic instability (no advanced heart failure refractory to medication; no need for intravenous drug or circulatory mechanical support) [94].

However, more research is needed to identify the responders to TEER and to refine the algorithms for selection of the right patients and the right device at the right time.

In conclusion, mitral regurgitation is a very heterogenous disease. Primary mitral regurgitation is a disease of a mitral valve apparatus and, in time, could lead

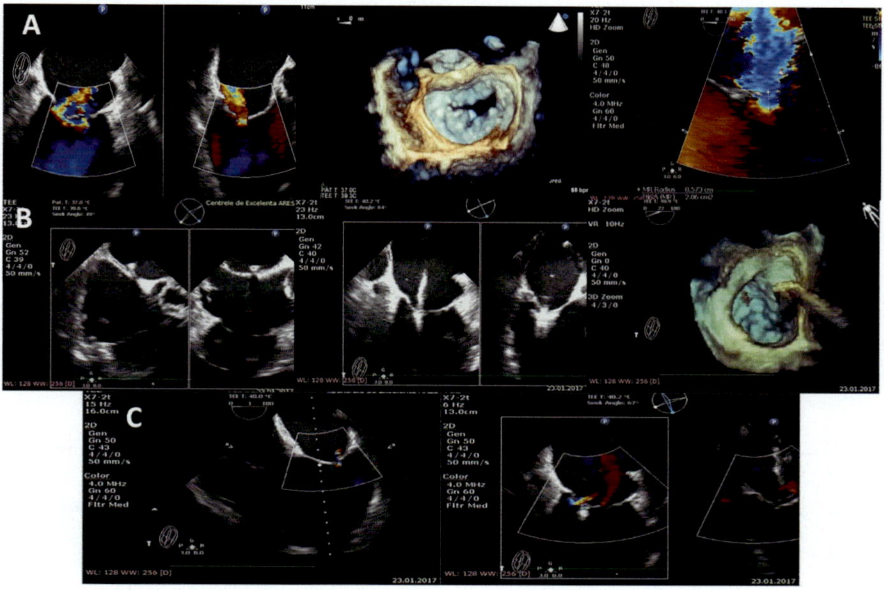

Fig. 6.8 MitraClip percutaneous implantation in a patient with severe secondary MR and depressed systolic function and prohibitive surgical risk. The patient had a history of CABG and CRT-D implant, in present with 75% stenosis of left main artery, oclusion of LAD, 90% stenosis of marginal 1 and oclusion RCA, with prohibitive surgical risk. (With courtesy of Dr. Silvia Deaconu). (**a**) 2D and 3 D TEE shows dilated left ventricle with severe systolic dysfunction EF 20% (LVTDV 180 ml); moderate to Severe functional mitral regurgitation (EORA 0,18 cm p, RegVol 35 ml) with dilated mitral ring 42 mm; severe functional tricuspid regurgitation; tricuspid ring 44 m and severe PHT (sPAP = 65mm hg with RV systolic dysfunction). (**b**) Implantation of MitraClip by transeptal puncture guided by 2D and 3D TEE; (**c**) optimal result of device: mild residual MR and no significant MV stenosis, improved NYHA status. The patient had also a percutaneous coronary revascularization. *CABG* coronary artery by-pass grafting, *CRT-D* cardiac resynchronization therapy—with defibrillator, *EF* ejection fraction, *EORA* effective orifice regurgitant area, *LAD* left descending artery, *LV* left ventricle, *NYHA* New York Heart Association, *MR* mitral regurgitation, *MV* mitral valve, *RCA* right coronary artery, *RegVol* regurgitant volume, *RV* right ventricle, *TEE* transesophageal echocardiography

to cardiac remodeling and dysfunction and to overt heart failure. Secondary mitral regurgitation, with ischemic or non-ischemic cause, is a disease of left ventricle or left atrium and heart failure is associated from the beginning. Understanding the mechanism and causes of primary and secondary forms, as well as defining the hemodynamic consequences are very important and needed a multi-imagistic technique approach. For treatment and optimal timing of interventions, discussions between members of expanded Heart Team are mandatory. In the era of new heart failure medication, new surgical procedures, such as repair, trans-apical approach, new chordae implantation and new trans-catheter techniques, such as mitral clip or mitral valve replacement, it is essential to choose the correct management—mitral valve surgery, with repair whenever is possible as a first line of treatment in primary mitral regurgitation and optimized medical treatment and cardiac resynchronization

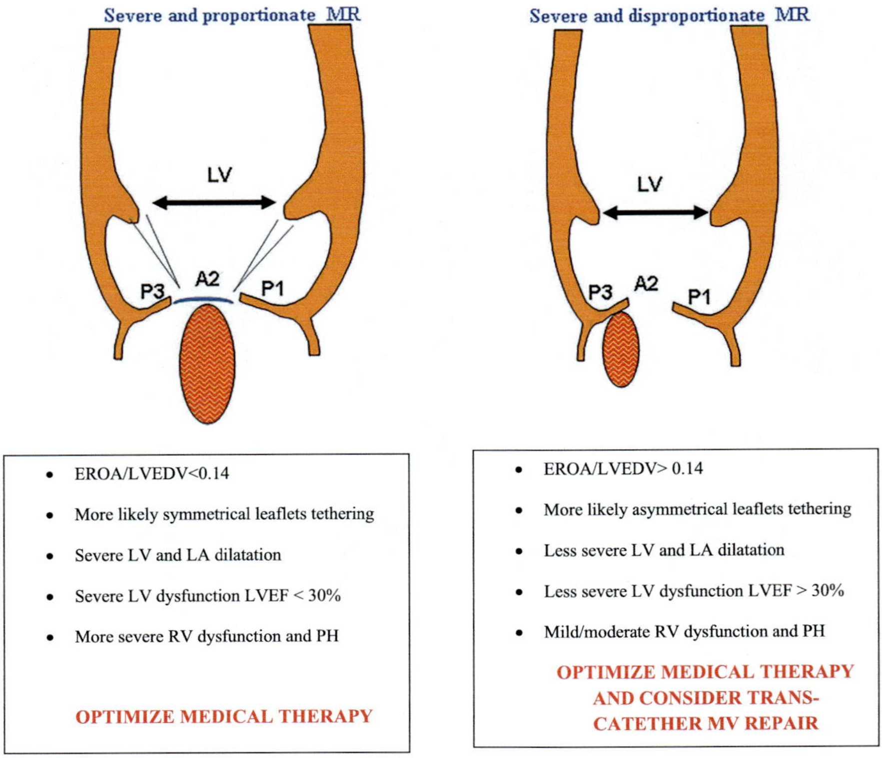

Fig. 6.9 Proportionality of secondary mitral regurgitation may dictate the optimal management. (Adapted from [14], no permission requested). *EROA* effective regurgitant orifice area, *LA* left atrium, *LV* left ventricle, *LVEF* left ventricular ejection fraction, *LVEDV* left ventricular end-diastolic volume, *PH* pulmonary hypertension, *RV* right ventricle

therapy in secondary mitral regurgitation. In selected patients necessitating coronary artery bass-grafting or other valvular intervention, mitral valve surgery should be indicated, with valve replacement in most of the cases and repair whenever risk of recurrence is low. In patients with severe secondary mitral regurgitation and heart failure with high surgical risk fulfilling the COAPT-criteria, trans-catheter intervention with mitral clip implantation should be recommended. Finally, in patients with severe secondary mitral regurgitation, end –stage cardiomyopathy and advanced heart failure, left ventricular assist device and heart transplant may by an option.

References

1. Grave C, Tribouilloy C, Tuppin P, Weill A, Gabet A, Juillere Y, et al. Fourteen-year temporal trends in patients hospitalized for mitral regurgitation: the increasing burden of mitral valve prolapse in men. J Clin Med. 2022;11:3289.

2. ReIung B, Delgado V, Rosenhek R, Price S, Prendergast B, Wendler O, The EORP VHD II Investigators. Contemporary presentation and management of valvular heart disease the EURObservational research program valvular heart disease II survey. Circulation. 2019;140:1156–69.
3. Shah M, Jorde UP. Percutaneous mitral valve interventions (repair): current indications and future perspectives. Front Cardiovasc Med. 2019;6:88.
4. Cioffi G, Tarantini L, De Feo S, Pulignano G, Del Sindaco D, Stefenelli C, et al. Functional mitral regurgitation predicts 1-year mortality in elderly patients with systolic chronic heart failure. Eur J Heart Fail. 2005;7:1112–7.
5. Benjamin EJ, Blaha MJ, Chiuve ES, Cushman M, Das RS, Deo R, et al. American Heart Association Statistics Committee and Stroke Statistics Subcommittee. Heart disease and stroke statistics-2017 update: a report from the American Heart Association. Circulation. 2017;135:e146–603.
6. Pecini R, Thune JJ, Torp-Pedersen C, Hassager C, Købber L. The relationship between mitral regurgitation and ejection fraction as predictors for the prognosis of patients with heart failure. Eur J Heart Fail. 2011;13:1121–5.
7. Coats AJS, Anker SD, Baumbach A, Alfieri O, von Bardeleben RS, Bauersachs J, et al. The management of secondary mitral regurgitation in patients with heart failure: a joint position statement from the Heart Failure Association (HFA), European Association of Cardiovascular Imaging (EACVI), European Heart Rhythm Association (EHRA), and European Association of Percutaneous Cardiovascular Interventions (EAPCI) of the ESC. Eur Heart J. 2021;42:1254–69.
8. Vahanian A, Beyersdorf F, Praz F, Milojevic M, Baldus S, Bauersachs J, et al. ESC/EACTS Scientific Document Group. 2021 ESC/EACTS Guidelines for the management of valvular heart disease. Developed by the Task Force for the management of valvular heart disease of the European Society of Cardiology (ESC) and the European Association for Cardio-Thoracic Surgery (EACTS). Eur Heart J. 2021;43:561–632.
9. Otto CM, Nishimura RA, Bonow RO, Carabello BA, Erwin JP III, Gentile F, et al. 2020 ACC/AHA Guideline for the management of patients with valvular heart disease. A report of the American College of Cardiology/American Heart Association Joint Committee on Clinical Practice Guidelines Developed in collaboration with and endorsed by the American Association for Thoracic Surgery, American Society of Echocardiography, Society for Cardiovascular Angiography and Interventions, Society of Cardiovascular Anesthesiologists, and Society of Thoracic Surgeons. J Am Coll Cardiol. 2021;77:e25–197.
10. Heidenreich PA, Bozkurt B, Aguilar D, Allen LA, Byun JJ, Colvin MM, et al. 2022 AHA/ACC/HFSA Guideline for the management of Heart Failure: a report of the American College of Cardiology/American Heart Association Joint Committee on Clinical Practice Guidelines. Circulation. 2022;145:e895–1032.
11. Topilsky Y. Mitral regurgitation: anatomy, physiology, and pathophysiology—lessons learned from surgery and cardiac imaging. Front Cardiovasc Med. 2020;7:84.
12. Vaca FS, Bordoni B. Anatomy, thorax, mitral valve. In Stat Pearls (internet) 2022. https://www.ncbi.nlm.nih.gov/books/NBK549884/. Accessed on 19 Aug 2023.
13. Dal-Bianco JP, Aikawa E, Bischoff J, Guerrero JL, Handschumacher MD, Sullivan S, et al. Active adaptation of the tethered mitral valve: insights into a compensatory mechanism for functional mitral regurgitation. Circulation. 2009;120:334–42.
14. Robinson S, Ring L, Augustine DX, Rekhraj S, Oxborough D, Harkness A, et al. The assessment of mitral valve disease: a guideline from the British Society of Echocardiography. Echo Res Pract. 2021;8:87–136.
15. Grewel J, Suri R, Mankad S, Tanaka A, Mahoney WD, Schaff VH, et al. Mitral annular dynamics in myxomatous valve disease. New insights with real-time 3-dimensional echocardiography. Circulation. 2010;121:1423–31.
16. Degandt AA, Weber PA, Saber HA, Duran CM. Mitral valve basal chordae: comparative anatomy and terminology. Ann Thorac Surg. 2007;84:1250–5.
17. O'Gara PT, Mack MJ. Secondary mitral regurgitation. N Engl J Med. 2020;383:1458–67.

18. Praz F, Grasso C, Taramasso M, Baumbach A, Piazza N, Tamburino C, et al. Mitral regurgitation in heart failure: time of rethink. Eur Heart J. 2019;40:2189–93.
19. Zoghbi WA, Adams D, Bonow RO, Enriquez-Sarano M, Foster E, Grayburn PA, et al. Recommendations for noninvasive evaluation of native valvular regurgitation. A report from the American Society of Echocardiography Developed in collaboration with the Society for Cardiovascular Magnetic Resonance. J Am Coll Cardiol. 2017;30:303–71.
20. Carpentier AF, Lessana A, Relland JY, Bell E, Mihaileanu S, Berrebi AJ, et al. The 'physio-ring': an advanced concept in mitral annuloplasty. Ann Thorac Surg. 1995;60:1177–86.
21. Zhou X, Otsuji Y, Yoshifuku S, Yuasa T, Zhang H, Takasaki K, et al. Impact of atrial fibrillation on tricuspid and mitral annular dilatation and valvular regurgitation. Circ J. 2002;66:913–6.
22. Gertz ZM, Raina A, Saghy L, Zado ES, Callans DJ, Marchlinski FE, et al. Evidence of atrial functional mitral regurgitation due to atrial fibrillation: reversal with arrhythmia control. J Am Coll Cardiol. 2011;58:1474–81.
23. Straw S, Gupta A, Johnosn K, Cole CA, Kneizeh K, Gierula J, et al. Atrial secondary mitral regurgitation: prevalence, characteristics, management, and long-term outcomes. Echo Res Pract. 2023;10:4–14.
24. Clavel MA, Mantovani F, Malouf J, Michelena HI, Vatury O, Jain MS, et al. Dynamic phenotypes of degenerative myxomatous mitral valve disease: quantitative 3-dimensional echocardiographic study. Circ Cardiovasc Imaging. 2015;l8:e002989.
25. Enriquez-Sarano M, Loulmet DF, Burkhoff D. The conundrum of functional mitral regurgitation in chronic heart failure. J Am Coll Cardiol. 2008;51:487–9.
26. Ross J Jr, Sonnenblick EH, Taylor RR, Spotnitz HM, Covell JW. Diastolic geometry and sarcomere lengths in the chronically dilated canine left ventricle. Circ Res. 1971;28:49–61.
27. Gaasch WH, Meyer TE. Left ventricular response to mitral regurgitation: implications for management. Circulation. 2008;118:2298–303.
28. Levine RA, Schwammenthal E. Ischemic mitral regurgitation on the threshold of a solution. From paradoxes to unifying concepts. Circulation. 2005;112:745–58.
29. Ciobanu AO, Vinereanu D. Chronic ischemic mitral regurgitation. In: Gherasim L, Oproiu AI, editors. Actualities in internal medicine. Editura Medicala; 2017.
30. Bertrand PB, Schwammenthal E, Levine RA, Vandervoort PM. Exercise dynamics in secondary mitral regurgitation: pathophysiology and therapeutic implications. Circulation. 2017;135:297–314.
31. Goliasch G, Bartko PE, Pavo N, Neuhold S, Wurm R, Mascherbauer J, et al. Refining the prognostic impact of functional mitral regurgitation in chronic heart failure. Eur Heart J. 2018;39:39–46.
32. Deferm S, Bertrand PB, Verbrugge FH, Verhaert D, Rega F, Thomas JD, et al. Atrial functional mitral regurgitation: JACC review topic of the week. J Am Coll Cardiol. 2019;73:2465–76.
33. Altes A, Vermes E, Levy F, Vancraeynest D, Pasquet A, Vincentelli A, et al. Quantification of primary mitral regurgitation by echocardiography: a practical approach. Front Cardiovasc Med. 2023;10:1–26.
34. Grigioni F, Tribouilloy C, Avierinos JF, Barbieri A, Ferlito M, Trojette F, et al. Outcomes in mitral regurgitation due to flail leaflets a multicenter European study. JACC Cardiovasc Imaging. 2008;1:133–41.
35. Sabbag A, Essayagh B, Barrera JDR, Basso C, Berni A, Cosyns B, et al. EHRA expert consensus statement on arrhythmic mitral valve prolapse and mitral annular disjunction complex in collaboration with the ESC Council on valvular heart disease and the European Association of Cardiovascular Imaging endorsed by the Heart Rhythm Society, by the Asia Pacific Heart Rhythm Society, and by the Latin American Heart Rhythm Society. Europace. 2022;24:1981–2003.
36. Mantovani F, Clavel MA, Vatury O, Suri RM, Mankad SV, Malouf J, et al. Cleft like indentations in myxomatous mitral valves by three-dimensional echocardiographic imaging. Heart. 2015;101:1111–7.

37. Landi A, Faletra FF, Pavon AG, Pedrazzini G, Valgimigli M. From secondary to tertiary mitral regurgitation: the paradigm shifts, but uncertainties remain. Eur Heart J Cardiovasc Imaging. 2021;22:835–43.
38. Kim KJ, Kim HK, Park JB, Hwang HY, Yoon YE, Kim YJ, et al. Transthoracic echocardiographic findings of mitral regurgitation caused by commissural prolapse. JACC Cardiovasc Imaging. 2018;11:925–6.
39. Kebed K, Kruse E, Addetia K, Ciszek B, Thykattil M, Guile B, et al. Atrial focused views improve the accuracy of two-dimensional echocardiographic measurements of the left and right atrial volumes: a contribution to the increase in normal values in the guidelines update. Int J Card Imaging. 2017;33:209–18.
40. Gaasch WH, Meyer TE. Left ventricular response to mitral regurgitation. Circulation. 2008;118:2298–303.
41. Galli E, Lancellotti P, Sengupta PP, Donal E. LV mechanics in mitral and aortic valve diseases: value of functional assessment beyond ejection fraction. JACC Cardiovasc Imaging. 2014;7:1151–66.
42. Bernard J, Altes A, Dupuis M, Toubal O, Mahjoub H, Tastet L, et al. Cardiac damage staging classification in asymptomatic moderate or severe primary mitral regurgitation. Struct Heart. 2022;6:100004.
43. van Wijngaarden AL, Mantegazza V, Hiemstra YL, Volpato V, van der Bijl P, Pepi M, et al. Prognostic impact of extra-mitral valve cardiac involvement in patients with primary mitral regurgitation. JACC Cardiovasc Imaging. 2022;15:961–70.
44. Florescu M, Benea DCCM, Rimbas RC, Cerin G, Diena M, Lanzzillo G, Enescu OA, et al. Myocardial systolic velocities and deformation assessed by speckle tracking for early detection of left ventricular dysfunction in asymptomatic patients with severe primary mitral regurgitation. Echocardiography. 2012;29:326–33.
45. Butcher SC, Essayagh B, Steyerberg EW, Benfari G, Antoine C, Grigioni F, et al. Factors influencing post-surgical survival in degenerative mitral regurgitation. Eur Heart J. 2023;44:871–81.
46. Petersen SE, Aung N, Sanghvi MM, Zemrak F, Fung K, Paiva JM, et al. Reference ranges for cardiac structure and function using cardiovascular magnetic resonance (CMR) in Caucasians from the UK biobank population cohort. J Cardiovasc Magn Reson. 2017;19:18.
47. Hagendorff A, Knebel F, Helfen A, Stöbe S, Haghi D, Ruf T, et al. Echocardiographic assessment of mitral regurgitation: discussion of practical and methodologic aspects of severity quantification to improve diagnostic conclusiveness. Clin Res Cardiol. 2021;110:1704–33.
48. Utsunomiya T, Ogawa T, Tang HA, Doshi R, Patel D, Quan M, et al. Doppler color flow mapping of the proximal isovelocity surface area: a new method for measuring volume flow rate across a narrowed orifice. J Am Soc Echocardiogr. 1991;4:338–48.
49. Mao W, Caballero A, Hahn RT, Sun W. Comparative quantification of primary mitral regurgitation by computer modeling and simulated echocardiography. Am J Physiol Heart Circ Physiol. 2020;318:547–57.
50. Moraldo M, Cecaro F, Shun-Shin M, Pabari PA, Davies JE, Xu XY, et al. Evidence-based recommendations for Pisa measurements in mitral regurgitation: systematic review, clinical and in-vitro study. Int J Cardiol. 2013;168:1220–8.
51. Goebel B, Heck R, Hamadanchi A, Otto S, Doenst T, Jung C, et al. Vena contracta area for severity grading in functional and degenerative mitral regurgitation: a transoesophageal 3d colour Doppler analysis in 500 patients. Eur Heart J Cardiovasc Imaging. 2018;19:639–46.
52. Coisne A, Aghezzaf S, Galli E, Mouton S, Richardson M, Dubois D, et al. Prognostic values of exercise echocardiography and cardiopulmonary exercise testing in patients with primary mitral regurgitation. Eur Heart J Cardiovasc Imaging. 2022;23:1552–61.
53. Garg P, Swift AJ, Zhong L, Carlhall CJ, Ebbers T, Westenberg J, et al. Assessment of mitral valve regurgitation by cardiovascular magnetic resonance imaging. Nat Rev Cardiol. 2020;17:298–312.

54. Vermes E, Altes A, Iacuzio L, Levy F, Bohbot Y, Renard C, et al. The evolving role of cardiovascular magnetic resonance in the assessment of mitral valve prolapse. Front Cardiovasc Med. 2023;10:109306.
55. Saiki Y, Kasegawa H, Kawase M, Osada H, Ootaki E. Intraoperative TEE during mitral valve repair: does it predict early and late postoperative mitral valve dysfunction? Ann Thorac Surg. 1998;66:1277–81.
56. Kwan J, Shiota T, Agler DA, Popovic ZB, Qin JX, Gillinov MA, et al. Geometric differences of the mitral apparatus between ischemic and dilated cardiomyopathy in with significant mitral regurgitation: real-time three dimensional echocardiography study. Circulation. 2003;107:1135–40.
57. Golba K, Mokrzycki K, Drozdz J, Cherniavsky A, Wrobel K, Roberts BJ, et al. Mechanisms of functional mitral regurgitation in ischemic cardiomyopathy determined by transesophageal echocardiography (from the Surgical Treatment for Ischemic Heart Failure Trial). Am J Cardiol. 2013;112:1812–8.
58. Grayburn PA, Sannino A, Packer M. Proportionate and disproportionate functional mitral regurgitation: a new conceptual framework that reconciles the results of the MITRA-FR and COAPT Trials. JACC Cardiovasc Imaging. 2019;12:353–62.
59. Detaint D, Messika-Zeitoun D, Avierinos J-F, Scott C, Chen H, Burnett JC Jr, et al. B-type natriuretic peptide in organic mitral regurgitation: determinants and impact on outcome. Circulation. 2005;111:2391–7.
60. Kim HM, Cho G-Y, Hwang I-C, Choi HM, Park JB, Yoon YE, et al. Myocardial strain in prediction of outcomes after surgery for severe mitral regurgitation. J Am Coll Cardiol Img. 2018;11:1235–44.
61. Antoine C, Benfari G, Michelena HI, Maalouf JF, Nkomo VT, Thapa P, et al. Clinical outcome of degenerative mitral regurgitation: critical importance of echocardiographic quantitative assessment in routine practice. Circulation. 2018;138:1317–26.
62. Gillinov AM, Mihaljevic T, Blackstone EH, George K, Svensson LG, Nowicki ER, et al. Should patients with severe degenerative mitral regurgitation delay surgery until symptoms develop? Ann Thorac Surg. 2010;90:481–8.
63. Lazam S, Vanoverschelde J-L, Tribouilloy C, Grigioni F, Suri RM, Avierinos JF, et al. Twenty-year outcome after mitral repair versus replacement for severe degenerative mitral regurgitation: analysis of a large, prospective, multicenter, international registry. Circulation. 2017;135:410–22.
64. David TE, David CM, Tsang W, Lafreniere-Roula M, Manlhiot CL. Long-term results of mitral valve repair for regurgitation due to leaflet prolapse. J Am Coll Cardiol. 2019;74:1044–53.
65. El-Eshmawi A, Castillo JG, Tang GHL, Adams DH. Developing a mitral valve center of excellence. Curr Opin Cardiol. 2018;33:155–66.
66. Dillon J, Yakub MA, Kong PK, Ramli MF, Jaffar N, Gaffar IF. Comparative long-term results of mitral valve repair in adults with chronic rheumatic disease and degenerative disease: is repair for "burnt-out" rheumatic disease still inferior to repair for degenerative disease in the current era? J Thorac Cardiovasc Surg. 2015;149:771–7.
67. Feldman T, Kar S, Elmariah S, Smart SC, Trento A, Siegel RJ, et al. Randomized comparison of percutaneous repair and surgery for mitral regurgitation: 5-year results of EVEREST II. J Am Coll Cardiol. 2015;66:2844–54.
68. Sorajja P, Vemulapalli S, Feldman T, Mack M, Holmes DR Jr, Stebbins A, et al. Outcomes with transcatheter mitral valve repair in the United States: an STS/ACC TVT registry report. J Am Coll Cardiol. 2017;70:2315–27.
69. Thourani VH. Current management strategies for mitral and tricuspid valve disease. https://www.youtube.com/watch?v=GLckm2s6gXU. Accessed on YouTube on 21 June 2023.
70. Hensey M, Brown RA, Lal S, Sathananthan J, Ye J, Cheung A, et al. Transcatheter mitral valve replacement: an update on current techniques, technologies, and future directions. J Am Coll Cardiol Intv. 2021;14:489–500.

71. Yousef S, Arnaoutakis GJ, Gada H, Conrad Smith AJ, Sanon S, Sultan I. Transcatheter mitral valve therapies: state of the art. J Card Surg. 2022;37:225–33.
72. Seferovic PM, Ponikowski P, Anker SD, Bauersachs J, Chioncel O, Cleland JGF, et al. Clinical practice update on heart failure 2019: pharmacotherapy, procedures, devices and patient management. An expert consensus meeting report of the Heart Failure Association of the European Society of Cardiology. Eur J Heart Fail. 2019;21:1169–86.
73. Crespo-Leiro MG, Metra M, Lund LH, Milicic D, Costanzo MR, Filippatos G, et al. Advanced heart failure: a position statement of the Heart Failure Association of the European Society of Cardiology. Eur J Heart Fail. 2018;20:1505–35.
74. Kang D-H, Park S-J, Shin S-H, Hong G-R, Lee S, Kim M-S, et al. Angiotensin receptor neprilysin inhibitor for functional mitral regurgitation. Circulation. 2019;139:1354–65.
75. Waagstein F, Stromblad O, Andersson B, Bohm M, Darius M, Delius W, et al. Increased exercise ejection fraction and reversed remodelling after long-term treatment with metoprolol in congestive heart failure: a randomized, stratified, double-blind, placebo controlled trial in mild to moderate heart failure due to ischemic or idiopathic dilated cardiomyopathy. Eur J Heart Fail. 2003;5:679–91.
76. Erlebacher JA, Barbarash S. Intraventricular conduction delay and functional mitral regurgitation. Am J Cardiol. 2001;88:83–6.
77. Mihos CG, Santana O, Yucel E, Capoulade R, Upadhyay GA, Orencole MP, et al. The effects of cardiac resynchronization therapy on left ventricular and mitral valve geometry and secondary mitral regurgitation in patients with left bundle branch block. Echocardiography. 2019;36:1450–8.
78. van Bommel RJ, Marsan NA, Delgado V, Borleffs CJ, van Rijnsoever EP, Schalij, et al. Cardiac resynchronization therapy as a therapeutic option in patients with moderate-severe functional mitral regurgitation and high operative risk. Circulation. 2011;124:912–9.
79. Castleberry AW, Williams JB, Daneshmand MA, Honeycutt E, Shaw LK, Samad Z, et al. Surgical revascularization is associated with maximal survival in patients with ischemic mitral regurgitation: a 20-year experience. Circulation. 2014;129:2547–56.
80. Campwala SZ, Bansal RC, Wang N, Razzouk A, Pai RG. Factors affecting regression of mitral regurgitation following isolated coronary artery bypass surgery. Eur J Cardiothorac Surg. 2005;28:783–7.
81. Goldstein D, Moskowitz AJ, Gelijns AC, Ailawadi G, Parides MK, Perrault LP, For the CTSN, et al. Two-year outcomes of surgical treatment of severe ischemic mitral regurgitation. N Engl J Med. 2016;374:344–53.
82. Petrus AHJ, Dekkers OM, Tops LF, Timmer E, Klautz RJM, Braun J. Impact of recurrent mitral regurgitation after mitral valve repair for functional mitral regurgitation: long-term analysis of competing outcomes. Eur Heart J. 2019;40:2206–14.
83. Harmel EK, Reichenspurner H, Girdauskas E. Subannular reconstruction in secondary mitral regurgitation: a meta-analysis. Heart. 2018;104:1783–90.
84. Acker MA, Parides MK, Perrault LP, Moskowitz AJ, Gelijns AC, Voisine P, CTSN, et al. Mitral-valve repair versus replacement for severe ischemic mitral regurgitation. N Engl J Med. 2014;370:23–32.
85. Aranda-Domene R, Canovas SJ. Going further of mitral ring annuloplasty: the role of surgery in atrial functional mitral regurgitation. J Thorac Dis. 2023;15:2381–4.
86. Farhan S, Silbiger JJ, Halperin JL, Zhang L, Dukkipati SR, Vogel B, et al. Pathophysiology, echocardiographic diagnosis, and treatment of atrial functional mitral regurgitation: JACC state-of-the-art review. J Am Coll Cardiol. 2022;80:2314–30.
87. Messika-Zeitoun D, Iung B, Armoiry X, Trochu JN, Donal E, Habib G, et al. Impact of mitral regurgitation severity and left ventricular remodeling on outcome after MitraClip implantation: results from the Mitra-FR Trial. JACC Cardiovasc Imaging. 2021;14:742–52.
88. Obadia JF, Messika-Zeitoun D, Leurent G, Iung B, Bonnet G, Piriou N, MITRA-FR Investigators, et al. Percutaneous repair or medical treatment for secondary mitral regurgitation. N Engl J Med. 2018;379:2297–306.

89. Stone GW, Lindenfeld J, Abraham WT, Kar S, Lim DS, Mishell JM, For the COAPT Investigators, et al. Transcatheter mitral-valve repair in patients with heart failure. N Engl J Med. 2018;379:2307–18.
90. Stone GW, Abraham WT, Lindenfeld J, Kar S, Grayburn PA, Lim DS, For the COAPT Investigators, et al. Five-year follow-up after transcatheter repair of secondary mitral regurgitation. N Engl J Med. 2023;388:20.
91. Iung B, Armoiry X, Vahanian A, Boutitie F, Mewton N, Trochu J-N, MITRA-FR Investigators. Percutaneous repair or medical treatment for secondary mitral regurgitation: outcomes at 2 years. Eur J Heart Fail. 2019;21:1619–1627.37-2048.
92. Kumbhani DJ. Cardiovascular outcomes assessment of the MitraClip percutaneous therapy for heart failure patients with functional mitral regurgitation—COAPT. ACC, 2023. acc.org/Latest-in-Cardiology/Clinical-Trials/2018/09/21/20/12/COAPT. Accessed on 16 Aug 2023.
93. Koell B, Orban M, Weimann J, Kassar M, Karam N, Neuss M, et al. Outcomes stratified by adapted inclusion criteria after mitral edge-to-edge repair. J Am Coll Cardiol. 2021;78:2408–21.
94. Adamo M, Fiorelli F, Melica B, D'Ortona R, Lupi L, Giannini C, et al. COAPT-like profile predicts long-term outcomes in patients with secondary mitral regurgitation undergoing MitraClip implantation. J Am Coll Cardiol Intv. 2021;14:15–25.

Chapter 7
Heart Failure and Aortic Stenosis: Intertwined Journeys

Sorin V. Pislaru and Vuyisile T. Nkomo

One of the memorable publications of the last century was the 1968 Ross and Braunwald opinion paper on natural evolution of patients with aortic stenosis (AS) [1]. The graphic suggesting a long latent period followed by very rapid decline after symptom onset is one of the most presented at cardiology meetings, and has driven clinical guidelines over the last 50 years (Fig. 7.1). While this idealized evolution is appealing in its logic, there is an abundance of data suggesting the connection between AS and heart failure (HF) is far more complex. Not only are we dealing with a different disease (AS in 2024 is dominated by calcific valvular degeneration in the elderly rather than due to rheumatic or bicuspid aortic valvulopathies of 1968), but there is enormous overlap of other conditions associated with the classic symptoms of angina, syncope and dyspnea. As such it is time to reevaluate the impact of AS and redefine therapeutic strategies and thresholds for intervention. In this chapter we will review recent progress in our understanding of AS.

AS and Heart Failure: Intertwined Epidemics of the Twenty-First Century

Calcific AS is the second most frequent valvular disease in developed countries, with a prevalence estimated at ~5% in patients age 75 or older [2, 3]. AS prevalence increases sharply with age, and as such the overall burden of AS is expected to rise

S. V. Pislaru (✉)
Division of Structural Heart Disease, Department of Cardiovascular Medicine, Mayo Clinic, Rochester, MN, USA
e-mail: Pislaru.sorin@mayo.edu

V. T. Nkomo
Department of Cardiovascular Medicine, Mayo Clinic, Rochester, MN, USA

M. Dorobanţu et al. (eds.), *Current Approach to Heart Failure*,
https://doi.org/10.1007/978-3-031-96562-3_7

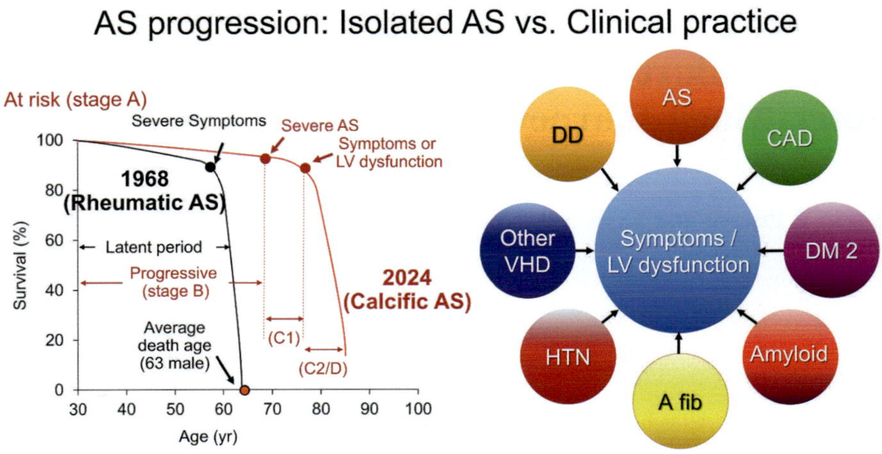

Fig. 7.1 **Stages of aortic stenosis**. (**Left**) The 1968 estimated progression of AS was based on post-mortem analysis of mostly rheumatic AS. The 2024 curve shows AS at a higher age consistent with calcific AS, but stages A-D follow the same paradigm of "isolated AS". (Adapted from Ref. [1]). (**Right**) In clinical practice symptoms or LV dysfunction in the elderly are most of the time due to a combination of comorbid conditions. *AS* aortic stenosis, *DD* diastolic dysfunction, *VHD* valvular heart disease, *HTN* hypertensionl, *A fib* atrial fibrillation, *DM2* diabetes mellitus, *CAD* coronary artery disease

in the context of an aging population. Furthermore, after the introduction of transcatheter aortic valve replacement (TAVR) the total number of valvular interventions has grown substantially, suggesting the burden of AS has been underestimated. Indeed, over less than a decade, the total number of aortic valve replacements (AVR) in older adults in the United States has increased over 60% [4]. Data from Edwards assessing the burden of AS in the European Union suggests approximately 70% of severe AS are not diagnosed and 80% do not undergo aortic valve replacement (Fig. 7.2) [5].

AS and heart failure (HF) are closely related, with up to 30% of patients with AS presenting with HF symptoms [6]. The concomitant presence of AS can contribute to adverse outcomes in patients with chronic heart failure, including increased rates of HF hospitalization and mortality [7]. This relationship is also observed in acute decompensated heart failure (ADHF), where AS is prevalent and associated with poor mortality outcomes [8].

The intertwined epidemic of AS and HF can be further explained by common pathogenesis. Indeed, pathological processes such as endothelial dysfunction, inflammation, fibrosis, and calcification are known to occur in both AS and systolic/diastolic HF [9]. Moreover, myocardial fibrosis, a common feature in patients with severe AS and HF, is an important determinant of postoperative clinical outcome and is not reversible after aortic valve replacement (AVR) [10].

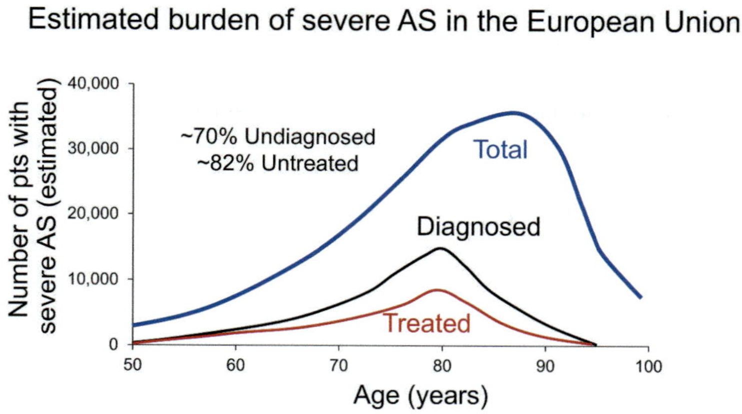

Fig. 7.2 Estimated burden of severe aortic stenosis. Data published in a recent review of AS suggests the vast majority of severe AS patients are not diagnosed, and a significant proportion of those with formal diagnosis are not undergoing aortic valve replacement. (Figure adapted from Ref. [5])

Staged Progression of Isolated Aortic Stenosis: Excellent Theoretical Concept But an Oversimplification of Clinical Practice

Current American College of Cardiology/American Heart Association valvular heart disease (VHD) guidelines emphasize a staged progression in disease severity, starting with patients at risk for development of VHD (stage A), going through a progressive stage where disease is mild to moderate and patients are asymptomatic (stage B), then an asymptomatic severe stage (stage C) and finally becoming symptomatic from severe VHD in stage D [11]. While this staged concept is appealing (obviously progression from no disease to severe disease has to go through different stages), it represents an oversimplification of the realities of clinical practice. In the "isolated AS" paradigm, patients cannot be symptomatic from VHD unless the disease is "severe", a concept that is challenged by recent data. In a study of Olmsted County residents with various degrees of AS, the classic triad of dyspnea, angina and syncope was present in 39% of patients with mild, 43% with moderate and 56% with severe AS [12]. This observation highlights the non-specific nature of the classic AS symptom triad and shows that the division into symptomatic and asymptomatic stages is more of a didactic nature. Indeed, AS hardly ever occurs in isolation; comorbidities are highly prevalent in the elderly population and make interpretation of the cause of symptoms challenging (Fig. 7.1).

Diastolic dysfunction is especially prevalent in this population. In a report from the PARTNER 2 Registry, 42% of patients had at least grade 2 diastolic dysfunction, and presence of DD prior to procedure was associated with an increase in death/rehospitalization at 1 year [13]. Conversely, improvement in DD was seen in 71% of patients after AVR and was independently associated with reduced CV death/rehospitalizations at 1 year. This association between diastolic dysfunction and AS is not confined to severe AS patients. In a cohort of 696 patients with moderate AS, presence of low ejection and stroke volume index was associated with increased mortality; in those with preserved ejection fraction an elevated E/e' was independently associated with excess mortality, highlighting the compound effect of non-severe AS and diastolic dysfunction in this elderly population [14].

Severe AS with Low Ejection Fraction: Burned-Out AS vs. Pre-existent Cardiomyopathy

There is no doubt that long-standing, untreated severe AS can lead to reduced ejection fraction. Support for this concept comes from the seminal work of John Ross describing the afterload mismatch and preload reserve when assessing ventricular function [15]. Chronic exposure to an ever-increasing afterload due to progressive AS leads to exhaustion of the preload reserve, and the afterload mismatch is expressed as a decrease in ejection fraction [16]. Relief of obstruction by AVRs a pure mechanical intervention and should not alter intrinsic myocardial contractility, yet ejection fraction frequently improves after valve replacement, often to normal range. The deleterious effects of afterload mismatch are well captured in the current guidelines, with an LVEF < 50% being a class I indication for AVR [11].

Recent work has highlighted an alternative pathway for progression to decreased ejection fraction in patients with severe AS. When looking backwards from the first echocardiographic diagnosis of severe AS, Ito et al. identified two distinct progression pathways in patients with and without depressed LVEF (Fig. 7.3) [17]. In both groups aortic valve area steadily decreased over the preceding years, with an accelerated drop in the last year prior to diagnosis. On the other hand, in patients with normal LVEF at first diagnosis of severe AS, earlier studies showed a remarkably steady value around 65%. In patients in whom LVEF was <50% at time of severe AS diagnosis, prior echocardiography demonstrated low normal LVEF (50–60%) but dropped significantly in the last year even <u>before</u> severe AS developed. This observation suggests some of these patients have undiagnosed, borderline LV systolic dysfunction with afterload mismatch and drop in LVEF developing at lower levels of valvular stenosis. Furthermore, when followed prospectively from the time of severe AS diagnosis, patients with LVEF of 50–60% fair worse than those >60%. These observations are now incorporated in the ACC/AHA guidelines that give a class IIb indication for AVR in patients with documented sustained decrease in LVEF < 60% [11].

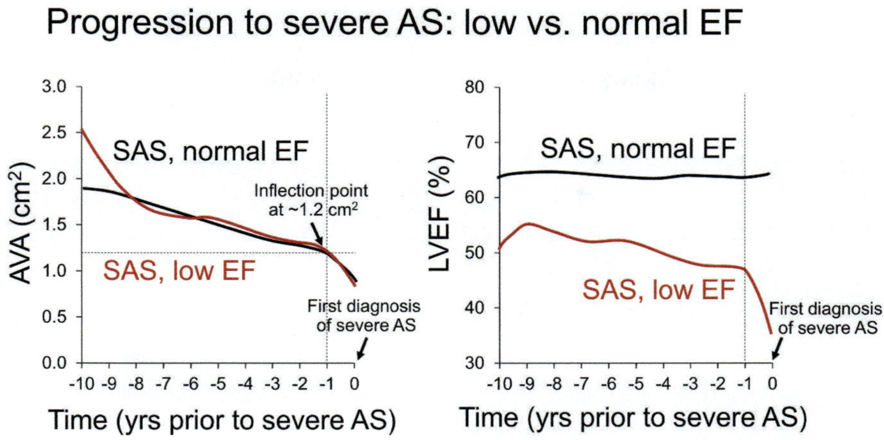

Fig. 7.3 Progression patterns to the first echocardiographic diagnosis of severe aortic stenosis. (**Left**) Aortic valve area decreases steadily and to similar extent in the 10 years preceding the first echocardiographic diagnosis of severe AS (time 0, right of the scale). Note an inflection point at about 1 year prior to diagnosis and a valve area of ~1.2 cm^2 after which decrease in valve area accelerates. (**Right**) In patients with normal EF at the time of first diagnosis of AS, LVEF remains remarkably constant in time, around 65%. In contrast, patients who have a low EF at their first diagnosis have a relatively steady borderline reduced LVEF around 50%; 1 year prior to diagnosis their LVEF drops sharply **before** severe AS is present, and parallels the accelerated progression seen on valve area. These patients should be considered for earlier AVR prior to development of severe AS. (Figure adapted from Ref. [17])

Concordant vs. Discordant Gradient-Valve Area in AS: A Complex Problem

Both European [18] and ACC/AHA [11] VHD guidelines definition of severe AS rely on demonstration of aortic valve velocity ≥ 4 m/s, mean gradient ≥ 40 mmHg or valve area ≤ 1 cm^2. When these parameters are all simultaneously present the diagnosis of severe AS is straightforward. However, frequently patients have discordant findings (Fig. 7.4); a comprehensive evaluation must be undertaken before decision on management.

The classic scenario of low-flow, low-gradient severe AS is that of patients with low LVEF. These patients have either true severe AS (low gradient caused by afterload mismatch with low stroke volume and low LVEF) or pseudo-severe AS (a separate cardiomyopathy causes low LVEF, and the low stroke volume fails to open the aortic valve). Low-dose dobutamine challenge has been validated as a method to distinguish between these entities [19]. An increase in stroke volume with no change in valve area but increase in gradients supports a diagnosis of severe AS, while no change in gradients but increase in valve area reflects pseudo-severe AS. Patients with no contractile reserve (no stroke volume increase to dobutamine) remain indeterminate and are at highest risk.

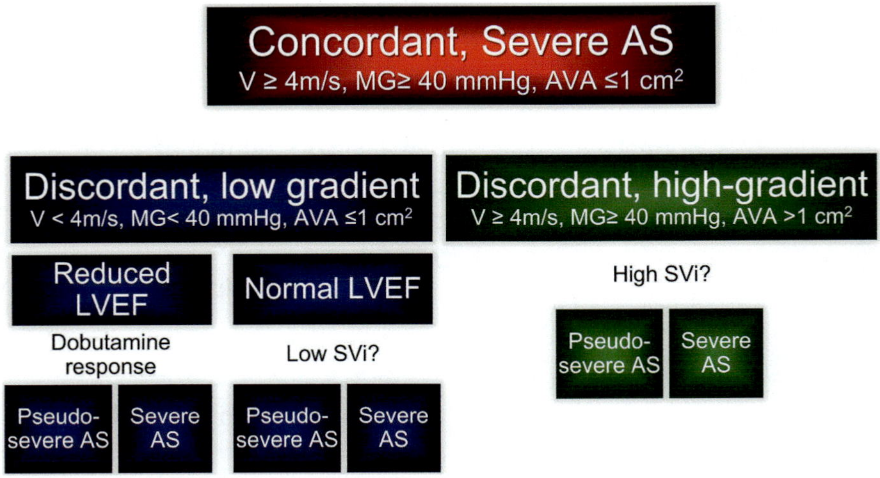

Fig. 7.4 Patterns of concordance/discordance in patients with aortic stenosis. (**Top**) Diagnosis of severe aortic stenosis is simple in patients with concordant abnormalities in peak aortic velocity, mean gradient and valve area. However, frequently these parameters are discordant. (**Left**) Discordant parameters with a low gradient and low valve area. Severe aortic stenosis can be separated from pseudosevere AS by either response to dobutamine (patients with low ejection fraction) or assessment of stroke volume index (patients with normal ejection fraction). (**Right**) The least described entity is discordance with high gradients but large valve area. These patients typically have bicuspid aortic valve with high gradients and large left ventricular outflow tract diameter. They must be differentiated from patients with high gradients caused by high cardiac output states. Stroke volume index is a potential marker, but a cutoff value has yet to be defined

Another common occurrence is presence of discordant low gradient and low valve area with normal ejection fraction. This paradoxically low-flow, low-gradient severe AS with preserved ejection fraction has been increasingly recognized [20]; the low stroke volume is typically caused by a small ventricular cavity in the context of concentric LV remodeling. Critical for an accurate diagnosis in these patients with discordant findings are meticulous review of echocardiographic measurements; notorious culprits are underestimation of true left ventricular outflow tract diameter (leading to lower aortic valve area calculations) and lack of systematic Doppler interrogation of velocity and gradients from multiple acoustic windows. Indeed, in a study of 100 consecutive patients with severe AS the acoustic window with the highest gradient was right parasternal (50%) followed by the apical window (39%); ignoring non-apical windows would have misclassified 8% of patients as "low-flow, low gradient AS" and 15% as moderate AS [21]. CT calcium scoring is particularly useful in this population as it provides an alternative method for AS diagnosis [22]. More importantly, it must be emphasized that any other coexistent comorbid condition leading to a reduction in stroke volume will result in discordant measurements of valve area and gradient. Typical examples are concomitant severe mitral or tricuspid valve disease, congenital heart disease with intracardiac shunts, uncontrolled hypertension, infiltrative or hypertrophic cardiomyopathies, constrictive pericarditis and atrial fibrillation [23].

Aortic Stenosis and Atrial Fibrillation

Given the high prevalence of both atrial fibrillation (AF) and AS in the elderly, it of no surprise the two diseases coexist in up to 50% of patients [24]. Atrial fibrillation is not necessarily a complication of AS in a significant proportion of these patients, but occurs independently before the development of significant AS. The combination is particularly troublesome both from a diagnostic and prognostic perspective due to a number of reasons.

First and foremost is the presence of beat-to-beat variability in stroke volume and gradients. The American Society of Echocardiography and the European Association of Cardiovascular Imaging endorse averaging signals from at least 5 consecutive cardiac cycles when assessing valve gradients in patients in AF or with other irregular rhythms [25]. Notably, averaging signals has been demonstrated superior to single cycle measurements in the evaluation of stroke volume and cardiac output. Whether averaging multiple cycles when reporting gradients in AS leads to more accurate diagnosis is completely unproven. On the contrary, there is mounting evidence that AS severity is underestimated in patients with AF, in part due to averaging.

In a series of 1541 consecutive AS patients with normal LVEF and valve area of ≤ 1 cm^2, patients were classified according to rhythm (SR vs. AF) and gradient (high, ≥ 40 mmHg, i.e. concordant area and gradient; low, <40 mmHg, i.e. discordant area and gradient) [26]. Regardless of rhythm, patients with concordant high gradient and low valve area were diagnosed with severe AS and commonly referred to AVR, while patients with low gradients (i.e., low flow, severe AS) were more likely misdiagnosed as "moderate AS" with fewer referred to AVR. Importantly, patients with AF with <u>low gradients</u> had similar CT calcium score as patients in SR with <u>high gradients</u>, suggesting AS severity is similar and differences in gradients are due to the lower flow status in AF. Furthermore, isolated cardiac cycles with aortic valve signals meeting gradient criteria for severe AS were frequently present in AF with low-gradient and were associated with higher aortic valve calcium scores. Overall these findings suggest that the practice of averaging gradients leads to underestimation of AS severity in AF. Further supporting the observation that averaging mean gradient underestimates disease severity comes from a series of patients who had echocardiographic AS assessment just before and after cardioversion [27]. The signal recorded from the cardiac cycle with the highest gradient during AF was similar to the average peak aortic velocity and mean gradient in SR; the averaged stroke volume, mean gradient and peak aortic velocity in AF were 10–17% lower than the values recorded in the same patient in SR.

Additional evidence that AS is under-diagnosed and under-referred or referred late to AVR comes from both surgical and transcatheter studies. In a series of 495 consecutive patients who underwent surgical AVR, the ratio of the weight of the explanted aortic valve (a measure of aortic valve calcification severity) and mean gradient was higher in AF than in SR patients, suggesting that at the same degree of calcification AF is associated with lower gradients [28]. This finding was corroborated by the lower stroke volume and transaortic flow rate noted in patients in AF. Similarly, in a series of 820 patients who underwent transcatheter AVR, CT calcium scores were significantly higher in both males and females with AF compared with SR despite similar valve areas and mean gradients [29]. Furthermore, disproportionately more patients had very high calcium score (>3000 AU units for males and >1600 AU in females) in AF than SR. Interestingly, the age difference at the time of AVR (AF patients were on average 2 years older) matches the estimated progression in valve calcification. Indeed, assuming an average progression in aortic valve calcium score of 152 units/year (Agatston method), the estimated AF distribution and median calcium score 2 years prior to TAVR matched the distribution of calcium scores in SR at time of TAVR. This observation suggests a ~2 year lag in severe AS diagnosis in patients in AF, and explains at least in part the observed higher mortality in AF when compared to patients in SR. Notably, outcomes in patients with AS and AF are uniformly worse than those with AS and SR, even in asymptomatic patients, raising concerns about a need for a different approach in these patients [30]. Worse yet are the additional structural and hemodynamic alterations associated with AF such as functional mitral and tricuspid valve regurgitation. Given all these observations, we have altered the practice in our echocardiography laboratory and we are reporting both the 5-cycle average gradient / velocity (as per current guidelines) and the highest single beat signal values.

Future Directions in Diagnosis and Management of AS and HF

From previous discussion it is obvious that AS and HF are major health problems of the twenty-first century. It is now clear that untreated AS is associated with excess mortality at all levels of stenosis severity, yet AS remains

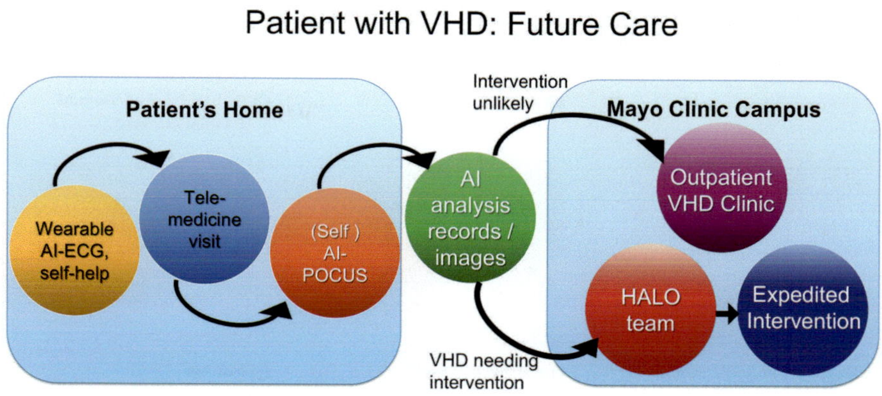

Fig. 7.5 **The future of care in VHD**. Development of powerful artificial intelligence tools coupled with technological advancement will drastically change the care of valvular heart disease patients. Initial prompt for evaluation will be AI-ECG base on wearable devices, triggering a telemedicine visit and a self examination with a point-of-care ultrasound tool. Initial records and images will be analyzed by AI driven tools. Patients in need of immediate intervention will have expedited care by a HALO team, while those with disease but in no need of intervention will come through the routine valvular heart disease clinic. *AI* artificial intelligence, *POCUS* point-of-care ultrasound, *HALO* high-acuity low-occurrence

under-diagnosed and referral to AVR is often delayed or not performed at all [31]. The questions is how to address these issues in the context of limited resources. Clearly the current paradigm of AS diagnosis based on clinical suspicion followed by echocardiographic testing is suboptimal. Recent advances using artificial intelligence tools hold great promise. Indeed, a signature of AS can be detected by standard 12 lead electrocardiography with good sensitivity and specificity [32], but the positive predictive value of 10.5% is suboptimal for mass deployment. Similarly, AI-ECG can identify patients with low ejection fraction [32] as well as presence of diastolic dysfunction [32–34]. The combination of AI-ECG with AI-assisted point-of-care ultrasound [35] may be an excellent solution for both AS and HF screening, and the future care of AS patients will look drastically different from today (Fig. 7.5). The promises of technological breakthroughs are vast—it is up to us to bring them to reality (Fig. 7.6).

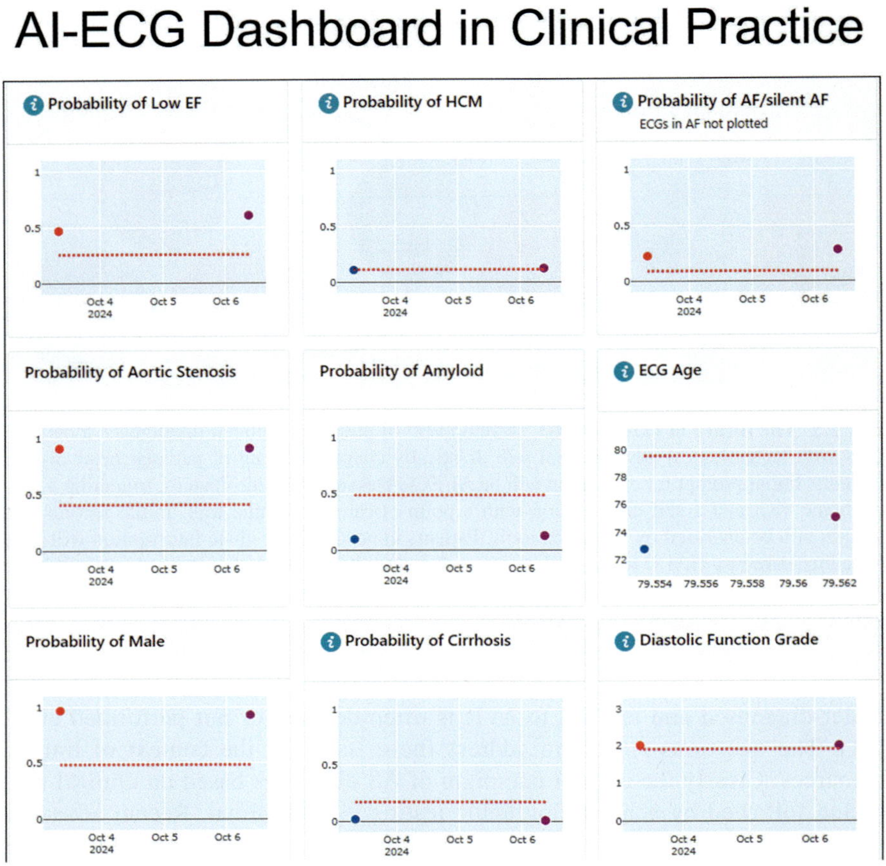

Fig. 7.6 Dashboard titled "AI-ECG Dashboard in Clinical Practice" featuring nine X-Y charts. Each chart displays probabilities or values over dates from October 4 to October 6, 2024. Categories include "Probability of Low EF," "Probability of HCM," "Probability of AF/silent AF," "Probability of Aortic Stenosis," "Probability of Amyloid," "ECG Age," "Probability of Male," "Probability of Cirrhosis," and "Diastolic Function Grade." Charts show data points and a red dotted line indicating a threshold or average

References

1. Ross J Jr, Braunwald E. Aortic stenosis. Circulation. 1968;38(1 Suppl):61–7. https://doi.org/10.1161/01.cir.38.1s5.v-61. PMID: 4894151.
2. Nkomo VT, Gardin JM, Skelton TN, Gottdiener JS, Scott CG, Enriquez-Sarano M. Burden of valvular heart diseases: a population-based study. Lancet. 2006;368(9540):1005–11. https://doi.org/10.1016/S0140-6736(06)69208-8. PMID: 16980116.
3. Coffey S, Roberts-Thomson R, Brown A, Carapetis J, Chen M, Enriquez-Sarano M, Zühlke L, Prendergast BD. Global epidemiology of valvular heart disease. Nat Rev Cardiol. 2021;18(12):853–64. https://doi.org/10.1038/s41569-021-00570-z. Epub 2021 Jun 25. PMID: 34172950.

4. Mori M, Gupta A, Wang Y, Vahl T, Nazif T, Kirtane AJ, George I, Yong CM, Onuma O, Kodali S, Geirsson A, Leon MB, Krumholz HM. Trends in transcatheter and surgical aortic valve replacement among older adults in the United States. J Am Coll Cardiol. 2021;78(22):2161–72. https://doi.org/10.1016/j.jacc.2021.09.855. PMID: 34823659.
5. Thoenes M, Bramlage P, Zamorano P, Messika-Zeitoun D, Wendt D, Kasel M, Kurucova J, Steeds RP. Patient screening for early detection of aortic stenosis (AS)—review of current practice and future perspectives. J Thorac Dis. 2018;10(9):5584–94. https://doi.org/10.21037/jtd.2018.09.02. PMID: 30416809; PMCID: PMC6196210.
6. Jean G, Mogensen NSB, Clavel MA. Aortic valvular stenosis and heart failure: advances in diagnostic, management, and intervention. Heart Fail Clin. 2023;19(3):273–83. https://doi.org/10.1016/j.hfc.2023.02.005.
7. Khan KR, Khan OA, Chen C, et al. Impact of moderate aortic stenosis in patients with heart failure with reduced ejection fraction. J Am Coll Cardiol. 2023;81(13):1235–44.
8. Sivaraj K, Arora S, Hendrickson M, et al. Epidemiology and outcomes of aortic stenosis in acute decompensated heart failure: the ARIC study. Circ Heart Fail. 2023;16(3):e009653.
9. Trimaille A, Hmadeh S, Matsushita K, et al. Aortic stenosis and the haemostatic system. Cardiovasc Res. 2023;119(6):1310–23. https://doi.org/10.1093/cvr/cvac192.
10. Weidemann F, Herrmann S, Störk S, et al. Impact of myocardial fibrosis in patients with symptomatic severe aortic stenosis. Circulation. 2009;120(7):577–84. https://doi.org/10.1161/CIRCULATIONAHA.108.847772.
11. Otto CM, Nishimura RA, Bonow RO, Carabello BA, Erwin JP 3rd, Gentile F, Jneid H, Krieger EV, Mack M, McLeod C, O'Gara PT, Rigolin VH, Sundt TM 3rd, Thompson A, Toly C. 2020 ACC/AHA Guideline for the Management of Patients with Valvular Heart Disease: a report of the American College of Cardiology/American Heart Association Joint Committee on Clinical Practice Guidelines. J Am Coll Cardiol. 2021;77(4):e25–e197. https://doi.org/10.1016/j.jacc.2020.11.018.
12. Malouf J, Le Tourneau T, Pellikka P, Sundt TM, Scott C, Schaff HV, Enriquez-Sarano M. Aortic valve stenosis in community medical practice: determinants of outcome and implications for aortic valve replacement. J Thorac Cardiovasc Surg. 2012;144(6):1421–7. https://doi.org/10.1016/j.jtcvs.2011.09.075. Epub 2012 Feb 14. PMID: 22336754.
13. Ong G, Pibarot P, Redfors B, Weissman NJ, Jaber WA, Makkar RR, Lerakis S, Gopal D, Khalique O, Kodali SK, Thourani VH, Anwaruddin S, McAndrew T, Zhang Y, Alu MC, Douglas PS, Hahn RT. Diastolic function and clinical outcomes after transcatheter aortic valve replacement: PARTNER 2 SAPIEN 3 registry. J Am Coll Cardiol. 2020;76(25):2940–51. https://doi.org/10.1016/j.jacc.2020.10.032. PMID: 33334422.
14. Ito S, Miranda WR, Nkomo VT, Boler AN, Pislaru SV, Pellikka PA, Crusan DJ, Lewis BR, Nishimura RA, Oh JK. Prognostic risk stratification of patients with moderate aortic stenosis. J Am Soc Echocardiogr. 2021;34(3):248–56. https://doi.org/10.1016/j.echo.2020.10.012. Epub 2020 Nov 5. PMID: 33161066.
15. Ross J Jr. Afterload mismatch and preload reserve: a conceptual framework for the analysis of ventricular function. Prog Cardiovasc Dis. 1976;18(4):255–64. https://doi.org/10.1016/0033-0620(76)90021-9. PMID: 128034.
16. Ross J Jr. Afterload mismatch in aortic and mitral valve disease: implications for surgical therapy. J Am Coll Cardiol. 1985;5(4):811–26. https://doi.org/10.1016/s0735-1097(85)80418-6. PMID: 3882814.
17. Ito S, Miranda WR, Nkomo VT, Connolly HM, Pislaru SV, Greason KL, Pellikka PA, Lewis BR, Oh JK. Reduced left ventricular ejection fraction in patients with aortic stenosis. J Am Coll Cardiol. 2018;71(12):1313–21. https://doi.org/10.1016/j.jacc.2018.01.045. PMID: 29566814.
18. Vahanian A, Beyersdorf F, Praz F, et al. 2021 ESC/EACTS Guidelines for the management of valvular heart disease. Eur Heart J. 2022;43(7):561–632. https://doi.org/10.1093/eurheartj/ehab395. PMID: 34453165.

19. Nishimura RA, Grantham JA, Connolly HM, Schaff HV, Higano ST, Holmes DR Jr. Low-output, low-gradient aortic stenosis in patients with depressed left ventricular systolic function: the clinical utility of the dobutamine challenge in the catheterization laboratory. Circulation. 2002;106(7):809–13. https://doi.org/10.1161/01.cir.0000025611.21140.34. PMID: 12176952.
20. Hachicha Z, Dumesnil JG, Bogaty P, Pibarot P. Paradoxical low-flow, low-gradient severe aortic stenosis despite preserved ejection fraction is associated with higher after-load and reduced survival. Circulation. 2007;115(22):2856–64. https://doi.org/10.1161/CIRCULATIONAHA.106.668681. Epub 2007 May 28. PMID: 17533183.
21. Thaden JJ, Nkomo VT, Lee KJ, Oh JK. Doppler imaging in aortic stenosis: the importance of the nonapical imaging windows to determine severity in a contemporary cohort. J Am Soc Echocardiogr. 2015;28(7):780–5. https://doi.org/10.1016/j.echo.2015.02.016. Epub 2015 Apr 6. PMID: 25857547.
22. Rosenhek R, Binder T, Porenta G, Lang I, Christ G, Schemper M, Maurer G, Baumgartner H. Predictors of outcome in severe, asymptomatic aortic stenosis. N Engl J Med. 2000;343(9):611–7. https://doi.org/10.1056/NEJM200008313430903. PMID: 10965007.
23. Pislaru SV, Pellikka PA. The spectrum of low-output low-gradient aortic stenosis with normal ejection fraction. Heart. 2016;102(9):665–71. https://doi.org/10.1136/heartjnl-2015-307893. Epub 2016 Jan 28. PMID: 26822426.
24. Tarantini G, Mojoli M, Urena M, Vahanian A. Atrial fibrillation in patients undergoing transcatheter aortic valve implantation: epidemiology, timing, predictors, and outcome. Eur Heart J. 2016;38:1285–93.
25. Baumgartner H, Hung J, Bermejo J, et al. Recommendations on the Echocardiographic Assessment of Aortic Valve Stenosis: a focused update from the European Association of Cardiovascular Imaging and the American Society of Echocardiography. J Am Soc Echocardiogr. 2017;30(4):372–92. https://doi.org/10.1016/j.echo.2017.02.009. PMID: 28385280.
26. Alsidawi S, Khan S, Pislaru SV, et al. High prevalence of severe aortic stenosis in low-flow state associated with atrial fibrillation. Circ Cardiovasc Imaging. 2021;14(7):e012453. https://doi.org/10.1161/CIRCIMAGING.120.012453. Epub 2021 Jul 12. PMID: 34250815.
27. Naser JA, Pislaru SV, Pislaru C, et al. Averaged transaortic mean gradient during atrial fibrillation does not accurately reflect aortic stenosis severity. J Am Soc Echocardiogr. 2022;35(8):885–7. https://doi.org/10.1016/j.echo.2022.05.003. Epub 2022 May 11. PMID: 35561958.
28. Alkurashi AK, Thaden JJ, Naser JA, El-Am EA, Pislaru SV, Greason KL, Negrotto SM, Clavel MA, Pellikka PA, Maleszewski JJ, Nkomo VT. Underestimation of aortic stenosis severity by Doppler mean gradient during atrial fibrillation: insights from aortic valve weight. J Am Soc Echocardiogr. 2023;36(1):53–9. https://doi.org/10.1016/j.echo.2022.10.007. Epub 2022 Oct 10. PMID: 36228839.
29. Masson R, Nkomo VT, Holmes DR Jr, Pislaru SV, Arsanjani R, Chao CJ, Klanderman M, Abraham B, Morsy M, Fortuin FD, Sweeney JP, Sell-Dotten K, Alsidawi S. Disproportionately high aortic valve calcium scores in atrial fibrillation: implications for transcatheter aortic valve replacement. Eur Heart J Cardiovasc Imaging. 2024;25(9):1264–75. https://doi.org/10.1093/ehjci/jeae113. PMID: 38669204.
30. Oguz D, Huntley GD, El-Am EA, et al. Impact of atrial fibrillation on outcomes in asymptomatic severe aortic stenosis: a propensity-matched analysis. Front Cardiovasc Med. 2023;10:1195123. https://doi.org/10.3389/fcvm.2023.1195123. PMID: 37408654; PMCID: PMC10318187.
31. Cohen-Shelly M, Attia ZI, Friedman PA, et al. Electrocardiogram screening for aortic valve stenosis using artificial intelligence. Eur Heart J. 2021;42(30):2885–96. https://doi.org/10.1093/eurheartj/ehab153. PMID: 33748852.
32. Attia ZI, Kapa S, Lopez-Jimenez F, McKie PM, Ladewig DJ, Satam G, Pellikka PA, Enriquez-Sarano M, Noseworthy PA, Munger TM, Asirvatham SJ, Scott CG, Carter RE, Friedman PA. Screening for cardiac contractile dysfunction using an artificial intelligence-enabled elec-

trocardiogram. Nat Med. 2019;25(1):70–4. https://doi.org/10.1038/s41591-018-0240-2. Epub 2019 Jan 7. PMID: 30617318.

33. Akerman AP, Porumb M, Scott CG, Beqiri A, Chartsias A, Ryu AJ, Hawkes W, Huntley GD, Arystan AZ, Kane GC, Pislaru SV, Lopez-Jimenez F, Gomez A, Sarwar R, O'Driscoll J, Leeson P, Upton R, Woodward G, Pellikka PA. Automated echocardiographic detection of heart failure with preserved ejection fraction using artificial intelligence. JACC Adv. 2023;2(6):100452. https://doi.org/10.1016/j.jacadv.2023.100452. PMID: 38939447; PMCID: PMC11198161.
34. Lee E, Ito S, Miranda WR, Lopez-Jimenez F, Kane GC, Asirvatham SJ, Noseworthy PA, Friedman PA, Carter RE, Borlaug BA, Attia ZI, Oh JK. Artificial intelligence-enabled ECG for left ventricular diastolic function and filling pressure. NPJ Digit Med. 2024;7(1):4. https://doi.org/10.1038/s41746-023-00993-7. PMID: 38182738; PMCID: PMC10770308.
35. Naser JA, Lee E, Pislaru SV, Tsaban G, Malins JG, Jackson JI, Anisuzzaman DM, Rostami B, Lopez-Jimenez F, Friedman PA, Kane GC, Pellikka PA, Attia ZI. Artificial intelligence-based classification of echocardiographic views. Eur Heart J Digit Health. 2024;5(3):260–9. https://doi.org/10.1093/ehjdh/ztae015. PMID: 38774376; PMCID: PMC11104471.

Further Reading

Généreux P, Sharma RP, Cubeddu RJ, et al. The mortality burden of untreated aortic stenosis. J Am Coll Cardiol. 2023;82(22):2101–9. https://doi.org/10.1016/j.jacc.2023.09.796. Epub 2023 Oct 24. PMID: 37877909.

Chapter 8
Assessment of Left Ventricular Contractile Reserve in Heart Failure

Serban Mihaileanu and Laura Antohi

What's well-conceived is easy to say, making the words to fully obey.

Nicolas Boileau

Abstract The goal of this chapter is to provide an integrated view of LV contractile function and reserve for clinicians involved in dynamic testing. LV contractile reserve (LVC) will be discussed by integrating:

- The Force-Frequency Relation (FFR) or the Bowditch treppe effect or the staircase effect
- The Gregg Effect
- Frank-Starling Law and the Anrep Effect
- The Metaboreflex
- Preload and Preload Reserve
  - Low preload reserve guided by echocardiographic indices, suggesting elevated LV filling pressure
  - Heart Rate and Preload
  - Left Ventricle Compliance and Preload Reserve:
- Afterload and afterload mismatch
  - Opposing force to LV ejection
  - Systolic Wall Stress as a reflection of the afterload on the LV myocardial wall

The original version of the chapter has been revised. A correction to this chapter can be found at https://doi.org/10.1007/978-3-031-96562-3_27

S. Mihaileanu (✉)
Institut Mutualiste Montsouris, Paris, France
e-mail: cardiologie@pm.me

L. Antohi
Emergency Institute for Cardiovascular Diseases 'C. C. Iliescu', Bucharest, Romania

University of Medicine 'Carol Davila', Bucharest, Romania

M. Dorobanţu et al. (eds.), *Current Approach to Heart Failure*,
https://doi.org/10.1007/978-3-031-96562-3_8

  - Can we consider wall stress as a contractility index?
  - Wall stress as a companion to fractional shortening/ejection fraction
  - Contractile function of the LV against a pressure overload

- Pharmacological tests used for LV contractile reserve investigation
- Exercise testing for LV contractile reserve
  - Maximal Myocardial Workload
  - Protocols for LV contractile reserve
  - The ABCDE protocol
  - Wall Motion Score Index (WMSI) and CR in non-ischemic cardiomyopathies
  - B-lines and stress echocardiography
  - Chronotropic Reserve (Heart Rate Reserve) and Chronotropic Incompetence
  - Studies on Contractile Reserve
- Left Ventricular Elastance (Ees) and Pressure-Volume Loops
  - End-Systolic Pressure-Volume Ratio (ESPVR) an elastance surrogate
- Arterial Effective Elastance (Ea)
- Ventriculo-Arterial Coupling (VAC)
  - Ventricular Efficiency
  - The potential energy (PE)
  - Avoiding the VAC simplified formula
  - VAC is more dynamic than EF
  - HFrEF
  - HFpEF
  - Various surrogates for VAC approximation
- Ejection Fraction and Stroke Volume
  - Components of the EF calculation and their relationship
  - Relationship of the EF to the VAC
  - Stroke Volume and Flow Reserve
- Cardiac Power Output and Reserve as a global hemodynamic index
- dP/dT
- LV longitudinal function
  - Doppler Tissue Imaging (DTI)
- LV myocardial strain(S) and strain rate (SR)
  - Ejection Fraction and Strain relationship
  - Pressure Strain Loops (PSL)

Keywords Contractile reserve · Preload · Afterload · Wall stress · Ejection fraction · Ventricular elastance · Arterial elastance · Ventriculo-arterial coupling · Cardiac power output · Left ventricular strain

Abbreviations

APMHR	Age Predicted Maximal Heart Rate
AS	Aortic Stenosis
AVA	Aortic Valve Area
AVG	Aortic Valve Gradient
BP	Blood Pressure
CAD	Coronary artery Disease
cESS	Circumferential End-Systolic Stress
CMR	Cardiac Magnetic Resonance
CO	Cardiac Output
CPI	Cardiac Power Index
CPO	Cardiac Power Output
CPOM	Cardiac Power Output normalised to LV mass
CR	Contractile Reserve
DTI	Doppler Tissue Imaging
Ea	Effective Arterial eEastance
EDV	End-diastolic Volume
Ees	Left Ventricular Elastance
ESPVR	End-Systolic Pressure-Volume Ratio
ESV	End-Systolic Volume
ET	Ejection Time
FFR	Force-Frequency Relation
GCS	Global Circumferential Strain
GCW	Global Constructed Work
GLS	Global Longitudinal Strain
GRS	Global Radial Strain
GWE	Global Work Efficiency
GWI	Global Work Index
GWW	Global Wasted Work
HF	Heart Failure
HFpEF	Heart Failure with Preserved Ejection Fraction
HFrEF	Heart Failure with Reduced Ejection Fraction
HR	Heart Rate
HRR	Heart Rate Reserve
HTN	Hypertension
ICT	Isovolumic Contraction Time
LA	Left Atrium
LLN	Lower Limit of Normal
LV	Left Ventricle
LVCR	Left Ventricle Contractile Reserve
LVEDP	Left Ventricular End-Diastolic Pressure
LVEF	Left Ventricular Ejection Fraction
LVESP	Left Ventricular End-Systolic Pressure

MAP	Mean Arterial Pressure
MR	Mitral Regurgitation
MRI	Magnetic Resonance Imaging
MRPP	Maximum Rate Pressure Product
mSF	Midwall Shortening Fraction
MW	Myocardial Work
PACS	Peak Atrial Contraction Strain
PALS	Peak Atrial Longitudinal Strain
PCWP	Pulmonary Capillary Wedge Pressure
PEP	Pre-Ejection Period
PET	Positron Emission Tomography
PSL	Pressure Strain Loops
PVL	Pressure-Volume Loop
RAP	Right Atrial Pressure
RV	Right Ventricle
SBP	Systolic Blood Pressure
SR	Strain Rate
STI	Systolic Time Intervals
STS	Society of Thoracic Surgeons
SV	Stroke Volume
SVi	Indexed Systolic Volume
SVR	Systemic Vascular Resistance
TAC	Total Arterial Compliance
TAVR	Transcatheter Aortic Valve Replacement
V0	zero-pressure volume
VAC	Ventriculo-Arterial Coupling
VO2	Maximal O2 consumption/min
VTI	Velocity Time Integral
WMSI	Wall Motion Score Index
WS	Wall stress
Zva	Valvulo-arterial impedance

Introduction

In order to survive, any biological system must be able to adapt to current circumstances and draw on its reserves. Every link in the circulatory system adapts, i.e. it has functional reserves. The heart is only one link in an extremely complex circulatory and metabolic system. Given the complexity of hemodynamics, especially in unstable patients and/or those with heart failure, understanding the role of the heart, particularly left ventricular (LV) contractility, remains a real diagnostic challenge. Is it the primary cause or not, and how can we determine this? What is the most appropriate method for daily practice? Most (if not all) of the formulas in use are approximations of a fundamental process, and there must be understanding of what is approximated. Investigation of LV contractile reserve (CR), in heart failure (HF), is an enthusiastic way to approach a very difficult situation. In clinical terms, CR means the ability of the LV to augment its performance, accordingly to inotropic enhancing. There are several ways, through different mechanisms, to stimulate the inotropic response. Choosing the most appropriate test is mandatory for the interpretation of the cardio-vascular response. However, LV contraction and its reserve are not the primary mechanism of hemodynamic adaptation, but just one link in a complex interacting system (Fig. 8.1).

An important issue is to familiarize clinical cardiologists with the fundamental relationship between left ventricular contraction and afterload, which is a governing principle in heart failure. J. Ross brought to light the concept of afterload mismatch, considered by some physiologists being as important as the Frank-Starling law. It is difficult to conceive the ventricular contraction, or the CR isolated from the ventriculo-arterial coupling (VAC). Is contraction more important than arterial elastance? CR is a virtual situation: the way to demonstrate it, using surrogates, needs to go through the basics.

In terms of global cardiac function, systole and diastole, are opposite temporal moments of a unique undulatory function. However, this chapter is dedicated to the systolic aspect—in terms of potential reserve. There are several clinical ways to explore LV function; this chapter will favor echo-Doppler examination which is the most widely used and popular.

Several important cardiac characteristics and physiopathological situations related to this subject will be briefly enumerated.

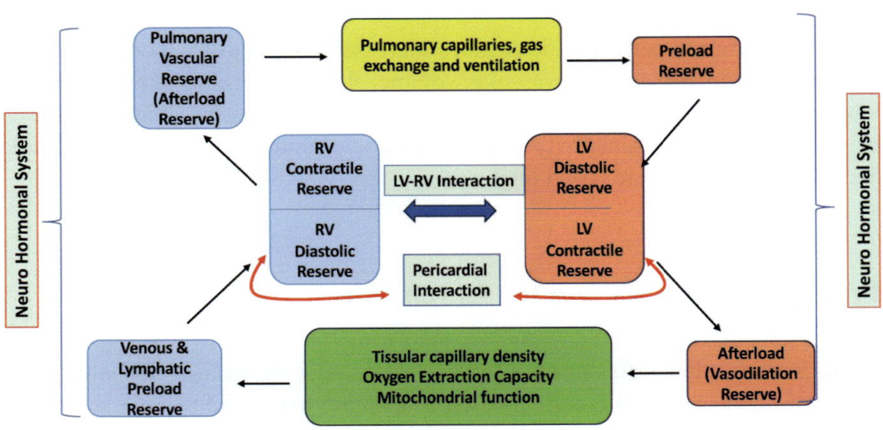

Fig. 8.1 Complex hemodynamic interactions in which the contractile reserve of the left ventricle is only one interconnected link

The Force-Frequency Relation (FFR) or the Bowditch Treppe Effect or the Staircase Effect

Increased heart rate (HR) delays the elimination of intra-cellular Ca^{++} and stimulates the sympathetic system, resulting in increased contractility. Increasing contraction force when heart frequency increases, is one of the main investigative ways for CR. This property of cardiac muscle is amplified by β-adrenergic stimulation, and, in a coordinated way, the neurohumoral state alters both frequency (acting on the sinoatrial node) as well as force generation (modifying ventricular myocytes). This synchronized tuning is needed to meet new metabolic demands [1]. Patients with HF with reduced ejection fraction (HFrEF) may have a negative treppe at HR > 100/min, suggesting that a correlation between myocardial disease and optimal contraction frequency may exist. The negative treppe can be shifted even much lower in advanced HF [2]. Many studies on contractility reserve are based on the FFR effect: increasing frequency—increases contractility. However, an expected positive effect may be negative. In a small study, pacing at 125 beats per minute, lowered mean LV end-diastolic pressure in both normal subjects and patients with HF with preserved ejection fraction (HFpEF), and volume loss was about twice as great in the HFpEF group than in controls [3]. In the RAPID-HF trial, Borlaug et al. showed that atrial pacing didn't significantly affect exercise cardiac output (CO) in HFpEF patients with chronotropic incompetence, despite increased HR, due to decreased stroke volume (SV) [4].

The Gregg Effect

Increased coronary perfusion determines increased contractility. Increased perfusion pressure increases microvascular volume, thereby opening stretch-activated ion channels, resulting in an increased intracellular Ca^{2+} transient, which is followed by an increase in Ca^{2+} sensitivity and higher muscle contractility [5]. Dipyridamole and adenosine testing are based on it.

Frank-Starling Law and the Anrep Effect

Frank-Starling's law states that the force of ventricular contraction depends on the length of fibers at rest. In a normal heart, an increase in preload by increasing fiber length in any of the four chambers will immediately promote a more forceful contraction, resulting in a greater SV to maintain circulatory balance. This relationship between preload and contractility operates within a limited range of fiber length. The rapid change in force is thought to be related to an increase in the Ca^{2+} responsiveness of the myofilaments. The same immediate response occurs when aortic resistance is increased as to avoid a decrease in SV. In the event of a significant increase in aortic resistance (afterload) lasting for more than 10–15 min, the normal heart will promote the slow force response to the change in length, described experimentally by Anrep. Physiologically, the Anrep effect is a powerful mechanism by which the heart adapts to an abrupt increase in afterload that occurs after the Frank-Starling law contribution [6].

The Metaboreflex

During physical exercise, the muscle metaboreflex is a cardiovascular reflex capable of eliciting marked increases in sympathetic activity during exercise. The efferent response to metaboreflex activation is an increase in sympathetic nerve activity that constricts the systemic vasculature and also stimulates parallel inotropic and chronotropic effects on the heart as to increase cardiac output [7]. Metaboreflex activation in patients with congestive HF will raise the blood pressure (BP), mostly due to an exaggerated increase of the systemic vascular resistances (SVR) but not by SV. The BP increase is achieved in those patients, by shifting from an output-increase to a vasoconstriction mediated mechanism. This shift may contribute to the early fatigue they experience [8]. In patients with HF, this shift may be due to an abnormal response to high sympathetic activity, causing coronary constriction and leading to impaired cardiac function and reduced CO [9]. Exercise testing in either HFrEF or HFpEF patients must consider that if a CR is still present, it may be blunted by an abnormally high SVR and/or exercise-induced myocardial ischemia. Patients with HFpEF have exaggerated cardiovascular responses to inspiratory muscle metaboreflex activation, compared to healthy individuals when tested with inspiratory resistive breathing tasks. This results in an approximately twofold increase in leg vascular resistance, coupled with a greater decrease in leg blood flow, resulting in a higher-than-normal increase in afterload triggered by the inspiratory muscle metaboreflex [10].

Preload and Preload Reserve

Preload represents the initial extent of stretch of the relaxed LV at end-diastole, before contraction and within physiological limits of the fiber length, and dictates the Frank-Starling law. No load no contraction—preload is the great promoter of the variable contractile states of the myocardium. Neither afterload nor contractility have a direct effect on the resting or stretched muscle length before contraction, whereas preload has no direct effect on the minimum muscle length after contraction [11]. Theoretically, it would be easy to calculate the end-diastolic wall stress according to Laplace's law: LV end-diastolic pressure × LV radius/2 * wall thickness. However, LV end-diastolic pressure is not linearly related to LV end-diastolic volume, and changes in pressure are not linearly related to changes in LV volume, SV, or stroke work. Myocardial distensibility cannot be derived from absolute LV volume. Pulmonary capillary wedge pressure (PCWP) has the additional limitation that it may underestimate LV end-diastolic pressure (LVEDP), but it is still the best clinical way to understand whether or not there is preload reserve. A low or normal range LVEDP (4–12 mmHg) suggests the presence of preload reserve, whereas an LVEDP >20 mmHg does not [11]. Keeping the preload at an optimal level is mandatory for LV contraction, when facing unstable hemodynamic situations or for the management of chronic congestive HF—where one needs to know if there is a preload reserve or not. The preload reserve is the major mechanism that allows SV and CO to adapt to acute changes in demand such as exercise. Fudim et al. in a comprehensive and remarkable review, draws attention to a sometimes overlooked problem, namely the venous system as a CO modulator and its dysfunction in HF induced by autonomic dysfunction [12]. Veins have a much greater capacitance than arteries, storing approximately 70% of total blood, while the splanchnic compartment contains 20–30%. Autonomic dysfunction in HF may lead to splanchnic venoconstriction, reducing its buffering function and overloading the central (less compliant) venous compartment, thereby exceeding the preload reserve. Conversely, impaired venous return, reducing preload reserve, may lead to vascular underfilling. Exercise limitation is caused by pooling of blood in venous reservoirs or the inability to recruit due to mechanical obstruction (transhepatic or large venous obstruction).

Preload reserve can be considered as the difference between the maximal value (where preload still has a positive inotropic effect) and the observed lower or not value. Preload reserve has important individual characteristics such as initial LV volume, LVEDP, LV compliance (a fibrotic LV vs. normal myocardium), afterload, right ventricle-LV interaction, pericardial restraint… Despite the absence of a perfect surrogate for measuring myocardial fiber stretch, variations of LV diastolic volume and mostly PCWP variations, can correctly guide, in clinical practice, the optimal vascular filling and/or diuretic/vasodilator strategy.

Low Preload Reserve Guided by Echocardiographic Indices, Suggesting Elevated LV Filling Pressure

Careful estimation of some echo-Doppler indices, especially in diseased hearts may correctly reflect the filling pressure.

Passive leg raising is a simple, basic method that creates an important venous transfer (≈150–300 ml) from the legs and splanchnic venous system to the central circulation, avoiding fluid overload, to predict preload responsiveness. This maneuver, described by Monnet and Teboul, is very valuable in critically ill patients and is considered positive for a 10–15% increase in SV or CO [13]. In a pooled metanalysis, comprising 653 patients, Bytyci et al. observed a strong correlation between PCWP (reflecting the atrial pressure) with peak atrial longitudinal strain

(PALS—reservoir strain), peak atrial contraction strain (PACS—pump strain) and less with the atrial volume [14]. A PCWP cutoff at > 15 mm Hg was correctly predicted by a PALS ≤ 19% (Sensitivity 80%, Specificity 77%). However, the reservoir strain may reflect a chronic evolution whereas the pump strain (if sinus rhythm) is a much better predictor of the filling pressure. Atrial strain is a much better predictor of LV filling pressure in patients with LVEF < 50% as compared to conventional measures (e.g. E/e').

For a PCWP cutoff > 15 mmHg and EF < 50%, a pump LA strain < 8% had the largest AUC (0.94), while the reservoir strain < 18% only had an AUC of 0.81 on the ROC curves [15]. In the same study, all patients with atrial fibrillation had a reservoir strain < 20%, regardless of the EF value, which means that atrial strain is of poor interest in atrial fibrillation.

Combining the LA strain with the classical indices E/A, E/e', LVEF, global LV longitudinal strain, LA indexed volume, tricuspid regurgitation velocity, can increase the accuracy of LV filling pressure estimation to more than 90%.

Heart Rate and Preload

The higher the HR, the shorter the LV filling time will be, which means a lower preload and a tendency to a lower SV. At the same time, the Bowditch effect will increase myocardial contraction, maintaining the same SV for a short period of time, but at higher HR, CO will no longer increase, and SV will decrease.

Left Ventricle Compliance and Preload Reserve

LV filling capacity is a function of LV filling time and compliance. An altered compliance implies a low to zero preload reserve, which occurs in several clinical situations: overstretching of myocardial fibers in dilated LV cardiomyopathies, pericardial restraint, ischemia, infiltrative diseases such as amyloid disease, increased myocardial stiffness commonly seen in HFpEF, acute or chronic right ventricular (RV) dilation. Passive leg raising during right heart catheterization creates an acute increased venous return during the next minute. Patients with HFpEF are unable to tolerate an increased venous return. A PCW of 19 mm Hg and above could be used to diagnose occult HFpEF with 100% accuracy, while a PCWP of less than 11 mm Hg could be used to rule out occult HFpEF [16]. In general, diastolic HF is associated with low preload reserve. In clinical practice, overtreatment of congestive HF (especially HFpEF) in an attempt to normalize wedge pressure may have a detrimental effect by excessively lowering preload, resulting in lower LV output. There is no mathematical formula, but clinical expertise must find a good compromise to maintain an efficient pressure gradient between wedge pressure and LVEDP.

Afterload and Afterload Mismatch

If the heart was to eject into a vascular system at a zero-opposing force, no pressure could be obtained, and no organ perfusion could be achieved. There is a distinction to be made: vascular mechanical load is the force opposing ventricular systolic flow, so it's a vascular force creating pressure, whereas LV afterload is the force opposing to the myocardial shortening during systole, so it's represented by the stress on the ventricular wall [17]. For example, aortic valve stenosis or LV outflow obstruction may increase afterload much more than vascular opposing force. On the other hand, in the absence of LV ejection obstruction, total systemic systolic load correctly reflects LV afterload. LV myocardial contraction-relaxation is an undulation of the same function, where myocardial fibre strain (wall stress) at end diastole is preload, whereas afterload is LV wall stress during systole. This is a non-linear function directly related to volume and pressure and inversely related to wall thickness according to Laplace's law. Variations in LV volume, wall thickness, and pressure during the cardiac cycle also determine variations in myocardial wall stress, i.e., the time-varying function. In an animal study (mammals and birds), maximum LV wall stress was calculated at end-diastolic volume against the systemic arterial diastolic BP [18]. Lower wall stress occurs in end-systole (lower volume, higher wall thickness). Basically, the higher wall stress occurs when the LV has the higher pressure against the higher volume and lower wall thickness—in humans during the isovolumic contraction. It might be tempting to apply Laplace's law for the afterload evaluation, LV Wall Stress = (Pressure × Radius)/(2 × wall thickness) but the Laplace principle applies to spheres while the LV may have very important geometry variations and variable wall thickness.

Opposing Force to LV Ejection

The arterial counterforce, the pulsatile load, represents a complex interaction between the arterial resistance (resistance of the smallest arteries and arterioles), the total arterial compliance and the characteristic arterial impedance—from which the three-element Windkessel model was created, which is the most widely used [19]. The three-element Windkessel is a lumped model and has a limited number of physiologically meaningful parameters, however, it can provide an adequate description of the pressure-flow relationships at the entrance to the arterial system.

A summary description of the elements composing the three-elements Windkessel model [20]:

- Ascending aortic characteristic impedance (Zc): (proximal aorta) governs load during early ejection.
- Systemic vascular resistance (SVR): a nonpulsatile component of afterload, depends on the number of arterioles in parallel (lesser resistance) and sensitive to arteriolar tone and rarefaction.

- Total arterial compliance (TAC): large arteries and, to a lesser extent, muscular arteries and small vessels, linearly proportional to vessel volume or radius and linearly and inversely proportional to wall stiffness.

The magnitude and timing of wave reflection (Fig. 8.2) are closely related to vascular stiffness. A high and/or early reflected wave will hit the downstream systolic flow and add additional afterload, which is detrimental in patients with HFpEF. At end-systole, when LV wall stress is lower, the myocardium may be more vulnerable. Late systolic load, even in subjects with normal EF, has been associated with LV hypertrophy and abnormal relaxation [20].

The relationship between volume, pressure, and fiber tension has been studied for more than a century. The maximum level at which myocardial fiber stretch still has a positive inotropic response represents the maximum preload reserve. During systole, the maximum level of fiber stretch still maintaining the same SV against the opposing arterial load has been called the maximum tolerable afterload [21]. However, according to the three-element Windkessel model, the only adaptive reserve is SVR. Vasodilation plays an important role in reducing afterload during exercise. Most therapeutic drugs (i.e. hypertension, HFrEF) are based on vasodilators. Higher aortic impedance, arterial stiffness, loss of peripheral arterioles and/or responsiveness will exhaust the adaptive mechanism.

John Ross defined this historic concept: "Afterload mismatch can be simply described as the inability of the left ventricle, operating at any stable level of inotropic state, to maintain a normal stroke volume against the prevailing systolic load on

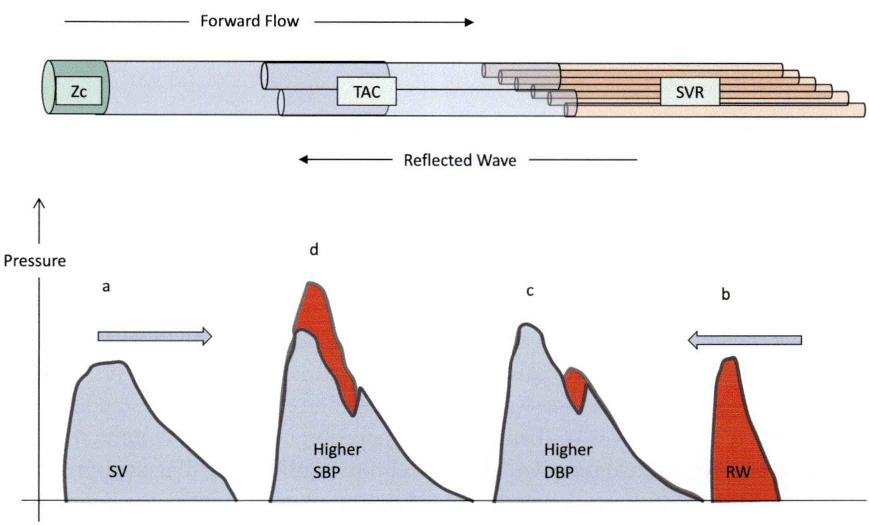

Fig. 8.2 (**a**) Virtual Stroke Volume pressure curve without reflected wave; (**b**) Reflected Wave; (**c**) Diastolic Blood Pressure elevation by a precocious RW; (**d**) Systolic Blood Pressure elevation by an even more precocious RW. *Zc* ascending aortic impedance, *TAC* total arterial compliance, *SVR* systemic vascular resistance

the ventricle, and it generally occurs in the setting of limited preload reserve" [22]. Limited or exhausted preload reserve is the situation where the LV can no longer benefit from the length-tension relationship, and no inotropy is added when preload is increased. Ross also defined the concept of ventricular afterload sensitivity in conditions of altered contractility and fully exploited preload reserve. In such situations, afterload mismatch can occur at different levels of systolic pressure and SV. In simple terms, when preload and contractile reserve are exhausted, LV function is largely determined by afterload status. Afterload mismatch is a core situation in HF that is well defined by the ventriculo-arterial coupling (VAC). In the presence of afterload mismatch, CR measured by volumetric tests (SV, EF) may not be detected by clinical stress tests, which may increase afterload beyond tolerable limits. Preload and afterload represent two different moments on the same undulatory function of the relation between load and fiber stretch. The approximation of the myocardial wall stress, diastolic or systolic, might be the closest approach to preload and afterload.

Let's say it as in a storytelling: in terms of tissue survival, the heart does not "decide" the level of CO required but is subject to the "decisions" of the circulatory and neurohormonal systems. A high level of wall stress is a detrimental "burning" situation for the myocardium, from which it will "escape" by contraction at a high energy cost, until the excessive wall stress is removed.

> It is my contention that preload and afterload should be consistently defined in terms of myocardial wall stress (or tension) and that the definitions should always include the major factors affecting wall tension for each, namely, chamber pressure, chamber radius, and wall thickness. If you keep wall stress or "wall tension" built into your definitions of preload and afterload, you will be better able, in my opinion, to help your students understand cardiovascular pathophysiology and the therapeutic approaches to heart disease. (Norton JM [23])

Systolic Wall Stress as a Reflection of the Afterload on the LV Myocardial Wall

Wall stress can be considered as a time-varying interaction between LV volume, geometry, wall thickness, afterload and contraction.

Wall stress calculation: There are two types of models, the thin layer model and the thick layer model. The latter, very complex, is closer to the LV anatomy. According to it, the LV wall is made up of several layers, the inner one with the higher stress and the outer one with a much lower stress. It is understandable why an uncorrected inner layer wall stress by the appropriate systolic volume reduction (i.e. EF) and wall thickening will keep a chronic subendocardial unappropriated fiber tension, high oxygen demands exceeding the oxygen supply, leading to myocardial alteration.

As a general mathematical assumption, Arts et al. note for the thin-layer cylindrical model that the dimensionless ratio of muscle fiber stress to left ventricular pressure appears to depend mainly on the dimensionless ratio of cavity volume to wall volume and is quite independent of other geometric parameters [24]. A good and simple approximation (±10%) of this relationship is:

$$WS / LVp = 1 + 3^{*} LVv / LVw$$

(WS: wall stress; LV pressure; LVv: LV volume; LVw: LV wall thickness).

Fiber stress in a thick layer model can be calculated by the formula:

$$WS = P / \left[1/3 \ln\left(1 + V_W / V_{LV}\right)\right]$$

(P = pressure, ln = natural logarithm, V_W = wall volume, and V_{LV} = ventricular cavity volume)

This formula takes into account the radial forces or forces generated within the wall that oppose fiber shortening, which vary significantly with cavity and wall thickness and can interfere with direct comparisons of myocardial stress at different times during ejection [25].

However, circumferential wall stress is strongly dependent on geometry and variable LV wall thickness. MRI with adapted software can propose a 3D regional curvature-based wall stress approach, applied to HF, dilated cardiomyopathy or hypertrophic cardiomyopathy [26].

Can We Consider Wall Stress a Contractility Index?

Fundamentally, the answer is no, but we can use it as a companion to volumetric indices. Wall stress is a measure of myocardial wall tension, in diastole or systole, reflecting preload (promoting contraction) or afterload (maintaining or increasing contraction). Systolic contraction reduces wall stress at end-systole, by increasing wall thickness and decreasing LV volume, i.e., contraction reduces wall stress. It is important to note that the contraction leading to LV cavity reduction will occur at a given wall stress level. To achieve the same EF at a high wall stress level, LV requires a more forceful contraction compared to a lower wall stress level. In patients with afterload mismatch (i.e., dilated cardiomyopathy) only the afterload reduction, shifting at a lower level the wall stress, may increase the EF. That's why wall stress, without being a contraction index by itself, can be used as a "companion" to volumetric indices, reflecting (but not measuring) the contraction level of the ventricle. De Simone et al. developed important concepts of midwall LV mechanics relating fractional shortening to end-systolic stress, with meridional end-systolic stress closely related to midwall circumferential end-systolic wall stress [27, 28]. The authors demonstrated that endocardial fractional shortening overestimates LV performance in hypertensive patients with circumferential remodeling. The relationship between midwall fractional shortening and midwall end-systolic stress identified 16.5% of hypertensive patients with normal fractional shortening but depressed LV myocardial function.

Wall Stress as a Companion to Fractional Shortening/ Ejection Fraction

Plotting midwall shortening fraction (mSF) or derived EF, against circumferential end-systolic stress (cESS) indicates the value of EF that is able to reduce end-systolic stress to normal limits, i.e., normal contraction, demonstrating a good contractile reserve. Conversely, it shows the situation where, despite an apparent normal EF, the cESS remains higher than normal, i.e., a weaker than necessary contraction to unload the myocardium from a high wall stress, demonstrating a depressed or exhausted contractile reserve. mSF is more sensitive than endocardial shortening fraction in patients with AS, where due to LV hypertrophy, EF may appear to be preserved despite underlying reduced contractility.

What Is the LV CR Required to Ensure Survival in a Patient with Aortic Stenosis (AS)? This is an important question; a situation close to the notion of "maximum tolerable afterload", whether or not the LV still has contractile reserve, whether or not there is myocardial damage due to chronic pressure overload.

Ito S, Pislaru C, Miranda W, et al. based on the mSF and cESS formulae of de Simone et al. retrospectively studied a group of patients with non-severe aortic stenosis (AS) that became severe at a 3-year interval [29]. Two groups were compared with a median follow-up of 3.4 years, with an EF cut-off of 60% and a cESS upper limit of 145 kDynes/cm. Contractility was quantified by calculating the percentage of predicted mFS relative to that of the normal population (stress-corrected mFS) at the same wall stress level. Interestingly, the study showed that in patients with severe AS, LVEF $< 60\%$ is associated with a poor prognosis and is associated with reduced contractility and/or high wall stress. Decreased contractility was also present in a subset of patients with EF $\geq 60\%$ (normal EF but elevated wall stress) providing additional prognostic value. These abnormalities were present before AVA reaches 1.0 cm^2. As to have the best survival prediction, mFS ($>15\%$) or the derived EF ($\geq 60\%$) has to be associated to a cESS < 145 kDynes/cm. This study demonstrates that increased wall stress needs, in terms of survival, a good contractile reserve able to increase the EF, above the standard values, as to lower the wall stress. The mSF, cESS formulas are based on simple measurements with long equations, that may be consulted in the publications of de Simone et al. [27] and Ito et al. [29].

Contractile Function of the LV Against a Pressure Overload

The LV in patients with AS must struggle with a large counterforce against contraction force. A simple formula for valvulo-arterial impedance (Zva) is the ratio of systolic BP (SBP) + mean aortic valve gradient (mean AVG) divided by indexed systolic volume (SVi):

$$Zva = (SBP + mean AVG) / SVi.$$

In the absence of aortic stenosis and when the mean gradient is negligible, the Zva formula becomes similar to the effective aortic elastance formula, Ea = (SBP * 0.9)/SV. A simple formula derived from Zva is the sum of pressures ignoring SV and provides a surrogate marker of cardiac contractile function against systemic afterload in patients with aortic stenosis. In a retrospective study of 974 patients undergoing transcatheter aortic valve replacement (TAVR), Chao et al. [30] found that augmented mean arterial pressure (Aug MAP1) was strongly associated with post-TAVR mortality and was superior to the STS risk score in predicting mortality. Several calculation variants of augmented pressure were used:

1. MAP = (SBP + 2 × DBP)/3 (MAP: mean arterial pressure)
2. Augmented SBP1 = mean AVG + SBP (AVG: mean aortic valve gradient; SBP: systolic blood pressure)
3. Augmented MAP1 = (AugSBP1 + 2 × DBP)/3 (DBP: diastolic blood pressure)
4. Augmented SBP2 = max instantaneous AVG + SBP
5. Augmented MAP2 = (AugSBP2 + 2 × DBP)/3
6. Augmented MAP3 = MAP + mean AVG
7. Zva = (SBP + mean AVG)/SVi

The best predictor was an AugMAP1 value of <102.5 mmHg, which was associated with a threefold increased risk of all-cause mortality at 1 year after TAVR. This simple index was more predictive than the STS score (ROC curve: area under the curve 0.700 vs. 0.587) and better than Zva (area under the curve: 0.700 vs. 0.559). In short, patients who survived were those who were able to maintain significantly higher blood pressure before TAVR (systolic, diastolic, and mean) compared to those who died.

Pharmacological Tests Used for LV CR Investigation

The most widespread pharmacological test uses Dobutamine, which is a potent inotrope, with weaker chronotropic activity, producing a mild decrease in SVR. Doses up to 15 μg/kg/min increase cardiac contractility without greatly affecting peripheral resistance; vasoconstriction progressively dominates at higher infusion rates [8]. Because of this property, the low-dose dobutamine infusion protocol is widely used for CR. The dobutamine infusion is usually started at 5 mg/kg/min but titrated upward in steps of 2.5–5 mg/kg/min every 5–8 min. After each increment in dobutamine dose, a period of 2–3 min before starting the image acquisition will allow the hemodynamic response to develop. At higher doses, tachycardia, arrhythmias, hypertension and possibly myocardial ischemia may blunt the result by reducing the contractile response. In patients with possible severe aortic valve stenosis, the maximal dose is usually 20 mg/kg/min; higher doses are less safe and probably unnecessary [31].

However, with low doses of dobutamine, the vasodilator effect may predominate over the contractile effect, so that a reduction in afterload may result in a favorable EF or SV outcome with little or no increased contraction—in other words, VAC improvement with little or no CR. On the other hand, beta-adrenergic receptors are downregulated in patients with advanced HF, but also in milder forms of HF, thus impairing the contractile response to dobutamine [32].

Dipyridamole and Adenosine
Based on the Gregg effect, a potent coronary vasodilator may be used to investigate contractile reserve [33]. Administration of dipyridamole: 0.84 mg/kg over 6 min or 10 min; or an initial dose of 0.56 mg/kg over 4 min sometimes followed by 4 min of no dose and additional 0.28 mg/kg over 2 min. Adenosine may be used at 140 mg/kg/min over 4–6 min to a maximum of 60 mg [31]. A head-to-head comparative study between Dobutamine and Dipyridamole in patients with dilated cardiomyopathy, based on EF and wall motion score, found no significant difference [34].

Exercise Testing for LV Contractile Reserve

Exercise is more physiological than dobutamine and can be quantified in METs, watts and blood pressure. The physiologic increase in cardiac load (pressure and volume) avoids the false results that can sometimes occur with dobutamine testing. When possible, exercise echocardiography appears to be superior to dobutamine testing. In the absence of ischemia, dobutamine reduces left ventricular volume, wall stress and peak systolic stress compared to exercise [35].

Maximal Myocardial Workload

Maximal exercise is a global hemodynamic capacity testing at high frequency rate, where the heart is volume-pressure overloaded. Whitman et al. revived the old "double product" (maximum HR × maximum systolic pressure: maximum rate pressure product: MRPP) by stress testing in 1080 patients with a follow-up of 5.3 years. MRPP (cut-off: 25,085) was the best predictor of cardiac events, compared with the percentage of maximal HR achieved or HR reserve [36]. Patients with an MRPP < 25,085 had almost 9 times more cardiovascular events at 10 years compared to those with an adequate myocardial workload (MRPP ≥ 25,085).

Protocols for LV Exercise Contractile Reserve

No standard protocol exists; upright, supine or semi-supine exercise is mostly used in Europe, while treadmill exercise is more popular in North America [31].

Treadmill (upright exercise) results in a higher HR than supine exercise, the latter producing a significant and early venous return (high preload). Echo-Doppler is technically difficult during upright exercise, but feasible during supine or semi-supine exercise. Semi-supine exercise offers a good compromise, allowing imaging during exercise. An exercise protocol for HFpEF was proposed by Erdei et al. [37]. The echo Doppler study must be combined with blood pressure monitoring, ECG, VO2 max measurement or at least O2 saturation.

The ABCDE Protocol

It is proposed as an integrated method for all types of physical or pharmacological stress modalities and allows a more integrated assessment of patient vulnerability beyond the detection of anatomic coronary artery disease (CAD): Step A, regional wall motion abnormalities (WMSI); Step B, B-lines; Step C, left ventricular contractile reserve; Step D, Doppler-based coronary flow velocity reserve in the left anterior descending coronary artery; and Step E, electrocardiogram-based HR reserve [38]. This approach to ABCDE-SE allows assessment of inducible myocardial ischemia (Step A), pulmonary congestion (Step B), contractile reserve (Step C), coronary microvascular dysfunction (Step D), and cardiac sympathetic reserve (Step E).

Wall Motion Score Index (WMSI) and CR in Non-ischemic Cardiomyopathies

WMSI is a widespread diagnostic method, mainly used in coronary artery disease (CAD) patients. Bach et al. described the heterogeneity of the LV wall in non-CAD dilated cardiomyopathy with EF < 30%, where 54% of the patients had an increased regional function in the basal lateral wall [39]. Segmental contraction scoring before and after exercise or pharmacological testing, is an affordable way to evaluate the contractile response. Otasevic et al. compared the predictability of several contractility indices at 5-year follow-up, using high-dose dobutamine stress testing (up to 40 μg/kg/min) in 63 patients with dilated cardiomyopathy [40]. The following cut-offs were identified at dobutamine echocardiography: WMSI $\geq$ 0.19, EF $\geq$ 6%,

CPO ≥ 0.44 W and ESPVR ≥ 0.33 as to predict a poor or favorable 5-years prognosis [40]. A multivariate Cox regression only identified dobutamine-induced change in WMSI as an independent predictor of cardiac mortality over the 5-year period.

B-Lines and Stress Echocardiography

During stress echocardiography, acute pulmonary congestion may occur due to high capillary hydrostatic pressure. Pulmonary echography can quantify stress-induced congestion by counting the number of B-lines which reflect extravascular lung water [41, 42]. The development of B-lines and their number indicates the severity of exercise-induced lung congestion, which has an important prognostic role.

Chronotropic Reserve (Heart Rate Reserve) and Chronotropic Incompetence

CO adapts to demand by varying SV and HR. The increase in HR is a fundamental response to the need to increase CO, controlled by increased sympathetic and/or decreased parasympathetic drive. During exercise, at low levels of stress, CO will increase by the increased preload, through the Starling law, but at higher levels, HR augmentation is required. Normal chronotropic reserve or HR reserve (HRR) means that the age-related maximum HR can be achieved, whereas chronotropic incompetence (CI) is the inability to achieve the predicted maximum HR. As exercise testing has gained much interest in patients at risk of or with HF, it is important to use the appropriate predictive HR formula. Maximal HR declines with age at a rate of ~0.7 beats min in healthy sedentary subjects [43]. Based on this inescapable age-related decline, the theoretical maximum HR is generally calculated using the formula 220 – age. Simple and widely used, this formula has serious limitations [44]. An alternative formula was described by Tanaka et al. (208–0.7 × age) becoming more accepted for determining age-predicted maximal HR and being recommended for apparently healthy persons [44, 45]. Brawner et al· developed a regression formula obtained on coronary artery disease patients on betablocker medication [46]:

$$\text{HR}(\max) = 164 - 0.7 \times \text{age}.$$

HR reserve (HRR) can be calculated as a simple percentage:

$$HRR = \left(\left[\text{peak}\,HR - \text{resting}\,HR\right] / \left[APMHR - \text{resting}\,HR\right] \times 100\right);$$

(APMHR: Age Predicted maximal Heart Rate)

In general, a HRR of <80% of the age-predicted HRR is used to consider chronotropic incompetence [47].

Studies on Contractile Reserve (CR)

Thein et al. performed a systematic review that identified 27 eligible studies (2425 patients) on LV contractile reserve (LVCR): 70% of the studies were performed with dobutamine, 15% with exercise, 7% with dipyridamole, 4% were invasive and 4% by magnetic resonance [48]. LV contractile reserve (LVCR) was assessed by volumetric indices in the majority of studies (55.5%: Δ EF 40.7%, ΔSV 11.1%, Δ fractional area 3.7%), 33.3% Δ wall motion score, 7.4% Δ global strain rate, 3.7% Δ cardiac output, 3.7% ΔS′. The majority of studies dedicated to LVCR are based on the variation of volumetric indices under low-dose dobutamine. Considering an increase in EF or SV as a sign of good CR is a reductive conclusion, since the volumetric effect obtained is the result of the interplay between preload reserve, systemic resistances (decreased or not by dobutamine, generally increased by exercise), and contraction force. Contractility, except in vitro studies, does not function in a stand-alone mode, and for a comprehensive approach it must be integrated into the ventriculo-arterial coupling (VAC), which is determined by the two opposing forces: ventricular systolic elastance (Ees) versus arterial elastance (Ea).

Left Ventricular Elastance (Ees) and Pressure-Volume Loops

Elastance is the opposite of compliance or distensibility and refers to elasticity. Both elastance and compliance are measured in units of pressure and volume: Elastance is expressed in mmHg/ml and, conversely, compliance is expressed in ml/mmHg. Pioneers in the study of contractility, Suga and Sagawa showed that the momentum corresponding to the end of contraction (maximum pressure) at the minimum LV volume (end-systolic), the end-systolic pressure-volume ratio (LVESP/LVESV = ESPVR), is rather insensitive to loading conditions but sensitive to inotropic interventions [49] (Fig. 8.3).

Multiple pressure-volume loops can be obtained relative to a variable such as contractility, afterload, or preload. Connecting the points from each curve, corresponding to the upper left corner, the end-systolic pressure-volume ratio, draws a linear relationship of the various ESPVR points characterized by the elastance slope

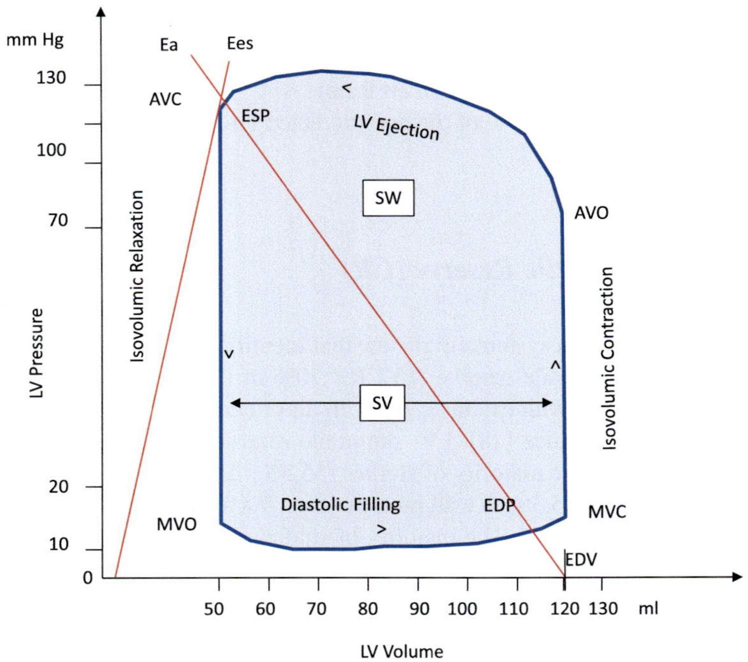

Fig. 8.3 The four phases of the cardiac cycle are displayed by plotting instantaneous pressure against volume, creating the pressure-volume loop. *MVO* mitral valve opening, *MVC* mitral valve closure, *AVO* aortic valve opening, *AVC* aortic valve closure, *ESP* end systolic pressure, *EDP* end diastolic pressure, *SV* stroke volume, *SW* stroke work

(Ees) (Fig. 8.4a) The point where this slope intercepts the zero-pressure line is the zero-pressure volume (V0). V0 is an extrapolated value, representing the unstressed LV volume intercept of the volume axis at a theoretical end-systolic pressure of 0 mmHg. Its value can be either positive or negative (Fig. 8.4b). The elastance formula is based on Ees = LVESP/(LVESV – Vo) where LVESV is the end-systolic volume and LVESP is the end-systolic pressure. V0 is a virtual non-physiologic volume, close to 0 ml in normal subjects, positive to highly positive in enlarged remodeled LV, and rather negative in small hearts [50]. Vo is approximated to be 0 mL in many studies for non-enlarged, non-remodeled left ventricles. Seven invasive studies in normal subjects demonstrated mean V0 values close to 0 mL: Starling, V0 = 1 ± 23 mL [51]; Maughan et al. 8 V0 = 5.5 ± 1.0 mL [52]; Senzaki et al. V0 = between +2.1 and −3.14 mL [53]; and Asanoi et al. V0 = 4 mL/m 2 (between −10 and +26 mL) [54]. However, even if the mean value for the normal subjects is near 0 mL, inside the groups, there are high individual variations [55]. Despite V0's virtual status, it's important to stress that V0 is not a simple volume, but a volume related to pressure which makes it a strong predictor of cardiac function.

Because end-systolic pressure-volume curves are nonlinear and time-varying, with different shapes depending on the contractile state, Ees and V0 intercept covary [49]. Ees is called time-varying elastance. The maximum value of elastance and the

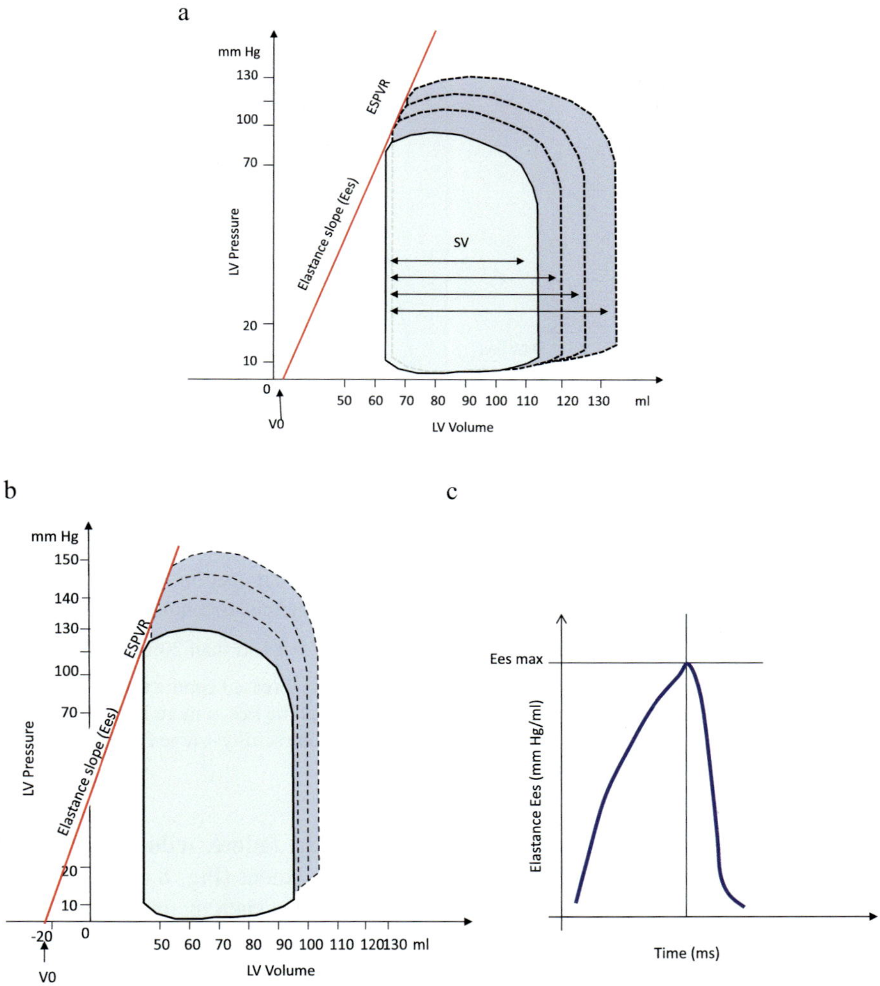

Fig. 8.4 (**a**) Serial pressure-volume loops obtained by preload augmentation. Connecting the points from each curve, corresponding to the upper left corner, the end-systolic pressure-volume ratio, draws a linear relationship of the various ESPVR points characterized by the elastance slope (Ees). (**b**) Hypertensive response to exercise. The Ees slope intercept the 0 mm Hg pressure line at a negative V0 value (−20 ml). (**c**) LV time-varying elastance. The maximum value of elastance and the time to reach it, characterize the instantaneous pressure-volume ratio curve

time taken to reach it characterise the instantaneous pressure-volume ratio curve [56] (Fig. 8.4c). Within physiological limits, Ees is a load-independent measure of left ventricular contraction (chamber stiffness at end systole). An increase in contractility is represented by an increase in slope and a leftward shift of the end-systolic pressure-volume relationship, i.e., more force of contraction increases pressure against the same volume [57] (Fig. 8.5). Reduced contractility will shift the slope to the right (Fig. 8.6a). In severe heart failure, where contractile force is

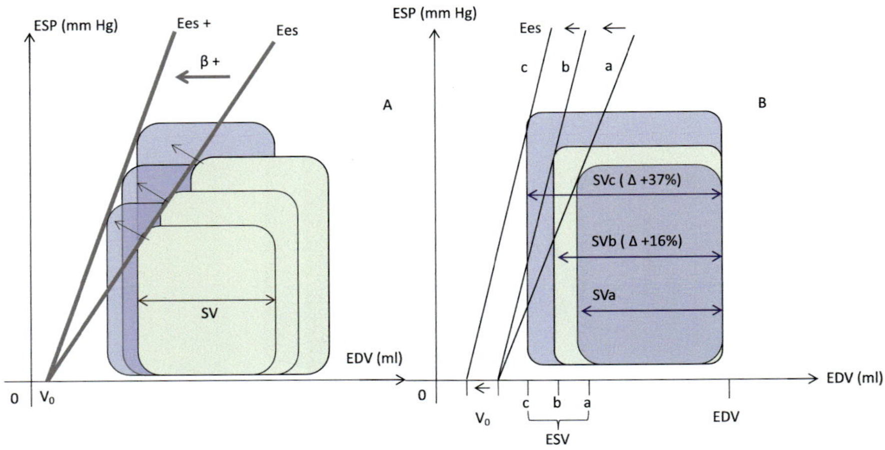

Fig. 8.5 (**a**) Influence of inotropic stimulation on pressure-volume loops resulting in higher end-systolic pressure-volume ratio (ESPVR). Multiple ESPVR points will draw the line of end-systolic elastance (Ees). Ees is shifted to the left by inotropic stimulation. (**b**) Sketch of stroke volume variation (flow reserve) during low-dose dobutamine echocardiography in a failing dilated LV. EDV was considered constant. *ESP* end systolic pressure, *EDV* end diastolic volume, ΔSV stroke volume variation, *a* basal Ees, *b* stimulated Ees by 10 μg/kg/min, *c* stimulated Ees by 20 μg/kg/min. $E_{es} = \frac{ESP}{ESV - V0}$. a→b: A moderate increase in +ΔSV but less than 20%, produced by a shift to the left (arrow) of the Ees and a steeper angle related to increased contractility. b→c variation shows the possible role of V0, obtaining a shift to the left of the Ees, a more important +ΔSV but due to a lower V0 volume and not by a further increase in contractility—note Ees (b) is parallel to Ees (c) without notable angle modification

exhausted and afterload is increased, as in acute heart failure, reducing afterload allows SV to increase regardless of elastance enhancement (Fig. 8.6b). However, Ees is also determined by structural myocardial changes such as myocardial stiffness or myocyte compliance or fibrosis. A concentric remodeling, a stiffer LV will need a higher Ees to eject into a stiffer aorta. Ees should therefore be considered as an integrated measure of left ventricular chamber performance that can be related to an integrated measure of arterial load (i.e., Ea). In their editorial, Chantler and Lakatta emphasized that because Vo and Ees are measured on a linear segment of a nonlinear function, the values of these parameters will covary with changes in inotropic or loading conditions [57]. However, if a serial measurement is performed in the same subject with unchanged LV structure, a shift in ESPVR clearly indicates a change in intrinsic myocardial contractility, emphasizing the appropriateness of acute studies such as administration of positive inotropes or exercise. What do we measure and what should we measure to evaluate CR, ESPVR or Ees? The simple ESPVR approach ignores V0, so the simple relationship between LVESP/LVESV (ESPVR) is related to Ees. Each new stage of inotropic intervention will create another point, drawing a line correlated (but not identical) to Ees.

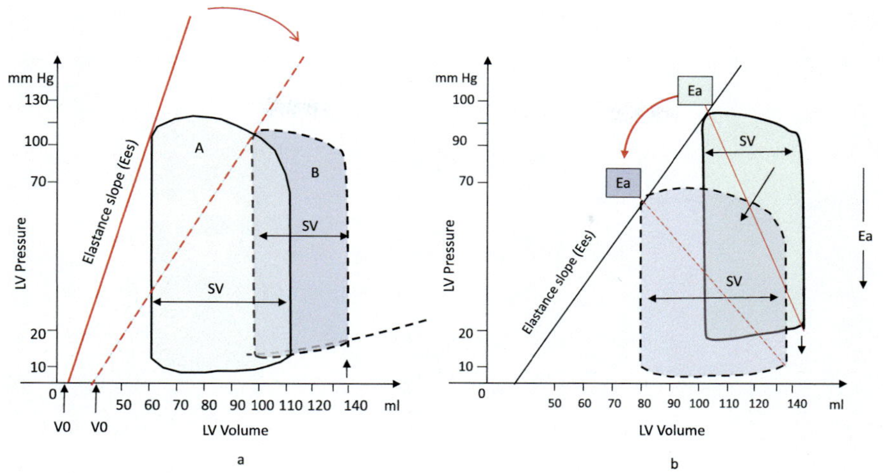

Fig. 8.6 (**a**) Acute heart failure with severe rightward PVL shift: higher EDP, higher V0, lower SV, lower ESP, and lower Ees. (**b**) Forceful afterload reduction (i.e., sodium nitroprusside) in a patient with acute heart failure and severe rightward PVL shift. Ees remains decreased, but the significant reduction in Ea will increase SV and decrease EDP. *EDP* end-diastolic pressure, *ESP* end-systolic pressure

As to offer a wider clinical application for non-invasive studies, several formulae for "single-beat Ees" estimation were proposed by: Senzaki [53], Shishido [58], Chen [59].

The mostly used formula was proposed by Chen et al. based on: systolic and diastolic pressure, SV, LVEF, pre-ejection time and total ejection time [59]:

$$\mathrm{Ees} = \left(\mathrm{DBP} - \left(\mathrm{End}\left(\mathrm{est}\right) \times \mathrm{SBP} \times 0.9\right)\right) / \mathrm{End}\left(\mathrm{est}\right) \times \mathrm{SV}$$

(DBP: diastolic blood pressure cuff estimation; SBP: systolic arterial pressure by cuff estimation; End(est): estimated normalized ventricular elastance at the onset of ejection; SV: Doppler-derived stroke volume)

$$\mathrm{End}\left(\mathrm{est}\right) = 0.0275 - 0.165 \times \mathrm{LVEF} + 0.3656 \times \left(\mathrm{DBP}/\mathrm{SBP} \times 0.9\right) + 0.515 \times \mathrm{End}\left(\mathrm{avg}\right)$$

$$\mathrm{End}\left(\mathrm{avg}\right) = 0.35695 - 7.2266 \times \mathrm{tNd} + 74.249 \times \mathrm{tNd}^2 - 307.39 \times \mathrm{tNd}^3 + 684.54 \times \mathrm{tNd}^4$$
$$-856.92 \times \mathrm{tNd}^5 + 571.95 \times \mathrm{tNd}^6 - 159.1 \times \mathrm{tNd}^7$$

tNd is the ratio of pre-ejection time (PEP) to total systolic time (TET). $E_{Nd(est)}$ is group-averaged value adjusted for individual contractile/loading effects, needing computation facilities.

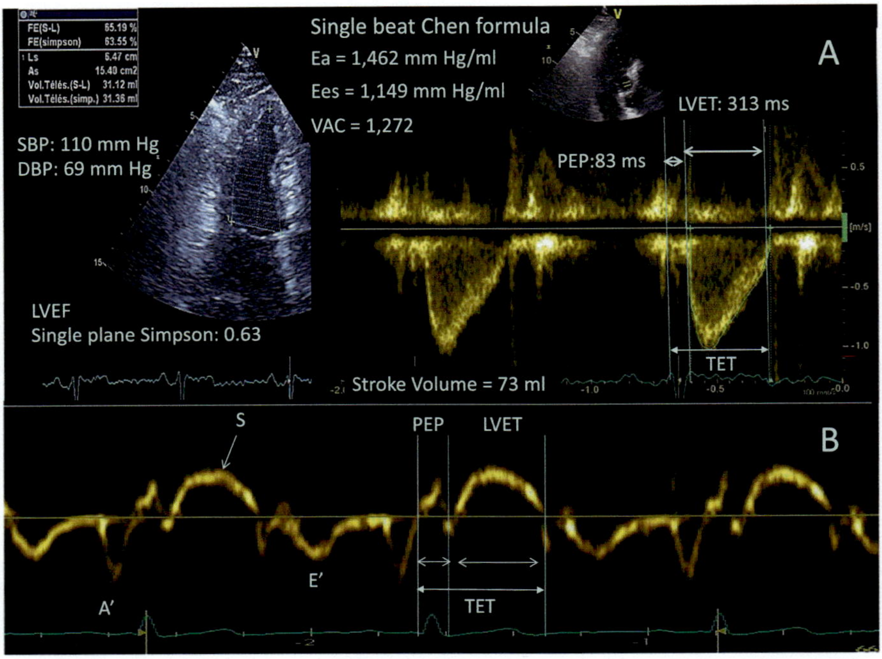

Fig. 8.7 Systolic time intervals can be measured by spectral pulsed Doppler or tissue Doppler at a high scrolling speed, at least 100 mm/s. *PEP* pre-ejection period, *LVET* left ventricle ejection time, *TET* total ejection time

This formula is highly sensitive to systolic time intervals, "tNd" being used from 1 to its 7th order! A 5 ms variation for the isovolumic contraction time can lead up to 9% variation of the calculated Es. LVESP is approximated from the brachial artery systolic pressure (greatest obtained value) where LVESP = 0.9 * SBP (brachial artery) [60]. Systolic time intervals can be measured by spectral pulsed Doppler or tissue Doppler (Fig. 8.7) at a high scrolling speed, at least 100 mm/s. Compared to the ESPVR, this formula is better correlated to Ees, while ESPVR overestimates Ees, especially for greater values. Another method of calculating "single beat Ees" was published by Shishido et al. which requires invasive measurement of LVEDP. [58]:

$$E_{es(SB)} = \left[P_{ad} + \left(P_{ad} - P_{ed}\right) / PEP \times ET \times \alpha - P_{es}\right] / SV$$

($Ees_{(SB)}$: single-beat estimation of Ees, P_{ad}: pressure at the end of isovolumic contraction, P_{ed}: end-diastolic pressure, P_{es}: end-systolic pressure, SV: stroke volume) $\alpha = -0.21 + 1.348 \times \text{LVEF} + 0.682 \times \text{ICT}/(\text{ICT} + \text{ET})$ (ICT: isovolumic contraction time: ET: ejection time).

Non-invasive estimation of LVESP is possible. A dobutamine echo study (5 and 10 μg/kg/min) in control subjects and dilated cardiomyopathy with low LVEF compared Chen's and Shishido's formulas [61]. LVEDP was derived from Doppler pulmonary venous diastolic deceleration time, LV volumes were calculated by 3D echocardiography, and LVSP was assessed by carotid tonometry. In normal subjects, mean Es values were 1.8 mmHg/ml (1.7–1.9) using Chen's formula and 2.18 mmHg/ml using Shishido's formula. Chen's formula showed considerable overlap between the two groups, whereas Shishido's formula showed no overlap and better reproducibility.

In an animal study, Wo et al. compared several single beat formulas with the multiple beat Ees calculation (considered the gold standard) and found that Shishido's formula had the best correlation [62]. All current methods performed better when afterload was increased. However, Chen's formula is the most widely used. As for any other single-beat formula, it is highly informative for individual variations.

In short, to get as close as possible to Ees with a single beat formula, 3 parameters are needed: pressure, volume and time. The systolic time intervals (STI), despite their high diagnostic value, have been forgotten in current practice. Time is an important determinant of contractile function. The longer the pre-ejection period (PEP) and the shorter the LV ejection time (LVET), the more the LV contraction is affected. Reant et al. in 134 heart failure patients and 43 control subjects, found a strong correlation between PEP/LVET with LVEF or Global Longitudinal Strain (GLS): R = −0.78 and 0.75 respectively [63].

PEP, LVET and/or total ejection time (TET = PEP + LVET) are used in Chen and Shishido's formulae. As an example of the high diagnostic value, the simple ratio SBP/PEP (SBP: systolic blood pressure) had a strong correlation with Chen's Ees formula (R = 0.92; R^2 = 0.84) [64]. In an attempt to make Chen's formula more understandable, the following formula was developed, using multiple regression, in a group of 33 patients with LVEF between 10% and 65%:

$$Ees\_d = \frac{SBP * 0.9}{SV * \left(0.553291 - 0.008988 * LVEF + 3.462988 * \frac{PEP}{TET}\right)}$$

(Where: Ees_d: derived Ees by multiple regression; SV: stroke volume; LVEF: LV ejection fraction;). Ees_d correlated, to Chen's Ees formula with R = 0.97 and R^2 = 0.95 meaning a 95% predictability with only 5% risk of error [64]. By this simple way of expressing the formula, it is easy to understand that SV, LVEF and STI, which are all load-dependent, have a large influence on the result, which means that Chen's Ees formula cannot be load-independent. In a very elaborate sensitivity analysis, Di Molfetta et al. showed that the Chen method, like all other single-beat methods, contains elements that are highly load-dependent, such as LV diastolic properties, LV stroke volume, ejection time, and pre-ejection time [65]. In addition, single beat elastance increases with higher LV end-systolic volume and decreases with higher SV, in contrast to the LV elastance definition. Single beat elastance was also found to be strongly dependent on cardiocirculatory parameters such as HR and arterial resistance [65].

In short, single-beat formulas are useful for detecting altered LV contraction but are less specific for dynamic CR because they are load dependent.

End-Systolic Pressure-Volume Ratio (ESPVR) an Elastance Surrogate

Easier to calculate in non-invasive studies, the variation of the End-Systolic Pressure-Volume Ratio (ESPVR) is well correlated to contractility being sensitive for contractile reserve testing. On this basis, Bombardini et al. studied the Force-Frequency Relation (FFR) based Δ ESPVR (: ESPVR mmHg/mL/m^2) in 400 in patients with left ventricular dysfunction (LVEF: 30 ± 9%) and negative stress echocardiography results [33]. The event-free survival was higher ($p < 0.001$) in patients with ΔESPVR ≥ 0.4 mmHg/mL/m^2. Same authors, in 10 echo studies on a total number of 1502 patients, calculated the predictive value for cardiac death (10/10 studies) heart failure or heart failure aggravation (6/10 studies). The positive predictive value was variable, sometimes rather weak (24% up to 77%), while the negative predictive value was very strong (84% up to 98%).

Reserve (ΔESPVR ≥ 0.4 mmHg/mL/m^2) was studied for its prognostic value of stress-induced in 891 patients with negative stress echocardiography (exercise, Dobutamine or Dipyridamole). Predictability of the ESPVR reserve was tested for death and heart failure hospitalization. Best results were found for exercise (AUC = 0.871) and dobutamine (AUC = 0.848) and in lesser degree the VAC reserve (AUC = 0.696) for dipyridamole [66].

Clinical outcome after cardiac resynchronization therapy (CRT) is contractility dependent. Echo-derived Δ ESPVR under dobutamine infusion has been used to predict improvement after CRT [67]. The cut-off value for Δ ESPVR was set to >0.72 mmHg/ml/m^2. Responder criteria for follow-up were clinical improvement and LVESV decrease >15%. Patients with higher ESPVR had better clinical improvement (86% vs. 46%, $P < .001$) and were better echocardiographic responders to CRT (79% vs. 40%, $P = .002$).

Considering that the complexity of the formulas hinders the dissemination of LVCR, the ESPVR in stress echocardiography was further simplified and referred to as "force" following the policy of "simplification for success". The term force refers to the force of contraction and not to the physical definition [68]. The author proposes to transform ESP/ESV into a simple dimensionless ratio SBP/ESV to provide an easily usable index during stress echocardiography without the correction of 0.9 for SBP or body mass index for ESV. LVCR is calculated as the peak to rest ratio of left ventricular force. LVCR values during dobutamine or exercise stress >2 indicate normal, 1.5–2.0 mild, 1.01–1.49 moderate, or ≤1.0 severe dysfunction. For vasodilators, normal values are lower: abnormal <1.1.

Arterial Effective Elastance (Ea)

The LV doesn't eject into a free space, its function is a component of a more complex system function described as VAC. Borlaug and Kass defines this relation as the optimal transfer of blood from heart to periphery without excessive changes in BP or a way to provide optimal cardiovascular flow reserve without compromising arterial pressure [69]. The LV is coupled to an arterial load composed of peripheral vascular resistance (largely determined by the small arteries), total arterial compliance (largely determined by the central elastic arteries), characteristic impedance, and systolic and diastolic time intervals. Sunagawa et al. in dogs and Kelly et al. in humans, grouped all the components of the arterial load in an all-in-one single entity named effective arterial elastance (Ea), measured in the same units as the Ees (mmHg/ml) as to compare LV contraction stiffness to the total arterial load [70, 71]. Ea = LVESP/SV, where LVESP may be estimated as 0.9 × Systolic brachial pressure. Ea is intended to integrate resistive and pulsatile components of the afterload.

Segers et al. based on a mathematical model, concluded that Ea has a linear relationship with R/T (R: peripheral vascular resistance; T: cycle length) and 1/C (C: compliance) E(a) = −0.127 + 1.02R/T + 0.31/C, indicating that R/T contributes about three times more to Ea than arterial stiffness (1/C) [72]. This relationship indicates that tachycardia by shortening the cardiac cycle length, sometimes associated with inadequate arterial dilation during exercise, may play an important role in increasing Ea. On the other hand, age-related arterial stiffening, by decreasing compliance (C), will cause a progressive and irreversible increase in Ea [73].

Segers formula can be calculated as follows:

$$\mathrm{Ea} = -0.127 + 1.02\mathrm{R} / \mathrm{T} + 0.314 / \mathrm{C} = -0.127 + 1.023 * \frac{(MAP - CVP) / CO}{T(cyclelength)} + \left(0.314 : \frac{SV}{PP}\right)$$

(where R: systemic resistance; T: time (cycle length); CVP: central venous pressure; C:vascular compliance). C can be approximated by the SV/PP ratio (SV: stroke volume; PP: pulse pressure) and CVP by the inferior vena cava collapsibility [74]. In a study of 33 patients, the Ea formula (LVESP * 0.9)/SV was compared with the Ea obtained by the Segers formula. No significant difference were found, and the correlation was almost perfect ($R^2 = 0.97$) [64].

Ventriculo-Arterial Coupling (Vac)

Ventriculo-arterial coupling (VAC = Ea/Ees) reflects the permanent instantaneous interplay between Ees and Ea to obtain the best possible relationship between LV stroke work and systemic circulation, providing optimal cardiac output at optimal pressure for tissular perfusion. As mentioned earlier, the Ea/Es ratio is related to many variables: LV end-diastolic volume, V0, LV end-systolic volume, systolic time intervals, systolic and diastolic blood pressure, arterial stiffness and total arterial resistance—thus integrating cardiovascular function. VAC is not a "per se" value.

Knowing the value of the VAC ratio is just as important as knowing what changes in the numerator and/or denominator produced the result. Abnormal VAC is a key understanding of HFrEF or unstable hemodynamic situations. In normal subjects the optimal range of Ea/Ees to cardiac efficiency and stroke work is generally ranging from 0.7 to 1.0 [54, 57, 75, 76] or 0.6 to 1.2 [69]. In healthy young subjects, during exercise, increased LV ejection force will act against a compliant aorta and arterial tree as to conduct higher blood volumes. For maintaining the VAC within the optimal limits Ea should diminish or remain stable or, at least, have a minimal augmentation compared to Ees.

Avoiding the VAC Simplified Formula

It might be tempting to simplify the VAC formula:

$$\text{Ea / Ees} = \frac{\dfrac{ESP(mmHg)}{SV(ml)}}{\dfrac{ESP(mmHg)}{ESV - VO(ml)}} = \frac{ESV - V0(ml)}{SV(ml)}$$

It can be observed that after the elimination of the common factor ESP, the numerator and the denominator are inverted, thus giving to V0 an opposite meaning: the higher the V0, the lower the VAC, which is wrong. If we consider V0 = 0 ml, then we obtain a simplistic volumetric ratio ESV/SV, far away from the physiological meaning of VAC. For the VAC value, both Ea and Ees must be calculated.

VAC Is More Dynamic Than EF

Subtle changes in Ea and/or Ees can result in a significant change in VAC without a change in LVEF. Discrete changes in Ea and/or Ees, when combined as a ratio, can provide significant hemodynamic information. Compared to EF, the VAC ratio Ea/

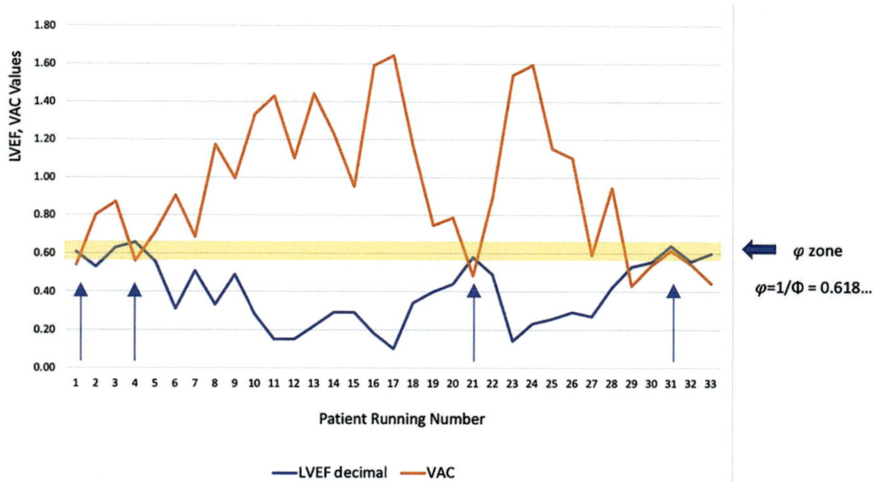

Fig. 8.8 Decimal LVEF (<1) correlated with the most used VAC formula (Ea/Ees). The blue line represents LVEF decimal, and the orange line represents VAC. The "ϕ zone" is the narrow interval very close to the optimal value (ϕ ≈ 0.618…), where LVEF = VAC = 0.62. The arrows show the four patients within this interval. Compared to the EF, the VAC variation is more important

Ees has greater percentage variations (Fig. 8.8). This is why coupling calculation is recommended in intensive care units where therapy-guided VAC hemodynamic monitoring is essential [77].

HFrEF

VAC reserve was studied by low doses Dobutamine echocardiography, in patients with dilated cardiomyopathy [78]. VAC, had much higher values in patients with DCM compared with controls (Ea/Ees: 2.49 ± 1.02 vs. 1.04 ± 0.21) [78]. The coupling reserve cut-off was defined as a > 0.29 Ea/Ees decrease, at 20 μg/kg/min dobutamine infusion [78]. Patients with good VA coupling reserve showed significantly favorable event-free survival compared those with poor VA coupling reserve [78].

Patients with HFrEF have an increased VAC ratio due to a concomitant decrease of contractility (Ees) and a parallel increase of Ea. Ky et al. in a non-invasive study (single-beat Ees estimation) on 466 patients with HFrEF found for VAC elevated values at 1.92 (median values; 25th, 75th percentile), by depressed Es (0.89) and elevated Ea (1.66) [79]. A very important finding published by the same authors needs to be developed: this group of 466 patients with chronic systolic heart failure (low LVEF) was studied for the combined endpoint of death, cardiac transplantation or ventricular assist device placement; and 2 cardiac hospitalization [79]. While Es was not found to be predictive, V0 (derived from the single-beat Chen formula) was the best predictor, followed by VAC calculated from Ea/Ees and ventricular size were associated with prognosis. In other words, they found that the most prognostic factors were LV remodeling (V0) and LV mismatch to afterload (Ees/Ea =VAC), but not contractility alone (Ees). There are several possible developments: in a most important position appears the principle of VAC, which shows that the afterload sensitivity and mismatch is the great ruler in the HF progress. Not the contractility (Ees) by itself, but its relation to the afterload (Ea) emerges as the governing principle. In the same study, V0 is more predictable than Ees. V0 reflects LV remodeling: dilation, geometry changes, wall thickness/cavity ratio, and indirectly (in some cases) fibrosis. Of course, reflecting such important structural changes, V0 is a strong predictor. As to avoid a virtual volume (V0) Ky et al. calculated the value of the intercept at 100 mmHg (V 100 = 100/Ees + V0) [78]. Intercepting the pressure axis at levels higher than 0 mmHg, a V0 surrogate should it be at 50 or 100 ml, results in less volume variation and eliminates the negative values [80].

Critically ill patients with low CO and altered LV contraction (Ees), increased Ea and VAC (Ea/Ees > 1), even if BP is low, will benefit from vasodilator infusion (i.e., sodium nitroprusside). The reduction in SVR (afterload reduction as assessed by Ea) lowers diastolic blood pressure, which is compensated by a higher pulse pressure, reflecting improved SV and resulting in higher forward flow and organ perfusion for a similar mean arterial pressure. The hemodynamic effects of vasodilator therapy are completely different when Ees is normal or only slightly reduced. In this group, with preserved ventriculoarterial coupling, afterload reduction has minimal effect on stroke volume [81].

In patients with HFrEF, the LV may have maintained some CR, but it cannot play a role alone and Ees must greatly exceed the increase in Ea to improve VAC. CR may be “hidden” by afterload mismatch, explaining why vasodilator therapy is the most effective energy-sparing way to improve VAC.

HFpEF

HFpEF patients may have normal or lower VAC values. In a historical study, Kawaguchi et al. compared HF patients with preserved ejection fraction with normotensive and hypertensive subjects [82]. Ees was higher in patients with HFpEF (4.7+/−1.5 mm Hg/mL) than in controls (2.1+/−0.9 mm Hg/mL in normotensives and 3.3+/−1.0 mm Hg/mL in hypertensives). Ea was also higher (2.6+/−0.5 versus 1.9+/−0.5 mm Hg/mL). Both Ees and Ea were significantly higher than in controls. Despite the elevated numerator and denominator, the Ea/Ees ratio was lower in HFpEF than in normal subjects: Ea/Ees = 0.55 vs. 0.90. Most strikingly, an exaggerated hypertensive response was observed during handgrip exercise (Fig. 8.9), accompanied by an increase in LV end-diastolic pressure. In summary (Figure legend), a brutal increase in LV end-systolic pressure, a much higher LV end-diastolic pressure, and a lower SV were observed during handgrip exercise despite a significant increase in ESPVR. The CR, measured by Ees variation at high resting values,

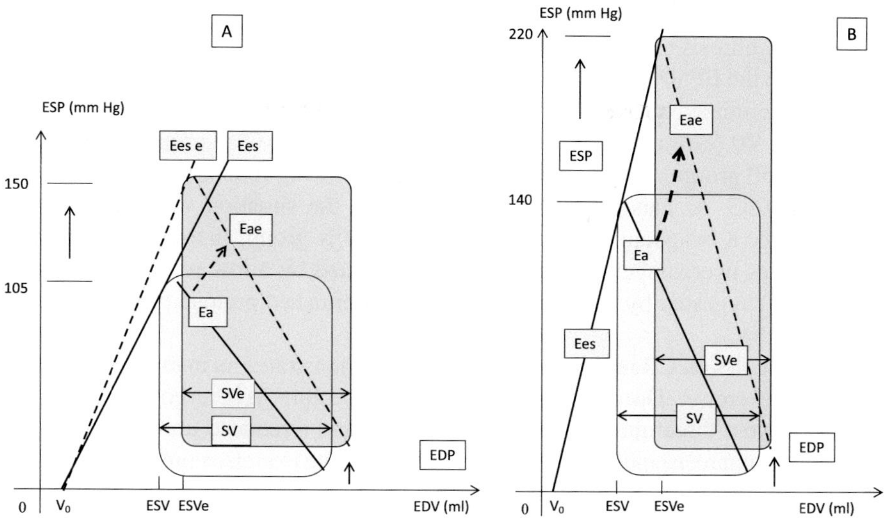

Fig. 8.9 Sketch of two possible ways to not increase SV during exercise. *ESP* end-systolic pressure, *EDP* end-diastolic pressure, *EDV* end-diastolic volume, *ESV* basal end-systolic volume, *ESVe* exercise end-systolic volume, *SV* basal stroke volume, *SVe* exercise stroke volume, *Ees* end-systolic elastance, *Ea* basal effective arterial elastance, *Eae* exercise effective arterial elastance, a. HFrEF and b. HFpEF. (**a**) Exercise blunting of contractile reserve by afterload sensitivity. Starting from a high ventriculo-arterial coupling (high afterload and depressed Ees), an increase in Ees during exercise is counterbalanced by a concomitant increase in Ea (high arterial resistances ± elevated HR), resulting in a null increase in SV (SV = SVe) and a concomitant increase in EDP, leading to dyspnea. (**b**) Inspired by (Kawaguchi et al. [82]). Low ventriculo-arterial coupling but high Ea and Ees. High resting contractility is required for basal circulatory demands, leaving little or no reserve to increase SV against very high exercise Ea, resulting in no increase or even a decrease in exercise SV (Sve < SV), accompanied by hypertension and elevated EDP. High resting Ees and Ea may predict a hypertensive response to exercise. (Kawaguchi et al. [82])

is somehow exhausted, leaving too little reserve for further inotropic stimulation to increase SV. The same study suggests that energy cost in HFpEF is >50% higher than in controls and may limit reserve in those with concomitant heart or coronary artery disease. Contractile reserve, measured by the Ees variation, when high rest values exist, is somehow exhausted, leaving to further inotropic stimulation to few reserve as to increase SV against a very elevated afterload. The same study considers that energy cost is predicted to be >50% higher in HFpEF versus controls and might limit reserve in those with concomitant heart or coronary artery disease. Borlaug and Kass made an important point: "Perhaps more important than the coupling ratio of ventricular and vascular stiffness are their absolute values" [69], which appears to be the core situation in HFpEF. Therefore, in HFpEF, the Ea/Ees ratio (VAC) may have less predictive value than Ees and Ea taken separately. Rosh et al. conducted an invasive study in conjunction with echocardiography and MRI in 56 patients with HFpEF [83]. The group was divided into HFpEF with EF between 50% and 60% (EF50%–60%) and HFpEF with EF >60% (EF > 60%). Preload was varied by vena cava occlusion and afterload by handgrip. Myocardial biopsy measured the degree of myocardial fibrosis: patients with EF50%–60% had more myocardial fibrosis (15.3%) than those with EF > 60% (11.3%). Baseline VAC was impaired in the EF50%–60% group, whereas in the EF > 60% group VAC was in the range of optimized stroke work (0.80 vs. 1.01). With preload variation, Ees was higher and V0 (estimated by V120) was lower in the EF>60% group compared to the EF50–60 group—very similar to the HFrEF showing reduced contractility and impaired VAC. At handgrip (afterload increase), the situation was the opposite, similar to the Kawaguchi article [82]: in the EF > 60% group, an excessive afterload increase was overcompensated by Ees, accompanied by a low relative contractile reserve, as suggested by the increase in V120, diminished preload reserve, leading to reduced SV.

Other studies on CR in HFpEF patients have demonstrated an inability to increase CO with exercise. During maximal exercise upright cycle ergometry, HFpEF patients have a threefold smaller increase in Ees and a reduced ability to decrease their peripheral resistance and increase their HR during exercise compared to hypertensive controls with left ventricular hypertrophy [22]. The higher the resting Ea and Ees, the more important is the exercise-induced increase in LV diastolic filling pressure. Exercise reserve is severely compromised in HFpEF patients, characterized by high Ees and Ea, low VAC ratio and low LV EF reserve. Ventricular and arterial elastance, alone or integrated into the VAC, allow today a better understanding of the pathology and a better choice of the method to be used for the investigation by a non-invasive approach. The fundamental advantage comes from the demonstrated influence of Ea and Ees abnormalities on SV, EF, preload pressure sensitivity, pressure lability, hypertension and some important aspects of cardiovascular reserve during exercise [33]. However, there are limitations [33]: Ea, influenced by HR, is not a pure arterial load index, being highly dependent on resistances and insensitive to changes in pulsatile load, and therefore does not measure arterial stiffness. Disadvantages of Ees come from the nonlinearity of ESPVR and from the fact that Ees is partially load dependent; finally, Ees doesn't assess myocardial properties (geometry, fibrosis). V0 becomes larger in dilated hearts and may have important variations. Extracting from a single beat Ees formula, instead of V0, a V0 volume at higher intercept pressures such as V30, V100 or V120, by reducing the extrapolation line, provides fewer odd values. Beyond these limitations, Ees, Ea, and Ea/Ees provided the best definitions in HF, allowing the understanding of contractile function and reserve integrated into VAC. If Chen's formula can be regarded as no more than an approximation of Ees, then the ratio ESP/ESV, appealing for its simplicity, is an even more far-reaching approximation. Nguyen et al. compared several non-invasive methods for Ees assessment in the ICU [84]. Their results do not support the use of ESP/ESV based method as a substitute for Chen method to measure and assess changes in VAC in cardiac intensive care patients.

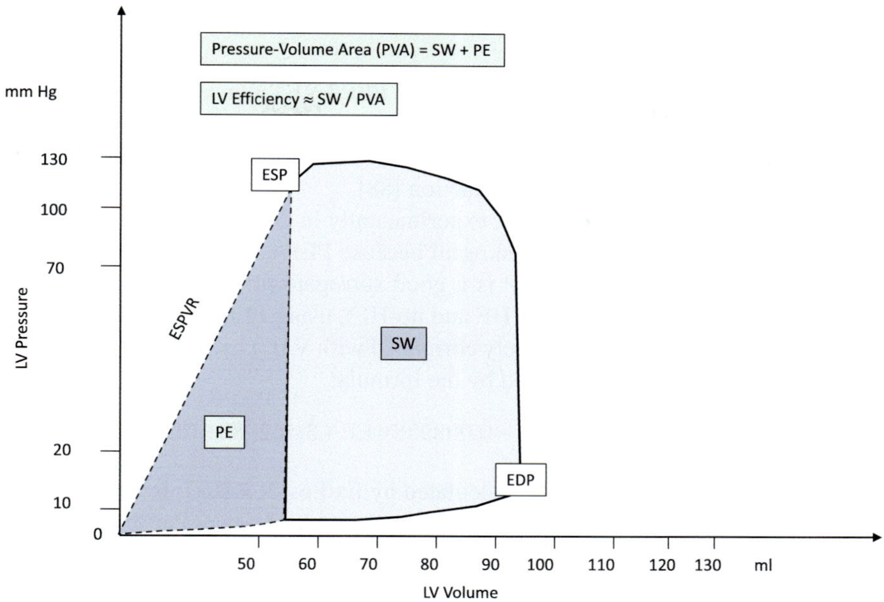

Fig. 8.10 Pressure-Volume Area (PVA) = SW + PE, LV Efficiency ≈ SW/PVA. *ESP* end-systolic pressure, *EDP* end-diastolic pressure, *SW* stroke work, *PE* potential energy

Ventricular Efficiency

Burkhoff and Sagawa defined the ventricular efficiency (Eff) as the ratio between external stroke work (SW) and MVo2 [85]. SW is obtained by integrating the PVL (Fig. 8.10). The SW is the useful fraction of ventricular energy that is delivered to the arterial system to maintain forward blood flow and provide adequate transport of oxygen and nutrients to the peripheral organs. O2 consumption is linearly related to the ventricular pressure-volume area [86, 87].

The Potential Energy (PE)

It is defined by the triangular area below the ESPVR line (Fig. 8.10) which represents the dissipated ventricular energy. Pressure-volume area (PVA) is the sum of SW + PE and correlates with myocardial oxygen consumption. Thus, pump efficiency can be calculated as the ratio of useful work to total O2 consumption: SW/PVA. Under resting conditions, cardiac function and arterial loading are adjusted to maximize ventricular efficiency rather than SW. At best efficiency (high work vs. low oxygen consumption), VAC (Ea/Ees) will be close to 0.5, whereas under stress conditions, higher oxygen consumption is required, which means lower efficiency, with VAC at its maximum at Ea = Ees = 1 [87].

Various Surrogates for VAC Approximation

VAC has a close relationship with STI. Using PEP/LVET> or =0.423 as cut point, the sensitivity and specificity to identify patients with altered VAC (Ea/Ees > 1.2) were 85.7% and 84.3%, respectively for the whole population, and 84.6% and 78.6%, for patients with systolic dysfunction [88].

Hayashi et al. described the VAC, experimentally in dogs, as a function of PEP/LVET and DBP/ESP, which is meaningful because PEP/LVET is a good surrogate for contractile function while DBP is a good surrogate for peripheral resistances [89, 90]. In a study of 33 patients (HF and no-HF), using PEP/TET as a good contractility surrogate and EF (negatively correlated with VAC) by multiple regression, VAC was almost perfectly predicted by the formula:

$$\text{VACestimated} = 0.553291 - 0.008988 * \text{EF} + 3.462988 * \text{PEP} / \text{TET}$$

(VAC estimated correlated to VAC calculated by Ea/Ees: $R = 0.97$; $R^2 = 0.95$) [64].

A consensus document of the ESC Working Group on Aorta & Periferal Vascular Diseases gives an extended description of the advantages and disadvantages of ventricular–arterial coupling assessment modalities [91].

Pugliese et al. derived a VAC surrogate from the relationship between aortic stiffness, as assessed by pulsed wave velocity (PWV) measured at the aortic arch or carotid-femoral level, and global longitudinal strain (GLS): PWV/GLS [92]. A significant correlation was obtained with peak VO2, but with very low predictability (R^2: 0.33 and 0.36, respectively). In his editorial comment, Chirinos developed several arguments: GLS is a load-dependent metric of myocardial deformation (active and passive); afterload is only partially reflected by large artery compliance; GLS/PWV should not be interpreted as a "load-corrected" metric of myocardial or LV performance or as VAC [93].

Ejection Fraction, Stroke Volume and VAC

Ejection fraction (EF) is the most widely used volumetric index of LV function. Wrongly considered an index of contractility and used as a definition for CHF, EF is currently unable to define more than 50% of HF cases.

LVEF is calculated as LVEF = SV/EDV or (EDV−ESV)/EDV, which can be mathematically expressed as: EF = 1 − (ESV/EDV) or indexed values EF = 1 − (ESVi/EDVi).

Components of the EF Calculation and Their Relationship

Looking at the dimensionless aspect of the LVEF, where the metric cannot express the magnitude of ESV and EDV, Kerkhof et al. proposed as a fundamental approach a 'volume regulatory state diagram in terms of ESV versus EDV as a cornerstone for more insightful analysis of ventricular function, linking therefore the LVEF to its constituents [94]. If the indexed values of EDV and ESV (EDVi, ESVi) have a strong linear correlation, EF to EDVi has a weak correlation, while EF to ESVi has a strong nonlinear logarithmic correlation ($R^2 = 0.9$). Their study shows that ESVi is the dominant factor for EF compared to EDVi. This is a reality in clinical practice where ESVi is by itself a LV function index with a strong prognostic value.

A normal EF does not guarantee of good systolic function. EF may remain unchanged despite significantly reduced LV function. Longitudinal shortening can vary significantly because it has less effect on EF than circumferential shortening. Wall thickness has a significant effect on EF, and in concentrically remodeled ventricles with thick walls and small cavities, EF remains high despite significantly reduced longitudinal and circumferential shortening [95]. The authors emphasized that EF is a function of 4 different variables: GLS, GCS, wall thickness, and EDV, situation which can be clinically defined as: the circumferential and longitudinal contraction acting on the EDV at a given wall thickness: 1% reduction in longitudinal shortening is compensated by a 0.5% increase in circumferential shortening, ~0.9-mm increased wall thickness, or a 6- to 9-ml reduction in EDV, depending on the operating range of the other variables.

In a simplified clinical view, if a highly dilated ESV will have a reduced EF, a small, hypertrophied LV will not guarantee a normal contractile function.

Relationship Between EF and VAC

VAC, calculated as Ea/Ees, is negatively correlated to EF. The formula: $Ea/Ees = 1/EF - 1$ is often found in the literature, which implies a simple linear relationship. It has been demonstrated that VAC and EF have a non-linear relationship and this formula is true only in a unique situation when VAC = EF = 0.618 = φ (EF 0.618 = 62%), suggesting that when V0 = 0 ml, it triggers the "perfect" situation where EF = Ea/Ees = 0.62 (62% for the EF) [55, 64]. Consistent with the mathematical demonstration Tona et al. in a 4-year follow-up of patients with systemic sclerosis, choosing a VAC cutoff at 0.63, showed that a VAC > 0.63 was associated with higher major adverse cardiovascular events and mortality (HR 2.5) compared to those with a VAC < 0.63 [96]. In a major epidemiologic study, Wehner et al. demonstrated that overall, adjusted hazard ratios for mortality have a U-shaped relationship with LVEF, with a nadir of risk at an LVEF of 60–65%, probably indicating the optimal relationship to VAC. Deviation of LVEF from 60% to 65% (lower or higher) is associated with worse survival, regardless of age, sex, or other relevant comorbidities such as heart failure [97].

Like the VAC, EF can be expressed as a ratio of elastances. LVEF formula can be rewritten in a way where all the components of the numerator and denominator are expressed in terms of elastances:

$$EF = \frac{SV}{EDV} = \frac{SV}{SV + ESV}$$

If, Ees = ESP/ (ESV – V0); then ESV = (ESP/Ees) + V0.
If, Ea = ESP/SV; then SV = ESP/Ea.

Leading to:

$$EF = \frac{ESP * Ees}{ESP\left(Ea + Ees\right) + Ea * Ees * V0} \tag{8.1}$$

If V0 = 0 ml, then: EF = Ees/(Ea + Ees).

Example:

ESP = 117 mm Hg (130 * 0.9); Ees = 1.6 mm Hg/ml; Ea = 1, VAC = 0.62 mm Hg/ml and
V0 = 5 ml ➔ EF = 60%
V0 variation: V0 = 0 ml ➔ EF 61%; V0 = +30 ml ➔ EF 53%; V0 = −25 ml ➔ EF 71%

There are two factors that reduce the EF, a positive V0 value and/or Ea:

- V0: if positive, it adds to the denominator the product of Ees and Ea multiplied by its value, which reduces the EF (i.e. remodeled dilated LV). For a negative value, it will increase the EF.
- Ea: for a constant ESP and constant V0 (+3 ml), a 10% increase in Ea will reduce the EF from 61% to 56% (−5%). To restore the EF back to 61%, the Ees must be increased by 24%.

This is a simple mathematical demonstration of the blunting effect of afterload on EF. (Fig. 8.9a, b) In pathological cases, some CR may be present, but the Ees cannot overcome the afterload counterforce, resulting in an absent or weak increase of the EF. For a marked increase in contractile force, a slight increase in arterial elastance, will blunt the effect on LVEF. In such cases, reducing afterload will improve volumetric indices (Fig. 8.6b). This simple numerical exercise attempts to promote the understanding that LVEF results from a permanent crosstalk between Ees and Ea, which is subordinate to VAC and may explain the reduced sensitivity of LVEF to contractility itself. This explains why LVEF is not a strong discriminator of contractility but considered as a composite result of Ees and Ea, LVEF is an excellent predictor in patients with HFrEF.

Using the actual formulas for Ees (ESP/(ESV − V0) and Ea (ESP/SV) Eq. 8.1 can be simplified to:

$$\mathrm{EF} = \frac{SV}{EDV + V0}$$

This shows that the V0 has an important role to play as long as we look at the EF in terms of the elastances.

Global function systolic measurements, commonly used, as ESV, SV, LVEF, dP/dT, global strain, are load dependent. Contractile reserve investigation in heart failure is confronted to two contrasted situations: high VAC in HFrEF (lower Ees and higher Ea) and low VAC in HFpEF (high Ees and high Ea). It is not yet clearly defined, what tests to use for different pathologies, ages or gender. Dobutamine and dipyridamole are widely used. Low dose dobutamine at steady HR, is appropriate to incite inotropy betting on a not-high peripheral response. On the other hand, exercise, adding or not the handgrip, by its physiological property to provoke an important peripheral response and therefore push to a "face-to-face" Ees-Ea relation, will provide excellent data on LV coupling to systemic circulation.

Leung et al. in a study using exercise echocardiography in patients with chronic mitral regurgitation found that an exercise LV end-systolic volume index > 25 ml/m^2 was the best predictor of postoperative dysfunction, with a sensitivity and specificity of 83% [98]. On exercise, this finding corresponded to an LVEF increase of 3%, which is less but also predictive. As mentioned above, this underlines the strong predictive role of LV end-systolic volume. A recent study in asymptomatic patients with severe mitral regurgitation (MR) suggested that asymptomatic patients with chronic severe (MR) may develop irreversible left LV dysfunction despite a normal resting LVEF, which may hide irreversible myocardial damage [99]. The difference between resting and post-exercise LVEF was defined as CR: a post-exercise LVEF increase of ≥ 4% was defined as CR+. In patients undergoing surgery, CR was an independent predictor of follow-up. Treadmill exercise echocardiography was performed in patients with severe aortic regurgitation. CR was considered positive (CR+) if an increase in LVEF was present at exercise. LV end-systolic volume was an independent predictor of CR+ [100]. Of great interest in this study was that patients with ≥75 mm LVED and ≥55 mm LVES, compared to those with ≤75 mm LVED and ≤55 mm LVES had a diminished LVEF (increment 0.67 ± 7.1 vs -3.9 ± 9.9; $p = 0.041$) accompanied by a higher blood pressure increment after treadmill exercise (181.6 ± 26.6 vs 202.2 ± 17.7, $p < 0.001$) suggesting a much heavier VAC alteration due to a more advanced systemic disease.

The cutoff for indices variation to consider contractile reserve has wide variation in different publications: EF 2–10%; Δ SV 20%; Δ WMSI ≥0.15–0.44 [48, 101].

The problem we have to face is that LVEF and volumes depend on the imaging method [102]. Compared with cardiac magnetic resonance (CMR) as the gold standard, LVEDV and LVESV measured by all echocardiographic methods were smaller and showed greater variability than those derived from CMR. In terms of agreement and reproducibility with CMR, all studies showed superiority of contrast-enhanced 2D echocardiography over non-contrast-enhanced 2D echocardiography and superiority of 3D echocardiography over 2D echocardiography [102]. In this study, 3D echo studies generally had no bias compared to CMR. Another difficulty with LVEF is the beat-to-beat variability, which has been reported to be as high as 5.8 ± 1.7%. In the absence of 3D echo facilities, LV volume in serial measurements for contractility reserve is at some risk because small tracing errors become cubic—Simpson's modified rule is based on the sum of a stack of cylinders. In stress echocardiography, the 2-chamber view may not be available due to pulmonary interposition, so a single section is calculated in volume, sometimes obscuring discrete variations. Measurement of SV seems to be mandatory for LVEF calculation as well as for small variations during stress echo Doppler examination. Considering that LV subaortic area doesn't change significantly with increasing blood flow, measurement of velocity time integral (VTI) variations, which indicate Δ SV, is a fair practical issue. If the clinical test doesn't significantly increase Ea, such as low-dose dobutamine in patients with low LVEF, the result (Δ SV and/or Δ LVEF) will be close enough to inotropy to detect contractile reserve and reveal an afterload mismatch. Following up with higher doses of dobutamine, or performing exercise testing, will bring into play a much more complex hemodynamic response: chronotropic response, hypertension, possibly myocardial ischemia, pulmonary arteriolar resistances, peripheral and myocardial oxygen consumption, or global energy reserve. An increase in afterload (Ea) may exacerbate the afterload mismatch but may also demonstrate the etiology of dyspnea or fatigue and provide evidence of an abnormal BP response.

Stroke Volume and Flow Reserve

Stroke volume (SV) is a simple and reliable method for estimating CR. Easy to use even in difficult clinical conditions or during stress echocardiography, SV variations (Δ) are a simple proof of the end product of all the aforementioned mechanisms. Based on the product between subaortic surface area and Doppler VTI measurement, it can be simplified to ΔVTI for serial measurements, since the subannular region doesn't have significant size variations with flow augmentation. Pibarot and Dumesnil prefer the term flow reserve rather than contractile reserve to avoid confounding contractility with afterload mismatch [103].

Monin et al. studied 45 patients with aortic stenosis with severe LV dysfunction and low transvalvular pressure gradients using low-dose dobutamine echo Doppler studies (5–20 μg/kg/min) [104]. This study was followed by the French multicenter study in 136 patients with the same pathology using the same methodology [105]. LV contractile reserve was considered positive (CR+) if an increase in SV of ≥20% was observed. CR+ patients had a low operative risk (5%) and a good long-term prognosis, whereas operative mortality was high (32%) in the absence of contractile reserve. Tribouilloy et al. studied 81 patients with low-flow/low-gradient symptomatic aortic stenosis (mean pressure gradient ≤ 40 mm Hg, LVEF ≤ 40%) without CR on dobutamine echocardiography, prospectively enrolled in 10 centers [106]. In patients with CR, aortic valve replacement was associated with a better outcome compared to medical management, suggesting that surgery should not be withheld based on this criterion alone. Maes et al. in a substudy of the TOPAS-TAVY registry, showed that transcatheter aortic valve replacement (TAVR) was associated with similar clinical outcomes in patients with low-flow, low-gradient aortic stenosis (LFLG-AS), and severe left ventricular dysfunction as in patients with milder left ventricular dysfunction [107]. TAVR was associated with a significant increase in LVEF regardless of the result of low-dose dobutamine testing of contractile reserve. This is a good example of EF and/or SV being blunted by the opposing force to ejection, where dobutamine may or may not reveal increased contraction.

In our personal series, we studied 52 patients with dilated cardiomyopathy with an end-diastolic diameter > 70 mm. Patients were listed or about to be listed for heart transplantation. Left ventricular remodeling (Batista procedure, now abandoned) was proposed as an alternative to heart transplantation. Given the high risk of the procedure, dobutamine echocardiography was used for patient selection. Because we considered this type of surgery to be very high risk, the Δ SV was set high (≥30%) and proved to be the most powerful predictive parameter for a good surgical outcome. Interestingly, patients who underwent the Batista procedure showed mild or no myocardial fibrosis on myocardial specimen. On the other hand, patients with <30% SV increase who were not candidates for the Batista procedure and who underwent heart transplantation showed diffuse moderate to severe myocardial fibrosis [108].

Cardiac Power Output (CPO) and Reserve as a Global Hemodynamic Index

Cardiac power output (CPO) is based on the product of cardiac output (CO) and mean arterial pressure (MAP), which describes hydraulic power. It is calculated in watts using the formula [109]:

$$\text{CPO}(\text{Watts}) = (\text{MAP} - \text{RAP}) \times \text{CO} \times 1/451 = (\text{MAP} - \text{RAP}) \times \text{CO} \times 2.22 \times 10^{-3}$$

(RAP: Right Atrial Pressure). The normal CPO value is around 1 W.

Example: (85 mm Hg (MAP) − 3 mm Hg (RAP)) × 5.2 l/min × 2.22 × 10^{-3} = 0.946 W.

The CPI is the CPO normalized to the body surface.

Let's consider the heart as a link in a long and complex chain. This index is not specifically related to LV contraction because it reflects the entire circulatory status: left and right heart systolic-diastolic function, chronotropy, systemic and pulmonary circulation, but it also measures the energy transfer from the LV to the aorta. Therefore, it should be considered a hemodynamic index. The CPO moves away from the cardiocentric approach to heart failure (i.e. EF) and proposes a more global index that is much better able to predict HF. Very useful in hemodynamically unstable situations, cardiogenic shock, a strong predictor of outcome in heart failure, the CPI is widely used as a baseline index and/or functional reserve. In patients with advanced heart failure, decreased CPI (<0.44 W/m^2) was associated with increased adverse outcomes, whereas CPI was able to stratify risk, independently of peak oxygen consumption [110].

CPO is often normalized to the LV mass (CPOM) and is calculated as follows:

$$\mathrm{CPOM}(\mathrm{W}/100\mathrm{g}) = 0.222 \times \left[(MAP - RAP) \times CO\right] / \mathrm{LVM}(\mathrm{g})$$

CPOM reflects the power-generating capacity per unit mass of LV myocardium, thus facilitating the comparison between individuals [111].

The power reserve is calculated as the difference between stress and rest:

$$\text{Power reserve} = \text{CPOM stress} - \text{CPOM rest}.$$

Resting CPO and reserve CPO during exercise were tested in patients with HFpEF compared to dyspneic patients without HF. Resting CPO did not discriminate between the two groups for 3-year event-free survival, but CPO reserve was a strong predictor of adverse outcome in patients with HFpEF and ΔCPO <0.49 W/100 g, compared to patients with HFpEF where ΔCPO >0.49 W/100 g [112]. The CPOM assessed at peak of dobutamine stress echocardiography allowed an effective prognostication in patients with ischemic cardiomyopathy. A peak-stress power/mass $\leq$ 50 W/100 g was strong and multivariable predictor of mortality [113].

In a group of 159 patients with chronic HFrEF, peak CPOM was the strongest independent predictor of all-cause death, ventricular assist device implantation, heart transplantation and hospitalization [114]. Patients were assessed by exercise echocardiography. Survival at 48 months was less than 40% for patients with peak CPOM $\leq$ 0.6 W/100 g, compared to nearly 90% for patients with peak CPOM between 0.6 and 1 W/100 g.

The cardiac power has a better prediction impact than EF. In a retrospective study on an impressive number of patients (24885) with normal EF, Anand et al. calculated the cardiac power by exercise echocardiography: CPOM at rest, at peak exercise and CPOM reserve: mean CPOM was 0.8 ± 0.2 W/100 g, increasing to 2.1 ± 0.7 W/100 g at peak exercise [111]. Mean CPOM reserve, (i.e. the power/mass developed from rest to exercise) was 1. 3 ± 0. 5 W/100 g. After more than 3 years of follow-up and adjusting for age, sex, achieved metabolic equivalents (METs), ischemia/infarction on stress test results, medication, and comorbidities, peak exercise power/mass and power reserve were independently associated with mortality and HF (highest vs. lowest quartile).

dP/dT

It is one of the oldest contractility indexes, measuring the ratio of pressure variation over time. dP/dT max is the maximum value of the rate of pressure change obtained during isovolumic contraction. dP/dT is load dependent: strongly positively correlated with preload, influenced by low afterload [115]. Commonly used in invasive

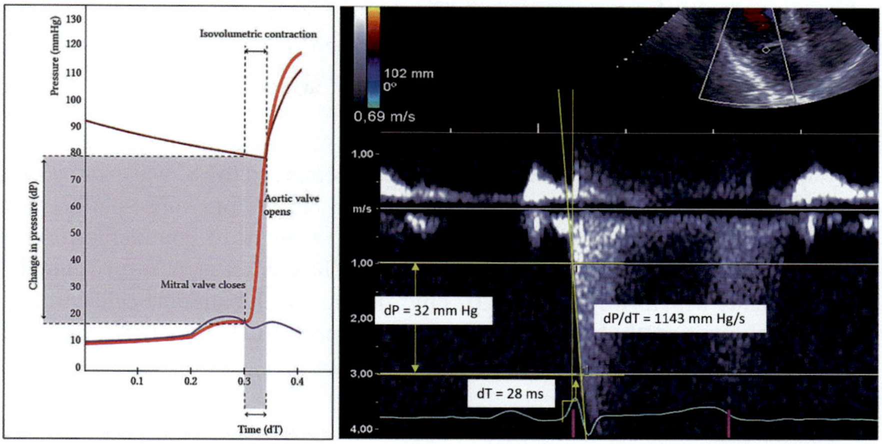

Fig. 8.11 dP/dT calculated based on mitral regurgitant flow. 32 mm Hg is the difference in gradient between 1 m/s (4 mm Hg) and 3 m/s (36 mm Hg). 32 mm Hg is divided by the time (ms) between 1 m/s and 3 m/s, i.e. dP/dT = (32/28) * 1000 = 1143 mm Hg/s. The increase in gradient between 1 m/s and 3 m/s occurs during the pre-ejection period. (The drawing is courtesy of: Alex Yartsev, Deranged Physiology)

studies, non-invasively dP/dT may be calculated by echo-Doppler in patient with mitral regurgitation (Fig. 8.11). Normal values are ≥1200 mm Hg/s [116]. Values below 800 mm Hg/s are definitely abnormal.

LV Longitudinal Function

Longitudinal contraction without being a global contraction index is highly sensitive to inotropy modifications and is a major determinant of the global systolic function. Considering the right-handed / left-handed helix arrangements of the fibers, it is preferably to speak about longitudinal contraction instead of longitudinal fibers. Sub-endocardial layer, the first to suffer in a broad spectrum of pathologies, has a strong impact on longitudinal contraction.

Doppler Tissue Imaging (DTI) is highly angle dependent: Comparing (in animal study) the S′ wave and LVEF against LV dP/dt, S′ wave had a much stronger correlation to dP/dt than LVEF (r = 0.665 vs. r = 0.40, respectively) [117]. At the same time S′ wave was associated to apical rotation (r = 0.674) leading to the conclusion that it is a more sensitive index of global LV contractility than is LVEF, reflecting both LV longitudinal shortening and torsional deformation [117]. Once again, it must be underlined that LVEF is not a pure contractility index. Meantime longitudinal contraction velocity is much closer to contractility. Without being a global index, it correlates well to global contractility, describing well enough two of the three contraction vectors, longitudinal and spiral. DTI will describe the contraction velocity at the place where the Doppler sample is located. Longitudinal contraction velocity recorded at the base of LV (mitral valve annulus) reflects well the LV contractility however as the contraction is unequal, postero-lateral higher versus antero-septal lower, more sampling zones need to be used as to obtain best reliable results. Simple to use, very affordable for Dobutamine or exercise testing, S′ wave is a good reliable tool for contractile reserve investigation. Ciampi et al. in a prospective study, on 89 patients with HFrEF (LVEF < 45%), compared the S′ wave variations, during Dobutamine and exercise echocardiography, to the pressure volume ratio (ESPVR)—which was considered for this study a standard of contractile reserve [118]. The cut-off for contractile reserve by ESPVR was set at Δ > 0.72 mmHg/mL/m. Patients with a Δ S′ wave > 2.02 cm/s during the Dobutamine echocardiography had a significantly higher ESPVR, a higher peak VO2 and a better diastolic filling with a lower E/E' ratio.

LV Myocardial Strain(S) and Strain Rate (SR)

2D speckle tracking echocardiography provides reliable deformation imaging data. S indicates relative shortening or lengthening of the myocardium without distinguishing between active and passive deformation. S is a tissular shortening or lengthening fraction measured in orthogonal planes. The SR is the contraction velocity, i.e. the change in length over time, and is therefore closer to the concept of contractility—but not widely used.

Compared to LVEF or SV, the S suffers from the same load and HR dependency, while SR is relatively independent of the HR [119]. S and SR are inversely correlated with longitudinal and circumferential wall stress; S is more dependent on afterload while SR much less [120]. S is image sensitive, whereas myocardial contrast agents blur the speckles. Narrow angles and high frame rates (>60/s; optimal 100/s) are required. When using S or SR in stress echocardiography, care must be taken to ensure image quality. Speckles are not "markers" of the myocardium, but simply interference between the ultrasound and the tissue, where the varying dimensions and shape of the LW wall related to HR may create a different pattern. A global 2D strain assessment requires three consecutive apical views, which implies equal cardiac cycle duration for each, while 3D strain requires a single acquisition. 3D strain is based on orthogonal vector calculation. 3D strain suffers from lower temporal and spatial resolution, which lowers tracking reliability. Multi-beat acquisition sometimes produces a stitching artifact between sub-volumes, leading to inaccurate speckle tracking analysis [121].

We have to face a disturbing situation: depending on the vendor, there are significant differences between 2D and 3D normal/abnormal strain values, making the comparison difficult.

Normal values published by Lang RM, Badano LP, Mor-Avi V, et al. in 2015 [122]:

GLS: Global longitudinal strain (2-D) (%), mean (range) −20% (−15.9% to −22.1%)

GCS: Global circumferential strain (2-D) (%), mean (range) −23% (−20.9% to −27.8%)
GRS: Global radial strain (2-D) (%), mean (range) +47% (+35.1% to +59.0%)

Normal Values and Lower Limits of Normal (LLN) Values, published by Wang et al. in 2020, based on a meta-analysis (44 studies; 8910 subjects), defines for the first time the LLN as the threshold beyond which strain measurements become abnormal. The following table shows a simplified result of their work [123]:

Strain (%)	Mean (%)	95% CI (%)	LLN (%)	95/ CI (%)
2D GLS	−20.1	−20.7, −19.6	−15.4	−16.0, −14.7
2D GCS	−21.9	−23.4, −20.3	−15.3	−16.9, −13.8
2D GRS	48.4	43.8, 53.0	25.5	17.8, 33.1
3D GLS	−18.5	−20.1, −16.9	−14.5	−16.8, −12.3
3D GCS	−25.0	−30.8, −19.3	−17.6	−22.6, −12.6
3D GRS	49.4	40.8, 58.0	27.9	16.8, 38.9

GLS global longitudinal strain, *GCS* global circumferential strain, *GRS* global radial strain, *LLN* lower limit of normal

Despite a very high heterogeneity, the 95% CI interval for LLN is a first step to compare results between studies.

Ejection Fraction and Strain Relationship

Longitudinal strain, as a measure of length variation, is closely related to the inner layer of the myocardial wall. The subendocardial myocardium is the first to suffer in most cardiac pathologies (i.e. dilated cardiomyopathy, ischemic, valvular…). While EF was still normal, numerous studies have demonstrated a reduction in GLS, which raises the question: what is the contribution of GLS to EF? Global Circumferential Strain (GCS) assesses circumferential myofibers, which are predominantly located in the mid-myocardial wall and are typically affected in more clinically significant myocardial disease [124].

Stokke et al. examined the relationship of EF to GLS and GCS. For EF ≥ 50%, GLS had a weak correlation (r = 0.42), but much stronger when EF < 50% (r = 0.8) [95]. This explains why a change in GLS can coexist with normal EF, reinforcing the diagnostic advantage of GLS over EF in an altered LV with still normal EF. The major contribution to EF comes from circumferential shortening as measured by GCS, whereas EF depends quadratically on circumferential shortening and only linearly on longitudinal shortening. They found that each percentage change in GCS had a 1.6-fold greater effect on LVEF than did GLS [95]. Thus, a decrease in GLS could be compensated by a smaller improvement in GCS to maintain LVEF at the same level.

Fung et al. compared contractile reserve in hypertensive (HTN) patients with normal subjects using low-dose dobutamine echocardiography [125]. Both groups had a comparable increase in EF > 5% under dobutamine, which could lead us to believe that HTN patients had a good contractile reserve. Meanwhile, HTN patients had impaired GLS at rest and with low-dose dobutamine. They had normal GCS at rest but impaired augmentation with low-dose dobutamine. Impaired CR correlated with LV wall thickness independently of prevailing blood pressure. Of note, EF augmentation with dobutamine was not due to contractile reserve but probably to reduced afterload. GLS is a widely used predictor of mortality or major cardiovascular events, while GCS or GRS are used primarily for research purposes [124].

In exercise echocardiography, global longitudinal strain (GLS) was found to be predictive of postoperative LV dysfunction in patients with degenerative mitral regurgitation [126]. Chronic LV overload due to mitral regurgitation is associated with an increase in LVEF, which may mask more severe than expected myocardial damage behind high or normal values. The predictive power of GLS has been tested in patients with > moderate mitral regurgitation [127]. Exercise improvement of GLS > 2% and LVEF ≥ +4% were defined as markers of contractile reserve (CR+) and compared with each other in terms of predictability. CR as assessed by LVEF was not predictive of 2-year event-free survival, whereas GLS was an independent strong predictor [127].

Longitudinal strain has a good but weak correlation with LVEF% ($r = -0.53$), which was improved when echogenicity was good ($r = -0.60$) [128]. A GLS < −14% allowed detection of LVEF ≤ 40% with a sensitivity of 95% and a specificity of 86%. In the same perspective, GLS was compared to LVEF in a group of patients undergoing cardiopulmonary exercise testing with peak VO2 measurement [129]. LVEF and GLS had the same good correlation with peak VO2 in all patients (LVEF: $r = 0.62$, $p < 0.001$ and LGS: $r = -0.63$, $p < 0.001$). However, in a subgroup of 37 patients identified with HFpEF, LVEF did not correlate with peak VO2, while LGS had a good correlation ($r = 0.50$, $p = 0.02$). A GLS value of −17.3% had an excellent sensitivity of 0.89 (95% CI 0.79–0.95) and specificity of 0.91 (95% CI 0.71–0.99) to identify patients with peak VO2 < 20 mL/kg/min. Eighty patients with heart failure and preserved ejection fraction (age 66 ± 8 years; 64% male) underwent exercise echocardiography and were followed for 3 years for all-cause mortality and/or heart failure [130]. Univariate predictors were: reduced resting left atrial ejection fraction, lower peak HR, increased E/e' ratio, reduced TDI myocardial velocities and impaired 2D global longitudinal strain during exercise. In the event group, GLS at rest increased from −17.5 ± 3.7% to −18.2 ± 3.9% (NS), whereas in the non-event group, GLS increased from −18.8 ± 2.9 to −21.4 ± 3.9%. On multivariate analysis, only impaired GLS remained an independent predictor of outcome. It appears that impaired subendocardial function during exercise is better reflected by speckle strain imaging than by other methods. HFpEF is associated with a wide range of comorbidities.

Lack of CR evaluated by less than 2 absolute points GLS increase at exercise, was an independent predictor of major cardiovascular events (HR: 1.98) in asymptomatic patients with severe aortic stenosis [131].

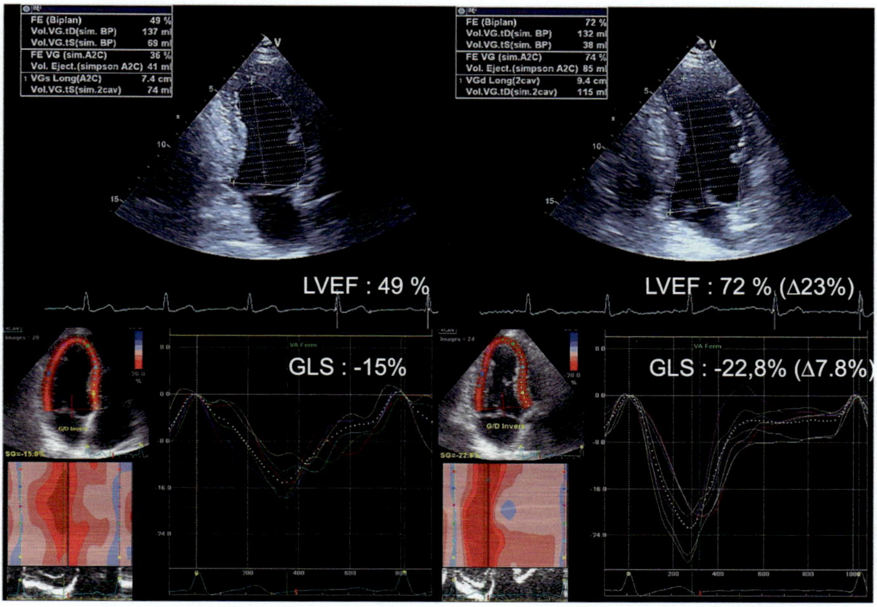

Fig. 8.12 Low-dose dobutamine (5, 10 µg/kg/min) echocardiography in a young male adult with mild reduction of LVEF (47%) and GLS (−15%), after myocarditis. Measurements: biplane LVED and LVES, subaortic diameter, subaortic VTI (Doppler), SBP, GLS (speckle tracking), HR. Calculations: SV, LV systolic pressure (SBP * 0.9), ESPVR (end-systolic pressure-volume ratio), arterial elastance (Ea) by (SBP * 0.9)/SV. V0 was ignored for two reasons: (1) No dilated, no remodeled LV, i.e. a V0 value close to 0 ml; (2) V0 variation (basal vs. dobutamine) cannot be significant. ESPVR was used as an approximation of Ees to estimate ventriculo-arterial coupling (Ea/Ees). LVEF was calculated using two formulae: (1) Simpson biplane and (2). the SV/LVED ratio. CR+ was demonstrated with an almost threefold increase in ESPVR, while Ea had only a very slight increase (+11%), leading to an important physiological reduction in the coupling ratio (Ea/Ees), thus optimising LV force to arterial load in order to increase SV at low energy cost. Note that GLS variation (Δ52%) was very close to the LVEF variation (Δ49%)

For borderline situations Fig. 8.12 shows a low-dose dobutamine echocardiogram in a young adult male with mild reduction in LVEF (47%), GLS (−15%) and LVES (34 ml/m^2) after myocarditis. High contractile reserve was demonstrated.

	Basal	Dobutamine (5–10 g/kg/min)—5 min
LVED	137 ml	132 ml
LVES	69 ml	38 ml
Systolic blood pressure	104 mmHg	169 mmHg
SV	64 ml	93 ml (+45%)
Ees = (SBP * 0.9)/LVES	1.356 mmHg/ml	4 mmHg/ml (×2.9)
Ea = (SBP * 0.9)/SV	1.462 mmHg/ml	1.635 mmHg/ml (×1.11)
VAC (Ea/Ees)	1.078	0.408 (−62%)
LVEF(SV/LVED)	47%	70% (Δ 23%)

(continued)

	Basal	Dobutamine (5–10 g/kg/min)—5 min
LVEF (Bi-plane Simpson)	49%	71% (Δ 22%)
HR	72/min	62/min
GLS	−15%	−22.8% (Δ 7.8%)

The presence of ischemia is associated with altered GLS. Segmental strain analysis is a good complementary tool to WMSI. Regional assessment of strain imaging quantitatively measures regional wall motion and can be used with resting and stress echocardiography [124]. High doses dobutamine or exercise echocardiography may add the GLS reserve to the WMSI (Fig. 8.13a, b).

Pressure Strain Loops (PSL)

The area of a pressure-volume loop (PVL) has been consistently shown in both animal and human studies to be an excellent predictor of myocardial oxygen consumption (MVO2), independent of loading conditions [132–134].

Pressure-strain loops (PSL) are delineated by the GLS variation during a cardiac cycle, approximating the shape of the PVL; their area represents a good surrogate for myocardial work (MW) [135]. For a PSL, the cyclic evolution of strain is not related to the variation of pressure, but to a single cuff measurement.

Analysis of myocardial work components [136]:

- Global work index (GWI): Total work; the PSL area loop calculated from mitral valve closure (MVC) to mitral valve opening (MVO) (Fig. 8.14a)
- Global constructive work (GCW): Total work contributing to pump function from aortic valve opening (AVO) to MVO, i.e., shortening of the myocytes during systole and lengthening during isovolumic relaxation.
- Global wasted work (GWW): Work that does not contribute to ejection; elongation of myocytes during systole and shortening against a closed AV.
- Global Work Efficiency (GWE) is the ratio: GWE = GCW/(GCW + GWW)

Non-invasive evaluation of global and segmental PSL was developed by the GE echocardiography vendor [137]. The initial study work from Russell et al. showed an excellent correlation between regional PSL and regional myocardial metabolism as evaluated using positron emission tomography (PET) [138]. The same authors also introduced the concept of global and segmental wasted work ratio (this is the ratio between the negative (meaning wasted work) and the positive (constructed work), having an immediate clinical relevance in assessing dyssynchrony [139]. When left bundle branch block occurs, while some segments are still contracting during systole (giving the positive constructed MW), the dyssinchronuos septum will begin relaxing and lengthen in late systole and create negative, wasted work [139]. The wasted work may thus be interpreted as a measure of contractile reserve, available after the successful correction of dyssynchrony (with CRT therapy), provided of course, that the segments are viable [139].

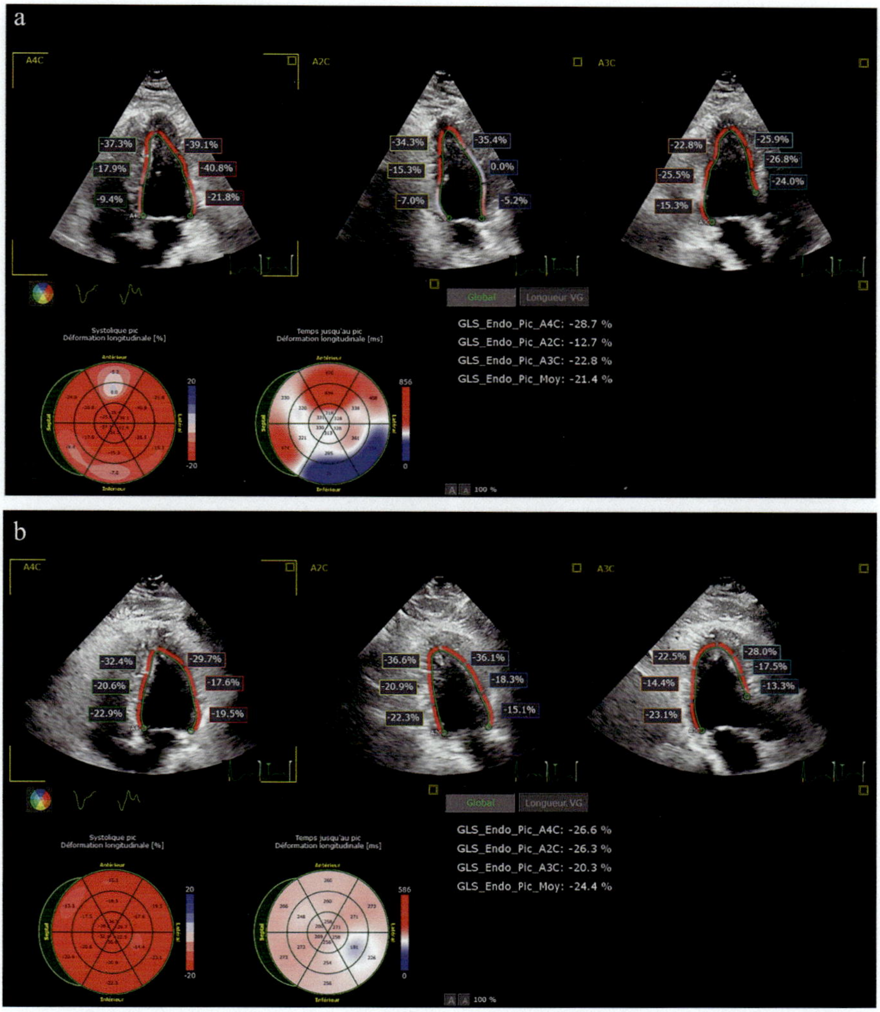

Fig. 8.13 (**a**) Exercise stress echocardiography in a patient with subendocardial infarction and 2-vessel PCI. Basal GLS: −21.4%; 4 segments with diminished longitudinal strain. (**b**) GLS calculated in the first minute of recovery after maximal exercise. GLS: −24.4% (Δ 3%) and quasi normalized strain

While a multitude of articles describing the application of this concept in clinical practice, were later published [140, 141], its role in further evaluating global and regional LV contractile reserve is less investigated. One Italian group showed only a poor determination coefficient of global MW indices using invasively the formula for LV stroke work index (= mean systemic arterial pressure–mean pulmonary artery wedge pressure) × stroke volume index × 0.0136) [142]; therefore, these indices should not be used interchangeably and have different physiological meaning.

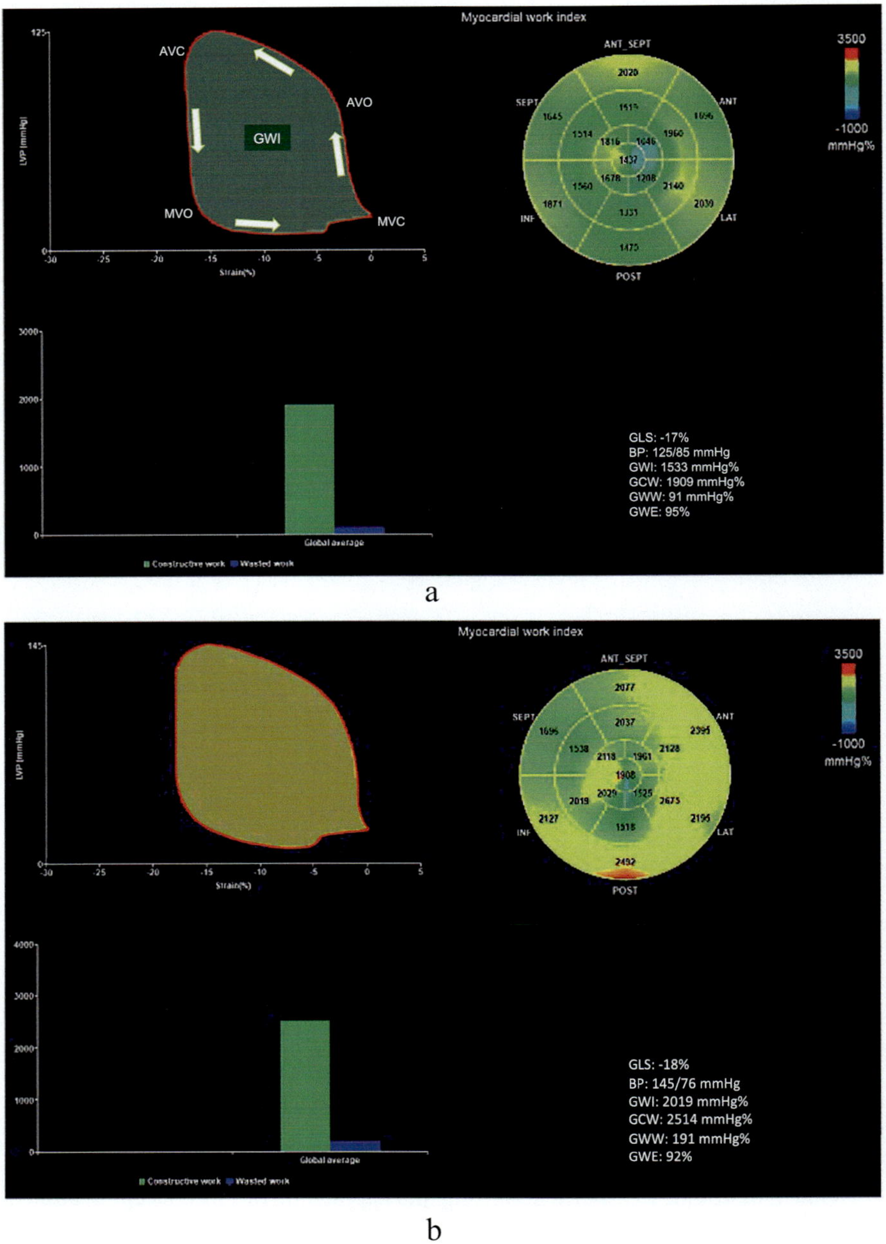

Fig. 8.14 37 young male, genetic DCM, without treatment, LVEF 50%, LVESVi 38 ml/m^2, LVEDVi 76 ml/m^2: (**a**) Basal Strain Loop. *MVO* mitral valve opening, *MVC* mitral valve closure, *AVO* aortic valve opening, *AVC* aortic valve closure. (**b**) Dobutamine 10 µg/kg/min. *GLS* less than 2% improvement; GWI: +32%; GCW: +32%; GWW: +110%; GWE: −3%. Less than 2% strain improvement indicates a low CR and/or afterload mismatch. GWE is blunted by doubling the GWW. In the case of dilated familial cardiomyopathy without LBBB, the increase in GWW suggests a positive dobutamine inotropy but a possible discrete subtle dyssynchrony

With ischemia, dobutamine stress testing can drive a positive regional work gain but this will be at least in part offset by an increase in wasted work (especially in the longitudinal strain direction) [143, 144]. Leitman et al. [145], showed that the use of dobutamine in low doses of 10 μg/kg/min (with unchanged BP) in a cohort of patients with normal dobutamine stress echocardiography resulted in a significant decrease of specific global MW index parameters, while global wasted work increased (global constructive work decreased from 2681.7 to 2152.6 mmHg%, $p = 0.001$, $p < 0.003$; global wasted work increased from 78.8 to 128.3 mmHg%) [145]. It therefore appears that the pattern of global MW indices in response to dobutamine, is greatly influenced by the amount of wasted work; the CR that may be recruited by the inotropic effect of dobutamine, will come with the price of more wasted work (the phenomenon may be understood as an extrapolation of the commonly recognized higher O2 consumption with dobutamine)—as depicted in (Fig. 8.14). The ability to explore regional mechanics by following the variability of regional MW indices may prove the more clinically relevant instrument.

A novel non-invasive index of LV systolic performance was derived from simultaneous registration of LV strain and brachial pressure waveforms [146]. The pressure-strain loop was obtained by integrating the pressure/time curve with the strain/time curve and was termed LV ejection work density (EWD). Older age, female sex, and hypertension were associated with higher EWD.

A Final Word Hemodynamics is a chaotic situation, which means that a huge number of non-linear variables are constantly interacting. Instead of focusing on a single parameter, we need an integrated view.

Future Directions and Developments

Today, in most departments, invasive cardiology is dedicated to interventional procedures, few centers continue to perform invasive hemodynamics. Even though magnetic resonance imaging outperforms echocardiography, echocardiography remains the everyday clinical tool. How can we bring the enormous amount of information and the huge number of sometimes very complex formulas, required for high-end diagnostics, into the everyday practice? Two directions seem promising:

1. Make echocardiographs more efficient for advanced hemodynamic studies. For example, pressure-volume loops could be a way forward by integrating 3D ventricular volume variations with an accompanying concomitant pressure curve (tonometer, sphygmomanometer). With a few pressure-volume loops, a strong Ees surrogate could be computed.
2. Integrate artificial intelligence into routine activities: which formula is more appropriate for a specific situation, what are its limitations, what could be the degree of approximation according to the patient's pathology, sex, age, comorbidities, etc.? A deep learning AI could have a significant impact on the feasibility and accuracy of diagnosis through multiple heterogeneous connections.

References

1. Puglisi JL, Negroni JA, Chen-Izu Y, Bers DM. The force-frequency relationship: insights from mathematical modeling. Adv Physiol Educ. 2013;37(1):28–34.
2. Inagaki M, Yokota M, Izawa H, Ishiki R, Nagata K, Iwase M, et al. Impaired force-frequency relations in patients with hypertensive left ventricular hypertrophy. A possible physiological marker of the transition from physiological to pathological hypertrophy. Circulation. 1999;99(14):1822–30.
3. Silverman DN, Rambod M, Lustgarten DL, Lobel R, LeWinter MM, Meyer M. Heart rate-induced myocardial Ca(2+) retention and left ventricular volume loss in patients with heart failure with preserved ejection fraction. J Am Heart Assoc. 2020;9(17):e017215.
4. Reddy YNV, Koepp KE, Carter R, Win S, Jain CC, Olson TP, et al. Rate-adaptive atrial pacing for heart failure with preserved ejection fraction: the RAPID-HF randomized clinical trial. JAMA. 2023;329(10):801–9.
5. Westerhof N, Boer C, Lamberts RR, Sipkema P. Cross-talk between cardiac muscle and coronary vasculature. Physiol Rev. 2006;86(4):1263–308.
6. Cingolani HE, Perez NG, Cingolani OH, Ennis IL. The Anrep effect: 100 years later. Am J Physiol Heart Circ Physiol. 2013;304(2):H175–82.
7. Boushel R. Muscle metaboreflex control of the circulation during exercise. Acta Physiol (Oxford). 2010;199(4):367–83.
8. Crisafulli A, Salis E, Tocco F, Melis F, Milia R, Pittau G, et al. Impaired central hemodynamic response and exaggerated vasoconstriction during muscle metaboreflex activation in heart failure patients. Am J Physiol Heart Circ Physiol. 2007;292(6):H2988–96.
9. Coutsos M, Sala-Mercado JA, Ichinose M, Li Z, Dawe EJ, O'Leary DS. Muscle metaboreflex-induced coronary vasoconstriction limits ventricular contractility during dynamic exercise in heart failure. Am J Physiol Heart Circ Physiol. 2013;304(7):H1029–37.
10. Smith JR, Hammer SM, Bruhn EJ, Borlaug BA, Olson TP. Abstract 10528: exaggerated inspiratory muscle metaboreflex in heart failure with preserved ejection fraction. Circulation. 2021;144(Suppl_1):A10528-A.
11. Peverill RE. Understanding preload and preload reserve within the conceptual framework of a limited range of possible left ventricular end-diastolic volumes. Adv Physiol Educ. 2020;44(3):414–22.
12. Fudim M, Sobotka PA, Dunlap ME. Extracardiac abnormalities of preload reserve: mechanisms underlying exercise limitation in heart failure with preserved ejection fraction, autonomic dysfunction, and liver disease. Circ Heart Fail. 2021;14(1):e007308.
13. Monnet X, Teboul JL. Passive leg raising: five rules, not a drop of fluid! Crit Care. 2015;19(1):18.
14. Bytyci I, Bajraktari G, Lindqvist P, Henein MY. Compromised left atrial function and increased size predict raised cavity pressure: a systematic review and meta-analysis. Clin Physiol Funct Imaging. 2019;39(5):297–307.
15. Inoue K, Khan FH, Remme EW, Ohte N, Garcia-Izquierdo E, Chetrit M, et al. Determinants of left atrial reservoir and pump strain and use of atrial strain for evaluation of left ventricular filling pressure. Eur Heart J Cardiovasc Imaging. 2021;23(1):61–70.
16. van de Bovenkamp AA, Wijkstra N, Oosterveer FPT, Vonk Noordegraaf A, Bogaard HJ, van Rossum AC, et al. The value of passive leg raise during right heart catheterization in diagnosing heart failure with preserved ejection fraction. Circ Heart Fail. 2022;15(4):e008935.
17. Crystal GJ, Assaad SI, Heerdt PM. 24—cardiovascular physiology: integrative function. In: Hemmings HC, Egan TD, editors. Pharmacology and physiology for anesthesia. 2nd ed. Philadelphia: Elsevier; 2019. p. 473–519.
18. Seymour RS, Blaylock AJ. The principle of Laplace and scaling of ventricular wall stress and blood pressure in mammals and birds. Physiol Biochem Zool. 2000;73(4):389–405.
19. Westerhof N, Lankhaar JW, Westerhof BE. The arterial Windkessel. Med Biol Eng Comput. 2009;47(2):131–41.

20. Chirinos JA, Segers P. Noninvasive evaluation of left ventricular afterload: part 1: pressure and flow measurements and basic principles of wave conduction and reflection. Hypertension. 2010;56(4):555–62.
21. Suma K, Tsuji T. Maximum tolerable afterload and afterload reserve for the evaluation of ventricular performance. Jpn Heart J. 1978;19(1):84–93.
22. Ross J Jr. The concept of afterload mismatch and its implications in the clinical assessment of cardiac contractility. Jpn Circ J. 1976;40(8):865–75.
23. Norton JM. Toward consistent definitions for preload and afterload. Adv Physiol Educ. 2001;25(1–4):53–61.
24. Arts T, Bovendeerd PH, Prinzen FW, Reneman RS. Relation between left ventricular cavity pressure and volume and systolic fiber stress and strain in the wall. Biophys J. 1991;59(1):93–102.
25. Chirinos JA, Segers P, Rietzschel ER, De Buyzere ML, Raja MW, Claessens T, et al. Early and late systolic wall stress differentially relate to myocardial contraction and relaxation in middle-aged adults: the Asklepios study. Hypertension. 2013;61(2):296–303.
26. Zhao X, Tan RS, Tang HC, Teo SK, Su Y, Wan M, et al. Left ventricular wall stress is sensitive marker of hypertrophic cardiomyopathy with preserved ejection fraction. Front Physiol. 2018;9:250.
27. de Simone G, Devereux RB, Roman MJ, Ganau A, Saba PS, Alderman MH, et al. Assessment of left ventricular function by the midwall fractional shortening/end-systolic stress relation in human hypertension. J Am Coll Cardiol. 1994;23(6):1444–51.
28. de Simone G, Devereux RB, Koren MJ, Mensah GA, Casale PN, Laragh JH. Midwall left ventricular mechanics. An independent predictor of cardiovascular risk in arterial hypertension. Circulation. 1996;93(2):259–65.
29. Ito S, Pislaru C, Miranda WR, Nkomo VT, Connolly HM, Pislaru SV, et al. Left ventricular contractility and wall stress in patients with aortic stenosis with preserved or reduced ejection fraction. JACC Cardiovasc Imaging. 2020;13(2 Pt 1):357–69.
30. Chao CJ, Agasthi P, Seri AR, Barry T, Shanbhag A, Wang Y, et al. Transcatheter aortic valve replacement prognostication with augmented mean arterial pressure. J Cardiovasc Dev Dis. 2023;10(5):192.
31. Lancellotti P, Pellikka PA, Budts W, Chaudhry FA, Donal E, Dulgheru R, et al. The clinical use of stress echocardiography in non-ischaemic heart disease: recommendations from the European Association of Cardiovascular Imaging and the American Society of Echocardiography. Eur Heart J Cardiovasc Imaging. 2016;17(11):1191–229.
32. Fowler MB, Laser JA, Hopkins GL, Minobe W, Bristow MR. Assessment of the beta-adrenergic receptor pathway in the intact failing human heart: progressive receptor down-regulation and subsensitivity to agonist response. Circulation. 1986;74(6):1290–302.
33. Bombardini T, Zoppe M, Ciampi Q, Cortigiani L, Agricola E, Salvadori S, et al. Myocardial contractility in the stress echo lab: from pathophysiological toy to clinical tool. Cardiovasc Ultrasound. 2013;11:41.
34. Pratali L, Otasevic P, Neskovic A, Molinaro S, Picano E. Prognostic value of pharmacologic stress echocardiography in patients with idiopathic dilated cardiomyopathy: a prospective, head-to-head comparison between dipyridamole and dobutamine test. J Card Fail. 2007;13(10):836–42.
35. Mehrotra P, Labib SB, Schick EC. Differential effects of dobutamine versus treadmill exercise on left ventricular volume and wall stress. J Am Soc Echocardiogr. 2012;25(8):911–8.
36. Whitman M, Jenkins C. Rate pressure product, age predicted maximum heart rate or heart rate reserve. Which one better predicts cardiovascular events following exercise stress echocardiography? Am J Cardiovasc Dis. 2021;11(4):450–7.
37. Erdei T, Smiseth OA, Marino P, Fraser AG. A systematic review of diastolic stress tests in heart failure with preserved ejection fraction, with proposals from the EU-FP7 MEDIA study group. Eur J Heart Fail. 2014;16(12):1345–61.

38. Ciampi Q, Zagatina A, Cortigiani L, Wierzbowska-Drabik K, Kasprzak JD, Haberka M, et al. Prognostic value of stress echocardiography assessed by the ABCDE protocol. Eur Heart J. 2021;42(37):3869–78.
39. Bach DS, Beanlands RS, Schwaiger M, Armstrong WF. Heterogeneity of ventricular function and myocardial oxidative metabolism in nonischemic dilated cardiomyopathy. J Am Coll Cardiol. 1995;25(6):1258–62.
40. Otasevic P, Popovic ZB, Vasiljevic JD, Pratali L, Vlahovic-Stipac A, Boskovic SD, et al. Head-to-head comparison of indices of left ventricular contractile reserve assessed by high-dose dobutamine stress echocardiography in idiopathic dilated cardiomyopathy: five-year follow up. Heart. 2006;92(9):1253–8.
41. Agricola E, Picano E, Oppizzi M, Pisani M, Meris A, Fragasso G, et al. Assessment of stress-induced pulmonary interstitial edema by chest ultrasound during exercise echocardiography and its correlation with left ventricular function. J Am Soc Echocardiogr. 2006;19(4):457–63.
42. Gargani L, Girerd N, Platz E, Pellicori P, Stankovic I, Palazzuoli A, et al. Lung ultrasound in acute and chronic heart failure: a clinical consensus statement of the European Association of Cardiovascular Imaging (EACVI). Eur Heart J Cardiovasc Imaging. 2023;24(12):1569–82.
43. Gulati M, Shaw LJ, Thisted RA, Black HR, Bairey Merz CN, Arnsdorf MF. Heart rate response to exercise stress testing in asymptomatic women: the St. James women take heart project. Circulation. 2010;122(2):130–7.
44. Brubaker PH, Kitzman DW. Chronotropic incompetence: causes, consequences, and management. Circulation. 2011;123(9):1010–20.
45. Tanaka H, Monahan KD, Seals DR. Age-predicted maximal heart rate revisited. J Am Coll Cardiol. 2001;37(1):153–6.
46. Brawner CA, Ehrman JK, Schairer JR, Cao JJ, Keteyian SJ. Predicting maximum heart rate among patients with coronary heart disease receiving beta-adrenergic blockade therapy. Am Heart J. 2004;148(5):910–4.
47. Zweerink A, van der Lingen ACJ, Handoko ML, van Rossum AC, Allaart CP. Chronotropic incompetence in chronic heart failure. Circ Heart Fail. 2018;11(8):e004969.
48. Thein PM, Mirzaee S, Cameron JD, Nasis A. Left ventricular contractile reserve as a determinant of adverse clinical outcomes: a systematic review. Intern Med J. 2022;52(2):186–97.
49. Sagawa K, Suga H, Shoukas AA, Bakalar KM. End-systolic pressure/volume ratio: a new index of ventricular contractility. Am J Cardiol. 1977;40(5):748–53.
50. Burkhoff D, Mirsky I, Suga H. Assessment of systolic and diastolic ventricular properties via pressure-volume analysis: a guide for clinical, translational, and basic researchers. Am J Physiol Heart Circ Physiol. 2005;289(2):H501–12.
51. Starling MR. Left ventricular-arterial coupling relations in the normal human heart. Am Heart J. 1993;125(6):1659–66.
52. Maughan WL, Sunagawa K, Burkhoff D, Sagawa K. Effect of arterial impedance changes on the end-systolic pressure-volume relation. Circ Res. 1984;54(5):595–602.
53. Senzaki H, Chen CH, Kass DA. Single-beat estimation of end-systolic pressure-volume relation in humans. A new method with the potential for noninvasive application. Circulation. 1996;94(10):2497–506.
54. Asanoi H, Sasayama S, Kameyama T. Ventriculoarterial coupling in normal and failing heart in humans. Circ Res. 1989;65(2):483–93.
55. Mihaileanu S, Antohi EL. Revisiting the relationship between left ventricular ejection fraction and ventricular-arterial coupling. ESC Heart Fail. 2020;7(5):2214–22.
56. Suga H, Sagawa K, Shoukas AA. Load independence of the instantaneous pressure-volume ratio of the canine left ventricle and effects of epinephrine and heart rate on the ratio. Circ Res. 1973;32(3):314–22.
57. Chantler PD, Lakatta EG. Arterial-ventricular coupling with aging and disease. Front Physiol. 2012;3:90.

58. Shishido T, Hayashi K, Shigemi K, Sato T, Sugimachi M, Sunagawa K. Single-beat estimation of end-systolic elastance using bilinearly approximated time-varying elastance curve. Circulation. 2000;102(16):1983–9.
59. Chen CH, Fetics B, Nevo E, Rochitte CE, Chiou KR, Ding PA, et al. Noninvasive single-beat determination of left ventricular end-systolic elastance in humans. J Am Coll Cardiol. 2001;38(7):2028–34.
60. Chen CH, Nevo E, Fetics B, Pak PH, Yin FC, Maughan WL, et al. Estimation of central aortic pressure waveform by mathematical transformation of radial tonometry pressure. Validation of generalized transfer function. Circulation. 1997;95(7):1827–36.
61. Gayat E, Mor-Avi V, Weinert L, Yodwut C, Lang RM. Noninvasive quantification of left ventricular elastance and ventricular-arterial coupling using three-dimensional echocardiography and arterial tonometry. Am J Physiol Heart Circ Physiol. 2011;301(5):H1916–23.
62. Wo N, Rajagopal V, Cheung MMH, Smolich JJ, Mynard JP. Assessment of single beat end-systolic elastance methods for quantifying ventricular contractility. Heart Vessel. 2019;34(4):716–23.
63. Reant P, Dijos M, Donal E, Mignot A, Ritter P, Bordachar P, et al. Systolic time intervals as simple echocardiographic parameters of left ventricular systolic performance: correlation with ejection fraction and longitudinal two-dimensional strain. Eur J Echocardiogr. 2010;11(10):834–44.
64. Antohi EL, Chioncel O, Mihaileanu S. Overcoming the limits of ejection fraction and ventricular-arterial coupling in heart failure. Front Cardiovasc Med. 2021;8:750965.
65. Di Molfetta A, Ferrari G, Cusimano V, Di Ruzza G, Mollo P, Boncompagni D, et al. Sensitivity analysis of single beat left ventricular elastance estimation by Chen method. Cardiovasc Eng Technol. 2022;13(1):139–46.
66. Bombardini T, Costantino MF, Sicari R, Ciampi Q, Pratali L, Picano E. End-systolic elastance and ventricular-arterial coupling reserve predict cardiac events in patients with negative stress echocardiography. Biomed Res Int. 2013;2013:235194.
67. Ciampi Q, Pratali L, Citro R, Villari B, Picano E, Sicari R. Clinical and prognostic role of pressure-volume relationship in the identification of responders to cardiac resynchronization therapy. Am Heart J. 2010;160(5):906–14.
68. Picano E, Bombardini T, Kovacevic Preradovic T, Cortigiani L, Wierzbowska-Drabik K, Ciampi Q. Left ventricular contractile reserve in stress echocardiography: the bright side of the force. Kardiol Pol. 2019;77(2):164–72.
69. Borlaug BA, Kass DA. Ventricular-vascular interaction in heart failure. Heart Fail Clin. 2008;4(1):23–36.
70. Sunagawa K, Maughan WL, Burkhoff D, Sagawa K. Left ventricular interaction with arterial load studied in isolated canine ventricle. Am J Phys. 1983;245(5 Pt 1):H773–80.
71. Kelly RP, Ting CT, Yang TM, Liu CP, Maughan WL, Chang MS, et al. Effective arterial elastance as index of arterial vascular load in humans. Circulation. 1992;86(2):513–21.
72. Segers P, Stergiopulos N, Westerhof N. Relation of effective arterial elastance to arterial system properties. Am J Physiol Heart Circ Physiol. 2002;282(3):H1041–6.
73. Redfield MM, Jacobsen SJ, Borlaug BA, Rodeheffer RJ, Kass DA. Age- and gender-related ventricular-vascular stiffening: a community-based study. Circulation. 2005;112(15):2254–62.
74. Chemla D, Hebert JL, Coirault C, Zamani K, Suard I, Colin P, et al. Total arterial compliance estimated by stroke volume-to-aortic pulse pressure ratio in humans. Am J Phys. 1998;274(2):H500–5.
75. Najjar SS, Schulman SP, Gerstenblith G, Fleg JL, Kass DA, O'Connor F, et al. Age and gender affect ventricular-vascular coupling during aerobic exercise. J Am Coll Cardiol. 2004;44(3):611–7.
76. Matsumoto K, Tanaka H, Ooka J, Motoji Y, Sawa T, Mochizuki Y, et al. Significant prognostic impact of improvement in ventriculo-arterial coupling induced by dobutamine stress on

cardiovascular outcome for patients with dilated cardiomyopathy. Eur Heart J Cardiovasc Imaging. 2016;17(11):1296–304.
77. Guinot P-G, Andrei S, Longrois D. Ventriculo-arterial coupling: from physiological concept to clinical application in peri-operative care and ICUs. Eur J Anaesthesiol Intensive Care. 2022;1(2):e004.
78. Ky B, French B, May Khan A, Plappert T, Wang A, Chirinos JA, et al. Ventricular-arterial coupling, remodeling, and prognosis in chronic heart failure. J Am Coll Cardiol. 2013;62(13):1165–72.
79. Antonini-Canterin F, Enache R, Popescu BA, Popescu AC, Ginghina C, Leiballi E, et al. Prognostic value of ventricular-arterial coupling and B-type natriuretic peptide in patients after myocardial infarction: a five-year follow-up study. J Am Soc Echocardiogr. 2009;22(11):1239–45.
80. Burkhoff D. Pressure-volume loops in clinical research: a contemporary view. J Am Coll Cardiol. 2013;62(13):1173–6.
81. Vanhentenrijk S, Verbrugge FH, Tang WHW, Menon V. PRO: vasodilators remain an indispensable treatment for acute heart failure. Eur Heart J Acute Cardiovasc Care. 2022;11(11):850–7.
82. Kawaguchi M, Hay I, Fetics B, Kass DA. Combined ventricular systolic and arterial stiffening in patients with heart failure and preserved ejection fraction: implications for systolic and diastolic reserve limitations. Circulation. 2003;107(5):714–20.
83. Rosch S, Kresoja KP, Besler C, Fengler K, Schober AR, von Roeder M, et al. Characteristics of heart failure with preserved ejection fraction across the range of left ventricular ejection fraction. Circulation. 2022;146(7):506–18.
84. Nguyen M, Berhoud V, Bartamian L, Martin A, Ellouze O, Bouhemad B, et al. Agreement between different non-invasive methods of ventricular elastance assessment for the monitoring of ventricular-arterial coupling in intensive care. J Clin Monit Comput. 2020;34(5):893–901.
85. Burkhoff D, Sagawa K. Ventricular efficiency predicted by an analytical model. Am J Phys. 1986;250(6 Pt 2):R1021–7.
86. Bastos MB, Burkhoff D, Maly J, Daemen J, den Uil CA, Ameloot K, et al. Invasive left ventricle pressure-volume analysis: overview and practical clinical implications. Eur Heart J. 2020;41(12):1286–97.
87. Monge Garcia MI, Santos A. Understanding ventriculo-arterial coupling. Ann Transl Med. 2020;8(12):795.
88. Cheng HM, Yu WC, Sung SH, Wang KL, Chuang SY, Chen CH. Usefulness of systolic time intervals in the identification of abnormal ventriculo-arterial coupling in stable heart failure patients. Eur J Heart Fail. 2008;10(12):1192–200.
89. Chaudhry R, Miao JH, Rehman A. Physiology, cardiovascular. [Updated 2022 Oct 16]. In: StatPearls [Internet]. Treasure Island: StatPearls Publishing; 2023. Available from: https://www.ncbi.nlm.nih.gov/books/NBK493197/.
90. Hayashi K, Shigemi K, Shishido T, Sugimachi M, Sunagawa K. Single-beat estimation of ventricular end-systolic elastance-effective arterial elastance as an index of ventricular mechanoenergetic performance. Anesthesiology. 2000;92(6):1769–76.
91. Ikonomidis I, Aboyans V, Blacher J, Brodmann M, Brutsaert DL, Chirinos JA, et al. The role of ventricular-arterial coupling in cardiac disease and heart failure: assessment, clinical implications and therapeutic interventions. A consensus document of the European Society of Cardiology Working Group on Aorta & Peripheral Vascular Diseases, European Association of Cardiovascular Imaging, and Heart Failure Association. Eur J Heart Fail. 2019;21(4):402–24.
92. Pugliese NR, Balletti A, Armenia S, De Biase N, Faita F, Mengozzi A, et al. Ventricular-arterial coupling derived from proximal aortic stiffness and aerobic capacity across the heart failure spectrum. JACC Cardiovasc Imaging. 2022;15(9):1545–59.
93. Chirinos JA. Ventricular-arterial coupling in heart failure: time to close the loop and catch the wave? JACC Cardiovasc Imaging. 2022;15(9):1560–2.

94. Kerkhof PLM, van de Ven PM, Yoo B, Peace RA, Heyndrickx GR, Handly N. Ejection fraction as related to basic components in the left and right ventricular volume domains. Int J Cardiol. 2018;255:105–10.
95. Stokke TM, Hasselberg NE, Smedsrud MK, Sarvari SI, Haugaa KH, Smiseth OA, et al. Geometry as a confounder when assessing ventricular systolic function: comparison between ejection fraction and strain. J Am Coll Cardiol. 2017;70(8):942–54.
96. Tona F, Zanatta E, Montisci R, Muraru D, Beccegato E, De Zorzi E, et al. Higher ventricular-arterial coupling derived from three-dimensional echocardiography is associated with a worse clinical outcome in systemic sclerosis. Pharmaceuticals (Basel). 2021;14(7):646.
97. Wehner GJ, Jing L, Haggerty CM, Suever JD, Leader JB, Hartzel DN, et al. Routinely reported ejection fraction and mortality in clinical practice: where does the nadir of risk lie? Eur Heart J. 2020;41(12):1249–57.
98. Leung DY, Griffin BP, Stewart WJ, Cosgrove DM 3rd, Thomas JD, Marwick TH. Left ventricular function after valve repair for chronic mitral regurgitation: predictive value of preoperative assessment of contractile reserve by exercise echocardiography. J Am Coll Cardiol. 1996;28(5):1198–205.
99. Lee R, Haluska B, Leung DY, Case C, Mundy J, Marwick TH. Functional and prognostic implications of left ventricular contractile reserve in patients with asymptomatic severe mitral regurgitation. Heart. 2005;91(11):1407–12.
100. Park SJ, Enriquez-Sarano M, Song JE, Lee YJ, Ha MR, Chang SA, et al. Contractile reserve determined on exercise echocardiography in patients with severe aortic regurgitation. Circ J. 2013;77(9):2390–8.
101. Waddingham PH, Bhattacharyya S, Zalen JV, Lloyd G. Contractile reserve as a predictor of prognosis in patients with non-ischaemic systolic heart failure and dilated cardiomyopathy: a systematic review and meta-analysis. Echo Res Pract. 2018;5(1):1–9.
102. Wood PW, Choy JB, Nanda NC, Becher H. Left ventricular ejection fraction and volumes: it depends on the imaging method. Echocardiography. 2014;31(1):87–100.
103. Pibarot P, Dumesnil JG. Low-flow, low-gradient aortic stenosis with normal and depressed left ventricular ejection fraction. J Am Coll Cardiol. 2012;60(19):1845–53.
104. Monin JL, Monchi M, Gest V, Duval-Moulin AM, Dubois-Rande JL, Gueret P. Aortic stenosis with severe left ventricular dysfunction and low transvalvular pressure gradients: risk stratification by low-dose dobutamine echocardiography. J Am Coll Cardiol. 2001;37(8):2101–7.
105. Monin JL, Quere JP, Monchi M, Petit H, Baleynaud S, Chauvel C, et al. Low-gradient aortic stenosis: operative risk stratification and predictors for long-term outcome: a multicenter study using dobutamine stress hemodynamics. Circulation. 2003;108(3):319–24.
106. Tribouilloy C, Levy F, Rusinaru D, Gueret P, Petit-Eisenmann H, Baleynaud S, et al. Outcome after aortic valve replacement for low-flow/low-gradient aortic stenosis without contractile reserve on dobutamine stress echocardiography. J Am Coll Cardiol. 2009;53(20):1865–73.
107. Maes F, Lerakis S, Barbosa Ribeiro H, Gilard M, Cavalcante JL, Makkar R, et al. Outcomes from transcatheter aortic valve replacement in patients with low-flow, low-gradient aortic stenosis and left ventricular ejection fraction less than 30%: a substudy from the TOPAS-TAVI registry. JAMA Cardiol. 2019;4(1):64–70.
108. Dreyfus G, Mihealainu S. The Batista procedure. Heart. 2001;85(1):1–2.
109. Lim HS. Cardiac power output revisited. Circ Heart Fail. 2020;13(10):e007393.
110. Grodin JL, Mullens W, Dupont M, Wu Y, Taylor DO, Starling RC, et al. Prognostic role of cardiac power index in ambulatory patients with advanced heart failure. Eur J Heart Fail. 2015;17(7):689–96.
111. Anand V, Kane GC, Scott CG, Pislaru SV, Adigun RO, McCully RB, et al. Prognostic value of peak stress cardiac power in patients with normal ejection fraction undergoing exercise stress echocardiography. Eur Heart J. 2021;42(7):776–85.
112. Takizawa D, Harada T, Obokata M, Kagami K, Sorimachi H, Yuasa N, et al. Pathophysiologic and prognostic importance of cardiac power output reserve in heart failure with preserved ejection fraction. Eur Heart J Cardiovasc Imaging. 2024;25(2):220–8.

113. Cortigiani L, Sorbo S, Miccoli M, Scali MC, Simioniuc A, Morrone D, et al. Prognostic value of cardiac power output to left ventricular mass in patients with left ventricular dysfunction and dobutamine stress echo negative by wall motion criteria. Eur Heart J Cardiovasc Imaging. 2017;18(2):153–8.
114. Pugliese NR, Fabiani I, Mandoli GE, Guarini G, Galeotti GG, Miccoli M, et al. Echo-derived peak cardiac power output-to-left ventricular mass with cardiopulmonary exercise testing predicts outcome in patients with heart failure and depressed systolic function. Eur Heart J Cardiovasc Imaging. 2019;20(6):700–8.
115. Kass DA, Maughan WL, Guo ZM, Kono A, Sunagawa K, Sagawa K. Comparative influence of load versus inotropic states on indexes of ventricular contractility: experimental and theoretical analysis based on pressure-volume relationships. Circulation. 1987;76(6):1422–36.
116. Chen C, Rodriguez L, Guerrero JL, Marshall S, Levine RA, Weyman AE, et al. Noninvasive estimation of the instantaneous first derivative of left ventricular pressure using continuous-wave Doppler echocardiography. Circulation. 1991;83(6):2101–10.
117. Seo JS, Kim DH, Kim WJ, Song JM, Kang DH, Song JK. Peak systolic velocity of mitral annular longitudinal movement measured by pulsed tissue Doppler imaging as an index of global left ventricular contractility. Am J Physiol Heart Circ Physiol. 2010;298(5):H1608–15.
118. Ciampi Q, Pratali L, Porta MD, Petruzziello B, Manganiello V, Villari B, et al. Tissue Doppler systolic velocity change during dobutamine stress echocardiography predicts contractile reserve and exercise tolerance in patients with heart failure. Eur Heart J Cardiovasc Imaging. 2013;14(2):102–9.
119. Weidemann F, Jamal F, Kowalski M, Kukulski T, D'Hooge J, Bijnens B, et al. Can strain rate and strain quantify changes in regional systolic function during dobutamine infusion, B-blockade, and atrial pacing—implications for quantitative stress echocardiography. J Am Soc Echocardiogr. 2002;15(5):416–24.
120. Murai D, Yamada S, Hayashi T, Okada K, Nishino H, Nakabachi M, et al. Relationships of left ventricular strain and strain rate to wall stress and their afterload dependency. Heart Vessel. 2017;32(5):574–83.
121. Nabeshima Y, Seo Y, Takeuchi M. A review of current trends in three-dimensional analysis of left ventricular myocardial strain. Cardiovasc Ultrasound. 2020;18(1):23.
122. Lang RM, Badano LP, Mor-Avi V, Afilalo J, Armstrong A, Ernande L, et al. Recommendations for cardiac chamber quantification by echocardiography in adults: an update from the American Society of Echocardiography and the European Association of Cardiovascular Imaging. Eur Heart J Cardiovasc Imaging. 2015;16(3):233–70.
123. Wang TKM, Desai MY, Collier P, Grimm RA, Griffin BP, Popovic ZB. Determining the thresholds for abnormal left ventricular strains in healthy subjects by echocardiography: a meta-analysis. Cardiovasc Diagn Ther. 2020;10(6):1858–73.
124. Luis SA, Chan J, Pellikka PA. Echocardiographic assessment of left ventricular systolic function: an overview of contemporary techniques, including speckle-tracking echocardiography. Mayo Clin Proc. 2019;94(1):125–38.
125. Fung MJ, Thomas L, Leung DY. Left ventricular function and contractile reserve in patients with hypertension. Eur Heart J Cardiovasc Imaging. 2018;19(11):1253–9.
126. Lancellotti P, Cosyns B, Zacharakis D, Attena E, Van Camp G, Gach O, et al. Importance of left ventricular longitudinal function and functional reserve in patients with degenerative mitral regurgitation: assessment by two-dimensional speckle tracking. J Am Soc Echocardiogr. 2008;21(12):1331–6.
127. Magne J, Mahjoub H, Dulgheru R, Pibarot P, Pierard LA, Lancellotti P. Left ventricular contractile reserve in asymptomatic primary mitral regurgitation. Eur Heart J. 2014;35(24):1608–16.
128. Benyounes N, Lang S, Soulat-Dufour L, Obadia M, Gout O, Chevalier G, et al. Can global longitudinal strain predict reduced left ventricular ejection fraction in daily echocardiographic practice? Arch Cardiovasc Dis. 2015;108(1):50–6.
129. Hasselberg NE, Haugaa KH, Sarvari SI, Gullestad L, Andreassen AK, Smiseth OA, et al. Left ventricular global longitudinal strain is associated with exercise capacity in fail-

ing hearts with preserved and reduced ejection fraction. Eur Heart J Cardiovasc Imaging. 2015;16(2):217–24.
130. Wang J, Fang F, Wai-Kwok Yip G, Sanderson JE, Feng W, Xie JM, et al. Left ventricular long-axis performance during exercise is an important prognosticator in patients with heart failure and preserved ejection fraction. Int J Cardiol. 2015;178:131–5.
131. Arbucci R, Lowenstein Haber DM, Rousse MG, Saad AK, Martinez Golleti L, Gastaldello N, et al. Long term prognostic value of contractile reserve assessed by global longitudinal strain in patients with asymptomatic severe aortic stenosis. J Clin Med. 2022;11(3):689.
132. Suga H, Goto Y, Nozawa T, Yasumura Y, Futaki S, Tanaka N. Force-time integral decreases with ejection despite constant oxygen consumption and pressure-volume area in dog left ventricle. Circ Res. 1987;60(6):797–803.
133. Takaoka H, Takeuchi M, Odake M, Yokoyama M. Assessment of myocardial oxygen consumption (Vo2) and systolic pressure-volume area (PVA) in human hearts. Eur Heart J. 1992;13(Suppl E):85–90.
134. Takaoka H, Takeuchi M, Odake M, Hayashi Y, Hata K, Mori M, et al. Comparison of hemodynamic determinants for myocardial oxygen consumption under different contractile states in human ventricle. Circulation. 1993;87(1):59–69.
135. Urheim S, Rabben SI, Skulstad H, Lyseggen E, Ihlen H, Smiseth OA. Regional myocardial work by strain Doppler echocardiography and LV pressure: a new method for quantifying myocardial function. Am J Physiol Heart Circ Physiol. 2005;288(5):H2375–80.
136. Papadopoulos K, Ozden Tok O, Mitrousi K, Ikonomidis I. Myocardial work: methodology and clinical applications. Diagnostics (Basel). 2021;11(3):573.
137. E. S. Evaluation of segmental myocardial work in the left ventricle. GE Healthcare website 2017. [Samset E. Evaluation of segmental myocardial work in the left ventricle. GE Healthcare website. https://www.gehealthcare.com/-/media/8cab29682ace4ed7841505f813001e33.pdf]. Available from: https://www.gehealthcare.com/-/media/8cab29682ace4ed7841505f813001e33.pdf
138. Russell K, Eriksen M, Aaberge L, Wilhelmsen N, Skulstad H, Remme EW, et al. A novel clinical method for quantification of regional left ventricular pressure-strain loop area: a non-invasive index of myocardial work. Eur Heart J. 2012;33(6):724–33.
139. Russell K, Eriksen M, Aaberge L, Wilhelmsen N, Skulstad H, Gjesdal O, et al. Assessment of wasted myocardial work: a novel method to quantify energy loss due to uncoordinated left ventricular contractions. Am J Physiol Heart Circ Physiol. 2013;305(7):H996–1003.
140. Marzlin N, Hays AG, Peters M, Kaminski A, Roemer S, O'Leary P, et al. Myocardial work in echocardiography. Circ Cardiovasc Imaging. 2023;16(2):e014419.
141. Moya A, Buytaert D, Penicka M, Bartunek J, Vanderheyden M. State-of-the-art: noninvasive assessment of left ventricular function through myocardial work. J Am Soc Echocardiogr. 2023;36(10):1027–42.
142. Landra F, Mandoli GE, Chiantini B, Barilli M, Merello G, De Carli G, et al. Correlation of left ventricular myocardial work indices with invasive measurement of stroke work in patients with advanced heart failure. Front Cardiovasc Med. 2022;9:946540.
143. Stendahl JC, Liu Z, Boutagy NE, Parajuli N, Lu A, Alkhalil I, et al. Multiaxial pressure-strain analysis of regional myocardial work in the setting of graded coronary stenoses and dobutamine stress. Am J Physiol Heart Circ Physiol. 2023;325(3):H492–509.
144. Edwards NFA, Scalia GM, Putrino A, Appadurai V, Sabapathy S, Anderson B, et al. Myocardial work and left ventricular contractile reserve during stress echocardiography: an angiographic validation. Echocardiography. 2021;38(10):1711–21.
145. Leitman M, Balboul Y, Burgsdorf O, Tyomkin V, Fuchs S. Myocardial work index during normal dobutamine stress echocardiography. Sci Rep. 2022;12(1):6813.
146. Cauwenberghs N, Tabassian M, Thijs L, Yang WY, Wei FF, Claus P, et al. Area of the pressure-strain loop during ejection as non-invasive index of left ventricular performance: a population study. Cardiovasc Ultrasound. 2019;17(1):15.

Chapter 9
Role of Cardiovascular Magnetic Resonance Imaging in Heart Failure

Sebastian Onciul

Abstract Cardiovascular magnetic resonance (CMR) imaging can provide a comprehensive assessment of cardiac morphology, structure and function. The guidelines for diagnosis and treatment of heart failure (HF) recommends a class I indication for CMR for the assessment of myocardial structure and function in patients with poor acoustic window. Due to its tissue characterization capacities CMR contributes to the etiological diagnosis of HF, discriminating among ischaemic and non-ischaemic causes of systolic dysfunction. Late Gadolinium enhancement (LGE) imaging can accurately quantify the extent and localize replacement fibrosis in LV walls. In this regard, CMR contributes to a better selection of patients for cardiac resynchronization therapy (CRT) and internal cardiac defibrillator (ICD) implantation for primary prevention of sudden cardiac death (SCD). In the context of cardiomyopathies, CMR provides important information, for phenotype characterization, therapy selection and prognostication.

Keywords Cardiovascular magnetic resonance · Heart failure · Cardiomyopathies · LGE · Myocardial fibrosis

CMR for Chamber Quantification

Cardiovascular magnetic resonance is currently the *gold standard* imaging modality for quantification of dimensions and function of the chambers of the heart. CMR provides accurate measurement of EF to guide pharmacotherapy that improves quality of life and prognosis of patients with HF with reduced ejection fraction (HFrEF), defined as signs and symptoms of heart failure and an ejection fraction below 40% [1].

S. Onciul (✉)
Carol Davila University of Medicine and Pharmacy, Bucharest, Romania
e-mail: sebastian.onciul@umfcd.ro

M. Dorobanţu et al. (eds.), *Current Approach to Heart Failure*,
https://doi.org/10.1007/978-3-031-96562-3_9

In clinical practice the CMR examination is often performed after a time interval after the first diagnosis of reduced EF by echocardiography. During the period between echocardiographic first diagnosis and CMR examination, majority of patients will have received guideline directed medical therapy with the aim of improving their EF. In this context, many of the patients will be diagnosed with *HF with improved EF* at the time of CMR exam. Nevertheless, these patients should always continue their HF treatment, independently of the EF, as studies clearly showed that stopping HF medication will result in a subsequent decrease in EF.

CMR for Etiological Diagnosis of Systolic Dysfunction

Besides the accurate quantification of LVEF, CMR is indicated for *etiological* diagnosis of both ischaemic and non-ischaemic cardiomyopathies. Assessment of the presence, pattern and localization of focal myocardial fibrosis provides the most important information for establishing the cause of systolic dysfunction. Gadolinium is the contrast agent of choice in CMR, because it is an extracellular agent accumulating in tissues with high extracellular space such as myocardial fibrosis/scar. Late Gadolinium enhancement (LGE) images are acquired 7–10 min after contrast injection and are the classical CMR method of visualizing myocardial fibrosis.

Focal myocardial fibrosis as detected by LGE is found in the great majority of patients with systolic dysfunction of *ischemic* origin. In comparison, patients with *non-ischemic* etiology of HF show less frequently focal fibrosis. This difference in the burden of myocardial fibrosis may explain at least partially the different outcomes and response to therapy between ischemic and non-ischemic patients.

Ischaemic cardiomyopathy is characterized by a subendocardial or transmural pattern of LGE related to the territory of a coronary artery (Fig. 9.1). On the other hand, in non-ischemic cardiomyopathies, LGE, when present, is located in the mid-myocardial or subepicardial layers of the myocardium. Of note, a substantial percentage of patients with non-ischaemic cardiomyopathy do not exhibit any LGE.

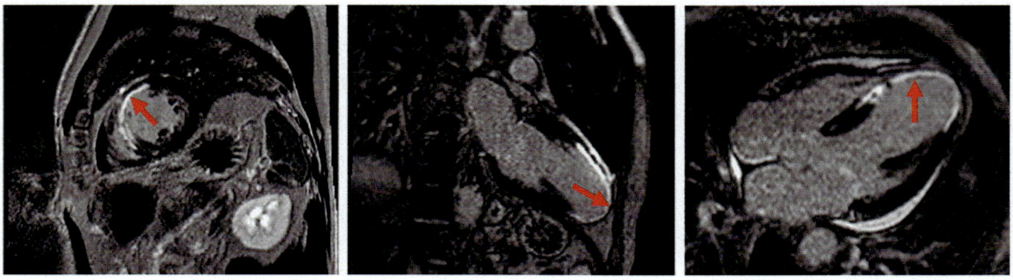

Fig. 9.1 Contrast enhanced cardiovascular magnetic resonance in a patient with a history of anterior myocardial infarction. From left to right: late Gadolinium enhancement imaging in short axis, 2 chambers and 4 chambers views respectively shows transmural scar in the left anterior descending territory suggesting no residual viable myocardium in the infracted area

Cardiovascular Magnetic Resonance can act as a gatekeeper to invasive coronary angiography (ICA) in patients presenting with HF of unknown etiology. When compared to ICA, LGE-CMR has equivalent sensitivity (100%), specificity (96%), and diagnostic accuracy (97%) for identifying ischemic cause of newly onset HF [2].

Several imaging phenotypes may be encountered in clinical practice when assessing patients with systolic dysfunction:

- extensive ischemic scar, proportional with the decrease in ejection fraction (LV systolic dysfunction can be explained solely by the ischemic scar) (Fig. 9.1).
- dilated cardiomyopathy (DCM) with systolic dysfunction but without any LGE—this is most probably non-ischemic DCM; although theoretically possible, significant coronary artery disease resulting in systolic dysfunction but without ischemic scarring should not be a common scenario in clinical practice.
- DCM with bystander infarct—these patients have systolic dysfunction which cannot be explained solely by a small infarction; frequently this is the case of non-ischemic DCM with severe systolic dysfunction, with a bystander segmental, usually embolic myocardial infarction.

Furthermore, CMR tissue characterization capacities allow for diagnosis of myocarditis, amyloidosis, sarcoidosis, Chagas disease, Fabry disease or arrhythmogenic cardiomyopathy.

Historically, the LGE value in predicting outcomes in HF was demonstrated from the beginnings of evidence-based therapies for HF. In the early 2000 it was demonstrated that in patients with HF with systolic dysfunction treated with ACEi/ARBs and beta-blockers there was an inverse relation between the extent of scarring and the likelihood of contractile improvement with treatment [3].

CMR for Cardiac Resynchronisation Therapy (CRT)

Several methods for assessing LV dyssynchrony with CMR have been described. In this regard it is important to note that the temporal resolution of CMR is inferior to that of echocardiography, thus favoring echocardiography for this specific purpose. However visual assessment of *septal flash* and *apical rocking* is an easy method for diagnosing intraventricular dyssinchrony.

Both LV dysssynchrony and the extent and location of scar tissue assessed by CMR are important predictors of response to CRT [4].

LGE imaging can accurately quantify the extent and localize replacement fibrosis in LV walls. In the context of CRT, the presence of myocardial scar at the place of LV lead deployment results in suboptimal resynchronization therapy. Leyva et al. showed that pacing scarred myocardium is associated with increased risk of cardiovascular death, hospitalization for HF, death from any cause or hospitalizations for major adverse cardiovascular events; on the other hand, pacing viable myocardium results in better reverse remodeling and favorable clinical outcomes [5]. Thus, a strategy of LGE-guided lead placement away from the scarred myocardium may be helpful in clinical practice for improving the results of CRT.

Recently, the impact of the myocardial substrate for the effect of left bundle branch area pacing (LBBAP) has been characterized [6]. Global, septal, and lateral scar burdens in the LV correlated negatively with reverse remodeling and displayed better performance beyond LBBB for predicting echocardiographic response in patients who underwent LBBAP-CRT [6].

CMR for ICD Primary Prophylaxis

Although the internal cardiac defibrillator (ICD) implantation is currently the most efficient strategy for primary prevention of sudden cardiac death (SCD) in both ischaemic (ICM) and non-ischaemic (NICM) cardiomyopathies, the parameters taken into account to decide implantation are lacking perfect accuracy. Despite ICD implantation being recommended in patients with echocardiographically measured LVEF < 35%, many of the SCD occur in patients with higher LVEF. Similarly, in patients with NICM, primary prevention with ICD implantation in patients with LVEF < 35%, did not result in a significant reduction in death of any cause compared with usual care, as was shown by the DANISH trial [7].

CMR proved additional prognostic stratification power when compared to transthoracic echocardiography in ICM and NICM patients evaluated for primary prevention ICD therapy [8]. Including LGE in the risk stratification algorithms results in better prediction of MACE as compared to LVEF only [8]. The presence of midwall LGE portends a higher risk of SCD in patients with DCM and a LVEF above 40% [9].

The DERIVATE study was a prospective, international, multicenter, observational registry of NICM and ICM patients with chronic HF and reduced LVEF who underwent clinical evaluation, transthoracic echocardiography and CMR [10]. The aim of the study was to establish the added value of CMR derived information in selecting patients for primary prevention with ICD implantation, over LVEF and NYHA classification. Primary end point of the study was all-cause mortality. Secondary end points were major adverse arrhythmic cardiac events [10]. The study included patients with HF and LVEF < 50% of both ischemic and non-ischemic cause.

Among CMR parameters, LV end-diastolic volume index, ejection fraction and LGE were independent predictors of major arrhythmic events in ICM. A score derived from these parameters resulted in net reclassification improvement for the indication of ICD implantation in ICM patients [11].

In the NICM cohort of the DERIVATE study, age and >3 segments with mid-wall fibrosis on LGE were the only independent predictors of all-cause mortality [12]. For major arrhythmic events, the independent predictors were male gender, left ventricular end-diastolic volume index and >3 segments with mid-wall fibrosis on LGE. The study resulted in a composite clinical and CMR-based risk score which proved incremental prognostic value beyond standard of care evaluation in NICM

[12]. Applying this risk score it was shown that almost one-third of NICM patients fulfilling the current criteria for primary prevention ICD implantation were having low risk of major arrhythmic events [12].

The Role of CMR in Non-ischemic Cardiomyopathies

The recent European Society of Cardiology (ESC) guideline on cardiomyopathies provided a new classification of cardiomyopathies comprising of 5 phenotypes: dilated cardiomyopathy (DCM), hypertrophic cardiomyopathy (HCM), restrictive cardiomyopathy (RCM), arrhythmogenic right ventricle cardiomyopathy (ARVC) and non-dilated left ventricular cardiomyopathy (NDLVC) [13].

Furthermore, the ESC guideline proposes a phenotype based integrated approach of cardiomyopathies which mandatory includes the presence or absence of myocardial fibrosis, besides the ejection fraction, genetic substrate and mendelian mode of inheritance.

As such, CMR received a class I indication for assessment of each patient with a suspected cardiomyopathy.

Hypertrophic Cardiomyopathy

Hypertrophic cardiomyopathy (HCM) is defined as the presence of increased wall thickness in any part of the left or right ventricular myocardium that is not solely explained by abnormal loading conditions [14]. CMR provides good quality images which permits accurate measurement of the thickness of any of the 17 LV segments and the right ventricle free wall, with higher accuracy than echocardiography. Patients with obstructive HCM and an indication for septal reduction therapies, should undergo CMR imaging for accurate anatomical description of the site of obstruction.

Left ventricular EF calculation by echocardiography is particularly difficult in the context of LV hypertrophy, and thus CMR may be essential in diagnosing mild degrees of systolic impairment with important prognostic implications in the context of HCM.

Tissue characterization capacities of CMR permit identification of HCM phenocopies such as cardiac amyloidosis or Anderson-Fabry disease, resulting in a great benefit for the patients receiving specific treatment.

Nevertheless, LGE imaging can identify and quantify HCM associated myocardial fibrosis, which may be present in some but not all HCM patients. When present, the typical appearance of LGE in HCM is that of patchy mid-myocardial hyperenhancement usually localized in the hypertrophied myocardium and the RV insertion points on the LV. The end-stage HCM (*burn-out* HCM) is characterized by extensive areas of myocardial fibrosis (Fig. 9.2).

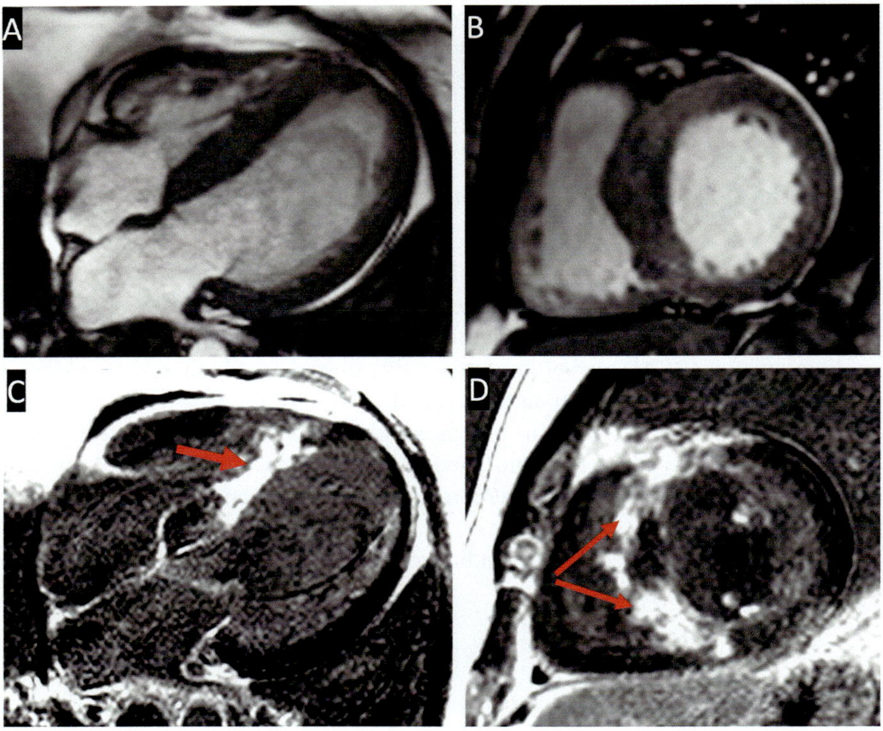

Fig. 9.2 Contrast enhanced CMR in a 35-years-old male with *burn-out* hypertrophic cardiomyopathy due to a pathogenic variant of MYBPC3 gene. (**a**, **b**) Diastolic frames of cine images in 4 chambers and short axis views respectively, showing a severely dilated left ventricle with severe LV systolic dysfunction (LVEF 22%), with basal interventricular septum hypertrophy with a maximum thickness of 25 mm. (**c**, **d**) Late Gadolinium enhancement (LGE) imaging in the corresponding 4 chambers and short axis views respectively, showing extensive myocardial fibrosis of the interventricular septum, anterior and inferior walls as well as the mitral papillary muscles

The presence of LGE is associated with an increased risk of SCD, all-cause mortality, cardiovascular mortality, and a trend for heart failure death [15]. The LGE amount may be used as a modulator of SCD risk prediction in clinical practice. The 2023 ESC guidelines on cardiomyopathies recommends extensive LGE (>15%) as a clinical risk factor to be considered in the shared decision-making process of prophylactic ICD implantation in patients who are in the low-risk category (<4% estimated 5-year risk of SCD, according to the HCM Risk-SCD calculator) [14].

Dilated Cardiomyopathy

Dilated cardiomyopathy is defined by the presence of LV dilatation and systolic dysfunction unexplained solely by abnormal loading conditions or coronary artery disease [14].

Besides accurate chamber quantification, CMR provides important information of tissue characteristics in patients with DCM. This is why patients with DCM should benefit a CMR examination at least once in their life. Not all DCM patients have focal myocardial fibrosis, but when present, fibrosis can be visualized and quantified by LGE imaging (Fig. 9.3). The presence of myocardial fibrosis is associated with an increased arrhythmic risk and lower chances of reverse remodeling despite optimal medical therapy. Fibrosis located in the interventricular septum is associated with a large increase SCD risk, and concomitant septal and LV free wall LGE is associated with the greatest SCD risk [16].

Thus, LGE imaging can contribute to risk stratification in patients with DCM, particularly when LVEF is greater than 35%. The 2023 ESC guideline on cardiomyopathies supports using LGE to guide ICD implantation in subgroups of patients with DCM [14].

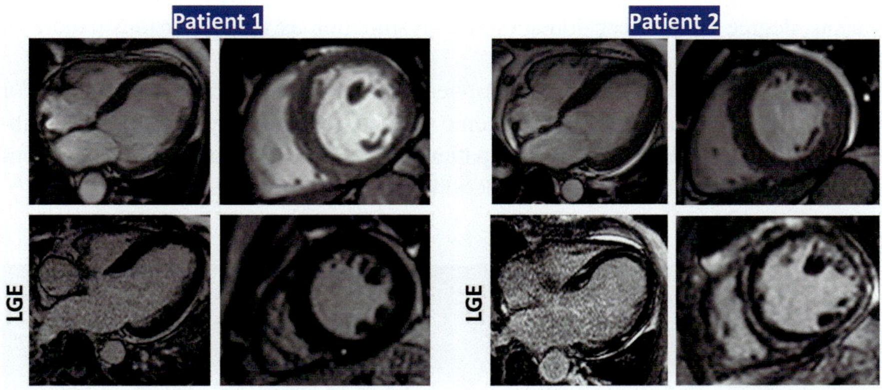

Fig. 9.3 Cardiovascular magnetic resonance in 2 patients with dilated cardiomyopathy (DCM) and similar native imaging phenotype but very different LGE appearance. On the upper row: Cine images in 4 chambers and short axis views showing the similarly dilated hearts, with similar LV wall thickness, and moderate LV systolic dysfunction (EF 35%). On the lower row, the LGE imaging in the corresponding views, shows no myocardial fibrosis in the first patient, but extensive focal mid-myocardial fibrosis with a *ring-like* pattern in the second patient. The presence of myocardial fibrosis is associated with an increased arrhytmic risk but also lower chances of reverse remodelling in despite optimal medical treatment

Non-dilated Left Ventricular Cardiomyopathy

The most recent cardiomyopathy phenotype proposed by the ESC guideline is the non-dilated left ventricular cardiomyopathy (NDLVC), which is defined as either:

- isolated LV dysfunction (regional or global) without scarring

or

- the presence of non-ischaemic LV scarring or fatty replacement regardless of the presence of global or regional wall motion abnormalities [13].

The second part of the above definition implies that for correct diagnosis of NDLVC, the contribution of CMR is mandatory due to its unique capacity of identifying myocardial scar. The NDLVC phenotype encompass a variety of genetic cardiomyopathies but also acquired post-myocarditis scarring. In this regard, according to the definition, a patient with a history of healed viral myocarditis that resulted in a subepicardial scar but without any wall motion abnormality will be classified as having NDLVC.

On the other hand, genetic causes of NDLVC include pathogenic variants in various genes such as: desmoplakin, LMNA, phospholamban, filamin C, titin, RBM20. These pathogenic variants result in CMR imaging phenotypes characterized by various degree of chamber dilatation and dysfunction as well as various pattern of fibrosis.

In some instances, some genotype-phenotype correlations cand be inferred. For example, desmoplakin (DSP) pathogenic variants result in a typical *ring-like* subepicardial fibrosis (Fig. 9.4). In these patients, the extent of fibrosis is disproportionate with the degree of systolic dysfunction which is not as severe as expected.

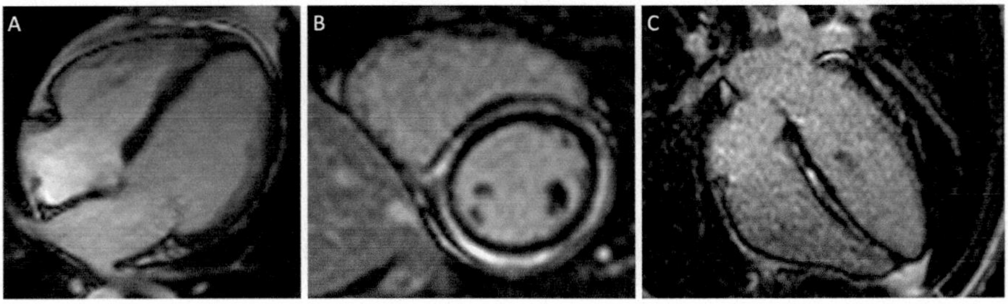

Fig. 9.4 Contrast enhanced CMR in a 49-years-old woman with non-dilated left ventricular cardiomyopathy (NDLVC) caused by a pathogenic variant in desmoplakin (DSP) gene. (**a**) B-SSFP cine frame in 4 chambers view showing non-dilated ventricles, with mild left ventricular systolic dysfunction. (**b**, **c**) Late Gadolinium Enhancement (LGE) imaging in short axis and 4 chambers views showing extensive subepicardial scarring with a ring-like pattern

Restrictive Cardiomyopathies

Restrictive cardiomyopathies (RCM) are defined as restrictive pathophysiology in the context of normal or reduced ventricular volumes and normal ventricular wall thickness [17]. The etiological spectrum of RCM includes genetic and non-genetic disorders classified in 4 general categories: infiltrative diseases, storage disorders, interstitial fibrosis and endomyocardial diseases.

CMR provides important information in each of these categories. The prototype of infiltrative diseases is cardiac amyloidosis, which is caused by extracellular accumulation of amyloid fibers. CMR has a unique capacity of assessing the myocardial extracellular space through 2 specific sequences. One of these sequences is LGE imaging in which amyloid deposition results in a specific pattern. As Gadolinium is an exclusively extracellular contrast agent, it will accumulate in tissues with expanded interstitium such as amyloid infiltrated myocardium. Consequently, LGE imaging in cardiac amyloidosis will show diffuse myocardial hyperenhancement, with a subendocardial localization in early stages and transmural in advanced stages of the disease (Fig. 9.5). The second sequence used for the assessment of the extracellular space is T1 mapping. By computing myocardial and blood pool T1 values before and after contrast administration, a value of extracellular volume fraction (ECV) is obtained. This parameter is a very accurate method for quantification of the amyloid deposition in the myocardium. Of note, in patients who cannot receive Gadolinium based contrast agents due to low glomerular filtration rate (<30 mL/min/1.73 m^2), native T1 mapping has proved high diagnostic accuracy for diagnosing cardiac amyloidosis. In the study conducted by Baggiano et al. a native T1 $<$ 1036 ms was associated with 98% negative predictive value for cardiac amyloidosis, whereas a native T1 $>$ 1164 ms was associated with 98% positive predictive value for cardiac amyloidosis [18].

On the other hand, the prototype of storage disorders is Anderson–Fabry disease (AFD) which is characterized by progressive intracellular accumulation of glycosphingolipids. Intra-myocyte lipids accumulation will result in reduction of native T1 signal as an early manifestation of cardiac involvement in AFD. On the other hand, long-term cardiac involvement in AFD results in LV hypertrophy and myocardial fibrosis typically manifest as the presence of posterolateral LGE (Fig. 9.6). More recently, a special phenotype with LV apical aneurysm was reported in nearly 10% of AFD patients with left ventricular hypertrophy [19]. The left ventricular apical aneurysm portends a higher risk for long-term adverse cardiovascular events [19].

Endomyocardial fibrosis (EMF) is characterized by diffuse thickening of the LV endocardium secondary to the injury produced by a large number of peripheral eosinophils [20].

Both left and right ventricle can be affected as well as the heart valves. Contrast enhanced CMR can identify endomyocardial fibrosis and associated thrombus (Fig. 9.7).

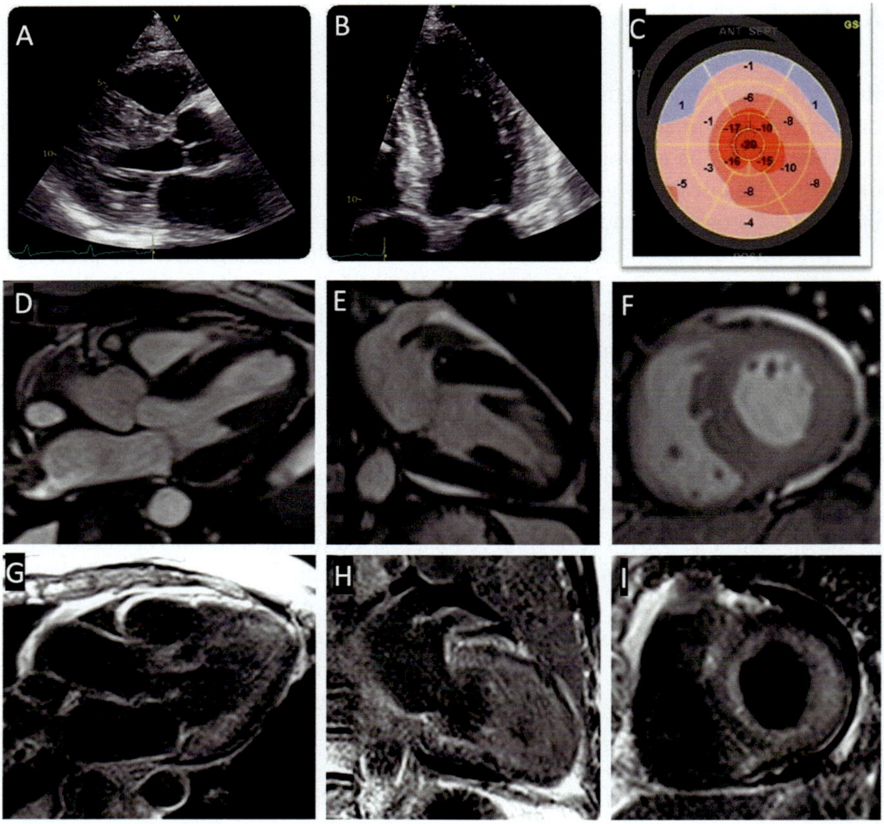

Fig. 9.5 Echocardiography and contrast enhanced cardiovascular magnetic resonance in a patient with cardiac amyloidosis. (**a**, **b**) Parasternal long axis and apical for chamber views showing thickening of the left ventricular (LV) walls. (**c**) Bull's eye representation of the global longitudinal strain showing the typical appearance of apical sparring. (**d**, **e**, **f**) b-SSFP images in 3, 2 chambers and short axis respectively confirming the thickening of the LV walls, and a small pericardial effusion. (**g**, **h**, **i**) Late Gadolinium enhancement (LGE) imaging in 3, 2 chambers and short axis respectively, showing diffuse hyperenhancement of the LV walls in a transmural pattern, with a dark blood pool. The hyperenhancement results from Gadolinium accumulation inn the expanded interstitial space secondary to amyloid deposition

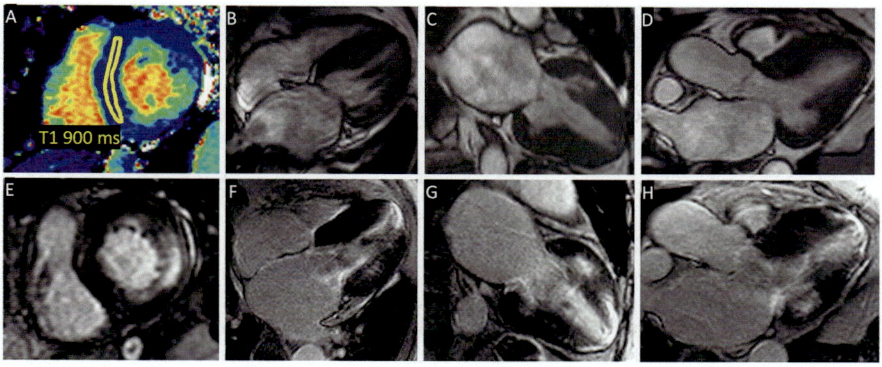

Fig. 9.6 Contrast enhanced cardiovascular magnetic resonance in a 61-year-old female with Anderson-Fabry disease secondary to a pathogenic missense variant c.44C > A, (p.Ala15Glu) of the GLA gene. (**a**) Native T1 mapping in short axis showing low native T1 values (900 ms). (**b**, **c**, **d**) b-SSFP in 4, 2 and 3 chambers views respectively showing asymmetric septal hypertrophy—maximum thickness of 20 mm in the medium inferoseptum. The LV was non-dilated with mild systolic dysfunction (LV EF 47%). The right ventricle had a normal ejection fraction and thin free wall. (**e**, **f**, **g**, **h**) Late Gadolinium enhancement (LGE) showing extensive mid-myocardial and transmural scar of the non-hypertrophic segments (the medio-basal segments of the infero-lateral, inferior and infero-septal walls) and the apex, respectively

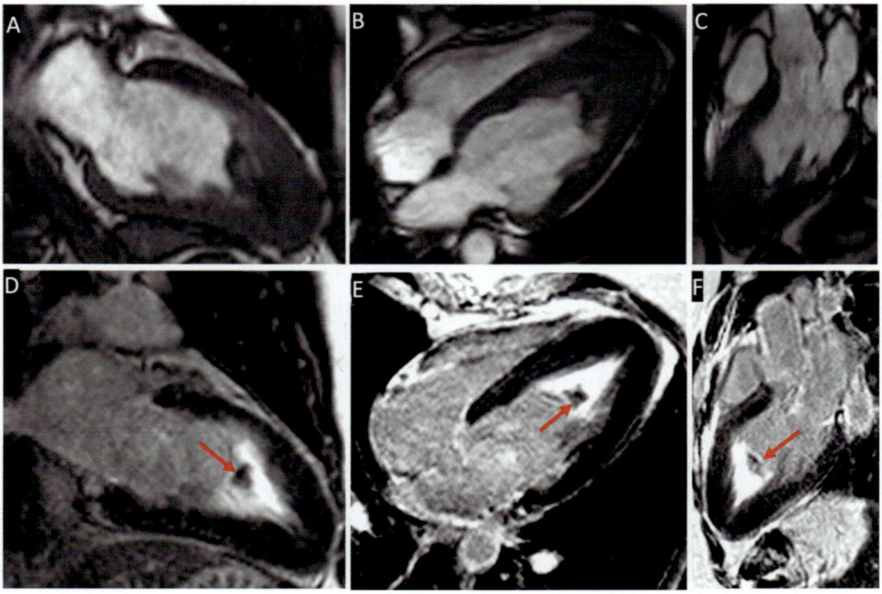

Fig. 9.7 Contrast enhanced CMR in a patient with endomyocardial fibrosis (EMF). (**a**, **b**, **c**) B-SSFP cine images in 2, 4 and 3 chambers views showing apical thickening of the LV walls and obliteration of LV cavity. (**d**, **e**, **f**) Late Gadolinium Enhancement (LGE) images in 2, 4 and 3 chambers views identifying fibrosis as the cause of LV obliteration, and also a thrombus located in the fibrotic mass (red arrow)

References

1. McDonagh TA, Metra M, Adamo M, Gardner RS, Baumbach A, Böhm M, et al. 2023 Focused Update of the 2021 ESC Guidelines for the diagnosis and treatment of acute and chronic heart failure: developed by the task force for the diagnosis and treatment of acute and chronic heart failure of the European Society of Cardiology (ESC) with the special contribution of the Heart Failure Association (HFA) of the ESC. Eur Heart J [Internet]. 2023;44(37):3627–39. Available from: https://doi.org/10.1093/eurheartj/ehad195
2. Assomull RG, Shakespeare C, Kalra PR, Lloyd G, Gulati A, Strange J, et al. Role of cardiovascular magnetic resonance as a gatekeeper to invasive coronary angiography in patients presenting with heart failure of unknown etiology. Circulation. 2011;124(12):1351–60.
3. Bello D, Shah DJ, Farah GM, Di Luzio S, Parker M, Johnson MR, et al. Gadolinium cardiovascular magnetic resonance predicts reversible myocardial dysfunction and remodeling in patients with heart failure undergoing β-blocker therapy. Circulation. 2003;108(16):1945–53.
4. Marsan NA, Westenberg JJM, Ypenburg C, van Bommel RJ, Roes S, Delgado V, et al. Magnetic resonance imaging and response to cardiac resynchronization therapy: relative merits of left ventricular dyssynchrony and scar tissue. Eur Heart J. 2009;30(19):2360–7.
5. Leyva F, Foley PWX, Chalil S, Ratib K, Smith REA, Prinzen F, et al. Cardiac resynchronization therapy guided by late gadolinium-enhancement cardiovascular magnetic resonance. J Cardiovasc Magn Reson. 2011;13(1):29.
6. Chen Z, Ma X, Gao Y, Wu S, Xu N, Chen F, et al. Cardiac magnetic resonance–derived myocardial scar is associated with echocardiographic response and clinical prognosis of left bundle branch area pacing for cardiac resynchronization therapy. EP Eur. 2023;25(11):euad326.
7. Køber L, Thune JJ, Nielsen JC, Haarbo J, Videbæk L, Korup E, et al. Defibrillator implantation in patients with nonischemic systolic heart failure. N Engl J Med. 2016;375(13):1221–30.
8. Pontone G, Guaricci AI, Andreini D, Solbiati A, Guglielmo M, Mushtaq S, et al. Prognostic benefit of cardiac magnetic resonance over transthoracic echocardiography for the assessment of ischemic and nonischemic dilated cardiomyopathy patients referred for the evaluation of primary prevention implantable cardioverter–defibrillator therapy. Circ Cardiovasc Imaging. 2016;9(10):e004956.
9. Halliday BP, Gulati A, Ali A, Guha K, Newsome S, Arzanauskaite M, et al. Association between midwall late gadolinium enhancement and sudden cardiac death in patients with dilated cardiomyopathy and mild and moderate left ventricular systolic dysfunction. Circulation. 2017;135(22):2106–15.
10. Guaricci AI, Masci PG, Lorenzoni V, Schwitter J, Pontone G. CarDiac MagnEtic resonance for primary prevention implantable CardioVerter DebrillAtor ThErapy international registry: design and rationale of the DERIVATE study. Int J Cardiol. 2018;261:223–7.
11. Pontone G, Guaricci AI, Fusini L, Baggiano A, Guglielmo M, Muscogiuri G, et al. Cardiac magnetic resonance for prophylactic implantable-cardioverter defibrillator therapy in ischemic cardiomyopathy: the DERIVATE-ICM international registry. JACC Cardiovasc Imaging. 2023;16(11):1387–400.
12. Guaricci AI, Masci PG, Muscogiuri G, Guglielmo M, Baggiano A, Fusini L, et al. CarDiac magnEtic resonance for prophylactic implantable-cardioVerter defibrillAtor ThErapy in non-ischaemic dilated CardioMyopathy: an international registry. EP Eur. 2021;23(7):1072–83.
13. Arbelo E, Protonotarios A, Gimeno JR, Arbustini E, Barriales-Villa R, Basso C, et al. 2023 ESC Guidelines for the management of cardiomyopathies: developed by the task force on the management of cardiomyopathies of the European Society of Cardiology (ESC). Eur Heart J. 2023;44(37):3503–626.
14. Arbelo E, Protonotarios A, Gimeno JR, Arbustini E, Barriales-Villa R, Basso C, et al. 2023 ESC Guidelines for the management of cardiomyopathies: developed by the task force on the management of cardiomyopathies of the European Society of Cardiology (ESC). Eur Heart J [Internet]. 2023;44(37):3503–626. Available from: https://doi.org/10.1093/eurheartj/ehad194

15. Weng Z, Yao J, Chan RH, He J, Yang X, Zhou Y, et al. Prognostic value of LGE-CMR in HCM: a meta-analysis. JACC Cardiovasc Imaging [Internet]. 2016;9(12):1392–402. Available from: https://www.sciencedirect.com/science/article/pii/S1936878X16304065
16. Halliday BP, Baksi AJ, Gulati A, Ali A, Newsome S, Izgi C, et al. Outcome in dilated cardiomyopathy related to the extent, location, and pattern of late gadolinium enhancement. JACC Cardiovasc Imaging [Internet]. 2019;12(8 Part 2):1645 LP–1655. Available from: http://imaging.onlinejacc.org/content/12/8_Part_2/1645.abstract
17. Rapezzi C, Aimo A, Barison A, Emdin M, Porcari A, Linhart A, et al. Restrictive cardiomyopathy: definition and diagnosis. Eur Heart J. 2022;43(45):4679–93.
18. Baggiano A, Boldrini M, Martinez-Naharro A, Kotecha T, Petrie A, Rezk T, et al. Noncontrast magnetic resonance for the diagnosis of cardiac amyloidosis. JACC Cardiovasc Imaging [Internet]. 2019:3055. Available from: http://imaging.onlinejacc.org/content/early/2019/06/07/j.jcmg.2019.03.026.abstract
19. Chang H, Kuo L, Sung S, Weng C, Chen C, Niu D, et al. Left ventricular apical aneurysm in Fabry disease: implications for clinical significance and risk stratification. J Am Heart Assoc [Internet]. 2023;12(1):e027041. Available from: https://doi.org/10.1161/JAHA.122.027041
20. Rapezzi C, Aimo A, Barison A, Emdin M, Porcari A, Linhart A, et al. Restrictive cardiomyopathy: definition and diagnosis. Eur Heart J [Internet]. 2022;43(45):4679–93. Available from: https://doi.org/10.1093/eurheartj/ehac543

Chapter 10
The Evolving Role of Multimodality Imaging in Heart Failure

Alessia Gimelli and Riccardo Liga

Abstract In patients with LV dysfunction, multimodality imaging offers the opportunity to obtain continued information on regional and global cardiac function, myocardial viability, coronary anatomy, and regional relative or absolute myocardial perfusion.

The different modalities may be performed separately and integrated/fused afterward (i.e. through hybrid imaging) or may be used in a single-step approach to defining HF etiology, the extent and severity of myocardial damage/ischemia, indicate and predict the response to targeted treatments (i.e. CRT, coronary revascularization) as well as to perform pre-interventional assessment (i.e. to program trans-catheter ablation of arrhythmias or valvular interventions.

Keywords Myocardial perfusion · Cardiac magnetic resonance · Cardiac resynchronisation therapy · Compute tomography coronary angiography · Global longitudinal strain · Multimodality imaging · Myocardial perfusion imaging · Myocardial functional imaging · Anatomical imaging · Metabolic imaging · Molecular imaging · Cardiac resynchronization · Arrhythmias · Cardio-oncology · Cardiac amyloidosis

Multi-modality imaging can be defined as the combination of anatomical, morphological, and functional data from non-invasive imaging techniques to enhance the diagnostic accuracy of single imaging modalities and guide targeted therapeutic interventions [1].

To this purpose, different imaging modalities may be performed separately and the information obtained integrated afterward or all the information can be obtained in a single-step approach using hybrid systems [2]. In the clinical context of heart

A. Gimelli (✉)
Fondazione Toscana Gabriele Monasterio, Pisa, Italy
e-mail: gimelli@ftgm.it

R. Liga
Cardio-thoracic and Vascular Department, University Hospital of Pisa, Pisa, Italy

M. Dorobanţu et al. (eds.), *Current Approach to Heart Failure*,
https://doi.org/10.1007/978-3-031-96562-3_10

failure (HF), multimodality and hybrid imaging can be best applied to define etiology, assess the severity of myocardial damage and ischemia, provide pre-interventional assessment, and guide revascularization [in coronary artery disease (CAD) patients] or electrophysiological procedures [i.e., cardiac resynchronization therapy (CRT)] [3]. More recently, molecular imaging techniques have proven valuable for early disease detection, better risk stratification, and ultimately targeted treatment interventions.

This chapter highlights recent observations using different imaging technologies (echocardiography, cardiac magnetic resonance [CMR], cardiac computed tomography [CT], single-photon emission computed tomography [SPECT], and positron emission tomography [PET], but also neuronal imaging with ^{123}I-metaiodobenzylguanidine [MIBG]) in the field of HF.

Imaging of Ischemia: Risk Area and Coronary Arteries

Hybrid SPECT-CT or PET-CT scanners offer the opportunity to perform an integrated evaluation of coronary anatomy and of the functional effects of coronary stenosis, combining the high diagnostic accuracy in detecting luminal narrowings of coronary CT angiography (CTCA) with the functional information provided by nuclear cardiac imaging, either with SPECT or PET, in the evaluation of stress and rest regional and global myocardial perfusion and thus in the evaluation of the area at risk of myocardial ischemia [3] (Fig. 10.1). In patients with HF, combined anatomical-functional imaging using SPECT-CT or PET-CT may be useful in identifying the aetiology of the underlying disease and, in the presence of obstructive CAD, indicating and guiding coronary revascularization. In this context, the 3D fusion of CTCA images with SPECT or PET perfusion data may allow the unique chance to reassign a specific perfusion defect to the pertinent coronary territory, univocally identifying the presence of hemodynamically significant CAD (i.e. a coronary stenosis with downstream significant myocardial ischemia downstream). Previous studies have demonstrated the existence of a huge inter-individual variability of coronary anatomy that may frequently prevent the correct allocation of a given myocardial perfusion defect to the specific coronary artery [4, 5]. Accordingly, hybrid imaging has been demonstrated to obviate the most frequent limitations that come from the side-by-side analysis of two different image modalities such as CT coronary angiography and myocardial perfusion imaging (MPI), by correctly ruling in and out the presence of hemodynamically significant CAD in the majority of patients [5]. While in the presence of a matched hybrid finding (i.e. a myocardial perfusion defect subtended by an anatomically significant—>50%—coronary luminal stenosis) coronary revascularization may be indicated to improve patients' symptomatic status and, in some circumstances (i.e., in the presence of a severe myocardial ischemic burden: >15% of the LV myocardium) [6], prognosis, a normal hybrid evaluation (i.e. absence of significant coronary stenosis as well as myocardial perfusion abnormalities) is associated with an excellent prognosis.

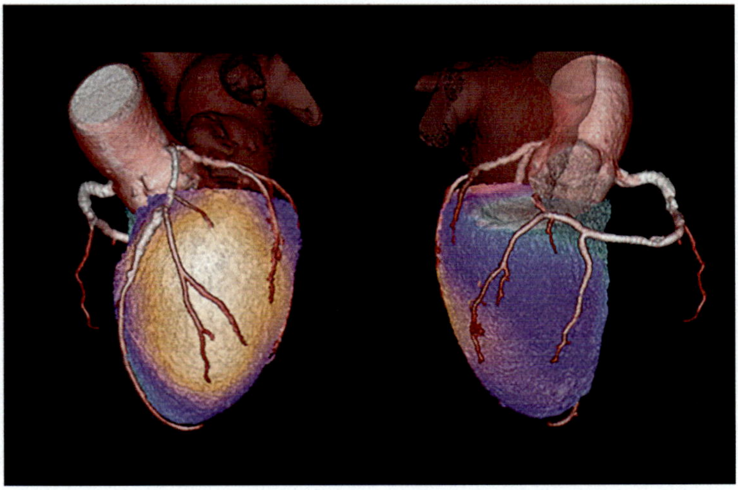

Fig. 10.1 A representative case of hybrid imaging. A 65-year-old gentleman with atypical anginal chest pain and an intermediate probability of CAD. He was submitted to computed tomography coronary angiography (CCTA) with evidence of three-vessel CAD with a long 80% mid-LAD calcific stenosis, a 75% mid-RCA mixed lesion, and a 50–70% distal LCX stenosis. Myocardial perfusion imaging with SPECT was then performed with evidence of extensive anterior distal to apical, as well as inferior to inferolateral reversible perfusion defect. On hybrid CCTA/SPECT imaging, the perfusion defects were reassigned to the LAD and the RCA coronary arteries, excluding the hemodynamic relevance of the LCX stenosis

Interestingly, patients presenting a mismatched hybrid finding at SPECT/CT or PET/CT (i.e. either anatomically significant coronary stenosis without evidence of myocardial ischemia at MPI or myocardial perfusion defects without evidence of significant CAD) show an intermediate long-term prognosis, further highlighting the need for aggressive medical treatment [7]. Those findings have been more recently confirmed by the long-term results of the "Evaluation of Integrated Cardiac Imaging for the Detection and Characterization of Ischemic Heart Disease" (EVINCI) study, showing that patients with CAD in whom early revascularization was performed in the presence of matched ischaemia and deferred in its absence had fewer adverse events than those managed non-adherently to imaging findings, similar to patients without CAD (HR 2.0, 95% CI 0.71–5.51; P = 0.195) [8].

In ischemic HF the indications for and relative benefits of revascularisation remain a source of contention [9, 10].

The relative effects of medical therapy and revascularization on the myocardial ischaemic burden and the independent prognostic significance of ischaemia changes following revascularization are still unclear [11–13]. In this regard, as elegantly suggested by the results of the nuclear sub-study of the COURAGE trial, the reduction of the global myocardial ischemic burden, by either percutaneous or surgical revascularization might not confer a relevant prognostic benefit, despite frequently having a significant symptomatic impact [13], findings more recently confirmed by the "International Study of Comparative Health Effectiveness with Medical and

Invasive Approaches" (ISCHEMIA), excluding a prognostic benefit of coronary revascularization in patients with moderate-to-severe ischemia at large [14]. While some data seem to suggest a possible prognostic benefit of ischemia-guided revascularization in patients with HF and moderately reduced LV ejection fraction (35–45%) [15], the management of patients with ischemia cardiomyopathy (ICM) at large is still contentious and mostly based on habits rather than evidence [16].

In this scenario, since ischemia is still one of the primary drivers of decisions regarding revascularization, clarification of these questions may have significant implications for both patient management as well as healthcare utilization.

Apart from myocardial ischemic burden, in the presence of left ventricular systolic dysfunction and stable CAD another relevant functional factor should be taken into account, the presence and location of residual hibernated myocardium. Those patients usually present a mixture of areas of necrotic myocardium interposed between regions of either prevalently hibernated or mainly ischemic heart muscle. In this context, to allow a targeted treatment, an appropriate multimodality cardiac imaging approach should be able to quantitate and localize the different "qualities" of the myocardium (i.e. scar, ischemic, hibernated, and normal) and define the pertinent coronary distribution. This information is particularly needed if a revascularization strategy, either surgical or percutaneous, is hypothesized since no benefit can be expected from the revascularization of necrotic or only partially viable myocardial regions [17].

PET imaging, through the use of widely established perfusion (i.e. ammonia and rubidium) and metabolic (FDG) tracers, still represents the reference standard for the combined evaluation of regional myocardial viability as well as ischemic burden, being particularly suited for the characterization of patients with post-ischemic left ventricular systolic dysfunction. Moreover, particularly when fused with the pertinent CT coronary angiography images, such as in the case of hybrid CT/MPI imaging, PET images may offer the chance to individuate the patients in whom a significant improvement of left ventricular systolic function can be expected after revascularization [18]. Nevertheless, despite the solid theoretical background, evidence in favor of viability-guided myocardial revascularization is, at best, scarce, and mostly based on retrospective appraisals, with most of the available prospective studies excluding a relevant impact of such treatment strategy on patients' prognosis [16], a finding more recently supported by the neutral results of the "REVascularization for Ischemic VEntricular Dysfunction (REVIVED)-BCIS2" study, whereby revascularization of hibernated myocardium (there performed with PCI rather than CABG) failed to provide a significant prognostic benefit to patients with ICM [19].

Metabolic Imaging

HF is associated with abnormal myocardial metabolism, including energy depletion and reduced mechanical efficiency [20].

These changes may play a role in the progression of HF and may potentially serve as therapeutic targets. In normal conditions, fatty acids represent the major source of cardiac substrate metabolism accounting for 60–90% of the energy production of a myocardial cell under the resting status. Conversely, in patients with heart failure, glucose becomes the preferred cardiac energy source, allowing deriving a significant quantity of energy despite the relatively contained amount of oxygen demand [21, 22]. However, while this metabolic switch may sustain the energetic needs of a failing heart in the short term, it becomes one of the most relevant counter-adaptive mechanisms in HF, significantly impairing cardiac metabolic reserve. Interestingly, recent evidence has shown how this metabolic adaptation of the failing heart may differ according to the patient's sex, with a relative predilection of the "female" heart for the metabolism of fatty acid even during HF [23].

PET imaging, mainly with the use of dedicated 11-carbon-labeled radiotracers (i.e. palmitate and acetate) may represent the ideal non-invasive imaging modality for the assessment of cardiac metabolism. However, the complex metabolism of fatty acids allows mainly semiquantitative measurements of substrate utilization with PET imaging of 11-carbon-labeled palmitate [24].

On the other hand, PET imaging of 11-carbon-labeled acetate allows the assessment of cardiac oxidative metabolism without the complexity of substrate interaction between glucose and fatty acids [25]. The early rapid clearance of acetate correlates closely with myocardial oxygen consumption, and the relationship of myocardial 11carbon-labeled acetate kinetics to cardiac work offers a noninvasive parameter for cardiac efficiency that can be used to demonstrate the effect of pharmacological and pacing interventions on cardiac energetics [26].

While the non-invasive investigation of fatty acid metabolism has never entered the clinical arena, 18fluorine-labeled fluorodeoxyglucose (^{18}F-FDG) still represents the backbone of metabolic imaging with PET, allowing tracing cellular glucose uptake and phosphorylation and quantifying regional and global left ventricular glucose metabolism [27]. In patients with idiopathic LV systolic dysfunction, glucose metabolism is enhanced as a result of an adaptive mechanism to the increased hemodynamic load. Interestingly, those patients may show significant regional heterogeneity in glucose oxidation, which may consistently vary in the different left ventricular walls [28]. This aspect may be particularly relevant in the case of patients showing a left bundle branch block (LBBB), in whom the dyssynchronous myocardial mechanical activation appears strictly parallelled by an inhomogeneous glucose utilization, lowest at the level of the left ventricular septum and highest in the lateral wall [28, 29].

However, while in patients with idiopathic left ventricular dysfunction ^{18}F-FDG PET may still give relevant pathophysiological information, the most important clinical role of this imaging modality relates to its ability to define the presence of viable tissue within malperfused segments in patients with post-ischemic left ventricular systolic dysfunction [30]. Still today, myocardial viability assessment with PET, either performed with combined perfusion/metabolism imaging [18, 31, 32] or with the hyperinsulinemic-euglycemic clamp technique [33], may represent the most accurate imaging modality for the evaluation of the indications for coronary revascularization, and for the prediction of patients outcome in post-ischemic left ventricular dysfunction [17, 34].

In the last years, the imaging armamentarium in the setting of chronic HF has been enriched by the introduction of a novel multimodal technology, hybrid cardiac PET/MR. In this respect, hybrid imaging with PET/MR dedicated devices combines almost simultaneous anatomic, functional, and metabolic imaging for the improved visualization of cardiac structure function and may provide new quantitative tools to study the pathophysiology of HF in vivo. In particular, the excellent tissue characterization offered by cardiac MR, combined with the superior metabolic information given by PET imaging can create a new reference standard for the non-invasive assessment of complex cardiac pathologies, such as chronic HF.

Hybrid PET/CMR tomographers were only recently introduced for clinical applications [35]. The integration of PET with structural and functional CMR imaging markers including wall thickness, contractile response to dobutamine, transmural late gadolinium enhancement, and perfusion has the potential to improve viability-based prediction of dysfunctional segments after revascularization and deserves to be evaluated in clinical studies.

Both MR and PET have independently gained wide acceptance for the assessment of myocardial perfusion and viability in different categories of patients [18, 36]. Thus, by combining the strengths of each modality, hybrid PET/MR imaging might ideally become the future "gold standard" for the evaluation of patients with LV systolic dysfunction, especially in the presence of CAD. Moreover, PET/MR may soon become the reference standard for the etiologic characterization of patients with non-ischemic LV systolic dysfunction, where the combined anatomic-functional assessment provided by hybrid imaging might easily identify patients with inflammatory cardiomyopathy [37], a category of patients that might benefit of targeted therapeutic (possibly immunosuppressive) approaches [38].

While PET/MR imaging offers a clear reduction of radiation exposure, by eliminating CT-based attenuation correction, it might consistently increase workflow complexity and operational costs. Above all, the combination of PET and MR technologies in a unique hybrid device poses the necessity to obtain reliable attenuation correction maps of PET photons, as a mandatory step for PET-based quantification of cardiac functional parameters.

In this respect, after an initial delay due to intrinsic technical limitations, methods for a reliable attenuation correction from MR data have been proposed, showing the ability to replicate the results obtained with the standard CT-base attenuation correction [39]. Ultimately, the great strength of PET/MR will lie in its ability to deliver multimodal quantitative imaging parameters based on dynamic data acquisition with both modalities, offering a simultaneous physiologic and biological quantitative characterization [40].

Moreover, relatively new acquisitions in the field of cardiac MR imaging seem to allow real-time metabolic imaging with extraordinary accuracy as well as spatial resolution. The introduction of MR spectroscopy with hyperpolarized molecules (i.e. carbon-13 pyruvate) in the clinical field might open new fields of the pathophysiological investigation centered on the in vivo evaluation of myocardial metabolic pathways (i.e. the Krebs cycle activity) through the quantification of the metabolic flux of key 13C-labelled molecules [41, 42].

While it is still not clear whether PET/MR will be able to offer added value or generate additional demand for imaging studies that PET/CT cannot satisfy, we can expect that the combination of molecular imaging with superb functional characterization of cardiac performance will help to better investigate cardiac pathophysiology and to develop predictive parameters for tissue recovery and response to therapy.

Molecular Imaging: The Evaluation of Cardiac Innervation

The cardiac autonomic nervous system comprises the parasympathetic and the sympathetic nervous systems (SNS), which are equally relevant and have specular actions on cardiac function and hemodynamics. The early effects of SNS activation include heart rate and blood pressure elevation as well as increased myocardial contractility. While those mechanisms may support cardiac systolic function in early phases, they become detrimental in the chronic setting.

The different functions of the SNS are primarily mediated by the synthesis and release of norepinephrine. Interestingly, after neuronal stimulation only a limited amount of norepinephrine is available to activate adrenergic receptors on the myocyte membranes since the majority of norepinephrine molecules are recycled into nerve terminals through dedicated transporters.

While these mechanisms ensure an optimal norepinephrine turnover at a normal neuronal stimulation frequency, they cannot compensate for the norepinephrine spillover in case of prolonged high stimulation frequencies, such as in patients with HF. In this situation, adrenergic terminals may become depleted of norepinephrine and the heart functionally denervated.

Unfortunately, despite its obvious clinical relevance, the status of cardiac SNS has been classically investigated indirectly, using surrogated, modestly reproducible, systemic measures (i.e. baroreceptor function or heart rate variability).

However, modern nuclear imaging offers the chance to shed light on cardiac sympathetic tone, through the use of a dedicated nervous radiotracer [123I-metaiodobenzylguanidine (123I-MIBG)]. In fact, since its introduction in clinical practice, 123I-MIBG imaging has become the reference radiotracer for the non-invasive evaluation of cardiac adrenergic nervous function using planar scintigraphy and SPECT imaging.

From planar images, 123I-MIBG uptake is semiquantitatively assessed by calculating the heart-to-mediastinum (H/M) ratio and the washout rate, which estimates cardiac global adrenergic receptor density and have been associated with adverse prognosis [43].

However, despite their excellent reproducibility, those planar scintigraphic measures are unable to unmask regional alterations of cardiac adrenergic tone, whose presence has been shown to associate with different cardiac pathologies, independently predicting patients' outcomes.

In this respect, SPECT imaging offers the chance to evaluate the presence of regional myocardial adrenergic innervation inhomogeneity, allowing, on the other hand, the comparison of regional cardiac innervation and perfusion obtained in the same patient with the same imaging format.

Not surprisingly, some studies have suggested how a regional 123I-MIBG defect score, derived from SPECT images, may be superior to the H/M ratio in predicting patient's adverse prognosis, highlighting the independent detrimental effect of regional adrenergic innervation heterogeneity [44].

Nevertheless, the combined assessment of myocardial innervation and perfusion has never gained wide clinical application, possibly because of the high radiation exposure and long acquisition time of this integrated imaging protocol. The use of new solid-state cardiac cameras with cadmium–zinc–telluride (CZT) detectors, characterized by a higher photon sensitivity and spatial resolution than standard cameras, can easily overcome these limitations and allow a comprehensive assessment of myocardial innervation and perfusion in a single imaging session and with a limited radiation burden. Accordingly, preliminary results obtained with this technique have shown the elevated image quality and possible clinical applications of combined innervation/perfusion CZT cardiac imaging in different patient categories, with and without cardiac pathologies [45, 46].

If SPECT imaging has made the clinical evaluation of cardiac sympathetic innervation feasible, PET still represents the reference standard for the non-invasive evaluation of myocardial adrenergic tone, allowing the absolute quantification of sympathetic nerve terminal activity. However, PET imaging also shows relevant technical disadvantages, mainly related to the short half-life of the Carbon-11 (^{11}C) labeled innervation tracers, which have limited the diffusion of this technique.

Specifically, the versatility of PET radiotracers allows to perform a combined investigation of both pre-synaptic and post-synaptic receptor density. Accordingly, the positron tracers [11C]hydroxyephedrine and [^{11}C]epinephrine permit quantification of the density of sympathetic nerve terminals [47], while postsynaptic-receptor density can be assessed with [^{11}C]CGP12177, which has been shown to independently predict adverse patients' prognosis, particularly related to the incidence of symptomatic HF.

Innervation Imaging of Arrhythmias

Structural heart diseases, such as post-ischemic LV dysfunction, are among the major predisposing factors for ventricular arrhythmias whose genesis relies on the combined presence of a triggering mechanism that initiates the arrhythmia and of an anatomic substrate that maintains the arrhythmia once it is initiated. While the anatomic substrate is mainly identified by the presence of isles of scar tissue (i.e. an old myocardial infarction or the results of myocarditis) interposed within bands of living myocardium, the triggering functional mechanism may vary. In this respect, cardiac MRI with late gadolinium enhancement technique represents the gold standard for the evaluation of the presence and extent of myocardial scar, allowing localizing myocardial fibrosis (i.e. sub-epicardial, sub-endocardial, or transmural) and defining the most likely etiology of the underlying disease (i.e. ischemic, inflammatory, infiltrative).

One of the most relevant factors that may trigger ventricular arrhythmias is represented by an abnormality of cardiac sympathetic tone [48].

In this context, due to an increase in the number of patients with heart failure and ventricular arrhythmias, ventricular tachycardia ablation has a growing clinical role. Long-term success rates remain suboptimal and require creating a detailed electroanatomic map during the procedure to identify fibrotic areas responsible for arrhythmias. In particular, areas of abnormal cardiac sympathetic innervation can be identified using ^{123}I MIBG SPECT imaging, which may help in identifying triggers that initiate ventricular tachycardia and also predict successful ablation sites within an otherwise normal myocardium [49]. In line with this evidence, recent proof-of-concept studies have shown the feasibility of "innervation" imaging-guided transcatheter ablation of symptomatic ventricular arrhythmias, where viable myocardial regions showing an impaired SNS activity [mismatch signal on "perfusion-innervation" (^{99m}Tc-tetrofosmin-123I-MIBG) SPECT] represented the most likely targets for a successful ablation [50–52].

Cardiac Resynchronization Therapy

In the last few decades, the evaluation of the presence of LV mechanical dyssynchrony has become a mandatory step in the functional assessment of patients with HF, since a dyssynchronous LV mechanical activation has been consistently associated with adverse patients' functional status and overall outcomes [53, 54]. From a theoretical point of view, LV mechanical dyssynchrony should be distinguished by electrical dyssynchrony, the first relating to the inability of the different myocardial walls to contract in unison, while the latter describing the delayed propagation of the electric impulse in a portion of the LV myocardium, such as in the case of a left-bundle branch block (LBBB). While different reports have shown how these two different entities (i.e. electrical and mechanical dyssynchrony) may be independent one from the other in predicting adverse cardiac morbidity—since significant mechanical dyssynchrony may develop even in patients with a normal QRS—[55], no convincing data exists on the clinical benefit derived by "treating" mechanical dyssynchrony in patients with a narrow QRS [56].

In the presence of LV mechanical dyssynchrony, cardiac resynchronization therapy (CRT), or biventricular pacing, aims at restoring a physiological myocardial mechanical activation by stimulating different positions of the LV (i.e. the septal and lateral walls).

All the available cardiac imaging modalities offer the opportunity to assess LV mechanical dyssynchrony with similar accuracy and reproducibility. In particular, 2D echocardiography has classically represented the standard imaging technique for the evaluation of patients with suspected myocardial dyssynchrony, and various indices, either based on mono-dimensional, two-dimensional, or Doppler imaging, have been proposed and validated in relatively small numbered studies. However, as clearly shown by the PROSPECT study, almost none of such echocardiographic measures of LV dyssynchrony [57, 58] shows acceptable reproducibility, failing to accurately predict the response to CRT.

Accordingly, in an attempt to overcome the intrinsic limitations of 2D echocardiography, novel indices derived from 3D imaging techniques have been developed, offering the opportunity to characterize LV contraction in a real-time three-dimensional manner. 3D echocardiography and single-photon emission computed tomography (SPECT) are undoubtedly the most diffused and clinically relevant techniques for the 3D estimation of LV mechanical dyssynchrony. On the one hand, 3-D echocardiography offers the opportunity to image the entire LV volume in real-time, allowing the derivation of a three-dimensional measure of global LV deformation (i.e. 3D LV strain) that may significantly better predict cardiac mechanics than 2D indices [59].

On the other hand, nuclear imaging has classically represented the reference standard for the assessment of LV mechanical dyssynchrony, allowing quantifying the degree of abnormal myocardial mechanical activation with "phase analysis" [60]. However, those indices of mechanical dyssynchrony (i.e. the phase standard deviation and the histogram bandwidth), initially derived from planar cardiac scintigraphy, have never gained wide clinical diffusion, probably because of the relative rudimentariness of the imaging technique.

SPECT imaging allows for obtaining superior measures of LV regional myocardial perfusion, still representing the backbone of the non-invasive evaluation of myocardial ischemia and viability. Moreover, gated SPECT analysis may provide absolute, highly reproducible, and validated, measures of LV structure and mechanics (i.e. LV volumes, ejection fraction, and mass) and quantitate the presence and extent of mechanical dyssynchrony in a three-dimensional manner [61]. SPECT-derived "phase analysis" represents an almost operator-independent technique to obtain a volumetric evaluation of LV mechanical dyssynchrony on top of the classical SPECT-derived perfusion analysis [62]. As expected, dyssynchrony analysis by SPECT has been shown to correctly identify patients that will benefit from CRT, allowing obtaining, particularly when performed with dedicated cardiac cameras equipped with cadmium-zinc-telluride (CZT) detectors, a comprehensive evaluation of myocardial perfusion and mechanics with an extremely low radiation burden [63, 64] (Fig. 10.2).

Nevertheless, despite the advancement of the different imaging modalities in the characterization of LV mechanical dyssynchrony, 30–40% of the patients having CRT do not respond to resynchronization therapy with improved clinical symptom and cardiac functions, posing a relevant problem of cos-effectiveness of the procedure [53]. Multimodal cardiac imaging offers the chance to overcome the limitations of single-modality imaging, offering the opportunity to characterize different predictors of CRT response, such as the presence and location of myocardial dyssynchrony (i.e. identification of the most delayed LV wall), myocardial viability burden, and coronary venous anatomy.

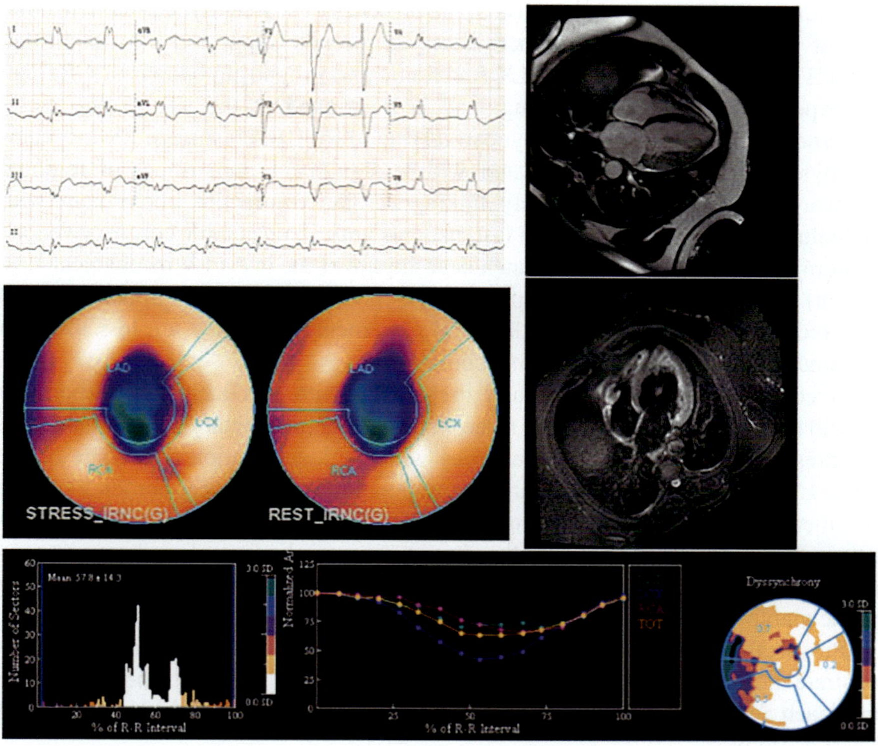

Fig. 10.2 Multimodality cardiac imaging in chronic heart failure. A male patient with post-ischemic left ventricular dysfunction and a previous anterior myocardial infarction treated with PCI on the mid LAD. On ECG a left-bundle branch-block was evident. Cardiac magnetic resonance showed the presence of a moderately dilated LV with depressed systolic function (EF 35%), while myocardial perfusion imaging at stress/rest SPECT revealed an anterior-distal and apical LV scar. Gated SPECT images demonstrated the presence of significant mechanical dyssynchrony with delayed activation of the lateral LV wall, suggesting the possible benefit of CRT therapy

It is capital for CRT response that the LV lead is placed away from a myocardial scar and at or near the site of the latest mechanical activation. Both echocardiographical and nuclear image-guided approaches for CRT have shown significant clinical value in assessing LV myocardial viability and mechanical dyssynchrony, recommending the optimal LV lead position, and navigating the LV lead to the target coronary venous site [65].

This is particularly true when imaging modalities that asses and quantitate the presence of LV mechanical dyssynchrony are combined with the non-invasive assessment of cardiac coronary sinus anatomy, as possible with computed tomography (CT) coronary venous angiography to preliminarily assess the anatomic feasibility of CRT implantation [66].

Specifically, patients with post-ischemic LV systolic dysfunction might benefit most from this multimodal approach. Those patients are least likely to respond to

CRT implantation, probably because of the presence of scared myocardium near the site of delayed LV mechanical activation, as recently supported by a dedicated SPECT study showing that both LV functional and prognostic benefit of CRT can be expected when the LV pacing lead is positioned at the site of the most-dyssynchronous but still viable myocardial region [67]. Interestingly, LV mechanical dyssynchrony is also associated with a significant impairment of regional myocardial SNS activity, possibly linking cardiac contractile impairment with arrhythmogenicity [46, 52, 68]. At last, patients with an unsuitable coronary venous anatomy (i.e. lacking a venous branch near the site of the latest LV mechanical activation) might be spared from the procedure of percutaneous CRT implantation and referred to trans-septal or epicardial lead placement, since they are less likely to respond to traditional implantation techniques.

Accordingly, the ideal approach to patients with mechanical dyssynchrony should theoretically include those three steps: (1) the preliminary 3D assessment of the presence of significant dyssynchrony with the identification of the site of the latest LV activation; (2) the definition of regional myocardial scar burden to define whether the abnormally contracting LV segments are viable and surrounded by significant viable myocardium; (3) the non-invasive evaluation of coronary venous anatomy to ascertain the presence of a suitable coronary venous branch in proximity to the viable dyssynchronous myocardial segments.

Prospective dedicated studies are needed to validate these techniques and demonstrate the clinical opportunity and cost-effectiveness of this multi-modal imaging approach for the management of patients with HF and signs of LV mechanical dyssynchrony.

Rheumatic Disease

Rheumatic diseases (RD) are the result of different pathophysiologic processes that derive from the development of systemic, myocardial, and vascular inflammation. At a cardiac level, RD is associated with early coronary atherosclerosis, abnormal coronary vasoreactivity resulting in cardiac ischemia, due to both micro and/or macrovascular lesions, and myocardial fibrosis [69]. On a functional level, patients with cardiac RD may present with myocardial, pericardial, and coronary artery diseases, and ultimately systolic and diastolic heart failure, as well as pulmonary arterial hypertension. The main effect of RD on cardiac structure is represented by the development of, primarily left-sided, valvular pathologies (i.e. mitral steno-insufficiency or aortic stenosis) that strongly condition the chronic phase of the disease and impact patients' clinical management.

In the initial phase, the symptoms of cardiac involvement in RD are usually subtle, particularly if compared to the prominent acute systemic involvement. On the other hand, cardiac-related symptoms dominate the chronic phase of the disease, underscoring the need for an accurate evaluation of cardiac structure and function through non-invasive imaging.

Echocardiography still represents the backbone of the non-invasive evaluation of patients with suspected or known RD offering the chance to individuate the initial signs of rheumatic manifestations also in the initial oligo-asymptomatic phase [70]. However, a normal echocardiogram cannot always exclude cardiac involvement and/or identify the acuity and pathophysiology of cardiac lesions. Therefore, cardiac magnetic resonance (CMR) imaging is a necessary adjunct, complementary to echocardiography, especially in the case of patients with new onset HF or when there are conflicting data from the initial evaluations. Moreover, CMR is the reference standard for the assessment of signs of pericarditis as well as myocarditis and can be used to quantify the degree of valvular regurgitation and stenosis in patients screened for surgical interventions [71].

Ultimately, cardiac SPECT/PET and coronary CT play a complementary role in patients with cardiac RD, ruling out the presence of other causes of myocardial ischemia in the case of chest pain and assessing the presence and severity of coronary microvascular involvement as a result of the chronic inflammatory process.

Management of Aortic Stenosis in HF

Aortic stenosis (AS) is the most frequent degenerative valvular heart disease in Western countries. While systolic HF, defined by the presence of reduced left ventricular ejection fraction, may be present in up to a quarter of patients with severe AS, most of the patients with significant AS primarily show signs of reduced LV compliance with various degrees of diastolic dysfunction that may consistently reduce effort tolerance even in the presence of a preserved ejection fraction [72].

Multimodality cardiac imaging has two prominent roles in the evaluation of patients with AS: assess coexistent myocardial and coronary pathology in patients with inconclusive symptoms (i.e. angina) or LV systolic dysfunction; perform an in-depth characterization of cardiac structure in a patient candidate for aortic valve replacement, either surgical or percutaneous [72].

In patients with apparently severe AS and LV systolic dysfunction, cardiac imaging can both confirm or exclude the severity of the valvular pathology and individuate other possible causes of HF.

Specifically, 3D imaging modalities, like cardiac CT or 3D echocardiography, may quantify the aortic annulus area and allow a better assessment of the real aortic valve area [72]. Moreover, the calcium score of the aortic valve, as an easy CT-derived measure, has been proposed as an indirect, though specific, sign of the anatomic severity of a given AS. Similarly, CT coronary angiography can evaluate the extent of underlying coronary artery disease, as a frequent, prognostically relevant, bystander in old patients with AS [73].

From the echocardiographic standpoint, LV deformation analysis through strain imaging has been proposed for the detection of early signs of contractile impairment in patients with still normal LV ejection fraction [74].

In patients that will undergo trans-catheter aortic valve implantation (TAVI) a comprehensive cardiac CT evaluation is currently performed to derive key cardiac and valvular parameters (i.e. annulus dimensions, degree of calcification, relationship with coronary ostia) as well as relevant satellite measures (i.e. anatomy of subclavian, iliac and femoral arteries) that will guide the intervention and define, for example, the best vascular access of the procedure [75].

In the last few years, molecular cardiac imaging has allowed a finer characterization of the mechanisms of AS progression. Studies with 123-I MIBG SPECT have demonstrated a consistently impaired SNS activity in patients with severe AS candidate to transcatheter aortic valve intervention (TAVI) with a significant association between the degree of LV hypertrophy (LVH) and the severity of regional myocardial sympathetic dys-innervation [52, 76]. Interestingly, despite the favorable effect of TAVI on LV mass, no changes in myocardial 123-I MIBG uptake were observed after the procedure [77], suggesting the existence of a complex interaction between AS, LVH, and sympathetic dysfunction.

Regarding PET imaging, ^{18}F-sodium fluoride (NaF) has a high affinity to microscopic calcified deposits and its signal can distinguish between areas of macro- and active microcalcification [78]. Consistent evidence has shown that in patients with aortic stenosis, ^{18}F-NaF uptake is correlated with progressive calcification and valvular dysfunction after a 2-year follow-up [79]. Similarly, in patients with bioprosthetic aortic valves increased ^{18}F-NaF uptake at baseline was associated with subsequent bioprosthetic degeneration over time [80].

Cardio-oncology and HF

Decades ago, myocardial biopsy was considered the most accurate method in identifying the myocardial damage induced by chemotherapy, detecting the ultrastructural alteration of cardiomyocytes as well as the alterations of cardiac interstitium [81].

Fortunately, during those years, non-invasive cardiac imaging modalities have emerged as the reference standards in monitoring cardiotoxicity in cancer patients. Nevertheless, despite different techniques and parameters that have been proposed, until recently the most diffused parameter for the serial evaluation of patients undergoing chemotherapy and for the early individuation of the presence of cardiotoxicity has been LV ejection fraction [82].

Despite current cardiac imaging modalities that may quantify the value of LV ejection fraction with excellent accuracy and reproducibility, it is now clear that the drop in LV ejection fraction represents a late phenomenon in the pathophysiology of chemotherapy-induced cardiotoxicity.

This evidence has led clinicians to look for other imaging methods that could evaluate cardiac function independently of the loading conditions, aiming to detect the earliest manifestation of cardiotoxicity and allowing for the appropriate management of the therapy.

Among the different parameters, the evaluation of LV "global longitudinal strain" (GLS) derived by myocardial deformation analysis through 2D-speckle tracking imaging has accumulated evidence supporting its introduction in the clinical evaluation and follow-up of patients with suspected chemotherapy-induced cardiotoxicity. Baseline and periodical evaluation of GLS is recommended by the recent guidelines by ASE/EACVI [83]. Promising techniques such as 3D-STE and tissue characterization performed by CMR are under investigation and could provide new insights into the future for the evaluation of chemotherapy-treated patients. Nuclear cardiac imaging with PET has a promising role in the evaluation of myocardial energy balance and metabolism that can be significantly impaired in patients treated with cardiotoxic chemotherapy and predict cardiac functional deterioration at follow-up [84]. Moreover, cardiac ^{18}F-fluorodeoxyglucose-PET can be used to assess for "immune checkpoint inhibitors"-mediated myocarditis in cases where CMR is either unavailable or inconclusive [85].

Cardiac Amyloidosis

Infiltrative heart disease represents a frequently underdiagnosed cause of congestive HF. Among the different etiologies, cardiac amyloidosis represents, by far, the most clinically relevant type of infiltrative heart disease, leading to restrictive cardiomyopathy.

The diagnosis of cardiac amyloidosis is based on multiple clinical, bio-humoral, imaging, and hysto-pathological findings. Among the different cardiac imaging modalities, CMR is probably the one-stop-shop for the non-invasive characterization of patients with suspected amyloidosis. Specifically, CMR can assess the presence and determine the distribution of myocardial infiltration, through the analysis of "late gadolinium enhancement" (LGE) data [86]. Accordingly, the temporal evolution of cardiac involvement can be tracked, with sub-endocardial LGE deposition in the earlier phases, and transmural fibrosis later. Moreover, innovative CMR techniques, such as mapping, and mapping analysis, can estimate myocardial extracellular volume, giving an idea of the global burden of infiltrative burden and predicting adverse patient outcome [87]. At the same time, through the analysis of the first-pass kinetics of gadolinium, CMR may assess the presence of regional myocardial perfusion inhomogeneities and early signs of coronary microvascular dysfunction that may develop in cardiac amyloidosis [88].

In addition to CMR, nuclear cardiac imaging now represents an essential tool for the characterization of patients with suspected or known cardiac amyloidosis, offering the chance for a non-invasive differential diagnosis of the major disease subtypes. On one hand, it has been shown that radiotracers traditionally used for bone scintigraphy, such as Technetium-99m-labelled 3,3-diphosphono-1,2-propanodicarboxylic acid (^{99m}Tc-DPD), has a specific affinity for cardiac amyloid deposits, particularly in the case of transthyretin amyloidosis [89], allowing an early

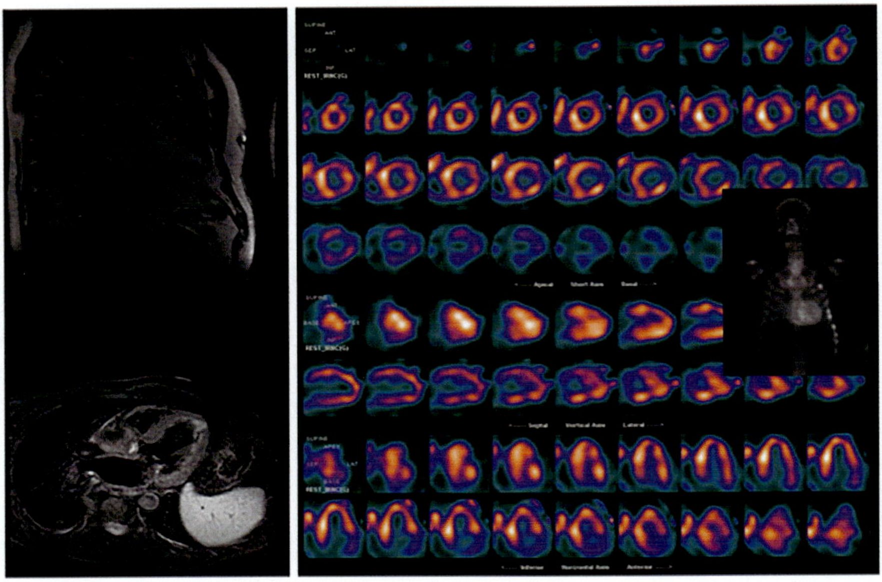

Fig. 10.3 Molecular imaging in heart failure. Representative images of an 85-year-old patient with congestive heart failure and preserved ejection fraction. Cardiac magnetic resonance showed the presence of a hypertrophic LV with a 50% ejection fraction and extensive, mainly intramyocardial, late-gadolinium enhancement (non-ischemic pattern). Because of the suspicion of cardiac infiltration, a technetium-99 m hydroxy diphosphonate whole body and cardiac SPECT scintigraphy was performed with evidence of extensive cardiac tracer uptake consistent with cardiac amyloid deposition

diagnosis of the disease even in the presence of inconsistent results from other clinical and/or imaging techniques [90] (Fig. 10.3). PET imaging with ^{18}F-fluoride has a similar ability to specifically identify myocardial deposits of transthyretin amyloidosis, offering an accurate differential diagnosis from other types of amyloidosis as well as from other "models" of LV hypertrophy [91].

On the other hand, PET imaging with ^{18}fluorine-labeled florbetapir can unmask the presence of light chain amyloidosis [92], possibly avoiding more invasive exams.

Quantitative Cardiac Imaging: The Need for an Absolute Measurement of Cardiac Parameters

Cardiac imaging, particularly when used in daily clinical practice, is generally used to provide qualitative measures of cardiac structure and function. For example, LV systolic function is described through a visual estimation of the ejection fraction, the presence and degree of LV hypertrophy is characterized with indirect measures (i.e. the interventricular septum thickness), and myocardial perfusion is evaluated in relative terms.

However, particularly in the setting of patients with HF, which frequently require periodic cardiac evaluations to modify targeted treatments (anti-hypertensives, diuretics), the accurate quantification of key LV parameters is necessary. Accordingly, the different cardiac imaging now allows the chance to precisely and reproducibly quantify measures of cardiac structure and function (i.e. LV ejection fraction and mass), LV mechanics (i.e. the global longitudinal strain), and cardiac perfusion (i.e. myocardial blood flow reserve).

Specifically, 3D-echocardiography may offer a to obtain an absolute evaluation of LV volumes, mass, and ejection fraction that parallels the results of CMR, showing a convincing reproducibility [93]. Moreover, the analysis of LV deformation through 2D (i.e. speckle tracking technique) or 3D echocardiography allows to obtain highly reproducible indices of regional and global LV function, such as the global longitudinal strain, that may additively characterize HF patients [94].

On the other hand, conventional nuclear imaging, particularly in the era of new dedicated cardiac devices equipped with CZT detectors, may become the one-stop-shop for the evaluation of patients with HF, offering the chance to obtain a rapid assessment of LV perfusion and regional viability and cardiac function and structure (i.e. LV mass, sphericity index, and dyssynchrony) within the same imaging session [62, 95]. Moreover, through dedicated molecular imaging, such as in the case of innervation imaging (i.e. 123I-MIBG SPECT) and amyloid imaging (i.e. 99mTc-DPD SPECT), current nuclear techniques allow a precise etiological characterization and risk assessment with contained costs and radiation burden [90].

Finally, when cardiac PET is considered, modern cardiac imaging allows a state-of-the-art evaluation of regional and global absolute myocardial blood flow (MBF) and MBF reserve, which still represent some of the most prognostically relevant cardiac functional measures, both in patients with idiopathic LV systolic dysfunction [96] and ischemic heart disease [97], as well as in those with primary (i.e. hypertrophic cardiomyopathy) [98] and secondary (i.e. amyloidosis) cardiomyopathies [99]. The recent diffusion of dedicated cardiac cameras equipped with CZT detectors has allowed quantifying MBF in a PET-like fashion [100] with obvious diagnostic [101, 102] and prognostic [103] implications.

Future Perspectives—Hybrid Imaging Using Molecular Targets

Cardiac imaging has been largely used to witness the functional and structural effects of a given pathology, being molecular imaging practically outside the possibilities of most of the imaging modalities. Nuclear cardiac imaging has traditionally represented the only chance to perform molecular imaging in the clinical field. Accordingly, cardiovascular molecular imaging aims at the visualization of specific molecules and pathways that precede or underlie changes in morphology, physiology, and function.

Examples are the use of neuronal imaging to identify subjects at risk for ventricular arrhythmia [104, 105], the development of compounds targeting plaque vulnerability before rupture and subsequent myocardial infarction [106, 107] or stroke [108]), and the analysis of the precocious mechanisms which precede left ventricular remodeling and heart failure development [109, 110], as well as aortic valve degeneration [111]. Additionally, molecular imaging has great potential to facilitate the discovery and development of novel therapies through improved target identification and implementation of more efficient endpoints, as well as visualization of cellular and subcellular target structures. Examples are the development of reporter gene imaging techniques [112], and the implementation of cell labeling for imaging of engraftment after transplantation [113]. This ability to visualize small amounts of molecular-targeted compounds in small target areas has clear translational potentials and may help to design dedicated imaging algorithms and instrumentations for dedicated molecular analysis. It also provides a strong rationale for hybrid imaging approaches, where the nuclear imaging component is used for molecular targeting and the CT is used for localization of the specific signal [114].

Conclusion

In patients with LV dysfunction, multimodality imaging offers the opportunity to obtain continued information on regional and global cardiac function (including mechanical dyssynchrony), myocardial viability and (sympathetic) innervation, coronary anatomy, and regional relative (SPECT) or absolute (PET) myocardial perfusion.

The different modalities may be performed separately and integrated/fused afterward (i.e. through hybrid imaging) or may be used in a single-step approach to defining HF etiology, the extent and severity of myocardial damage/ischemia, indicate and predict the response to targeted treatments (i.e. CRT, coronary revascularization) as well as to perform pre-interventional assessment (i.e. to program trans-catheter ablation of arrhythmias or valvular interventions).

References

1. Berman DS. Fourth Annual Mario S. Verani, MD Memorial Lecture: noninvasive imaging in coronary artery disease: changing roles, changing players. J Nucl Cardiol. 2006;13:457–73.
2. Gaemperli O, Bengel FM, Kaufmann PA. Cardiac hybrid imaging. Eur Heart J. 2011;32:2100–8.
3. Flotats A, Knuuti J, Gutberlet M, Marcassa C, Bengel FM, Kaufmann PA, et al. Hybrid cardiac imaging: SPECT/CT and PET/CT. A joint position statement by the European Association of Nuclear Medicine (EANM), the European Society of Cardiac Radiology (ESCR) and the European Council of Nuclear Cardiology (ECNC). Eur J Nucl Med Mol Imaging. 2011;38:201–12.

4. Javadi MS, Lautamäki R, Merrill J, Voicu C, Epley W, McBride G, et al. Definition of vascular territories on myocardial perfusion images by integration with true coronary anatomy: a hybrid PET/CT analysis. J Nucl Med. 2010;51:198–203.
5. Liga R, Vontobel J, Rovai D, Marinelli M, Caselli C, Pietila M, et al. Multicentre multi-device hybrid imaging study of coronary artery disease: results from the EValuation of INtegrated Cardiac Imaging for the Detection and Characterization of Ischaemic Heart Disease (EVINCI) hybrid imaging population. Eur Heart J Cardiovasc Imaging. 2016;17:951–60.
6. Miller RJH, Bonow RO, Gransar H, Park R, Slomka PJ, Friedman JD, et al. Percutaneous or surgical revascularization is associated with survival benefit in stable coronary artery disease. Eur Heart J Cardiovasc Imaging. 2020;21(9):961–70.
7. Pazhenkottil AP, Nkoulou RN, Ghadri JR, Herzog BA, Buechel RR, Küest SM, et al. Prognostic value of cardiac hybrid imaging integrating single-photon emission computed tomography with coronary computed tomography angiography. Eur Heart J. 2011;32:1465–71.
8. Neglia D, Liga R, Caselli C, Carpeggiani C, Lorenzoni V, Sicari R, et al. Anatomical and functional coronary imaging to predict long-term outcome in patients with suspected coronary artery disease: the EVINCI-outcome study. Eur Heart J Cardiovasc Imaging. 2020;21(11):jez24.
9. Ghali JK. CABG in patients with left ventricular dysfunction. N Engl J Med. 2011;365:468.a.
10. O'Connor CM, Velazquez EJ, Gardner LH, Smith PK, Newman MF, Landolfo KP, et al. Comparison of coronary artery bypass grafting versus medical therapy on long-term outcome in patients with ischemic cardiomyopathy (a 25-year experience from the Duke cardiovascular disease databank). Am J Cardiol. 2002;90:101–7.
11. Hachamovitch R, Rozanski A, Shaw LJ, Stone GW, Thomson LEJ, Friedman JD, et al. Impact of ischaemia and scar on the therapeutic benefit derived from myocardial revascularization vs. medical therapy among patients undergoing stress-rest myocardial perfusion scintigraphy. Eur Heart J. 2011;32:1012–24.
12. Farzaneh-Far A, Borges-Neto S. Ischemic Burden, treatment allocation, and outcomes in stable coronary artery disease. Circ Cardiovasc Imaging. 2011;4:746–53.
13. Shaw LJ, Berman DS, Maron DJ, Mancini GBJ, Hayes SW, Hartigan PM, et al. Optimal medical therapy with or without percutaneous coronary intervention to reduce ischemic burden: results from the Clinical Outcomes Utilizing Revascularization and Aggressive Drug Evaluation (COURAGE) trial nuclear substudy. Circulation. 2008;117:1283–91.
14. Maron DJ, Hochman JS, Reynolds HR, Bangalore S, O'Brien SM, Boden WE, et al. Initial invasive or conservative strategy for stable coronary disease. N Engl J Med. 2020;382:1395–4.
15. Lopes RD, Alexander KP, Stevens SR, Reynolds HR, Stone GW, Piña IL, et al. Initial invasive versus conservative management of stable ischemic heart disease in patients with a history of heart failure or left ventricular dysfunction: insights from the ISCHEMIA trial. Circulation. 2020;142(18):1725–35.
16. Liga R, Colli A, Taggart DP, Boden WE, De Caterina R. Myocardial revascularization in patients with ischemic cardiomyopathy: for whom and how. J Am Heart Assoc. 2023;12(6):e026943.
17. Abraham A, Nichol G, Williams KA, Guo A, DeKemp RA, Garrard L, et al. 18F-FDG PET imaging of myocardial viability in an experienced center with access to 18F-FDG and integration with clinical management teams: the Ottawa-FIVE substudy of the PARR 2 trial. J Nucl Med. 2010;51:567–74.
18. Beanlands RSB, Ruddy TD, DeKemp RA, Iwanochko RM, Coates G, Freeman M, et al. Positron emission tomography and recovery following revascularization (PARR-1): the importance of scar and the development of a prediction rule for the degree of recovery of left ventricular function. J Am Coll Cardiol. 2002;40:1735–43.
19. Perera D, Clayton T, O'Kane PD, Greenwood JP, Weerackody R, Ryan M, et al. Percutaneous revascularization for ischemic left ventricular dysfunction. N Engl J Med. 2022;387(15):1351–60.

20. Ashrafian H, Frenneaux MP, Opie LH. Metabolic mechanisms in heart failure. Circulation. 2007;116:434–48.
21. Lionetti V, Guiducci L, Simioniuc A, Aquaro GD, Simi C, De Marchi D, et al. Mismatch between uniform increase in cardiac glucose uptake and regional contractile dysfunction in pacing-induced heart failure. Am J Physiol Heart Circ Physiol. 2007;293:H2747–56.
22. Neglia D, De Caterina A, Marraccini P, Natali A, Ciardetti M, Vecoli C, et al. Impaired myocardial metabolic reserve and substrate selection flexibility during stress in patients with idiopathic dilated cardiomyopathy. Am J Physiol Heart Circ Physiol. 2007;293:H3270–8.
23. Kadkhodayan A, Lin CH, Coggan AR, Kisrieva-Ware Z, Schechtman KB, Novak E, et al. Sex affects myocardial blood flow and fatty acid substrate metabolism in humans with nonischemic heart failure. J Nucl Cardiol. 2017;24(4):1226–35.
24. Schwaiger M, Hicks R. The clinical role of metabolic imaging of the heart by positron emission tomography. J Nucl Med. 1991;32(4):565–78.
25. Buxton DB, Schwaiger M, Nguyen A, Phelps ME, Schelbert HR. Radiolabeled acetate as a tracer of myocardial tricarboxylic acid cycle flux. Circ Res. 1988;63:628–34.
26. Beanlands RSB, Nahmias C, Gordon E, Coates G, DeKemp R, Firnau G, et al. The effects of β1-blockade on oxidative metabolism and the metabolic cost of ventricular work in patients with left ventricular dysfunction: a double-blind, placebo-controlled, positron-emission tomography study. Circulation. 2000;102:2070–5.
27. Gambhir SS, Schwaiger M, Huang SC, Krivokapich J, Schelbert HR, Nienaber CA, et al. Simple noninvasive quantification method for measuring myocardial glucose utilization in humans employing positron emission tomography and fluorine-18 deoxyglucose. J Nucl Med. 1989;30:359–66.
28. Morita K, Katoh C, Yoshinaga K, Noriyasu K, Mabuchi M, Tsukamoto T, et al. Quantitative analysis of myocardial glucose utilization in patients with left ventricular dysfunction by means of 18F-FDG dynamic positron tomography and three-compartment analysis. Eur J Nucl Med Mol Imaging. 2005;32:806–12.
29. Masci PG, Marinelli M, Piacenti M, Lorenzoni V, Positano V, Lombardi M, et al. Myocardial structural, perfusion, and metabolic correlates of left bundle branch block mechanical derangement in patients with dilated cardiomyopathy: a tagged cardiac magnetic resonance and positron emission tomography study. Circ Cardiovasc Imaging. 2010;3:482–90.
30. Tillisch J, Brunken R, Marshall R, Schwaiger M, Mandelkern M, Phelps M, et al. Reversibility of cardiac wall-motion abnormalities predicted by positron tomography. N Engl J Med. 1986;314:884–8.
31. D'Egidio G, Nichol G, Williams KA, Guo A, Garrard L, deKemp R, et al. Increasing benefit from revascularization is associated with increasing amounts of myocardial hibernation. A substudy of the PARR-2 trial. JACC Cardiovasc Imaging. 2009;2:1060–8.
32. Lautamaki R, Schuleri KH, Sasano T, Javadi MS, Youssef A, Merrill J, et al. Integration of infarct size, tissue perfusion, and metabolism by hybrid cardiac positron emission tomography/computed tomography evaluation in a porcine model of myocardial infarction. Circ Cardiovasc Imaging. 2009;2:299–305.
33. Chareonthaitawee P, Schaefers K, Baker CS, Turkheimer F, Stegger L, Banner NR, et al. Assessment of infarct size by positron emission tomography and [18F]2-fluoro-2-deoxy-D--glucose: a new absolute threshold technique. Eur J Nucl Med. 2002;29:203–15.
34. Pagano D, Bonser RS, Townend JN, Ordoubadi F, Lorenzoni R, Camici PG. Predictive value of dobutamine echocardiography and positron emission tomography in identifying hibernating myocardium in patients with postischaemic heart failure. Heart. 1998;79:281–8.
35. Rischpler C, Nekolla SG, Dregely I, Schwaiger M. Hybrid PET/MR imaging of the heart: potential, initial experiences, and future prospects. J Nucl Med. 2013;54:402–15.
36. Greenwood JP, Maredia N, Younger JF, Brown JM, Nixon J, Everett CC, et al. Cardiovascular magnetic resonance and single-photon emission computed tomography for diagnosis of coronary heart disease (CE-MARC): a prospective trial. Lancet. 2012;379:453–60.

37. Chen W, Jeudy J. Assessment of myocarditis: cardiac MR, PET/CT, or PET/MR? Curr Cardiol Rep. 2019;21:76–8.
38. Tung R, Bauer B, Schelbert H, Lynch JP, Auerbach M, Gupta P, et al. Incidence of abnormal positron emission tomography in patients with unexplained cardiomyopathy and ventricular arrhythmias: the potential role of occult inflammation in arrhythmogenesis. Heart Rhythm. 2015;12(12):2488–98.
39. Vontobel J, Liga R, Possner M, Clerc OF, Mikulicic F, Veit-Haibach P, et al. MR-based attenuation correction for cardiac FDG PET on a hybrid PET/MRI scanner: comparison with standard CT attenuation correction. Eur J Nucl Med Mol Imaging. 2015;42:1574–80.
40. Ratib O, Nkoulou R, Schwaiger M. Cardiovascular clinical applications of PET/MRI. Clin Translat Imaging. 2013;1:65–71.
41. Aquaro GD, Frijia F, Positano V, Menichetti L, Santarelli MF, Ardenkjaer-Larsen JH, et al. 3D CMR mapping of metabolism by hyperpolarized 13C-pyruvate in ischemia-reperfusion. JACC Cardiovasc Imaging. 2013;6:743–4.
42. Dodd MS, Atherton HJ, Carr CA, Stuckey DJ, West JA, Griffin JL, et al. Impaired in vivo mitochondrial krebs cycle activity after myocardial infarction assessed using hyperpolarized magnetic resonance spectroscopy. Circ Cardiovasc Imaging. 2014;7:895–904.
43. Bristow MR. The adrenergic nervous system in heart failure. N Engl J Med. 1984;311:850–1.
44. Hachamovitch R, Nutter B, Menon V, Cerqueira MD. Predicting risk versus predicting potential survival benefit using 123I-m IBG imaging in patients with systolic dysfunction eligible for implantable cardiac defibrillator implantation: analysis of data from the prospective ADMIRE-HF study. Circ Cardiovasc Imaging. 2015;8(12):e003110.
45. Gimelli A, Liga R, Giorgetti A, Genovesi D, Marzullo P. Assessment of myocardial adrenergic innervation with a solid-state dedicated cardiac cadmium-zinc-telluride camera: first clinical experience. Eur Heart J Cardiovasc Imaging. 2014;15:575–85.
46. Gimelli A, Liga R, Genovesi D, Giorgetti A, Kusch A, Marzullo P. Association between left ventricular regional sympathetic denervation and mechanical dyssynchrony in phase analysis: a cardiac CZT study. Eur J Nucl Med Mol Imaging. 2014;41:946–55.
47. Caldwell JH, Link JM, Levy WC, Poole JE, Stratton JR. Evidence for pre- to postsynaptic mismatch of the cardiac sympathetic nervous system in ischemic congestive heart failure. J Nucl Med. 2008;49:234–41.
48. Arora R, Ferrick KJ, Nakata T, Kaplan RC, Rozengarten M, Latif F, et al. I-123 MIBG imaging and heart rate variability analysis to predict the need for an implantable cardioverter defribillator. J Nucl Cardiol. 2003;2003(10):121–31.
49. Duell J, Dilsizian V, Smith M, Chen W, Dickfeld T. Nuclear imaging guidance for ablation of ventricular arrhythmias. Curr Cardiol Rep. 2016;18(2):19.
50. Gimelli A, Liga R, Giorgetti A, Kusch A, Pasanisi EM, Marzullo P. Relationships between myocardial perfusion abnormalities and poststress left ventricular functional impairment on cadmium-zinc-telluride imaging. Eur J Nucl Med Mol Imaging. 2015;42(7):994–1003.
51. Gimelli A, Menichetti F, Soldati E, Liga R, Scelza N, Zucchelli G, et al. Predictors of ventricular ablation's success: viability, innervation, or mismatch? J Nucl Cardiol. 2021;28(1):175–83.
52. Gimelli A, Liga R, Agostini D, Bengel FM, Ernst S, Hyafil F, et al. The role of myocardial innervation imaging in different clinical scenarios: an expert document of the European Association of Cardiovascular Imaging and Cardiovascular Committee of the European Association of Nuclear Medicine. Eur Heart J Cardiovasc Imaging. 2021;22:480–90.
53. McDonagh TA, Metra M, Adamo M, Baumbach A, Böhm M, Burri H, et al. 2021 ESC Guidelines for the diagnosis and treatment of acute and chronic heart failure. Eur Heart J. 2021;42(36):3599–726.
54. Cleland JGF, Daubert JC, Erdmann E, Freemantle N, Gras D, Kappenberger L, et al. The effect of cardiac resynchronization on morbidity and mortality in heart failure. N Engl J Med. 2005;352:1539–49.

55. Yu CM, Chan YS, Zhang Q, Yip GWK, Chan CK, Kum LCC, et al. Benefits of cardiac resynchronization therapy for heart failure patients with narrow QRS complexes and coexisting systolic asynchrony by echocardiography. J Am Coll Cardiol. 2006;48:2251–7.
56. Tayal B, Gorcsan J, Bax JJ, Risum N, Olsen NT, Singh JP, et al. Cardiac resynchronization therapy in patients with heart failure and narrow QRS complexes. J Am Coll Cardiol. 2018;71(12):1325–33.
57. Fornwalt BK, Sprague WW, Carew JD, Merlino JD, Fyfe DA, León AR, et al. Variability in tissue doppler echocardiographic measures of dyssynchrony is reduced with use of a larger region of interest. J Am Soc Echocardiogr. 2009;22:478–85.
58. Chung ES, Leon AR, Tavazzi L, Sun JP, Nihoyannopoulos P, Merlino J, et al. Results of the predictors of response to crt (prospect) trial. Circulation. 2008;117:2608–16.
59. Seo Y, Ishizu T, Kawamura R, Yamamoto M, Kuroki K, Igarashi M, et al. Three-dimensional propagation imaging of left ventricular activation by speckle-tracking echocardiography to predict responses to cardiac resynchronization therapy. J Am Soc Echocardiogr. 2015;28:606–14.
60. Marzullo P, Parodi O, Schelbert HR, L'Abbate A. Regional myocardial dysfunction in patients with angina at rest and response to isosorbide dinitrate assessed by phase analysis of radionuclide ventriculograms. J Am Coll Cardiol. 1984;3:1357–66.
61. Boogers MM, Van Kriekinge SD, Henneman MM, Ypenburg C, Van Bommel RJ, Boersma E, et al. Quantitative gated SPECT-derived phase analysis on gated myocardial perfusion SPECT detects left ventricular dyssynchrony and predicts response to cardiac resynchronization therapy. J Nucl Med. 2009;50:718–25.
62. Gimelli A, Liga R, Giorgetti A, Favilli B, Pasanisi EM, Marzullo P. Determinants of left ventricular mechanical dyssynchrony in patients submitted to myocardial perfusion imaging: a cardiac CZT study. J Nucl Cardiol. 2016;23:728–36.
63. Einstein AJ, Blankstein R, Andrews H, Fish M, Padgett R, Hayes SW, et al. Comparison of image quality, myocardial perfusion, and left ventricular function between standard imaging and single-injection ultra-low-dose imaging using a high-efficiency SPECT camera: the MILLISIEVERT study. J Nucl Med. 2014;55:1430–7.
64. Acampa W, Buechel RR, Gimelli A. Low dose in nuclear cardiology: state of the art in the era of new cadmium-zinc-telluride cameras. Eur Heart J Cardiovasc Imaging. 2016;17:591–5.
65. Boogers MJ, Chen J, Van Bommel RJ, Borleffs CJW, Dibbets-Schneider P, Van Der Hiel B, et al. Optimal left ventricular lead position assessed with phase analysis on gated myocardial perfusion SPECT. Eur J Nucl Med Mol Imaging. 2011;38:230–8.
66. Bakos Z, Markstad H, Ostenfeld E, Carlsson M, Roijer A, Borgquist R. Combined preoperative information using a bullseye plot from speckle tracking echocardiography, cardiac CT scan, and MRI scan: targeted left ventricular lead implantation in patients receiving cardiac resynchronization therapy. Eur Heart J Cardiovasc Imaging. 2014;15:523–31.
67. Liga R, Startari U, Spadafora D, Michelotti E, Gimelli A. Prognostic impact of cardiac resynchronization therapy guided by phase analysis: a CZT study. Eur Heart J Imaging Methods Pract. 2023;1(1):qyad004.
68. Gimelli A, Liga R, Menichetti F, Soldati E, Bongiorni MG, Marzullo P. Interactions between myocardial sympathetic denervation and left ventricular mechanical dyssynchrony: a CZT analysis. J Nucl Cardiol J Nucl Cardiol. 2019;26(2):509–18.
69. Mavrogeni SI. "How many times must a man look up before he can really see the sky?" Rheumatic cardiovascular disease in the era of multimodality imaging. World J Methodol. 2015;5:136–43.
70. Pardos-Gea J, Avegliano G, Evangelista A, Vilardell M, Ordi-Ros J. Cardiac manifestations other than valvulopathy in antiphospholipid syndrome: long-time echocardiography follow-up study. Int J Rheum Dis. 2015;18:76–83.
71. Mavrogeni S, Sfikakis PP, Gialafos E, Bratis K, Karabela G, Stavropoulos E, et al. Cardiac tissue characterization and the diagnostic value of cardiovascular magnetic resonance in systemic connective tissue diseases. Arthritis Care Res. 2014;66:104–12.

72. Kamperidis V, Delgado V, Van Mieghem NM, Kappetein AP, Leon MB, Bax JJ. Diagnosis and management of aortic valve stenosis in patients with heart failure. Eur J Heart Fail. 2016;18:469–81.
73. Cueff C, Serfaty JM, Cimadevilla C, Laissy JP, Himbert D, Tubach F, et al. Measurement of aortic valve calcification using multislice computed tomography: correlation with haemodynamic severity of aortic stenosis and clinical implication for patients with low ejection fraction. Heart. 2011;97:721–6.
74. Monin JL, Quéré JP, Monchi M, Petit H, Baleynaud S, Chauvel C, et al. Low-gradient aortic stenosis. Operative risk stratification and predictors for long-term outcome: a multicenter study using dobutamine stress hemodynamics. Circulation. 2003;108:319–24.
75. Petronio AS, De Carlo M, Bedogni F, Marzocchi A, Klugmann S, Maisano F, et al. Safety and efficacy of the subclavian approach for transcatheter aortic valve implantation with the CoreValve revalving system. Circ Cardiovasc Interv. 2010;3:359–66.
76. Liga R, Gimelli A, Marzullo P, Ambrosio G, Cameli M, Cerbai E, et al. Myocardial 123I-metaiodobenzylguanidine imaging in hypertension and left ventricular hypertrophy. J Nucl Cardiol. 2018;25(2):461–70.
77. Liga R, Gimelli A, De Carlo M, Marzullo P, Pedrinelli R, Petronio AS. Cardiac sympathetic dysfunction in left ventricular hypertrophy caused by arterial hypertension and degenerative aortic stenosis. J Nucl Cardiol. 2022;29(1):337–47.
78. De Azevedo D, Geers J, Gheysens O, Dweck M, Vancraeynest D. 18F-sodium fluoride PET/CT in assessing valvular heart and atherosclerotic diseases. Semin Nucl Med. 2023;53(2):241–57.
79. Jenkins WSA, Vesey AT, Shah ASV, Pawade TA, Chin CWL, White AC, et al. Valvular 18F-fluoride and 18F-fluorodeoxyglucose uptake predict disease progression and clinical outcome in patients with aortic stenosis. J Am Coll Cardiol. 2015;66(10):1200–1.
80. Cartlidge TRG, Doris MK, Sellers SL, Pawade TA, White AC, Pessotto R, et al. Detection and prediction of bioprosthetic aortic valve degeneration. J Am Coll Cardiol. 2019;73(10):110.
81. Mason JW, Bristow MR, Billingham ME, Daniels JR. Invasive and noninvasive methods of assessing adriamycin cardiotoxic effects in man: superiority of histopathologic assessment using endomyocardial biopsy. Cancer Treat Rep. 1978;62(6):857–64.
82. Gulati G, Heck SL, Ree AH, Hoffmann P, Schulz-Menger J, Fagerland MW, et al. Prevention of cardiac dysfunction during adjuvant breast cancer therapy (PRADA): a 2 × 2 factorial, randomized, placebo-controlled, double-blind clinical trial of candesartan and metoprolol. Eur Heart J. 2016;37(21):1671–80.
83. Plana JC, Galderisi M, Barac A, Ewer MS, Ky B, Scherrer-Crosbie M, et al. Expert consensus for multimodality imaging evaluation of adult patients during and after cancer therapy: a report from the American Society of Echocardiography and the European Association of Cardiovascular Imaging. Eur Heart J Cardiovasc Imaging. 2014;27:911–39.
84. Sarocchi M, Bauckneht M, Arboscello E, Capitanio S, Marini C, Morbelli S, et al. An increase in myocardial 18-fluorodeoxyglucose uptake is associated with left ventricular ejection fraction decline in Hodgkin lymphoma patients treated with anthracycline. J Transl Med. 2018;16:295.
85. Čelutkienė J, Pudil R, López-Fernández T, Grapsa J, Nihoyannopoulos P, Bergler-Klein J, et al. Role of cardiovascular imaging in cancer patients receiving cardiotoxic therapies: a position statement on behalf of the Heart Failure Association (HFA), the European Association of Cardiovascular Imaging (EACVI) and the Cardio-Oncology Council of the European Society of Cardiology (ESC). Eur J Heart Fail. 2020;22(9):1504–24.
86. Fontana M, Pica S, Reant P, Abdel-Gadir A, Treibel TA, Banypersad SM, et al. Prognostic value of late gadolinium enhancement cardiovascular magnetic resonance in cardiac amyloidosis. Circulation. 2015;132:1570–9.
87. Fontana M, Banypersad SM, Treibel TA, Maestrini V, Sado DM, White SK, et al. Native T1 mapping in transthyretin amyloidosis. JACC Cardiovasc Imaging. 2014;7(2):157–65.

88. Li R, Yang ZG, Wen LY, Liu X, Xu HY, Zhang Q, et al. Regional myocardial microvascular dysfunction in cardiac amyloid light-chain amyloidosis: assessment with 3T cardiovascular magnetic resonance. J Cardiovasc Magn Reson. 2016;18:16.
89. Hutt DF, Quigley AM, Page J, Hall ML, Burniston M, Gopaul D, et al. Utility and limitations of 3,3-diphosphono-1, 2-propanodicarboxylic acid scintigraphy in systemic amyloidosis. Eur Heart J Cardiovasc Imaging. 2014;15:1289–98.
90. Longhi S, Guidalotti PL, Quarta CC, Gagliardi C, Milandri A, Lorenzini M, et al. Identification of TTR-related subclinical amyloidosis with 99mTc-DPD scintigraphy. JACC Cardiovasc Imaging. 2014;7:531–2.
91. Andrews JPM, Trivieri MG, Everett R, Spath N, MacNaught G, Moss AJ, et al. 18F-fluoride PET/MR in cardiac amyloid: a comparison study with aortic stenosis and age- and sex-matched controls. J Nucl Cardiol. 2022;29(2):741–9.
92. Cuddy SAM, Bravo PE, Falk RH, El-Sady S, Kijewski MF, Park MA, et al. Improved quantification of cardiac amyloid burden in systemic light chain amyloidosis: redefining early disease? JACC Cardiovasc Imaging. 2020;13(6):1325–36.
93. Macron L, Lim P, Bensaid A, Nahum J, Dussault C, Mitchell-Heggs L, et al. Single-beat versus multibeat real-time 3d echocardiography for assessing left ventricular volumes and ejection fraction: a comparison study with cardiac magnetic resonance. Circ Cardiovasc Imaging. 2010;3:450–5.
94. Toro-Salazar OH, Ferranti J, Lorenzoni R, Walling S, Mazur W, Raman SV, et al. Feasibility of echocardiographic techniques to detect subclinical cancer therapeutics-related cardiac dysfunction among high-dose patients when compared with cardiac magnetic resonance imaging. J Am Soc Echocardiogr. 2016;29:119–31.
95. Giorgetti A, Masci PG, Marras G, Rustamova YK, Gimelli A, Genovesi D, et al. Gated SPECT evaluation of left ventricular function using a CZT camera and a fast low-dose clinical protocol: comparison to cardiac magnetic resonance imaging. Eur J Nucl Med Mol Imaging. 2013;40:1869–75.
96. Neglia D, Michelassi C, Giovanna Trivieri M, Sambuceti G, Giorgetti A, Pratali L, et al. Prognostic role of myocardial blood flow impairment in idiopathic left ventricular dysfunction. Circulation. 2002;105:186–93.
97. Tio RA, Dabeshlim A, Siebelink HMJ, De Sutter J, Hillege HL, Zeebregts CJ, et al. Comparison between the prognostic value of left ventricular function and myocardial perfusion reserve in patients with ischemic heart disease. J Nucl Med. 2009;50:214–9.
98. Cecchi F, Olivotto I, Gistri R, Lorenzoni R, Chiriatti G, Camici PG. Coronary microvascular dysfunction and prognosis in hypertrophic cardiomyopathy. N Engl J Med. 2003;349:1027–35.
99. Dorbala S, Vangala D, Bruyere J, Quarta C, Kruger J, Padera R, et al. Coronary microvascular dysfunction is related to abnormalities in myocardial structure and function in cardiac amyloidosis. JACC Heart Fail. 2014;2:358–67.
100. Zavadovsky KV, Mochula AV, Maltseva AN, Shipulin VV, Sazonova SI, Gulya MO, et al. The current status of CZT SPECT myocardial blood flow and reserve assessment: tips and tricks. J Nucl Cardiol. 2022;29(6):3137–51.
101. Zavadovsky KV, Mochula AV, Maltseva AN, Boshchenko AA, Baev AE, Andreev SL, et al. The diagnostic value of SPECT CZT quantitative myocardial blood flow in high-risk patients. J Nucl Cardiol. 2022;29(3):1051–63.
102. Zavadovsky KV, Mochula AV, Boshchenko AA, Vrublevsky AV, Baev AE, Krylov AL, et al. Absolute myocardial blood flows derived by dynamic CZT scan vs invasive fractional flow reserve: correlation and accuracy. J Nucl Cardiol. 2021;28(1):249–59.
103. Liga R, Neglia D, Kusch A, Favilli B, Giorgetti A, Gimelli A. Prognostic role of dynamic CZT imaging in CAD patients: interaction between absolute flow and CAD burden. JACC Cardiovasc Imaging. 2022;15(3):540–2.
104. Jacobson AF, Senior R, Cerqueira MD, Wong ND, Thomas GS, Lopez VA, et al. Myocardial iodine-123 meta-iodobenzylguanidine imaging and cardiac events in heart failure. Results of

the prospective ADMIRE-HF (AdreView Myocardial Imaging for Risk Evaluation in Heart Failure) study. J Am Coll Cardiol. 2010;55:2212.
105. Sasano T, Abraham MR, Chang KC, Ashikaga H, Mills KJ, Holt DP, et al. Abnormal sympathetic innervation of viable myocardium and the substrate of ventricular tachycardia after myocardial infarction. J Am Coll Cardiol. 2008;51:2266–7.
106. Elkhawad M, Rudd JHF. Radiotracer imaging of atherosclerotic plaque biology. Cardiol Clin. 2009;27:345–54.
107. Bengel FM. Atherosclerosis imaging on the molecular level. J Nucl Cardiol. 2006;13:111–8.
108. Fletcher AJ, Tew YY, Tzolos E, Joshi SS, Kaczynski J, Nash J, et al. Thoracic aortic 18F-sodium fluoride activity and ischemic stroke in patients with established cardiovascular disease. JACC Cardiovasc Imaging. 2022;15(7):1274–88.
109. Gaemperli O, Liga R, Spyrou N, Rosen SD, Foale R, Kooner JS, et al. Myocardial-adrenoceptor down-regulation early after infarction is associated with long-term incidence of congestive heart failure. Eur Heart J. 2010;31(14):1722–9.
110. Kramer CM, Sinusas AJ, Sosnovik DE, French BA, Bengel FM. Multimodality imaging of myocardial injury and remodeling. J Nucl Med. 2010;51(Suppl. 1):107S–21S.
111. Pawade TA, Cartlidge TRG, Jenkins WSA, Adamson PD, Robson P, Lucatelli C, et al. Optimization and reproducibility of aortic valve 18F-fluoride positron emission tomography in patients with aortic stenosis. Circ Cardiovasc Imaging. 2016;9(10):e005131.
112. Avril N, Bengel FM. Defining the success of cardiac gene therapy: how can nuclear imaging contribute? Eur J Nucl Med Mol Imaging. 2003;30:757–71.
113. Wu JC, Abraham MR, Kraitchman DL. Current perspectives on imaging cardiac stem cell therapy. J Nucl Med. 2010;51(Suppl 1):128S–36S.
114. Wagner B, Anton M, Nekolla SG, Reder S, Henke J, Seidl S, et al. Noninvasive characterization of myocardial molecular interventions by integrated positron emission tomography and computed tomography. J Am Coll Cardiol. 2006;48:2107–15.

Part III
New Approaches to the Treatment of Heart Failure

Chapter 11
Approach to Ventricular Arrhythmia in Heart Failure

Elena Sauer and Thomas Deneke

Abstract Overall, ventricular tachycardias (VTs) may occur at all stages of HF, whereas monomorphic VT usually is driven by a stable substrate; polymorphic, pleomorphic and rarely monomorphic VT may be induced by worsening HF. Ventricular tachycardias (VT) complicating the evolution of patients with documented heart failure (HF) are associated with a high mortality. The management of patients with HF and VT is multimodal based on pharmacological, device and respectively interventional therapy. Frequently a VT episode is the first clinical event which reveals an underlying structural heart disease (SHD). Therefore, in every patient presenting with a VT, the multimodal, comprehensive clarification of the underlying SHD is of paramount importance for planning the therapeutical strategy and prognostic evaluation. On the other hand, in patients with already known SHD and recurrent VT episodes, beyond optimal HF therapy and device therapy, the most effective long-term strategy is represented by catheter ablation (CA) or antiarrhythmic medication. As VT target areas and substrate usually are colocalized, cardiac imaging has evolved as a very helpful tool not only for planning the technical approach based on substrate distribution (endocardial, epicardial, intramural) but also for preprodurally substrate distribution and ablation targets.

Keywords Heart failure · Structural heart disease · Sustained ventricular tachycardia

E. Sauer (✉) · T. Deneke
Cardiology Clinic II with Interventional Electrophysiology, Rhön Klinikum Campus Bad Neustadt, Bad Neustadt an der Saale, Germany

Clinic for Arrhythmology, University Hospital Nuremberg, South Campus, Nuremberg, Germany

M. Dorobanţu et al. (eds.), *Current Approach to Heart Failure*, https://doi.org/10.1007/978-3-031-96562-3_11

The Multimodal Approach in Management of Patients with Heart Failure and VT

Sustained VT episodes represent the main cause of sudden cardiac death in patients with HF. Whereas prevention of VT in patients identified to be at high risk is crucial management of VT in HF patients must focus on two main aspects:

1. acute approach to VT for rhythm stabilization
2. Chronic approach to VT having as main goals: prevention of SCD, reduction of VT episodes and consequently ICD therapies

According to the recommendations of the current ESC guidelines for diagnosis and treatment of patients with heart failure, a minimum of investigations by first documentation of heart failure is represented by standard 12 leads EKG, 24 h Holter monitoring, exercise test and completed by special procedures including coronary angiography (based on data from history, results of non—invasive tests, cardiovascular risk score) and magnetic resonance imaging [1]. A clear identification of potential reversible causing factors of HF and their specific treatment is extremely important as an increasingly better LVEF is associated with lower risk of SCD. Figure 11.1a, b presents a flow chart for diagnostic approach respectively management in a patient with HF and VT. Also, Case Presentations # 1 and # 2 illustrates the practical approach in management of patients with HF and VT. A first presentation of VT should prompt investigation into potential underlying causes including structural heart disease [2].

The risk of sudden cardiac death (SCD) due to malignant arrhythmias is increased in patients with LVEF < 35%, irrespective of etiology. As a consequence, after initiation of HF standard pharmacological therapy and specific treatment of other causes (for example myocardial revascularization, surgical or interventional treatment of relevant valvular heart diseases), this category of patients may receive a wearable cardioverter defibrillator usually for the next 3 months until the final decision to implant an ICD as primary prophylaxes is confirmed [3].

Based on the results of relatively old studies, the degree of LVEF reduction was used over decades as only risk predictor factor for malignant arrhythmias in patients with different etiologies of HF [4–6]. However, depending on the etiology of the underlying SHD, more recently other risk factors for malignant arrhythmias have been identified: positive familial history of SCD, documented non sustained VT on EKG Holter (for example in cases of laminopathy or malignant mitral valve prolapse), scar burden derived from MRI scan, genetic testing but also type of underlying non-ischemic cardiomyopathy. The degree of scar burden identified on standard MRI is superior in predicting the risk for malignant arrhythmias both in ischemic and in dilative non ischemic cardiomyopathy (DNICM) respectively hypertrophic cardiomyopathy [7–10]. At least the scar burden in NIDCM has strong and incremental prognostic value for SCD risk stratification [9]. Also, the scar distribution pattern plays an important role in SCD risk stratification, the association between intramural septal and epicardial lateral scar being associated with highest risk of

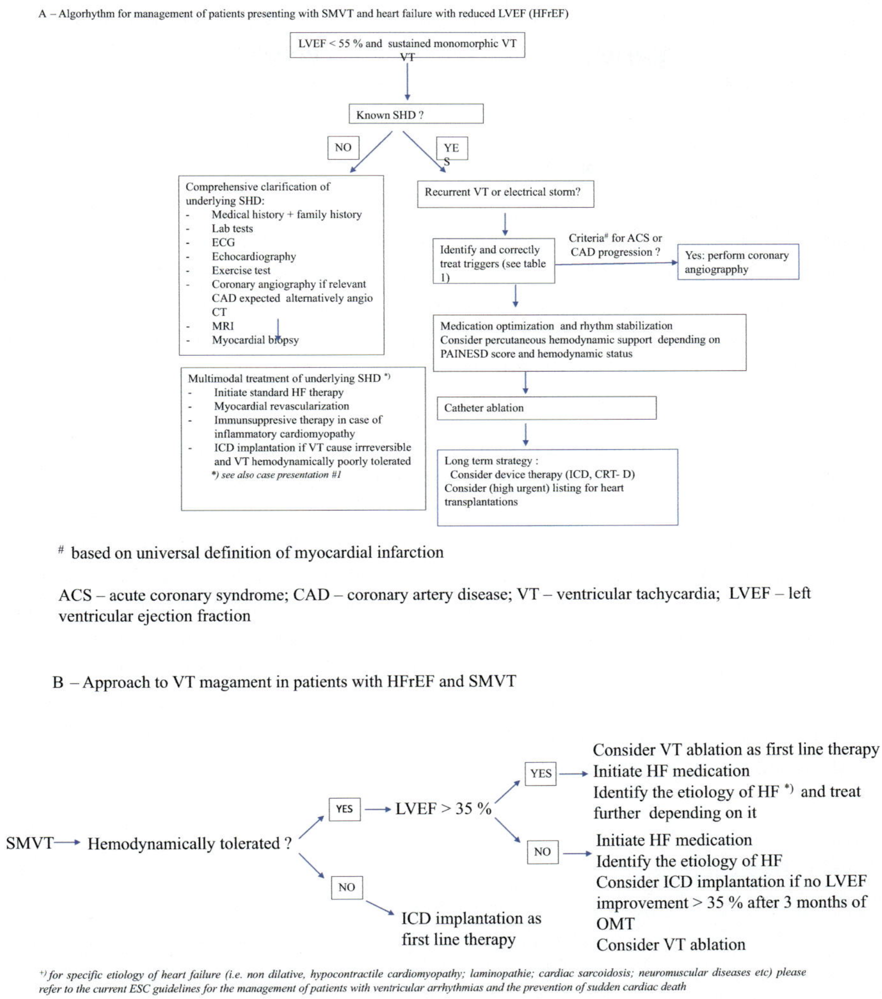

Fig. 11.1 (**a**) Algorithm for management of patients presenting with SMVT and heart failure with reduced LVEF (HFrEF). # based on universal definition of myocardial infarction. *ACS* acute coronary syndrome, *CAD* coronary artery disease, *VT* ventricular tachycardia, *LVEF* left ventricular ejection fraction. (**b**) Approach to VT management in patients with HFrEF and SMVT

SCD [11]. A very promising technology in SCD risk stratification is represented by modelling of VT inducibility and MRI-derived scar geometry [12]. Based on this currently available data, cardiac imaging industry invests in developing better predictability models as a digital twin of the heart [13].

In patients with NI(D)CM with moderately reduced LVEF 36–50% associated with other 2 risk factors from: (1). unexplained syncope; (2). pathogenic mutation of LMNA (phospholamban, filamin C or RNA-binding motif protein 20); (3). proof of LGE on cardiac MRI respectively (4). inducible VT at programmed ventricular stimulation, ICD implantation may be considered as primary prophylaxe [1].

In the same category of patients, the identification of LMNA on genetic testing associated with a 5 years risk of VA ≥ 10% and one of the following: (1) LVEF < 50%; (2). AV conduction delay or (3). NSVT on EKG Holter monitoring should also prompt an ICD implantation [1].

Different automatic algorithms have been developed for calculation of 5-years risk of VA/SCD and could be accessed online (i.e. https://lmna-risk-vta.fr, https://doc2do.com/hcm/webHCM.html, in pediatric population https://hcmriskkids.org).

Programmed ventricular stimulation (PVS) using up to 3 extrastimuli and two different cycle lengths of the driving train in risk stratification for risk of malignant arrhythmias has regained increasing value over the past years. The current main indications for PVS are:

1. In patients with ICM and history of remote MI (i.e. older than 6 weeks) a PVS is indicated in case of unexplained syncope or documented NSVT; in case of inducibility of sustained monomorphic VT, an ICD implantation should be considered. The ongoing study PROTECT-ICD in whom patients with acute coronary syndromes (STEMI or NSTEMI) with an LVEF < 40% assessed on day 2 after admission, will answer the question whether the ICD implantation based on inducibility of sustained VTs on PVS will be associated with lower rate of SCD [14].
2. In patients with NI(D)CM and with family history of DCM/HNDCM with moderately reduced LVEF 36–50% and unexplained syncope. In patients with left ventricular non compaction with scar of MRI, the VT inducibility on PVS is associated with VT recurrence [15].

Case Presentation # 1

A 52 y/o old female was referred for further investigations due to recurrent syncopes. One year ago, she had an episode of broad QRS complex tachycardia without syncope. An acute coronary syndrome was ruled out at that time—on angiography normal coronary arteries.

Negative family history for cardiovascular diseases and SCD.

Initial lab tests were in normal limits.

Investigations on admission (see also algorithm Fig. 11.1***—left arm):***

- EKG—see Fig. 11.2
- transthoracal echocardiography—firstly documented severe LV systolic dysfunction due to hypokinesia of anterior lV wall, no relevant heart valve disease

Completed by

- MRI—see Fig. 11.3
- PET CT—see Fig. 11.4
- Electrophysiological study and VT ablation due to incessant character of VTs

Treatment:

- Standard pharmacological therapy for HF

  Bisoprolol 5 mg bid
  Sacubitril/Valsartan 24/26 mg bid
  Rivaroxaban 20 mg
  Dapaglifozin 10 mg

- Immusuppresive therapy

  Prednisolon 1 mg/KgC for 1 months, 10 mg doses reduction/months
  Azathioprine 50 mg bid

- ICD implantation as secondary prophylaxe (recurrent VTs despite VT ablation, high scar burden on MRI)

Follow—up:

Improvement of LVEF from 35% at admission to 50% 1 month later
No VT recurrence

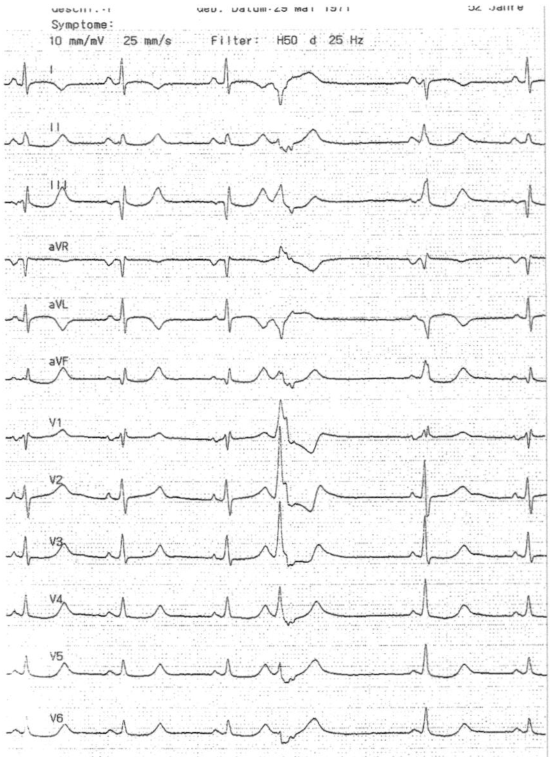

Fig. 11.2 Case#1: EKG on admission: sinus rhythm, incomplete right bundle branch block, PQ respectively QTc intervals within normal limits, deep Q waves in DIII and aVF associated with negative T waves in DI, aVL and a non outflow tract PVC all suggestive of underlying myocardial scar

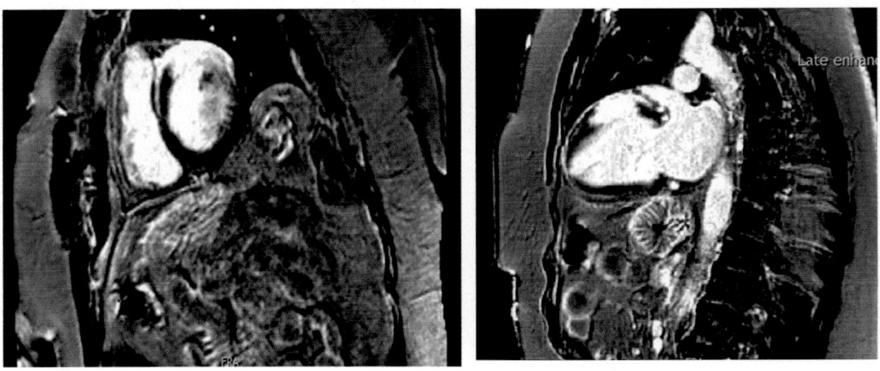

Fig. 11.3 Case#1: MRI scan with LGE—large transmural scar area interventricular septum and anterior wall from basal to midventricular. *LGE* late gadolinium enhancement, *MRI* magnetic resonance imaging

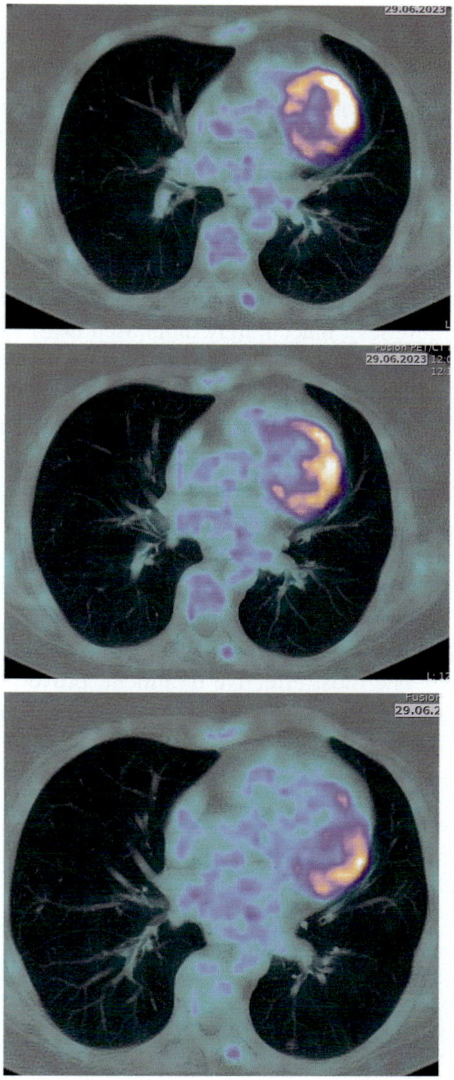

Fig. 11.4 Case#1: PET CT showing segmental increased uptake of F-18-FDG on the anterior wall of LV compatible with cardiac sarcoidosis, *F-18-FDG* Fluor-18 2-Fluor-2-Deoxy-D--Glucose, *PET CT* positron emission computer tomography

Electrical Storm—Effective Treatment Requires Precise Algorithms

Electrical storm (ES) is defined as at least 3 episodes of sustained VT/VF occurring within 24 h requiring a specific form of therapy for termination (i.e. cardioversion/defibrillation/ICD-intervention—shocks/ATPs). The episodes are separated by at least one or more sinus beats (or 1–5 min). ES is an independent midterm (5.4× in secondary preventive ICD, 17.3× in primary preventive ICD) and long-term predictor of mortality (long-term mortality 54% at 2 years) as shown in the MADIT II study [16]. In the majority of cases monomorphic VT is the determining arrhythmia mechanism in ES and only in a minority polymorphic VTs or VF.

ES is a very severely event complicating the natural history of patients with HF and known structural heart diseases. Seldomly, it appears as an inaugural event in a patient with firstly diagnosed HF apparently without known SHD as for example in patients with fulminant myocarditis.

ES is usually not an isolated event and in more than 50% of cases triggers maybe identified. In our daily experience, in order of frequency, the commonest triggers are: infections (mostly pneumonia, urinary tract infections or bacteriemia, rarely endocarditis); electrolytes imbalances (mostly hypokalemia due to excessive use of diuretics); inaccurately diagnosed heart valves diseases (frequently underestimated mitral valve insufficiency); unrecognized and/or underevaluated progression of heart failure—see Case Presentation #3 associating the last 2 ones.

The main goal of acute management in patients with ES is hemodynamic stabilization in order to avoid the deleterious effects of cardiogenic shock and consecutively multiorgan failure. The essential part of hemodynamic stabilization resides in rhythm stabilization. As shown above, the ES is not a singular event and frequently a trigger can be identified. In consequence, rhythm stabilization means rapid identification and correct treatment of potential triggers. Figure 11.5 summarizes the algorithms for acute management of ES. In Case Presentation #2 a step-by-step approach, guided by the algorithm presented in Fig. 11.5 is shown.

The most effective treatment, proven to effectively reduce the VT recurrences and adequate ICD therapies is the catheter ablation—class I level of evidence A in

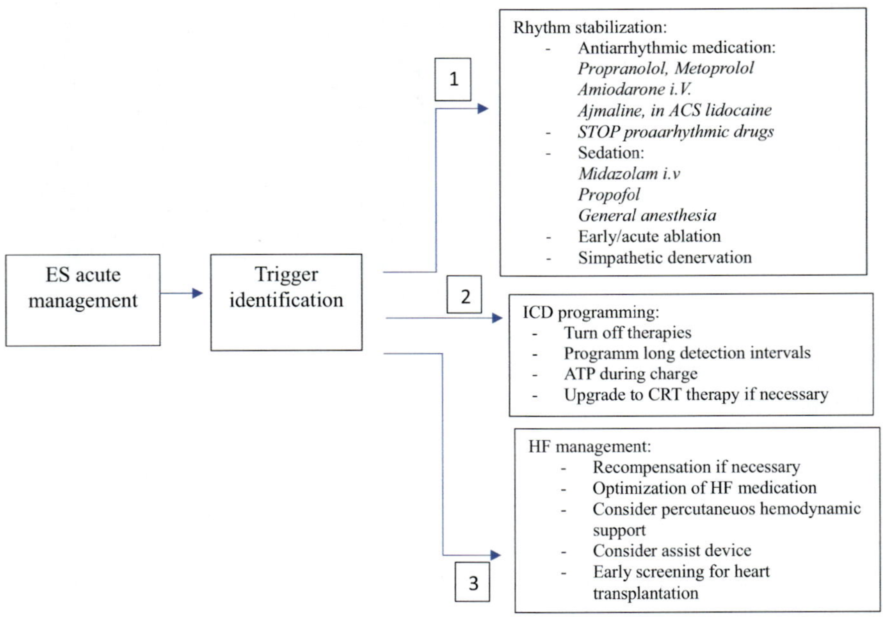

Fig. 11.5 Essential steps in management of patients with electrical storm

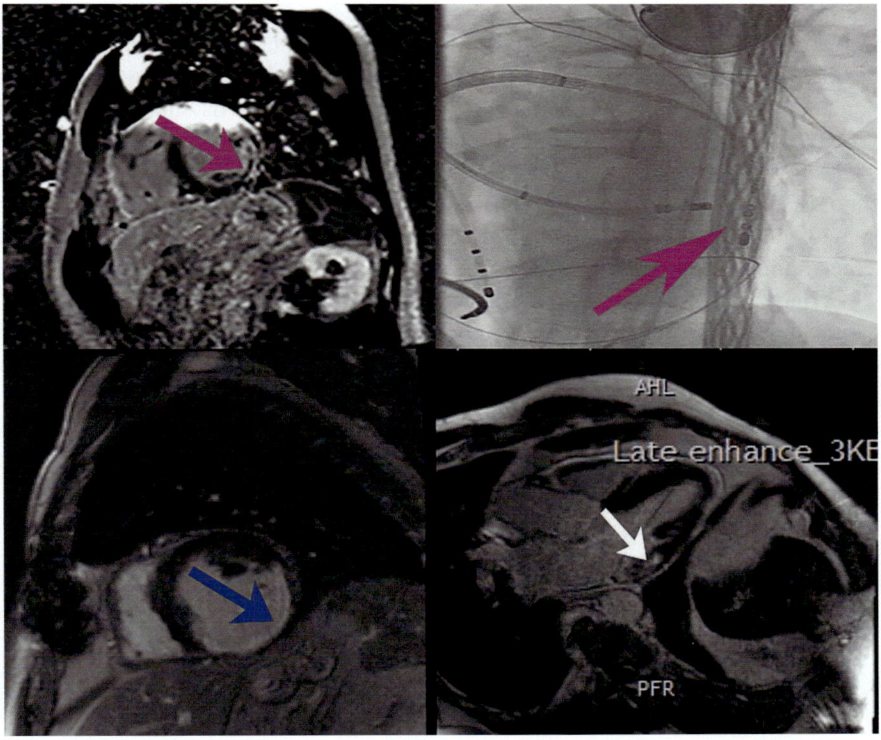

Fig. 11.6 Upper raw: "sandwich" like intramural substrate on lateral aspect of LV in MRI with LGE requiring an bipolar epi/endocardial ablation approach for successful elimination of VT (magenta arrows); bottom left: subendocardial till transmural inferior and infero-lateral substrate distribution requiring an endocardial approach for VT ablation (blue arrow); bottom right—sub-epicardial till intramural basal lateral substrate distribution (white arrow)

the current ESC guidelines [3]. The results of VANISH, SURVIVE and PARTITA studies strongly support an early referral for VT ablation even after the first ICD shock [17–19]. A dedicated VT unit and specialized VT ablation centers may improve management and outcome of structural VT patients. An accurate characterization of scar distribution pattern (i.e. endocardial, intramural, epicardial) and pre-procedural identification of ablation targets based on preprocedural cardiac MRI or CT are extremely helpful, help in planning of ablation strategy and is associated with better long term outcomes after VT ablation—see Fig. 11.6 [20].

The preferred timing for CA should be as early as possible (i.e. during index admission) but after rhythm stabilization and correct trigger treatment (i.e. within the next 8 h after admission). Acute CA is associated with a high risk of recurrences and acute hemodynamic deterioration and should be used only as bailout emergency strategy in order to avoid the deleterious consequences of cardiogenic shock due to recurrent VTs/VF episodes which cannot be eliminated despite maximal conventional therapy [21]. In patients with advanced forms of HF, the risk of periprocedural hemodynamic deterioration should be incorporated into a standardized approach [22] and protected CA procedure may be performed under percutaneous hemodynamic support (protected VT ablation). However, the devices used for percutaneous hemodynamic support should be left in place as short as clinically possible in order to avoid related complications (vascular access complications like bleeding or acute limb ischemia, embolic events, infections, hemolysis) which should worsen the patients' outcome—see Case Presentation #3. Weaning off the hemodynamic support may be problematic in severely heart failure patients and expertise in HF management is needed.

Certain etiologies like arrhythmogenic RV cardiomyopathy, Chagas cardiomyopathy, post myocarditis NI(D)CM are associated with a predominantly epicardial distribution of substrate. Therefore, an epicardial VT ablation in specialized centers should be planned.

The acute outcome of VT ablation is ideally represented by abolition of all LAVAs and non-inducibility of any but at least the clinical VT. This scenario is associated with the best long-term outcome in terms of VT recurrences [23].

Case Presentation # 2

56 y/o male with ICM and severely reduced LVEF 20% was referred for catheter ablation in context of ES (13S-ICD shocks in 3 days).

Medical history:

- *12/2015 anterior wall MI—primary PTCA*
- *03/2016S-ICD implantation as primary prevention*
- *08/2018 substrate based VT ablation*
- *12/2018 last coronary angiographie no progression*

At admission on VT Unit—ICU

S-ICD Interrogation—adequate shocks, but batterie capacity only 32%

After 24 h—neu ES-3 extern defibrillation & ALS—VT under programmed detection zones S-ICD (see Fig. 11.5—EKG documentation of clinical VT)

Step by step management:

1. S-ICD deactivation
2. Sedation—Midazolam i.v.
3. Amiodarone 300 mg i.v. as bolus after 2. schock
4. Potassium i.v. suppl—target 4,5 mmol

Sustained VTs still recurrent:

5. Ajmaline i.v. perfusion
6. HF therapy optimization:

(continued)

- Metoprolol high doses
- Sacubitril/Valsartan
- SOTALOL stopped

After 1.5 h ALS—patient completely stable
CT MT performed before catheter ablation after patient's stabilization—see Fig. 11.6
After 48 h from admission—CT based VT ablation—see Fig. 11.7
Follow up—no inducibility with 4 extrastimuli after VT ablation

- No in hospital recurrence of VT
- No VT recurrence after 1 year

ALS—advanced life support; *ES*—electrical storm; ICU—intermediate care unit; MI—myocardial infarction S—ICD—subcutaneous implantable cardiodefibrillator.

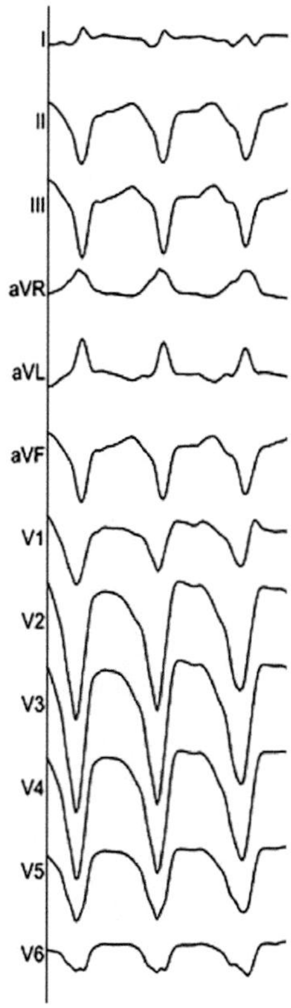

Fig. 11.7 12 lead EKG morphology of clinical VT–HR 180 bpm, LBBB—morphology, superior QRS axis', negative concordance V1–V6 suggesting an apical septal origin from LV

Case Presentation # 3
A 65 y/o female was referred for CA in context of ES.

History:

Severely reduced LVEF 10%
Anterior wall MI—chronic total obstruction of LAD (2011)
2 chamber ICD implantation (2021)—ineffective CRT-D upgrade due to CS dissection (05/2023)
Catheter ablation of His Bundle unclear indication 07/2023
Embolic Stroke of right posterior cerebral artery
Persistent atrial fibrillation
Renal insufficiency AKIN III

Evaluation at admission:
Clinical status: NYHA IV class, no weaning possible from Dobutamine
Severely reduced LVEF 5%
Undiagnosed relevant aspects before transfer in our institution:

- Severe, functional mitral regurgitation
- Slow, incessant VT which run approx. 1 week, under the programmed detection zone, most probably due to Amiodarone therapy
- Prolonged cardiogenic shock

Relevant data from right heart catheterization:

Severe postcapillary pulmonary hypertension (PA syst 65 mmHg, PA diast 27 mmHg, PA mid 47 mmHg)
PCWPm 40 mmHg
PWR 4 Wood
Severely reduced cardiac index 1.3 l/min/m^2

Management plan—see Fig. 11.1***—right arm:***

Recompensation (loop diuretics i.v. under catecholamine)
Impella CP 5.5 (right subclavian artery) implant for LV unloading—PAINESD Score = 28
Protected VT ablation under Impella CP 5.5—see Fig. 11.8
LVAD Screening

Procedures performed during index hospital admission:

Impella CP 5.5 Implantation
VT ablationunder Impella CP 5.5—see Figs. 11.9, 11.10 respectively 11.11, 11.12 and 11.13.
LVAD Heartmate III implantation (severe lung oedema after Impella explanation)

(continued)

Follow—up:

No VT inducible at noninvasive programmed ventricular stimulation 2 days after VT ablation

No VT recurrence at 2 months follow-up after before and after LVAD implantation

Fig. 11.8 3D reconstruction of LV and scar area with different colors coded levels of myocardial thinning based on computer tomography with myocardial thinning (red—1 mm myocardial thinning, yellow—5 mm myocardial thinning); supplementary reconstruction of coronary arteries in red, coronary sinus in blue and left phrenic nerve in green

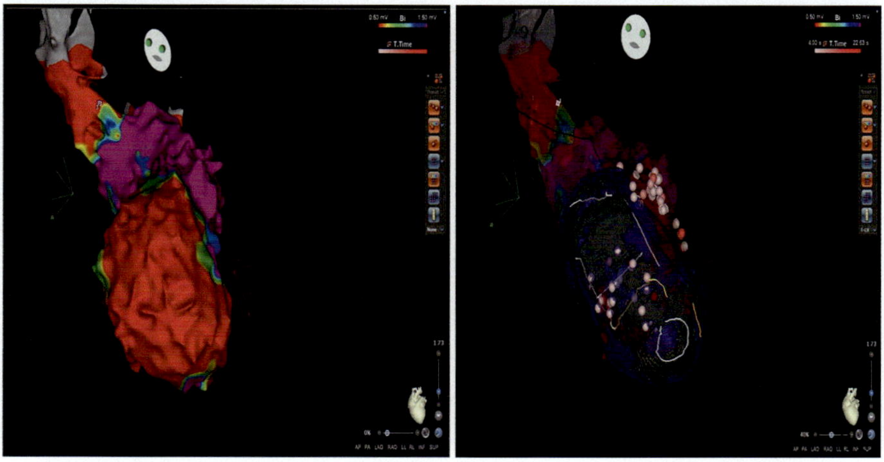

Fig. 11.9 (Left) Substrate mapping showing an extensive scar area over anterior wall of LV from lateral to septal and from basal till apical. (Right) Catheter ablation based on in CT MT preidentified conducting channels (white lines)

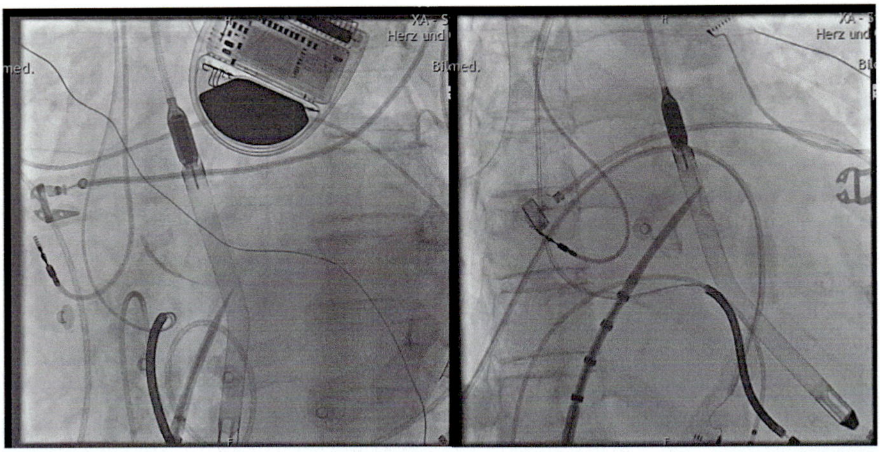

Fig. 11.10 LAO (left) and RAO (right) X-ray projections during the VT ablation procedure showing correct position of Impella inflow canula in the LV

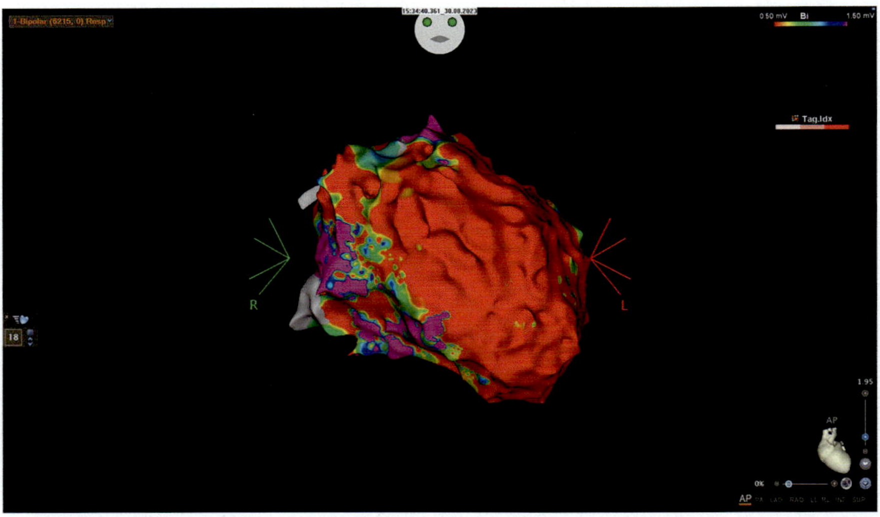

Fig. 11.11 Endocardial substrate mapping showing extensive scar area located on the anterior wall of LV from apical to basal segments and from lateral to septal respectively (red area)

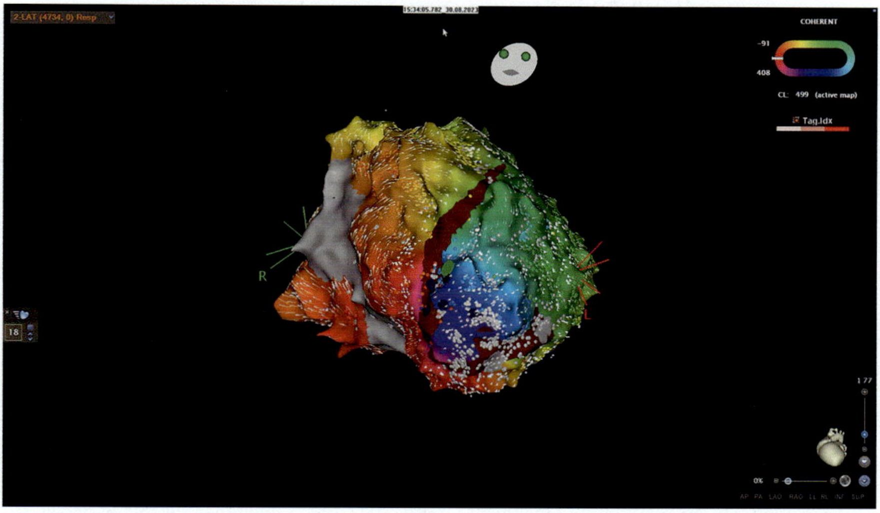

Fig. 11.12 Activation mapping during the clinical VT showing a zone of very slow conduction (brown area) corresponding to the critical isthmus of the clinical VT

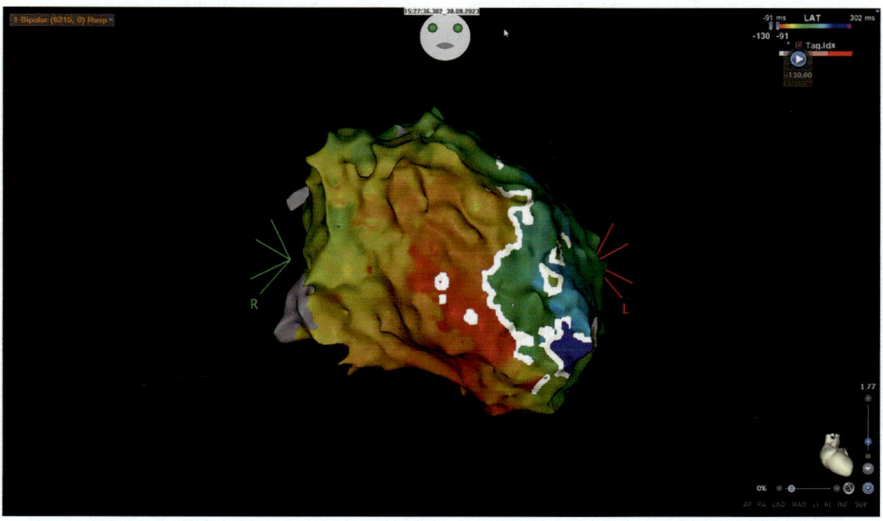

Fig. 11.13 Propagation mapping showing a reentry mechanism around the LV apex—early meets late corresponding to the critical isthmus depicted in Fig. 11.10

Summary

Management of patients with HF and VTs is a multidisciplinary process.

Critical parts of acute management include: rhythm stabilization focused on trigger identification and therapy, pharmacological and device therapy optimization, exact diagnosis of underlying structural heart disease in cases with unclear etiology and early referral for VT ablation in specialized centers.

References

1. McDonagh TA, Metra M, Adamo M, Gardner RS, Baumbach A, Böhm M, Burri H, Butler J, Čelutkienė J, Chioncel O, Cleland JGF, Coats AJS, Crespo-Leiro MG, Farmakis D, Gilard M, Heymans S, Hoes AW, Jaarsma T, Jankowska EA, Lainscak M, Lam CSP, Lyon AR, McMurray JJV, Mebazaa A, Mindham R, Muneretto C, Piepoli MF, Price S, Rosano GMC, Ruschitzka F, Skibelund AK, ESC Scientific Document Group. 2021 ESC Guidelines for the diagnosis and treatment of acute and chronic heart failure. Eur Heart J. 2021;42(36):3599–726.
2. Ghannam M, Siontis KC, Cochet H, Jais P, Juhoor M, Attili A, Sharaf-Dabbagh G, Latchamsetty R, Jongnarangsin K, Morady F, Bogun F. Risk stratification in patients with nonischemic cardiomyopathy and ventricular arrhythmias based on quantification of intramural delayed enhancement on cardiac magnetic resonance imaging. J Cardiovasc Electrophysiol. 2020;31(7):1762–9.
3. Zeppenfeld K, Tfelt-Hansen J, de Riva M, Winkel BG, Behr ER, Blom NA, Charron P, Corrado D, Dagres N, de Chillou C, Eckardt L, Friede T, Haugaa KH, Hocini M, Lambiase PD, Marijon E, Merino JL, Peichl P, Priori SG, Reichlin T, Schulz-Menger J, Sticherling C, Tzeis S, Verstrael A, Volterrani M, ESC Scientific Document Group. 2022 ESC Guidelines for the management of patients with ventricular arrhythmias and the prevention of sudden cardiac death. Eur Heart J. 2022;43(40):3997–4126.
4. Bardy GH, Lee KL, Mark DB, Poole JE, Packer DL, Boineau R, Domanski M, Troutman C, Anderson J, Johnson G, McNulty SE, Clapp-Channing N, Davidson-Ray LD, Fraulo ES, Fishbein DP, Luceri RM, Ip JH, Sudden Cardiac Death in Heart Failure Trial (SCD-HeFT) Investigators. Amiodarone or an implantable cardioverter-defibrillator for congestive heart failure. N Engl J Med. 2005;352(3):225–37.
5. Kadish A, Dyer A, Daubert JP, Rebecca Quigg NA, Estes M, Anderson KP, Calkins H, Hoch D, Goldberger J, Shalaby A, Sanders WE, Schaechter A, Levine JH, Defibrillators in Non-Ischemic Cardiomyopathy Treatment Evaluation (DEFINITE) Investigators. Prophylactic defibrillator implantation in patients with nonischemic dilated cardiomyopathy. N Engl J Med. 2004;350(21):2151–8.
6. Moss AJ, Wojciech Zareba W, Hall J, Klein H, Wilber DJ, Cannom DS, Daubert JP, Higgins SL, Brown MW, Andrews ML, Multicenter Automatic Defibrillator Implantation Trial II Investigators. Prophylactic implantation of a defibrillator in patients with myocardial infarction and reduced ejection fraction. N Engl J Med. 2002;346(12):877–83.
7. Gouda S, Abdelwahab A, Salem M, Hamid MA. Scar characteristics for prediction of ventricular arrhythmia in ischemic cardiomyopathy. Pacing Clin Electrophysiol. 2015;38(3):311–8.
8. Scott PA, Morgan JM, Carroll N, Murday DC, Roberts PR, Peebles CR, Harden SP, Curzen NP. The extent of left ventricular scar quantified by late gadolinium enhancement MRI is associated with spontaneous ventricular arrhythmias in patients with coronary artery disease and implantable cardioverter-defibrillators. Circ Arrhythm Electrophysiol. 2011;4(3):324–30.
9. Klem I, Klein M, Khan M, Yang EY, Nabi F, Ivanov A, Bhatti L, Hayes B, Graviss EA, Nguyen DT, Judd RM, Kim RJ, Heitner JF, Shah DJ. Relationship of LVEF and myocardial scar to

long-term mortality risk and mode of death in patients with nonischemic cardiomyopathy. Circulation. 2021;143(14):1343–58.
10. Greulich S, Seitz A, Herter D, Günther F, Probst S, Bekeredjian R, Gawaz M, Sechtem U, Mahrholdt H. Long-term risk of sudden cardiac death in hypertrophic cardiomyopathy: a cardiac magnetic resonance outcome study. Eur Heart J Cardiovasc Imaging. 2021;22(7):732–41.
11. Halliday BP, John Baksi A, Gulati A, Ali A, Newsome S, Izgi C, Arzanauskaite M, Lota A, Tayal U, Vassiliou VS, Gregson J, Alpendurada F, Frenneaux MP, Cook SA, Cleland JGF, Pennell DJ, Prasad SK. Outcome in dilated cardiomyopathy related to the extent, location, and pattern of late gadolinium enhancement. JACC Cardiovasc Imaging. 2019;12(8 Pt 2):1645–55.
12. Trayanova NA, Pashakhanloo F, Wu KC, Halperin HR. Imaging-based simulations for predicting sudden death and guiding ventricular tachycardia ablation. Circ Arrhythm Electrophysiol. 2017;10(7):e004743.
13. Zhang Y, Zhang K, Prakosa A, James C, Zimmerman SL, Carrick R, Sung E, Gasperetti A, Tichnell C, Murray B, Calkins H, Trayanova N. Predicting ventricular tachycardia circuits in patients with arrhythmogenic right ventricular cardiomyopathy using genotype-specific heart digital twins. medRxiv [Preprint], Aug 1:2023.05.31.2329058; 2023.
14. Zaman S, Taylor AJ, Stiles M, Chow C, Kovoor P. Programmed ventricular stimulation to risk stratify for early cardioverter-defibrillator implantation to prevent tachyarrhythmias following acute myocardial infarction (PROTECT-ICD). Heart Lung Circ. 2016;25(11):1055–62.
15. Gunda S, Ghannam M, Liang JJ, Attili A, Dabbagh GS, Cochet H, Lathkar-Pradhan S, Latchamsetty R, Jongnarangsin K, Morady F, Bogun F. The value of cardiac magnetic resonance imaging and programmed ventricular stimulation in patients with ventricular noncompaction and ventricular arrhythmias. J Cardiovasc Electrophysiol. 2021;32(3):745–54.
16. Sesselberg HW, Moss AJ, McNitt S, Zareba W, Daubert JP, Andrews ML, Hall WJ, McClinitic B, Huang DT, MADIT-II Research Group. Ventricular arrhythmia storms in postinfarction patients with implantable defibrillators for primary prevention indications: a MADIT-II substudy. Heart Rhythm. 2007;4(11):1395–402.
17. Sapp JL, Wells GA, Parkash R, Stevenson WG, Blier L, Sarrazin J-F, Thibault B, Rivard L, Gula L, Leong-Sit P, Essebag V, Nery PB, Tung SK, Raymond J-M, Sterns LD, Veenhuyzen GD, Healey JS, Redfearn D, Roux J-F, Tang ASL. Ventricular tachycardia ablation versus escalation of antiarrhythmic drugs. N Engl J Med. 2016;375(2):111–21.
18. Arenal Á, Ávila P, Jiménez-Candil J, Tercedor L, Calvo D, Arribas F, Fernández-Portales J, Merino JL, Hernández-Madrid A, Fernández-Avilés FJ, Berruezo A. Substrate ablation vs antiarrhythmic drug therapy for symptomatic ventricular tachycardia. J Am Coll Cardiol. 2022;79(15):1441–53.
19. Della Bella P, Baratto F, Vergara P, Bertocchi P, Santamaria M, Notarstefano P, Calò L, Orsida D, Tomasi L, Piacenti M, Sangiorgio S, Pentimalli F, Pruvot E, De Sousa J, Sacher F, Tritto M, Rebellato L, Deneke T, Romano SA, Nesti M, Gargaro A, Giacopelli D, Peretto G, Radinovic A. Does timing of ventricular tachycardia ablation affect prognosis in patients with an implantable cardioverter defibrillator? Results from the multicenter randomized PARTITA trial. Circulation. 2022;145(25):1829–38.
20. Ghannam M, Bogun F. Improving outcomes in ventricular tachycardia ablation using imaging to identify arrhythmic substrates. Card Electrophysiol Clin. 2022;14(4):609–20.
21. Carbucicchio C, Santamaria M, Trevisi N, Maccabelli G, Giraldi F, Fassini G, Riva S, Moltrasio M, Cireddu M, Veglia F, Bella PD. Catheter ablation for the treatment of electrical storm in patients with implantable cardioverter-defibrillators: short- and long-term outcomes in a prospective single-center study. Circulation. 2008;117(4):462–9.
22. Santangeli P, Eduardo Rame J, Birati EY, Marchlinski FE. Management of ventricular arrhythmias in patients with advanced heart failure. J Am Coll Cardiol. 2017;69(14):1842–60.
23. Silberbauer J, Oloriz T, Maccabelli G, Tsiachris D, Baratto F, Vergara P, Mizuno H, Bisceglia C, Marzi A, Sora N, Guarracini F, Radinovic A, Cireddu M, Sala S, Gulletta S, Paglino G, Mazzone P, Trevisi N, Bella PD. Noninducibility and late potential abolition: a novel combined prognostic procedural end point for catheter ablation of postinfarction ventricular tachycardia. Circ Arrhythm Electrophysiol. 2014;7(3):424–35.

Chapter 12
Approach to Atrial Fibrillation and Heart Failure

Ştefan Bogdan

Abstract Atrial fibrillation and heart failure are significant challenges in cardiovascular medicine, often coexisting and exacerbating each other's impact on patient health, leading to increased morbidity and mortality rates. Managing patients with both AF and HF is complicated because many medications effective for AF are not suitable when HF is present, especially in cases of HF with reduced ejection fraction. However, recent research supports the use of catheter ablation in patients with both conditions.

AF is the prevailing sustained cardiac arrhythmia in adults and is becoming more prevalent due to improved survival rates in cardiovascular disease and an aging population. It occurs in approximately 25% of HF cases. Despite extensive research, the most effective long-term strategies for managing HF and AF together remain unclear. Treatment for AF in HF patients is intricate and may improve over time with advancements in catheter-based techniques or HF medications. Current literature emphasizes the negative impact of AF on left-ventricular function and the advantages of a rhythm-controlled approach. Clinical trials in patients with AF and HF demonstrate that rhythm control through catheter ablation, specifically pulmonary vein isolation, can enhance symptoms, quality of life, and left-ventricular ejection fraction (LVEF). Increasing evidence indicates improvements in critical outcomes such as mortality and HF hospitalization with rhythm control, especially when applied early and through pulmonary vein isolation. However, catheter ablation should be used selectively, considering the patient's comorbidities and risk factors.

If sinus rhytm cannot be restored and AF becomes permanent, discussing the option of AV-node ablation and CRT implantation with the patient in a timely manner is essential. Future research efforts should focus on high-power short-duration ablation, pulsed field ablation, and hybrid/convergent AF ablation strategies for individuals with AF and HF.

Ş. Bogdan (✉)
Cardiology Department—Elias University Emergency Hospital, "Carol Davila" University of Medicine and Pharmacy, Bucharest, Romania

M. Dorobanţu et al. (eds.), *Current Approach to Heart Failure*,
https://doi.org/10.1007/978-3-031-96562-3_12

Keywords Atrial fibrillation · Heart failure · Rate control · Rhythm control · Catheter ablation · PVI · AV-node ablation

Introduction

Atrial fibrillation (AF) and heart failure (HF) represent two major epidemics in the field of cardiovascular medicine, often coexisting and mutually influencing each other's progression, resulting in heightened morbidity and mortality rates. The management of patients experiencing both AF and HF poses a significant challenge. Many medications effective for AF in the absence of HF become contraindicated when HF is present, particularly in cases of HF with reduced ejection fraction. However, recent years have seen a rise in data supporting the use of catheter ablation in patients with both AF and HF.

Globally, AF stands as the most prevalent cardiac arrhythmia, significantly impacting public health and healthcare economies. Treatment for AF adopts a multidisciplinary approach, focusing on stroke prevention and symptom alleviation. Currently, two primary therapeutic strategies are employed: rhythm control, aiming to maintain sinus rhythm, and rate control, targeting the reduction of ventricular rate. Subsequent advancements, especially the routine use of catheter-based pulmonary vein isolation (PVI) in symptomatic AF patients, have significantly enhanced the safety and efficacy of rhythm-control strategies. Unlike earlier studies, recent evidence suggests that rhythm control, particularly through catheter ablation, leads to improved outcomes, especially in HF patients.

The present review explores the physiological connection between heart failure and atrial fibrillation, pharmacological methods for managing heart rate and rhythm including recent developments in catheter ablation techniques and the optimization of cardiac resynchronization therapy.

Epidemiology of Atrial Fibrillation in Heart Failure

Atrial fibrillation (AF) is the predominant sustained cardiac arrhythmia in adults and presents a growing health challenge due to enhanced survival rates in cardiovascular disease and aging of population. AF is the most prevalent sustained arrhythmia in HF, occurring in approximately 25% of cases [1]. Despite extensive research on HF and AF, the most effective long-term strategies remain unclear. The widely accepted concept is that AF can lead to HF, and vice versa, due to shared pathophysiological mechanisms and risk factors. This dual affliction amplifies the risk of stroke, dementia, HF-related hospitalizations, and all-cause mortality. AF and HF share common risk factors like hypertension, obesity, diabetes mellitus, and ischemic heart disease [2]. Atrial cardiomyopathy can develop due to structural, architectural, contractile, and electrophysiological changes in the atria, driven by these comorbidities and AF itself. Early intervention is vital to impede the progression of both diseases and enhance prognosis [3]. Recent guidelines from the European Society of Cardiology stress the importance of treating underlying conditions comprehensively. Therefore, identifying and addressing risk factors are fundamental components of AF treatment, particularly in HF patients, where AF detrimentally impacts prognosis [2].

Pathophysiology (Relationship Between Atrial Fibrillation and Heart Failure)

AF can impact HF through various pathways. Loss of atrial contraction lowers cardiac output, and increased heart rate and shorter diastolic filling time further diminish it. Irregular ventricular response reduces output by 25%, as filling during long cycles fails to compensate for reduced filling in short cycles. AF with rapid ventricular response and irregularity can cause tachycardia-mediated reversible cardiomyopathy [4].

Conversely, HF can lead to AF through mechanisms like atrial pressure overload, altered myocardial conduction, maladaptive gene expression, and structural remodeling. HF elevates the risk of AF by acutely and chronically iBncreasing left atrial pressures. Elevated atrial pressure and distension cause scarring and fibrosis, leading to conduction abnormalities, decreased atrial conduction velocities, and anisotropy. In HF, atrial tissue stretching induces triggered activity, promoting AF [5].

Differences in atrial remodeling exist between HFrEF and HFpEF. HFrEF exhibits greater eccentric left atrial remodeling, while HFpEF shows increased left atrial stiffness [5]. AF is more likely to precede HF, especially in HFpEF, possibly due to similar underlying mechanisms like myocardial inflammation and fibrosis leading to atrial fibrosis. AF might be less tolerated in HFpEF patients, triggering clinical recognition. The temporal relationship of AF and HF affects patient outcomes, with higher mortality in HFrEF patients developing new AF compared to HFpEF patients [6].

These pathophysiological processes can also lead to sinus node dysfunction. AF can lead to HF decompensation or be the primary stimulus for HF development. Irregularity in atrial systole and variable diastole timing elevates left atrial pressures, reducing blood pressure, stroke volume, and cardiac output [4]. While atrial pathology often takes the spotlight in discussions about atrial fibrillation (AF), it could be better understood as a symptom of a systemic disease. If AF is driven by systemic inflammation, treatments targeting only the heart might not effectively address the high recurrence rate [7]. Inflammation serves as both a trigger for the initial development of AF and a factor that perpetuates the arrhythmia. Many comorbid conditions shared by heart failure (HF) and AF, such as hypertension, diabetes, obesity, and coronary artery disease, involve chronic inflammation leading to structural and electrical remodeling [8].

Oxidative stress and consequent myocardial injury are potential targets for therapeutic intervention in HF-AF treatment [9]. The SToP AF (Statin Therapy for the Prevention of Atrial Fibrillation) trial investigated the impact of atorvastatin on AF recurrence following cardioversion. Although certain inflammatory markers like C-reactive protein and interleukin-6 were significantly reduced, others like tumor necrosis factor-a and interleukin-1b remained unchanged. Statins, while affecting specific inflammatory markers, do not influence systemic oxidative stress that drives AF recurrence [10]. Despite observational studies suggesting reduced AF with statin therapy, meta-analysis of randomized data shows no benefit [11].

The synergy between HF and AF adversely affects quality of life, exercise capacity, and frequency of hospitalizations. AF can directly lead to the development of left ventricular (LV) dysfunction and HF through tachycardia-induced cardiomyopathy. This condition, diagnosed by excluding other causes, manifests as atrial or ventricular dysfunction due to persistent tachycardia, resolving with appropriate treatment for the underlying tachycardia. Although any tachyarrhythmia can cause this form of cardiomyopathy, AF is the most common trigger. Recent studies suggest that tachycardia-induced cardiomyopathy continues to negatively impact LV remodeling even after the normalization of ejection fraction (EF), prompting questions about whether patients with this condition harbor a subclinical cardiomyopathy that becomes evident under tachycardic conditions [12].

In lone AF, functional mitral regurgitation (MR), known as atrial functional MR (AFMR) gains attention as a significant cause of heart failure. Mitral annular dilatation due to left atrial (LA) dilatation stands out as an original cause of AFMR, although the exact cascade of etiologies remains unclear. In contrast, secondary MR (i.e., functional MR) typically results from papillary muscle displacement and mitral leaflet tethering-tenting due to LV systolic dysfunction and remodeling in patients with ischemic heart disease or dilated cardiomyopathy. The concept of AFMR differs substantially from that of traditional ventricular functional MR (VFMR). It's crucial to distinguish the original cause of atrial functional MR from ventricular functional MR. Atrial dilatation in patients with AF accounts for "atrial" functional MR, while LV dysfunction and/or dilatation in ischemic heart disease or dilated cardiomyopathy cause traditional "ventricular" functional MR. Nevertheless, a relationship exists between LV dilatation and worsening AFMR, as well as between LA dilatation and worsening VFMR. Ultimately, both LV and LA dilatation contribute to the worsening of both types of functional MR, despite their distinct initial causes [13].

HF-AF Subtypes and Impact of AF on Global Cardiac Function

HF-AF Subtypes

Up to now, the majority of research efforts have concentrated on atrial fibrillation (AF) occurring in the context of heart failure with reduced ejection fraction (HFrEF). However, it is widely acknowledged that heart failure with preserved ejection fraction (HFpEF) accounts for at least half of clinical heart failure cases. AF appears to be more common among individuals with higher ejection fraction (EF), although the rates of adverse events in patients with AF and heart failure are comparable across all HF classes. Similar risk factors, such as diabetes, obstructive sleep apnea, smoking, coronary artery disease, hypertension, and obesity, predispose individuals to AF in both HFpEF and HFrEF cases [14, 15].

The distribution of AF types (paroxysmal, persistent, and long-standing persistent) varies significantly based on the studied population. Long-standing persistent or permanent AF is the most frequently diagnosed type in general population studies, accounting for 40–50% of cases. Paroxysmal and persistent AF are distributed more evenly, each comprising 20–30% of cases. Recent analyses from studies like PARADIGM-HF and ATMOSPHERE have shown that 30% of patients exhibit paroxysmal AF. Persistent AF appears to be the predominant type encountered in both the general population and the HF-AF group. Due to the shared risk factors between AF and HF, distinguishing which condition occurs first, how one exacerbates the other, or whether they represent different expressions of the same underlying pathophysiology often proves challenging [16].

Impact of AF on Atrial Function

The influence of AF on atrial (LA) function has been extensively examined. Permanent AF results in intracellular oxidative stress, leading to calcium overload and initiation of the inflammation cascade. This process perpetuates the arrhythmia and remodels the LA, causing fibrosis. This continuous process is termed "atrial failure" in the literature [17]. It's crucial to note that atrial fibrosis detected by cardiac MRI significantly affects the success of rhythm-control strategies, particularly catheter ablation [18]. The DECAAF II trial, investigating the targeted ablation of fibrotic areas versus pulmonary vein isolation (PVI) alone, holds great anticipation as its outcomes might shape future therapeutic approaches [19].

Impact of AF on Left-Ventricular Function

Although the effects of AF on LA myocytes have been extensively studied, even on a cellular level, the impact of AF on ventricular myocardium remains inadequately understood. MR-guided studies have shed light on the adverse effects of AF on LV function [20]. These studies revealed that patients with AF scheduled for pulmonary vein isolation (PVI), regardless of preserved or impaired LV function, exhibited significantly longer T1 relaxation times compared to a healthy matched control group. Three to six months after catheter ablation and the restoration of stable sinus rhythm, the T1 time returned to normal values, indicating the potential for reversing LV remodeling by establishing a stable sinus rhythm. T1 relaxation time serves as an early marker for LV fibrosis, underscoring AF's detrimental effects on the LV [21]. Research by Soulat-Dufour et al. demonstrated that restoring sinus rhythm led to improvements in echocardiographic remodeling parameters, such as the index volume of both atria and the end-systolic right ventricular volume, as well as enhanced four-chamber function. Additionally, studies have shown that the positive impact of beta-blockers on mortality in HF patients diminishes when the patient is in AF rather than sinus rhythm, even if the AF is rate-controlled. This could be attributed to AF-induced remodeling directly counteracting the positive effects of beta-blockers [22].

General Management Approach

In individuals diagnosed with both atrial fibrillation (AF) and heart failure (HF), the primary approach involves optimizing HF treatment through recommended medical and device therapies, including implantable cardioverter-defibrillators with or without cardiac resynchronization therapy, based on guidelines. A key consideration is the presence of AF symptoms, especially if they persist despite adequate rate control. Identifying AF symptoms in HF patients can be challenging due to overlapping symptoms like breathlessness and reduced exercise capacity. Practically, assessing symptomatic AF in HF patients often involves comparing symptom improvement in normal sinus rhythm versus AF, which may necessitate attempting cardioversion and evaluating symptoms afterward. In some cases, a connection can be established where AF onset precedes HF worsening, suggesting a rhythm control approach.

Another crucial factor is evaluating the likelihood of achieving successful rhythm control with minimal risk to the patient. This assessment takes into account the patient's age, existing health conditions, kidney function, left atrial size, AF type and duration, New York Heart Association (NYHA) class, and ejection fraction. The third factor involves shared decision-making with the patient, which entails a comprehensive discussion about the advantages and disadvantages of various management options. Patients need to be informed that multiple AF ablation procedures might be necessary for about one-third of HF patients undergoing ablation.

Additionally, when considering antiarrhythmic medications, discussions should encompass both short- and long-term side effects of these drugs.

Prevention of Thromboembolism

The coexistence of heart failure (HF) and atrial fibrillation (AF) significantly elevates the risk of stroke, irrespective of HF subtype [23]. Recently, the options for oral anticoagulation (OAC) to prevent stroke have expanded, including warfarin and four approved non-vitamin K antagonist oral anticoagulants (NOACs). NOACs are generally preferred due to their favorable bleeding profile and ease of use, especially for patients already taking multiple medications, as they do not require frequent monitoring. The choice of NOAC depends on individual patient factors such as concurrent medications, kidney function, and the familiarity of the prescribing physician. Notably, the specific subtype of heart failure does not dictate the recommended type of oral anticoagulant [23].

Research has established HF as an independent risk factor for stroke in AF, and the combination of HF and AF intensifies the severity of strokes and overall mortality. Although strokes in HF are commonly associated with AF, there is evidence indicating that HF alone, even without AF, increases the risk of abnormal blood clot formation. Recent meta-analyses comparing outcomes between patients with AF and reduced ejection fraction (HFrEF) versus preserved ejection fraction (HFpEF) revealed no significant differences in stroke risk between the two subtypes. These findings underscore that the presence of heart failure, rather than its subtype, primarily influences the risk of stroke, a conclusion supported by real-world observational data [23].

Additionally, meta-analyses of key randomized trials have affirmed the effectiveness of NOACs in HF subgroups, demonstrating a significant reduction in the risk of stroke with single/high-dose NOAC regimens compared to warfarin. Low-dose NOACs showed similar efficacy in preventing stroke as warfarin, with a nonsignificant decrease in major bleeding risk [24]. Guidelines recommend oral anticoagulation for patients with both AF and HF, acknowledging the synergistic adverse effects of these conditions [2].

Considering that most atrial fibrillation (AF)-related blood clots in the left atrium (LA) are found in the LA appendage (LAA), closing off the LAA can be a potential strategy for preventing strokes in AF patients who cannot undergo long-term anticoagulant treatment, for instance, due to conditions like intracranial bleeding without a reversible cause. This approach is now a class IIb recommendation with a level B evidence in current atrial fibrillation guidelines [2]. The implantation of LAA closure (LAAC) devices in individuals with non-valvular AF and congestive heart failure (CHF) is safe. It's important to note that the higher mortality rate observed in patients with CHF, compared to those without, in long-term follow-ups is primarily due to the additional health issues associated with CHF [25].

However, it's worth mentioning that LAA occlusion can lead to an increase in heart failure (HF) events, even after a successful procedure. Therefore, it is crucial to evaluate the risk of developing HF in patients who have undergone LAAO. Factors such as a patient's history of HF, LA function, and diastolic function should be carefully taken into account before considering LAAO [26].

Acute Management of Atrial Fibrillation in Acute Heart Failure

The presence of AF or HF often influences the occurrence of the other, with acute HF posing the highest risk for the development of AF. Additionally, AF can worsen left ventricular (LV) dysfunction, leading to AF-induced cardiomyopathy. Around 35% of AHF patients also have AF [2].

There are four primary scenarios of AF in AHF:

1. AF is the primary cause of AHF, marked by a rapid ventricular rate of 130–160 bpm and typically discovered for the first time. Episodes of AF with rapid ventricular response may lead to AHF presentation.
2. AF results from AHF, with a rapid ventricular rate, and AHF treatment is paramount.
3. AF being an incidental finding in AHF; another factor triggers AHF, such as a myocardial infarction.
4. The initial assessment does not allow clear classification of AF's role in AHF's pathophysiology. Additional triggers like myocardial infarction and systemic infection need active investigation [27].

Studies indicate that new-onset AF or HF significantly worsens prognosis compared to longstanding disease. A higher admission heart rate (HR) is independently linked to worse outcomes in HF patients, regardless of rhythm. In the Beta-blocker Evaluation of Survival Trial (BEST), new-onset AF in patients with HFrEF led to a twofold increase in mortality and a 4.5-fold increase in all-cause or HF-related hospitalizations compared to those without AF [28]. Another study found that AF on admission, especially if newly diagnosed, independently correlated with adverse hospital outcomes and longer stays. Therefore, in AHF patients, AF is associated with a poorer prognosis [29].

It's crucial to identify and rectify all reversible causes of AF and AHF whenever feasible. Detecting and treating acute coronary syndrome (ACS) is essential. Potential reversible causes of advanced AHF include severe valve stenosis or regurgitation, pericardial disease, reversible cardiomyopathy, and contributing factors like severe anemia, thyroid issues, and sleep apnea. Many of these conditions can both trigger and worsen AF. Identifying the underlying causes typically involves a comprehensive medical history, physical examination, electrocardiography (ECG), basic laboratory tests, and echocardiography [27].

Improving Pre-hospital Outcomes

Acute heart failure (AHF) is a complex syndrome that requires collaboration among cardiologists, emergency physicians, intensivists, and other healthcare providers for prompt patient care. In the pre-hospital setting, it is crucial to swiftly transfer AHF patients with atrial fibrillation (AF) to the nearest hospital, preferably one equipped with a cardiology department and/or coronary care unit. Within minutes of medical contact, non-invasive monitoring, including pulse oximetry, arterial blood pressure, respiratory rate, and continuous ECG, should be initiated. Immediate attention is necessary if hemodynamic instability is detected, requiring urgent cardioversion. Medical treatment should be initiated based on arterial blood pressure and the degree of congestion. Notably, for patients with AHF and AF, we recommend intravenous (IV) administration of amiodarone to rapidly control the ventricular rate. If amiodarone alone does not achieve rate control, IV digoxin could be considered as an option. However, it is important to note that cardiac glycosides have limited heart rate-reducing effects during AF in AHF, where sympathetic nerve activity is generally heightened. Upon arrival at the emergency department or coronary care unit, immediate clinical examination, further investigations, and treatment should be initiated [30].

Rate Control in AHF

Before initiating rate control, it is essential to evaluate and address underlying causes of elevated heart rate, such as ischemia, infection, anemia, and pulmonary embolism. The choice of drug and target heart rate depends on patient characteristics, symptoms, left ventricular function, and hemodynamics. For AHF patients, IV amiodarone could be a suitable option. If amiodarone fails to achieve rate control, digitalis (digoxin) may be added for acute ventricular rate control, although there is controversy surrounding digoxin use in patients with AF or HF [2]. Meta-analyses and retrospective analyses have shown that digoxin use in AF patients is associated with an increased risk of mortality, [31, 32] although neutral effects have also been reported [33]. Beta-blockers are usually contraindicated in acute situations, and calcium channel blockers are always contraindicated. The optimal target heart rate for AHF patients has not been extensively studied but is generally maintained at <100 bpm based on hemodynamic and symptomatic improvement. Urgent cardioversion is appropriate for unstable patients [34].

Rhythm Control in AHF

In AF associated with AHF, rhythm control might be the preferred approach. Before considering rhythm control, underlying causes of AHF and AF must be identified and treated. Rate control should be initiated first, and urgent cardioversion could be used for unstable patients if necessary [2]. If rhythm control becomes necessary, all antiarrhythmic drugs (AADs) are contraindicated except for amiodarone. Amiodarone's rhythm-converting effect is slower compared to electrical cardioversion. In the short term, electrical cardioversion restores sinus rhythm more rapidly and effectively, leading to a shorter length of stay in the emergency department compared to pharmacological cardioversion with amiodarone. However, pharmacological cardioversion does not require sedation and also slows heart rate, potentially contributing to improved hemodynamics [35].

The effectiveness of non-antiarrhythmic drugs in acute heart failure (AHF) patients remains unknown, necessitating the extrapolation of data from chronic heart failure (HF) and HFpEF patients. Studies involving chronic HF patients and those with hypertensive LV hypertrophy suggest that angiotensin-converting enzyme inhibitors (ACEIs) or angiotensin receptor blockers (ARBs) may decrease the risk of new-onset AF. Neprilysin inhibition did not show additional benefits. In individuals with reduced ejection fraction (HFrEF) and sinus rhythm, beta-blockers (BBs) were found to reduce the occurrence of new-onset AF compared to placebo and decrease symptomatic AF recurrences after cardioversion [36]. The EMPHASIS-HF study indicated a lowered incidence of new-onset AF with eplerenone use. However, there isn't enough data to support widespread use of mineralocorticoid receptor antagonists (MRAs) solely for AF prevention [37].

Rate Control: Pharmacological and Interventional Treatments

Pharmacologic management of heart rate in patients with atrial fibrillation involves the use of various medications to achieve rate control. Options for atrioventricular (AV) nodal blockers include beta blockers, nondihydropyridine calcium channel blockers (such as diltiazem and verapamil), and cardiac glycosides (like digoxin). However, nondihydropyridine calcium channel blockers are not suitable for patients with reduced ejection fraction due to increased mortality rates [2]. Therefore, beta blockers are considered the primary choice for rate control in patients with heart failure and reduced ejection fraction (HFrEF) [38, 39]. Digoxin, while an option, is not as effective as beta blockers or calcium channel blockers and is not recommended as a first-line treatment. It primarily slows ventricular rate by inhibiting AV nodal conduction through vagotonic effects, making it more effective at rest and less so during exercise when sympathetic tone is high.

Studies have shown that beta blockers significantly reduce all-cause mortality in patients with sinus rhythm but not necessarily in those with atrial fibrillation (AF).

However, specific trials like AF-CHF have indicated that beta blockers are associated with lower mortality in patients with HFrEF and AF [40]. The optimal target heart rate for patients with AF and heart failure remains uncertain. While some studies suggest strict rate control has no impact on outcomes, guidelines from organizations like the American College of Cardiology and American Heart Association recommend a target ventricular rate of 80–90 bpm at rest and 110–130 bpm with moderate exercise [41]. The European Society of Cardiology, on the other hand, suggests lenient rate control as an acceptable initial approach, regardless of heart failure status [2]. Stricter rate control is only reserved for specific cases like tachycardia-induced cardiomyopathy or when symptomatic patients require higher biventricular pacing percentages. Individualized decisions on rate control targets should be made based on patients' symptoms, suspicion of tachycardia-mediated cardiomyopathy, and activity levels, with the use of ambulatory monitors like Holter monitors to assess the level of rate control [42].

Atrioventricular Node Ablation for Definitive Rate Control

At the opposite end of the treatment spectrum from catheter ablation for rhythm control is the strategy known as "ablate and pace." This approach involves atrioventricular (AV) node ablation accompanied by permanent pacemaker placement and is considered for patients with permanent atrial fibrillation (AF) and systolic dysfunction, experiencing rapid ventricular rates despite medical interventions. Unfortunately, this strategy results in permanent reliance on a pacemaker. AV node ablation should be approached cautiously and only considered if other methods of rate and rhythm control have proven ineffective [2]. This strategy, involving AV node ablation with right ventricular pacing, has been employed for many years and is a viable option when pharmacological treatments are insufficient or not tolerated.

In a comprehensive analysis involving 1181 patients assessing outcomes and survival following AV node ablation and right ventricular pacing in medically refractory AF, significant enhancements were observed in various aspects, including quality of life, exercise capacity, and healthcare utilization [43]. Research such as the APAF-CRT trial has demonstrated that combining cardiac resynchronization therapy (CRT) with AV node ablation outperforms pharmacological rate control in patients with symptomatic permanent AF and narrow QRS complexes [44].

According to the 2019 American College of Cardiology Foundation/American Heart Association/Heart Rhythm Society guidelines, CRT can be advantageous for patients with heart failure with reduced ejection fraction (HFrEF) and left ventricular ejection fraction (LVEF) of 35% or lower who are on guideline-directed medical therapy and undergoing AV node ablation, as they require 100% ventricular pacing [40]. For patients with HFrEF and LVEF between 36% and 50% undergoing AV node ablation, considering biventricular pacing or conduction system pacing is deemed reasonable [45].

Studies such as the BLOCK HF trial have indicated improved outcomes in patients with AV block and LVEF less than 50% undergoing biventricular pacing compared to right ventricular-only pacing. Additionally, a systematic review of non-randomized data revealed that AV node ablation in patients with CRT and AF led to reduced all-cause mortality, cardiovascular mortality, and enhanced New York Heart Association functional class compared to medical therapy [46]. Furthermore, a randomized trial demonstrated CRT's superiority over right apical pacing in reducing heart failure events in patients with permanent AF undergoing AV nodal ablation [47].

However, it's important to note that the AV node ablation and pacing strategy does not restore normal sinus rhythm. Studies such as the PABA-CHF trial emphasize the benefits of restoring sinus rhythm, especially when comparing the ablate-and-pace approach to catheter ablation. In the PABA-CHF trial, pulmonary vein isolation was found to be superior to AV node ablation with biventricular pacing in improving ejection fraction, exercise capacity, and patient-reported quality of life [48]. Nevertheless, atrioventricular node ablation with pacemaker placement remains a crucial option for certain patients with permanent AF complicated by rapid ventricular conduction that does not respond to medical therapies.

Conduction system pacing (CSP), utilizing His bundle pacing (HBP) or left bundle branch area pacing (LBBAP), has emerged as an alternative to traditional pacing methods like right ventricular pacing (RVP) or biventricular pacing. HBP offers simultaneous stimulation of both His bundle branches, creating a physiological contraction pattern and ensuring intra and interventricular synchrony. However, its widespread use is limited by technical challenges such as a higher capture threshold, leading to decreased pacemaker battery life, and a significant threshold increase during follow-up, potentially resulting in loss of capture in certain cases.

LBBAP, which targets the left branch of the His bundle, has emerged as a promising alternative for physiological pacing. Compared to RVP pacing, LBBAP is linked to reduced long-term heart failure hospitalizations and mortality rates [49]. Additionally, LBBAP offers more favorable pacing parameters, including lower and more stable capture thresholds. Notably, among patients undergoing subsequent atrioventricular nodal ablation (AVNA), LBBAP demonstrates higher success rates and a reduced incidence of acute and chronic lead-related complications when compared to HBP [50].

At the moment, there is a lack of studies comparing the clinical outcomes of conventional pacing (CP) versus CSP in this context. Currently, the PACE-FIB trial aims to evaluate the long-term patient prognosis of heart rhythm regularization through CSP (specifically LBBAP) and AVN ablation in this patient population, comparing it with optimal pharmacological heart rate control [51].

Rhythm Control: Pharmacological and Interventional Treatment

For a considerable time, it was widely believed, following the AFFIRM trial, that controlling heart rate was as effective as maintaining normal heart rhythm in patients with heart failure (HF). However, recent studies have challenged this notion, leading to a Class I recommendation for atrial fibrillation (AF) ablation in a majority of HF patients in the recent ESC-AF guidelines [2].

One of the studies that significantly influenced the guidelines was the CASTLE-AF trial. In this prospective study, 363 patients with AF and a left-ventricular ejection fraction (LVEF) of ≤35% were randomized into two groups: an interventional arm receiving rhythm control through catheter ablation and a conservative treatment arm using antiarrhythmic drugs. The primary endpoint was a combination of death and hospitalization. During the follow-up period, this endpoint occurred in 51 patients (28.5%) in the interventional arm. In contrast, almost twice as many patients (44.6%) in the conservative arm reached the endpoint. Catheter ablation reduced the absolute risk by 16.1%. Additionally, there was an improvement in LVEF in the ablation group, whereas LVEF remained almost unchanged in the control group. Notably, this effect was not significant in the subgroup of patients with an LVEF ≤ 25%, a population for which the study was not powered [52].

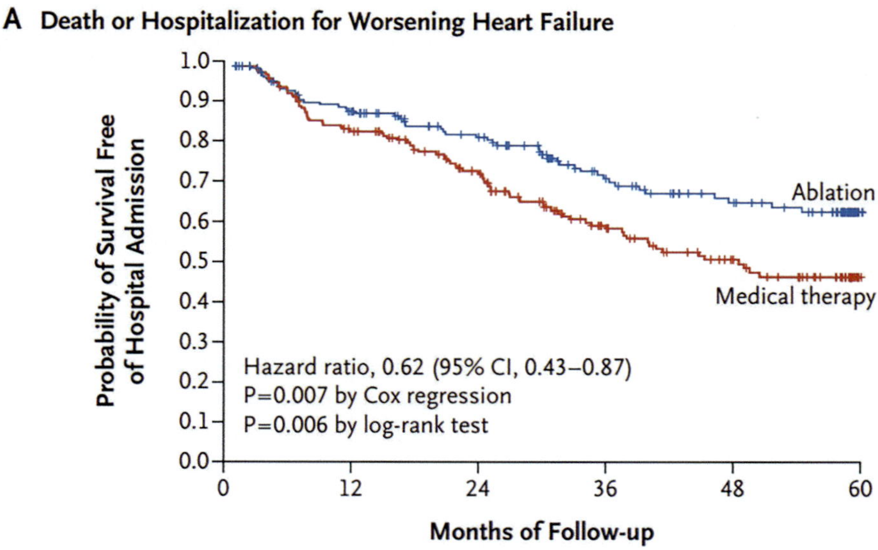

No. at Risk

	0	12	24	36	48	60
Ablation	179	141	114	76	58	22
Medical therapy	184	145	111	70	48	12

Fig. 12.1 The primary outcome in subgroups of interest in CASTLE-AF [52]

More recently, in the CASTLE-HTx trial, patients diagnosed with atrial fibrillation and advanced heart failure, the use of catheter ablation in conjunction with guideline-recommended medical treatment, compared to using medical therapy alone, was linked to a reduced probability of experiencing a combination of outcomes, including all-cause mortality, the need for a left ventricular assist device implantation, or an urgent heart transplantation [53] (Fig. 12.1).

The CAMERA-MRI study, published in 2017, reached a similar outcome. In this research, 66 patients with atrial fibrillation (AF) and a left-ventricular ejection fraction (LVEF) of ≤35% were randomly assigned to either catheter ablation or rate control. Over a 6-month follow-up period, the ablation group showed a significant enhancement in LVEF compared to patients with rate-controlled AF [54]. After 4 years, the LVEF was further boosted by, in contrast to the LVEF in the conventional treatment group [55].

Additionally, a sub-study from the CABANA trial demonstrated a notable decrease in all-cause mortality and a reduction in atrial fibrillation (AF) burden within the subgroup of patients with heart failure (HF) and AF. However, it's essential to consider the study design and implementation limitations when interpreting the results of the CABANA trial [56].

The EAST-AFNET 4 trial, published in 2021, explored the most effective approach for recently diagnosed atrial fibrillation (AF) patients. This prospective, randomized study involved a total of 2789 individuals diagnosed with AF within the past 12 months, conducted between 2011 and 2016. Participants were evenly divided into two groups: rate control (control arm) or rhythm control (therapy arm) in a 1:1 ratio. The primary endpoint included a combination of cardiovascular death, stroke, hospitalization for heart failure, or acute coronary syndrome. After a median follow-up period of 5.1 years, the study was halted after the third interim analysis due to a significant difference favoring the therapy arm. Rhythm control therapy lowered the risk of reaching the primary endpoint by 22%. Notably, amiodarone usage was relatively low (not exceeding 20%), with preference given to catheter ablation, indicating that the positive impact of rhythm maintenance became evident with the introduction of catheter ablation [57]. This mortality benefit from a rhythm-control-based strategy was further confirmed in the heart failure subgroup, comprising 798 patients [58] (Fig. 12.2).

In contrast to the CASTLE-AF and CAMERA-MRI trials, which compared catheter ablation with antiarrhythmic drug therapy, the recently published RAFT trial investigated catheter ablation versus a rate-control strategy. Conducted between 2011 and 2018, the study randomized 411 patients into these therapy arms. The primary outcome, a composite of all-cause mortality and heart failure events, was followed for a minimum of 2 years. Although catheter ablation significantly improved left ventricular ejection fraction (LVEF), the 6-min walk distance, and quality of life, the trial was prematurely halted due to futility as the primary endpoint did not reach significance. At that point, the primary endpoint occurred in 23.4% patients in the ablation-based rhythm-control group compared to 32.5% patients in the rate-control group. Despite the study's early termination, it remains a topic of scientific discussion, especially due to the borderline significance of the

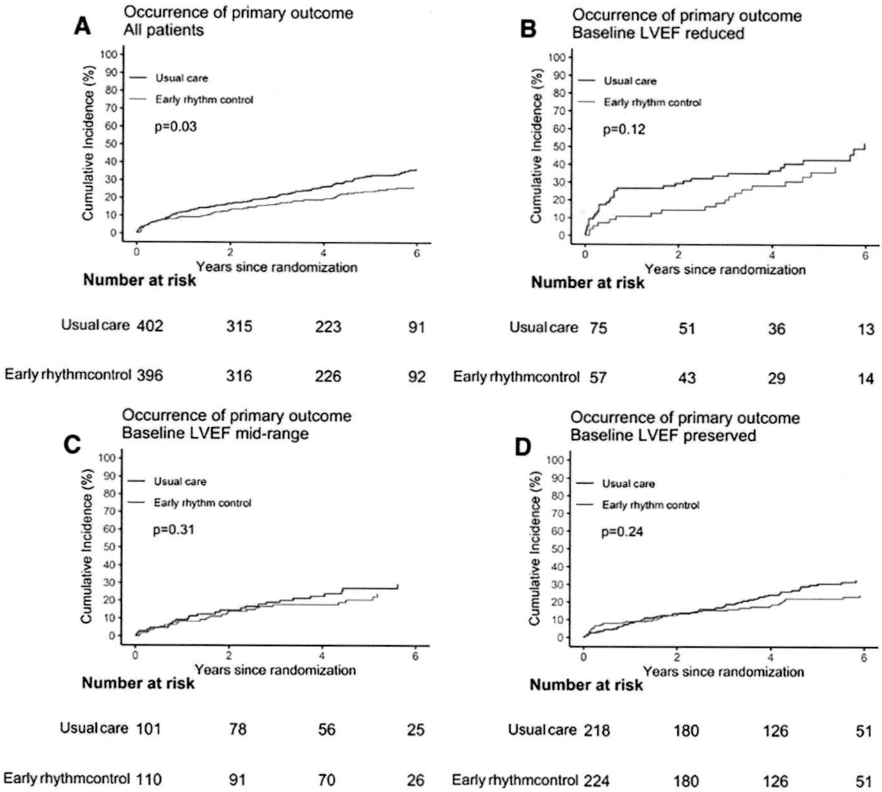

Fig. 12.2 Primary outcome in EAST-AFNET4 patients with heart failure by randomized groups. Aalen-Johansen cumulative-incidence curves for the effects of early rhythm control on the primary outcome. Primary outcome is defined as a composite of death from cardiovascular causes, stroke, or hospitalization with worsening of heart failure or acute coronary syndrome. (**a**) All patients with heart failure. (**b**) Heart failure with reduced ejection fraction. (**c**) Heart failure with midrange ejection fraction. (**d**) Heart failure with preserved ejection fraction. EAST-AFNET4 indicates Early Treatment of Atrial Fibrillation for Stroke Prevention Trial; and LVEF, left ventricular ejection fraction [57]

primary endpoint and the lower-than-expected recruitment rate. One possible explanation is that 19% of patients with an LVEF $\geq$ 45% were carriers of cardiac resynchronization therapy (CRT), and 60 patients in the rate-control group received atrioventricular (AV) node ablation and possibly CRT implantation (not reported) during the treatment [59]. This is noteworthy as demonstrated in the APAF-CRT trial, where AV-node ablation and CRT implantation for rate control proved superior to conventional drug-based rate control in patients with heart failure and permanent AF. In this study, involving 133 patients, the trial was prematurely terminated due to efficacy after a median follow-up of 29 months [44].

Ablation Strategy

Pulmonary vein isolation (PVI) stands as the fundamental approach for catheter ablation in atrial fibrillation (AF), given that no additional ablation techniques have demonstrated significant benefits thus far. Moreover, in most trials, additional ablation methods such as posterior wall isolation, linear lines, or complex fractionated atrial electrograms ablation were left to the operator's discretion and were not systematically studied [60].

Presently, there are ongoing trials involving HF patients, employing a PVI-only approach using single-shot devices. For instance, the Cryoballoon Ablation vs Medical Therapy in Patients With Heart Failure and Atrial Fibrillation (RACE-8-HF) and the Ablation of Atrial Fibrillation in Heart Failure Patients (CONTRA-HF) both utilize cryoballoon ablation for PVI, in comparison to nonspecific guideline-directed medical therapy.

High-power short-duration ablation, a technique involving brief applications at higher wattage, significantly reduces procedure time. This approach may enhance the feasibility of extensive left atrial ablations, addressing advanced substrate in HF patients. While long-term follow-up appears promising, these methods require evaluation in large randomized HF trials [61]. Additionally, there are various surgical AF ablation techniques, such as thoracoscopic (minimally invasive using radiofrequency clamps on the pulmonary veins), convergent (pericardioscopic epicardial posterior wall isolation), and hybrid ablation (a combination of endocardial and epicardial ablation). However, the complications associated with these invasive procedures must be carefully considered [62]. Clearly, future research efforts should focus on high-power short-duration ablation, pulsed field ablation, and hybrid/convergent AF ablation strategies for individuals with AF and HF.

Patient Selection

Patient selection criteria for catheter ablation involve addressing underlying cardiovascular conditions and managing risk factors. Eligibility for catheter ablation depends on the etiology and severity of heart failure (HF). Currently, a limited number of HF patients are referred for catheter ablation due to concerns about higher complication rates and unsatisfactory ablation outcomes. Recent trials, however, indicate that AF ablation can be conducted safely, leading to long-term prognosis improvement, particularly in patients with tachycardiomyopathy without other detectable heart disease.

Nevertheless, specific patient characteristics can guide the decision regarding who would benefit from catheter ablation. A post-hoc analysis of CASTLE-AF suggests that patients with NYHA I/II classification and non-ischaemic HF etiology derive the most benefit, indicating that early intervention might be advantageous [63]. When considering the selection of patients likely to benefit the most, the

Table 12.1 Analysis of rate versus rhythm control trials in atrial fibrillation (AF) treatment within the context of heart failure (HF) using drug therapy (no ablation therapy)

Study	No of patients	Mean age	Women	Persistent AF	Inclusion criteria	Endpoint	Comparison	Comorbidity treatment	Follow-up (years)	Outcome
DIAMOND-CHF	1518	70	26.6%	100%	NYHA III/IV and LVEF < 35%	Mortality	Dofetilide versus placebo	Not specified	1.5	No effect on mortality (p = ns)
RACE-HF	261	69	35%	100%	NYHA II/III	Composite of mortality and hospitalisation	Rate versus rhythm	Not specified	2.3	Rate control is not inferior to rhythm control (p = ns)
AFFIRM-HF	788	N/A	25%	Recurrent AF	LVEF < 50%	ACM	Rate versus rhythm	Not specified	3.5	No effect on mortality (p = ns)
AF-CHF	1376	67	18%	68.5%	LVEF < 35%	Cardiovascular death	Rate versus rhythm	Not specified	3.1	No effect on mortality (p = ns)
CAFÉ-II	61	72	16%	100%	NYHA ≥ II and systolic dysfunction	QOL	Rate versus rhythm	Not specified	1.0	Sinus rhythm may improve QOL (p = 0.019) and LV function (p = 0.014)

Table 12.2 Summary of ablation studies for treating atrial fibrillation in patients with heart failure

Study	No of patients	Mean age	Women	Inclusion criteria	Endpoint	Comparison	PVI	Comorbidity treatment	Follow-up (years)	Outcome
PABA-CHF	81	60	8%	NYHA III/IV and LVEF < 40%	Composite of QOL, LVEF, 6-MWT	PVI versus AVN ablation	51%	Not specified	0.5	PVI was superior ($p < 0.001$)
MacDonald et al	41	63	22%	NYHA II (11%)/III (89%) and LVEF < 35%	Change in LVEF	PVI versus rate control (digoxin)	54%	Not specified	0.5 or 0.75	PVI did not improve LVEF (p = ns)
ARC-HF	52	63	13%	NYHA II–IV and LVEF < 35%	12-month change in peak oxygen consumption	PVI versus rate control	50%	Not specified	1.0	PVI was superior ($p = 0.018$)
CAMTAF	50	57	4%	NYHA II (46%)/III (54%) and LVEF < 50%	Difference in LVEF	PVI versus rate control	52%	Not specified	1.0	PVI was superior ($p = 0.015$)
AATAC	203	61	26%	NYHA II–IV and LVEF < 40%	Recurrence of AF	PVI versus amiodarone	50%	Not specified	2.0	PVI was superior ($p < 0.0001$)
CAMERA-MRI	68	61	9%	LVEF < 45%	Change in LVEF	PVI versus rate control	50%	Not specified	0.5	PVI was superior ($p < 0.0001$)
CASTLE-AF	363	64	14%	NYHA I–IV (11%, 58%, 27%, 1%) and LVEF < 35%	Composite of ACM of HF hospitalisation	PVI versus medical therapy (rhythm or rate control)	49%	Not specified	3.1	PVI was superior ($p = 0.007$)
CABANA-HF (post-hoc)	778	68	44%	NYHA II–IV (76%, 23%, 1%)	Composite of ACM, stroke, bleeding, CA	PVI versus medical therapy (rhythm or rate control)	49%	Not specified	4.0	PVI was superior (p = significant)

RACE 3	245	64	21%	HFrEF = NYHA I–III and LVEF < 45%. HFpEF = NYHA II–III and LVEF>45%	Sinus rhythm on 7-day Holter	Targeted therapy of underlying conditions versus conventional(causal treatment of AF and HF + rhythm control)	N/A	Targeted therapy	1.0	Targeted therapy was superior (p = 0.042) at 1 year; no differences at 5 years
EAST-AFNET 4	2789	70	46%	Stable heart failure (n = 798 (28.6%))	Composite of death from CV causes, stroke, hospitalisation for HF or ACS	Early rhythm control or usual care (initial rate control, in case of symptoms mitigation to rhythm control)	13%	According to guidelines	5.1	Early rhythm control was superior (p = 0.005)
CASTLE HTx	194	62	12%	End-stage heart failure and symptomatic AFib: stable NYHA II–IV, LVEF < 35%	Composite of death from any cause, implantation of a left ventricular assist device, or urgent heart transplantation	Catheter ablation with GDMT vs. GDMT alone	84%	GDMT	1.5	Catheter ablation was superior (HR 0.24; P < 0.001)

GDMT guidelines-directed medical therapy

EAST-AFNET 4 trial emphasizes the importance of early AF cases [58]. Additionally, atrial enlargement, a surrogate marker for atrial cardiomyopathy and advanced disease, makes patients with enlarged atria or fibrosis on CMR less suitable candidates for catheter ablation [56]. In situations where uncertainty exists about whether patients would benefit from returning to sinus rhythm, a trial of cardioversion, often coupled with a short period of amiodarone use, can be attempted to assess whether sinus rhythm restoration leads to improvements in functional class and LVEF (Tables 12.1 and 12.2).

References

1. Lardizabal JA, Deedwania PC. Atrial fibrillation in heart failure. Med Clin North Am. 2012;96(5):987–1000.
2. Hindricks G, Potpara T, Kirchhof P, Kühne M, Ahlsson A, Balsam P, et al. 2020 ESC Guidelines for the diagnosis and management of atrial fibrillation developed in collaboration with the European Association for Cardio-Thoracic Surgery (EACTS): the Task Force for the diagnosis and management of atrial fibrillation of the European Society of Cardiology (ESC) developed with the special contribution of the European Heart Rhythm Association (EHRA) of the ESC. Eur Heart J [Internet]. 2021 [cited 2023 Oct 30];42(5):373–498. Available from: https://doi.org/10.1093/eurheartj/ehaa612
3. Nerheim P, Birger-Botkin S, Piracha L, Olshansky B. Heart failure and sudden death in patients with tachycardia-induced cardiomyopathy and recurrent tachycardia. Circulation [Internet]. 2004 [cited 2023 Oct 30];110(3):247–52. Available from: https://www.ahajournals.org/doi/abs/10.1161/01.CIR.0000135472.28234.CC
4. Deedwania PC, Lardizabal JA. Atrial fibrillation in heart failure: a comprehensive review. Am J Med [Internet]. 2010 [cited 2023 Oct 30];123(3):198–204. Available from: http://www.amjmed.com/article/S00029343090009516/fulltext
5. Melenovsky V, Hwang SJ, Redfield MM, Zakeri R, Lin G, Borlaug BA. Left atrial remodeling and function in advanced heart failure with preserved or reduced ejection fraction. Circ Heart Fail [Internet]. 2015 [cited 2023 Oct 30];8(2):295–303. Available from: https://pubmed.ncbi.nlm.nih.gov/25593126/
6. Santhanakrishnan R, Wang N, Larson MG, Magnani JW, McManus DD, Lubitz SA, et al. Atrial fibrillation begets heart failure and vice versa: temporal associations and differences in preserved versus reduced ejection fraction. Circulation [Internet]. 2016 [cited 2023 Oct 30];133(5):484–92. Available from: https://www.ahajournals.org/doi/abs/10.1161/CIRCULATIONAHA.115.018614
7. Hu YF, Chen YJ, Lin YJ, Chen SA. Inflammation and the pathogenesis of atrial fibrillation. Nat Rev Cardiol 2015;124 [Internet]. 2015 [cited 2023 Oct 30];12(4):230–43. Available from: https://www.nature.com/articles/nrcardio.2015.2
8. Boos CJ, Anderson RA, Lip GYH. Is atrial fibrillation an inflammatory disorder? Eur Heart J [Internet]. 2006 [cited 2023 Oct 30];27(2):136–49. Available from: https://doi.org/10.1093/eurheartj/ehi645
9. Van Wagoner DR. Oxidative stress and inflammation in atrial fibrillation: role in pathogenesis and potential as a therapeutic target. J Cardiovasc Pharmacol [Internet]. 2008 [cited 2023 Oct 30];52(4):306–13. Available from: https://pubmed.ncbi.nlm.nih.gov/18791466/
10. Negi S, Shukrullah I, Veledar E, Bloom HL, Jones DP, Dudley SC. Statin therapy for the prevention of atrial fibrillation trial (SToP AF trial). J Cardiovasc Electrophysiol [Internet]. 2011 [cited 2023 Oct 30];22(4):414–9. Available from: https://onlinelibrary.wiley.com/doi/full/10.1111/j.1540-8167.2010.01925.x

11. Bang CN, Greve AM, Abdulla J, Køber L, Gislason GH, Wachtell K. The preventive effect of statin therapy on new-onset and recurrent atrial fibrillation in patients not undergoing invasive cardiac interventions: a systematic review and meta-analysis. Int J Cardiol. 2013;167(3):624–30.
12. Gorenek B, Halvorsen S, Kudaiberdieva G, Bueno H, Van Gelder IC, Lettino M, et al. Atrial fibrillation in acute heart failure: a position statement from the Acute Cardiovascular Care Association and European Heart Rhythm Association of the European Society of Cardiology 894255A Position paper. Eur Heart J Acute Cardiovasc Care [Internet]. 2020 [cited 2023 Oct 30];2020(4):348–57. Available from: https://doi.org/10.1177/2048872619894255
13. Abe Y, Takahashi Y, Shibata T. Functional mitral regurgitation, updated: ventricular or atrial? J Echocardiogr [Internet]. 2020 [cited 2023 Oct 30];18(1). Available from: https://pubmed.ncbi.nlm.nih.gov/31728977/
14. Sartipy U, Dahlström U, Fu M, Lund LH. Atrial fibrillation in heart failure with preserved, mid-range, and reduced ejection fraction. JACC Heart Fail. 2017;5(8):565–74.
15. Patel RB, Vaduganathan M, Shah SJ, Butler J. Atrial fibrillation in heart failure with preserved ejection fraction: insights into mechanisms and therapeutics. Pharmacol Ther. 2017;176:32–9.
16. Zoni-Berisso M, Lercari F, Carazza T, Domenicucci S. Epidemiology of atrial fibrillation: European perspective. Clin Epidemiol [Internet]. 2014 [cited 2023 Oct 30];6(1):213–20. Available from: https://www.dovepress.com/epidemiology-of-atrial-fibrillation-european-perspective-peer-reviewed-fulltext-article-CLEP
17. Sohns C, Marrouche NF. Atrial fibrillation and cardiac fibrosis. Eur Heart J [Internet]. 2020 [cited 2023 Oct 30];41(10):1123–31. Available from: https://doi.org/10.1093/eurheartj/ehz786
18. Bisbal F, Baranchuk A, Braunwald E, Bayés de Luna A, Bayés-Genís A. Atrial failure as a clinical entity: JACC review topic of the week. J Am Coll Cardiol. 2020;75(2):222–32.
19. Marrouche NF, Greene T, Dean JM, Kholmovski EG, Boer LM de, Mansour M, et al. Efficacy of LGE-MRI-guided fibrosis ablation versus conventional catheter ablation of atrial fibrillation: the DECAAF II trial: study design. J Cardiovasc Electrophysiol [Internet]. 2021 [cited 2023 Oct 30];32(4):916–24. Available from: https://onlinelibrary.wiley.com/doi/full/10.1111/jce.14957
20. Kowallick JT, Staab W, Schuster A, Backhaus SJ, Weber-Krüger M, Bauer L, et al. Reverse left ventricular structural remodeling after catheter ablation of atrial fibrillation in patients with preserved left ventricular function: insights from cardiovascular magnetic resonance native T1 mapping. Heart Rhythm [Internet]. 2019 [cited 2023 Oct 30];16(3):424–32. Available from: http://www.heartrhythmjournal.com/article/S1547527118309391/fulltext
21. Prabhu S, Costello BT, Taylor AJ, Gutman SJ, Voskoboinik A, McLellan AJA, et al. Regression of diffuse ventricular fibrosis following restoration of sinus rhythm with catheter ablation in patients with atrial fibrillation and systolic dysfunction: a substudy of the CAMERA MRI trial. JACC Clin Electrophysiol [Internet]. 2018 [cited 2023 Oct 30];4(8):999–1007. Available from: https://pubmed.ncbi.nlm.nih.gov/30139501/
22. Soulat-Dufour L, Lang S, Addetia K, Ederhy S, Adavane-Scheuble S, Chauvet-Droit M, et al. Restoring sinus rhythm reverses cardiac remodeling and reduces valvular regurgitation in patients with atrial fibrillation. J Am Coll Cardiol. 2022;79(10):951–61.
23. Agarwal M, Apostolakis S, Lane DA, Lip GYH. The impact of heart failure and left ventricular dysfunction in predicting stroke, thromboembolism, and mortality in atrial fibrillation patients: a systematic review. Clin Ther [Internet]. 2014 [cited 2023 Oct 30];36(9):1135–44. Available from: https://pubmed.ncbi.nlm.nih.gov/25146364/
24. Kotecha D, Chudasama R, Lane DA, Kirchhof P, Lip GYH. Atrial fibrillation and heart failure due to reduced versus preserved ejection fraction: a systematic review and meta-analysis of death and adverse outcomes. Int J Cardiol [Internet]. 2016 [cited 2023 Oct 30];203:660–6. Available from: https://pubmed.ncbi.nlm.nih.gov/26580351/
25. Saad M, Osman M, Hasan-Ali H, Abdel Ghany M, Alsherif MA, Risha O, et al. Atrial appendage closure in patients with heart failure and atrial fibrillation: industry-independent single-centre study. ESC Heart Fail. 2022;9(1):648–55.

26. Kim DY, Kim MJ, Seo J, Cho I, Shim CY, Hong GR, et al. Predictors of subsequent heart failure after left atrial appendage closure. Circ J [Internet]. 2022 [cited 2023 Oct 30];86(7):1129–36. Available from: https://pubmed.ncbi.nlm.nih.gov/34880153/
27. Mueller C, Christ M, Cowie M, Cullen L, Maisel AS, Masip J, et al. European Society of Cardiology-Acute Cardiovascular Care Association Position paper on acute heart failure: a call for interdisciplinary care. Eur Heart J Acute Cardiovasc Care [Internet]. 2017 [cited 2023 Oct 30];6(1):81–6. Available from: https://pubmed.ncbi.nlm.nih.gov/26124458/
28. Aleong RG, Sauer WH, Davis G, Bristow MR. New-onset atrial fibrillation predicts heart failure progression. Am J Med [Internet]. 2014 [cited 2023 Oct 30];127(10):963–71. Available from: https://pubmed.ncbi.nlm.nih.gov/24931393/
29. Mountantonakis SE, Grau-Sepulveda M V., Bhatt DL, Hernandez AF, Peterson ED, Fonarow GC. Presence of atrial fibrillation is independently associated with adverse outcomes in patients hospitalized with heart failure an analysis of get with the guidelines-heart failure. Circ Heart Fail [Internet]. 2012 [cited 2023 Oct 30];5(2):191–201. Available from: https://www.ahajournals.org/doi/abs/10.1161/circheartfailure.111.965681
30. Mebazaa A, Yilmaz MB, Levy P, Ponikowski P, Peacock WF, Laribi S, et al. Recommendations on pre-hospital and early hospital management of acute heart failure: a consensus paper from the Heart Failure Association of the European Society of Cardiology, the European Society of Emergency Medicine and the Society of Academic Emergency Medicine—short version. Eur Heart J. 2015;36(30):1958–66.
31. Vamos M, Erath JW, Benz AP, Lopes RD, Hohnloser SH. Meta-analysis of effects of digoxin on survival in patients with atrial fibrillation or heart failure: an update. Am J Cardiol [Internet]. 2019 [cited 2023 Oct 30];123(1):69–74. Available from: https://pubmed.ncbi.nlm.nih.gov/30539748/
32. Mulder BA, Van Veldhuisen DJ, Crijns HJGM, Tijssen JGP, Hillege HL, Alings M, et al. Digoxin in patients with permanent atrial fibrillation: data from the RACE II study. Hear Rhythm [Internet]. 2014 [cited 2023 Oct 30];11(9):1543–50. Available from: https://pubmed.ncbi.nlm.nih.gov/24924587/
33. Chamaria S, Desai AM, Reddy PC, Olshansky B, Dominic P. Digoxin use to control ventricular rate in patients with atrial fibrillation and heart failure is not associated with increased mortality. Cardiol Res Pract [Internet]. 2015 [cited 2023 Oct 30];2015. Available from: https://pubmed.ncbi.nlm.nih.gov/26788401/
34. Van Gelder IC, Rienstra M, Crijns HJGM, Olshansky B. Rate control in atrial fibrillation. Lancet (London, England) [Internet]. 2016 [cited 2023 Oct 30];388(10046):818–28. Available from: https://pubmed.ncbi.nlm.nih.gov/27560277/
35. Bellone A, Etteri M, Vettorello M, Bonetti C, Clerici D, Gini G, et al. Cardioversion of acute atrial fibrillation in the emergency department: a prospective randomised trial. Emerg Med J [Internet]. 2012 [cited 2023 Oct 30];29(3):188–91. Available from: https://pubmed.ncbi.nlm.nih.gov/21422032/
36. McMurray JJV, Packer M, Desai AS, Gong J, Lefkowitz MP, Rizkala AR, et al. Angiotensin-neprilysin inhibition versus enalapril in heart failure. N Engl J Med [Internet]. 2014 [cited 2023 Oct 30];371(11):132–3. Available from: https://pubmed.ncbi.nlm.nih.gov/25176015/
37. Swedberg K, Zannad F, McMurray JJV, Krum H, Van Veldhuisen DJ, Shi H, et al. Eplerenone and atrial fibrillation in mild systolic heart failure: results from the EMPHASIS-HF (Eplerenone in Mild Patients Hospitalization and SurvIval Study in Heart Failure) study. J Am Coll Cardiol [Internet]. 2012 [cited 2023 Oct 30];59(18):1598–603. Available from: https://pubmed.ncbi.nlm.nih.gov/22538330/
38. Cadrin-Tourigny J, Shohoudi A, Roy D, Talajic M, Tadros R, Mondésert B, et al. Decreased mortality with beta-blockers in patients with heart failure and coexisting atrial fibrillation: an AF-CHF substudy. JACC Heart Fail. 2017;5(2):99–106.
39. Kotecha D, Holmes J, Krum H, Altman DG, Manzano L, Cleland JGF, et al. Efficacy of β blockers in patients with heart failure plus atrial fibrillation: an individual-patient data meta-analysis. Lancet. 2014;384(9961):2235–43.

40. Atrial fibrillation and congestive heart failure—American College of Cardiology [Internet]. [cited 2023 Oct 30]. Available from: https://www.acc.org/Latest-in-Cardiology/Clinical-Trials/2013/05/22/13/10/AFCHF
41. January CT, Wann LS, Calkins H, Chen LY, Cigarroa JE, Cleveland JC, et al. 2019 AHA/ACC/HRS focused update of the 2014 AHA/ACC/HRS Guideline for the management of patients with atrial fibrillation: a report of the American College of Cardiology/American Heart Association Task Force on Clinical Practice Guidelines and the Heart Rhythm Society in Collaboration With the Society of Thoracic Surgeons. Circulation [Internet]. 2019 [cited 2023 Oct 30];140(2):e125–51. Available from: https://www.ahajournals.org/doi/abs/10.1161/CIR.0000000000000665
42. Van Gelder IC, Rienstra M, Crijns HJGM, Olshansky B. Rate control in atrial fibrillation. Lancet. 2016;388(10046):818–28.
43. Wood MA, Brown-Mahoney C, Kay GN, Ellenbogen KA. Clinical outcomes after ablation and pacing therapy for atrial fibrillation. Circulation [Internet]. 2000 [cited 2023 Oct 30];101(10):1138–44. Available from: https://www.ahajournals.org/doi/abs/10.1161/01.cir.101.10.1138
44. Brignole M, Pokushalov E, Pentimalli F, Palmisano P, Chieffo E, Occhetta E, et al. A randomized controlled trial of atrioventricular junction ablation and cardiac resynchronization therapy in patients with permanent atrial fibrillation and narrow QRS. Eur Heart J [Internet]. 2018 [cited 2023 Oct 30];39(45):3999–4008. Available from: https://pubmed.ncbi.nlm.nih.gov/30165479/
45. Kusumoto FM, Schoenfeld MH, Barrett C, Edgerton JR, Ellenbogen KA, Gold MR, et al. 2018 ACC/AHA/HRS Guideline on the evaluation and management of patients with bradycardia and cardiac conduction delay: executive summary: a report of the American College of Cardiology/American Heart Association Task Force on Clinical Practice Guidelines, and the Heart Rhythm Society. J Am Coll Cardiol [Internet]. 2019 [cited 2023 Oct 30];74(7):932–87. Available from: https://pubmed.ncbi.nlm.nih.gov/30412710/
46. Curtis AB, Worley SJ, Adamson PB, Chung ES, Niazi I, Sherfesee L, et al. Biventricular pacing for atrioventricular block and systolic dysfunction. N Engl J Med [Internet]. 2013 [cited 2023 Oct 30];368(17):1585–93. Available from: https://pubmed.ncbi.nlm.nih.gov/23614585/
47. Ganesan AN, Brooks AG, Roberts-Thomson KC, Lau DH, Kalman JM, Sanders P. Role of AV nodal ablation in cardiac resynchronization in patients with coexistent atrial fibrillation and heart failure a systematic review. J Am Coll Cardiol [Internet]. 2012 [cited 2023 Oct 30];59(8):719–26. Available from: https://pubmed.ncbi.nlm.nih.gov/22340263/
48. Khan MN, Jaïs P, Cummings J, Di Biase L, Sanders P, Martin DO, et al. pulmonary-vein isolation for atrial fibrillation in patients with heart failure. https://doi.org/101056/NEJMoa0708234 [Internet]. 2008 [cited 2023 Oct 30];359(17):1778–85. Available from: https://www.nejm.org/doi/full/10.1056/NEJMoa0708234
49. Sharma PS, Patel NR, Ravi V, Zalavadia DV, Dommaraju S, Garg V, et al. Clinical outcomes of left bundle branch area pacing compared to right ventricular pacing: results from the Geisinger-Rush Conduction System Pacing Registry. Heart Rhythm [Internet]. 2022 [cited 2023 Nov 1];19(1):3–11. Available from: https://pubmed.ncbi.nlm.nih.gov/34481985/
50. Hua W, Fan X, Li X, Niu H, Gu M, Ning X, et al. Comparison of left bundle branch and his bundle pacing in bradycardia patients. JACC Clin Electrophysiol [Internet]. 2020 [cited 2023 Nov 1];6(10):1291–9. Available from: https://pubmed.ncbi.nlm.nih.gov/33092757/
51. Rodríguez Muñoz D, Crespo-Leiro MG, Fernández Lozano I, Zamorano Gómez JL, Peinado Peinado R, Manzano Espinosa L, et al. Conduction system pacing and atrioventricular node ablation in heart failure: the PACE-FIB study design. ESC Hear Fail [Internet]. 2023 [cited 2023 Nov 1]; Available from: https://onlinelibrary.wiley.com/doi/full/10.1002/ehf2.14488
52. Marrouche NF, Brachmann J, Andresen D, Siebels J, Boersma L, Jordaens L, et al. Catheter ablation for atrial fibrillation with heart failure. N Engl J Med [Internet]. 2018 [cited 2023 Oct 30];378(5):417–27. Available from: https://www.nejm.org/doi/full/10.1056/nejmoa1707855

53. Sohns C, Fox H, Marrouche NF, Crijns HJGM, Costard-Jaeckle A, Bergau L, et al. Catheter ablation in end-stage heart failure with atrial fibrillation. N Engl J Med. 2023;89(15):1380–9.
54. Prabhu S, Taylor AJ, Costello BT, Kaye DM, McLellan AJA, Voskoboinik A, et al. Catheter ablation versus medical rate control in atrial fibrillation and systolic dysfunction: the CAMERA-MRI study. J Am Coll Cardiol. 2017;70(16):1949–61.
55. Sugumar H, Prabhu S, Voskoboinik A, Young S, Gutman SJ, Wong GR, et al. Atrial remodeling following catheter ablation for atrial fibrillation-mediated cardiomyopathy: long-term follow-up of CAMERA-MRI study. JACC Clin Electrophysiol. 2019;5(6):681–8.
56. Packer DL, Piccini JP, Monahan KH, Al-Khalidi HR, Silverstein AP, Noseworthy PA, et al. Ablation versus drug therapy for atrial fibrillation in heart failure. Circulation [Internet]. 2021 [cited 2023 Oct 30];143(14):1377–90. Available from: https://www.ahajournals.org/doi/abs/10.1161/CIRCULATIONAHA.120.050991
57. Kirchhof P, Camm AJ, Goette A, Brandes A, Eckardt L, Elvan A, et al. Early rhythm-control therapy in patients with atrial fibrillation. N Engl J Med [Internet]. 2020 [cited 2023 Oct 30];383(14):1305–16. Available from: https://www.nejm.org/doi/10.1056/NEJMoa2019422
58. Rillig A, Magnussen C, Ozga AK, Suling A, Brandes A, Breithardt G, et al. Early rhythm control therapy in patients with atrial fibrillation and heart failure. Circulation [Internet]. 2021 [cited 2023 Oct 30];144(11):845–58. Available from: https://www.ahajournals.org/doi/abs/10.1161/CIRCULATIONAHA.121.056323
59. Parkash R, Wells GA, Rouleau J, Talajic M, Essebag V, Skanes A, et al. Randomized ablation-based rhythm-control versus rate-control trial in patients with heart failure and atrial fibrillation: results from the RAFT-AF trial. Circulation [Internet]. 2022 [cited 2023 Oct 30];145(23):1693–704. Available from: https://www.ahajournals.org/doi/abs/10.1161/CIRCULATIONAHA.121.057095
60. Verma A, Jiang C, Betts TR, Chen J, Deisenhofer I, Mantovan R, et al. Approaches to catheter ablation for persistent atrial fibrillation. N Engl J Med [Internet]. 2015 [cited 2023 Oct 30];372(19):1812–22. Available from: https://pubmed.ncbi.nlm.nih.gov/25946280/
61. Mulder BA, Luermans JGLM, Hindricks G, Blaauw Y. Innovations and paradigm shifts in atrial fibrillation ablation. Europace [Internet]. 2021 [cited 2023 Oct 30];23(23 Suppl 2):II23–7. Available from: https://pubmed.ncbi.nlm.nih.gov/33837757/
62. Al-Jazairi MIH, Rienstra M, Klinkenberg TJ, Mariani MA, Van Gelder IC, Blaauw Y. Hybrid atrial fibrillation ablation in patients with persistent atrial fibrillation or failed catheter ablation. Neth Heart J [Internet]. 2019 [cited 2023 Oct 30];27(3):142–51. Available from: https://pubmed.ncbi.nlm.nih.gov/30715671/
63. Noseworthy PA, Van Houten HK, Gersh BJ, Packer DL, Friedman PA, Shah ND, et al. Generalizability of the CASTLE-AF trial: catheter ablation for patients with atrial fibrillation and heart failure in routine practice. Hear Rhythm [Internet]. 2020 1 [cited 2023 Oct 30];17(7):1057. Available from: https://www.pmc/articles/PMC7648571/

Chapter 13
Cardiac Implantable Electronic Devices for Heart Failure

Michael Glikson and Ştefan Bogdan

Abstract Cardiac resynchronization therapy (CRT) has become a standard of care for symptomatic heart failure patients with reduced left ventricular ejection (LVEF) in the setting of electrical conduction disease. Successfully delivered CRT corrects left ventricular electromechanical dyssynchrony resulting in LVEF increase, reverse remodeling, improved quality of life, and better survival. The development of conduction system pacing during the last decade has emerged as an alternative and complementary technique to classic CRT. In the following chapter we will analyze the pathophysiology of dyssynchrony and dyssynchrony assessment, the extent of clinical evidence in cardiac resynchronization therapy, the issue of non-response to CRT, how to improve patient selection and CRT delivery, as well as the role of conduction system pacing for CRT according to clinical evidence and current guidelines.

Keywords Cardiac resynchronization therapy · Heart failure · Reduced ejection fraction · Non-response · Conduction system pacing

Introduction

Since Cazeau's first case of cardiac resynchronization therapy (CRT) in 1994 showing the beneficial effects of four-chamber pacing in a 54-year-old dilated cardiomyopathy patient [1], cardiac resynchronization therapy (CRT) has come a long way. Targeting cardiac electro-mechanical dyssynchrony correction, it has become a well-established treatment for symptomatic heart failure patients with reduced left

M. Glikson (✉)
Jesselson Integrated Heart Center, Shaare Zedek Medical Center and Hebrew University, Jerusalem, Israel
e-mail: mglikson@szmc.org.il

Ş. Bogdan
Cardiology Department—Elias University Emergency Hospital, "Carol Davila" University of Medicine and Pharmacy, Bucharest, Romania

M. Dorobanţu et al. (eds.), *Current Approach to Heart Failure*,
https://doi.org/10.1007/978-3-031-96562-3_13

ventricular ejection fraction (HFrEF) and wide QRS (>130 ms). Evidence from multiple large randomized trials has shown the clinical (symptoms improvement; mortality reduction) as well as structural (left ventricular reverse remodeling with ejection fraction increase and mitral regurgitation reduction) benefits of CRT and represent the basis for current guidelines [2, 3]. However, response to CRT is uneven and some patients will have a lesser or even absent benefit following CRT. Understanding nonresponse and predicting response has to do with understanding the interrelationship between electro-mechanical dyssynchrony and the underlying heart disease. To improve response, efforts have been made for better patient selection by clinical, electrocardiographic, and imaging techniques, as well as better CRT delivery—with new evidence suggesting that conduction system pacing (CSP) may play an important role.

Pathophysiology of Cardiac Dyssynchrony and Dyssynchrony Assessment

Cardiac mechanical dyssynchrony refers to a difference in the contraction/relaxation timing (lack of synchrony) between different heart areas, which usually occurs in the setting of electrical conduction disease (electrical dyssynchrony). Large differences in contraction timing can result in reduced cardiac efficiency and are correlated to heart failure [4]. Cardiac imaging by advanced echocardiography and cardiac magnetic resonance plays an important role in mechanical dyssynchrony assessment. Other imaging techniques, including radionuclide imaging, have been used for cardiac dyssynchrony evaluation.

Three main types of dyssynchrony can be corrected by CRT: atrioventricular, interventricular, and intraventricular (Table 13.1).

Atrioventricular dyssynchrony occurs because of a loss of timing between atrial and ventricular contractions, in the presence of prolonged PR interval, QRS widening, or both [5]. The hemodynamic consequence is an impairment of the left ventricular (LV) filling secondary to a shortening of the diastole. Using pulsed-wave Doppler echocardiography, atrioventricular dyssynchrony can be evaluated by measuring the LV filling time from transmitral flow recordings. In the presence of prolonged atrioventricular interval, the early (E wave) and late (A wave) diastolic waves are fused with a shortening of the ventricular filling time. A ratio of the LV filling time (ms)/RR interval (ms) <40% indicates atrioventricular dyssynchrony [5]. An opposite type of AV dyssynchrony may occur following pacemaker implantation, after programming a too-short AV delay so that the atrial systole is truncated (resulting in one wave) [6, 7].

Inter-ventricular dyssynchrony occurs because of a delay between right ventricular and left ventricular contractions, in the setting of wide QRS. This delay affects cardiac output by creating a paradoxical septal motion that reduces contraction efficacy. One of the first indexes used to assess inter-ventricular dyssynchrony was the

Table 13.1 Cardiac dyssynchrony: types, setting, consequence

Dyssynchrony	Electric disease	Consequence
Atrioventricular	Prolonged PR	Diastolic impairment
Inter-ventricular	Wide QRS	Systolic impairment
Intra-ventricular LV	Wide QRS	Systolic and diastolic impairment Mitral regurgitation

Wide QRS QRS duration > 120 ms, *LV* left ventricle

inter-ventricular mechanical delay (IVMD), obtained by calculating the difference between aortic and pulmonary pre-ejection intervals (time from QRS onset to flow onset) with pulsed-wave Doppler echocardiography [5]. Using a cut-off value >40 ms for defining inter-ventricular dyssynchrony, the CARE-HF trial showed a correlation between IVMD and response to CRT [8].

Intra-ventricular dyssynchrony of the left ventricle (LV dyssynchrony) occurs because of delayed contraction of certain LV segments (usually the postero-lateral wall that is last to contract while the inter-ventricular septum contracts first). This phenomenon is associated with but not limited to the setting of prolonged QRS duration—typically left bundle branch block (LBBB). The difference in activation timing results in contraction delay, loss of contraction efficiency, and reduced stroke volume. In prolonged LV contraction, while the atria relax and atrial pressure falls, the LV pressure might exceed the atrial pressure resulting in diastolic mitral regurgitation. Dis-coordinated papillary muscle function can also cause or further aggravate mitral regurgitation. These dyssynchrony-related changes promote adverse LV remodeling [9].

While all types of cardiac dyssynchrony can be corrected by dedicated cardiac implantable electronic devices, only the intra-left ventricular dyssynchrony correction, in the setting of LBBB, was proven in randomized controlled trials to improve prognosis in patients with HFrEF.

Imaging in Cardiac Resynchronization Therapy

Imaging in CRT is important as it serves several roles: establish CRT indication according to left ventricular ejection fraction (LVEF) ($\leq$35%), assess mechanical dyssynchrony, myocardial scar burden and viability, identify the best location for LV lead implantation to maximize response, and evaluate structural response upon follow-up. Lead location is the most complex element, which combines identification of the latest contracting segment as well as localization of scars that should be avoided as pacing in a scar area is associated with poor response [10].

It is mainly LV dyssynchrony that has been shown in several milestone studies to be an independent predictor of response to CRT in HF patients following CRT. Pitzalis et al. introduced a reliable, easy-to-use, and reproducible M-mode echocardiography parameter for LV dyssynchrony measurement [11]. Using the parasternal short-axis LV view, the operator measures the time difference between the maximal systolic inward movement of the septum and posterior wall resulting in the septal-to-posterior-wall-motion-delay (SPWMD). A SPWMD ≥130 ms is correlated with significant LV dyssynchrony [11]. This initial approach was limited due to the non-uniform pattern of contraction in different segments of the LV, and the limited imaging by M-mode. Several other echocardiographic parameters have since been used for LV dyssynchrony evaluation besides M-mode, including tissue Doppler imaging, speckle tracking that is commonly used as it is considered superior to conventional echo-Doppler techniques [12], and more recently 3D echocardiography (Table 13.2). It is conceivable that a technique that includes scar imaging in addition to dyssynchrony in the same test has an advantage in the site selection of the LV lead.

Special attention has been given to the assessment of rotational dyssynchrony. Left ventricular fibers have a helical configuration: right-hand orientation from the base toward the apex in the endocardial layers and left-hand orientation in the epicardial layers [21]. This spiral architecture of the cardiac fibers causes the LV to

Table 13.2 Echocardiographic measurement of intra-ventricular LV dyssynchrony

Parameter	Echo technique	Cut-off
Septal to posterior wall motion delay [11]	M-mode	≥130 ms
Septal flash	M-mode	Non-quantifiable[a]
Apical rocking	2D apical 4 chambers	Non-quantifiable[b]
Basal septal to lateral Ts delay [13]	Tissue Doppler imaging	≥60 ms
Max delay in Ts in 4 basal LV segments [14]	Tissue Doppler imaging	>65 ms
SD of Ts of 6 basal LV segments [15]	Tissue Doppler imaging	≥34.4 ms
Max delay in Ts in 12 basal and mid LV segments [16]	Tissue Doppler imaging	≥100 ms
SD of Ts in 12 basal and mid LV segments (Dyssynchrony index; Yu index) [17]	Tissue Doppler imaging	≥32.6 ms
SD of time-to-peak longitudinal strain in 12 basal and mid-LV segments [18]	Tissue Doppler imaging	>60 ms
Antero-septal to posterior time to peak strain difference (radial strain) [19]	2D speckle tracking	≥130 ms
SD of time to minimum systolic volume of 16 LV segments (systolic dyssynchrony index) [20]	3D echocardiography	>5.6%

Ts time-to-peak systolic velocity, *SD* standard deviation, *LV* left ventricular, *2D* two dimensional, *3D* three dimensional

[a]Septal flash = early septal systolic thickening and thinning resulting in a short inward motion of the septum

[b]Apical rocking = the initial septal systolic thickening that causes the apex to move septally is followed by delayed activation of the lateral wall that pulls the apex laterally while stretching the septum, resulting in a typical motion pattern of the apex defined as "apical rocking"

make a wringing motion as a result of the opposite rotation of the LV apex and base (counterclockwise and clockwise, respectively, when viewed from the LV apex) [22]. Twist, that is the difference in rotation between apex and base, contributes to LV systolic function [23] and in patients with heart failure, it is reduced [24]. Two-dimensional speckle tracking can assess the LV rotational motion and has demonstrated that twist can be affected by right ventricular pacing (the experimental model of LBBB) [25, 26]. While LV twist is the net difference at isochronal time points between the apex and base in the rotation angle along the LV longitudinal axis, LV torsion represents the LV twist indexed to the distance between the LV apex and the LV base (LV length) [21, 22]. LV torsion can be assessed in a standardized way by using three-dimensional speckle-tracking echocardiography [27]. The use of two-dimensional speckle-tracking echocardiography has proven its clinical utility in the field of CRT [28].

With the advent of cardiac magnetic resonance (CMR), several CMR-derived dyssynchrony parameters [29]—such as regional vector variance (RVV), cross-correlation delay, uniformity of strain, time to maximum strain, and standard deviation of time to maximum strain, have been analyzed in the setting of HF with low left ventricular ejection fraction (LVEF) and wide QRS. Some, such as RVV, may provide an additive value for the prediction of response to CRT [30]. Cardiac magnetic resonance has the potential to become an alternative to echocardiography for assessing cardiac dyssynchrony. Image acquisition is less operator-dependent and it has the advantages of high spatial resolution, highly reproducible wall motion tracking, and the capability to assess LV scar, volumes, systolic function, velocity, strain, and torsion [31]. The current limitation is the fact that MRI-derived dyssynchrony parameters have been investigated in rather a small sample size population and cut-off values for derived indices have yet to be established. Its use in patients with existing devices is limited by safety issues as well as by the quality of imaging that may be distorted by the device.

Phase analysis of gated single-photon emission computed tomography (SPECT) myocardial perfusion imaging (MPI) has been used for evaluating LV dyssynchrony using radionuclide imaging [32]. Phase analysis is based on the partial volume effect, which indicates that LV regional maximal counts in SPECT MPI images are proportional to the regional wall thickness. Phase analysis approximates the variation of regional maximal counts over the cardiac cycle with the first Fourier harmonic function to measure the onset of mechanical contraction [32]. Quantitative gated SPECT-derived phased analysis on gated myocardial perfusion SPECT was able to detect left ventricular dyssynchrony (strong correlation with tissue Doppler imaging dyssynchrony parameters) and was able to accurately predict response to CRT [33]. Phase analysis of SPECT MPI has several advantages over other imaging techniques such as automated calculation, better reproducibility, and the ability to simultaneously assess myocardial scar location and severity for CRT optimization. However, in the presence of normal coronary artery and LBBB, SPECT can display perfusion defects in the septal and apical segments. These perfusion abnormalities are due to the relative septal hypoperfusion, compared to the lateral wall, and can be disclosed by the measure of the absolute regional myocardial perfusion at positron emission tomography [34]. Other limitations include reduced availability and the small number of centers with clinical experience in relatively small sample size populations [31].

Cardiac imaging can play an important role in the assessment of myocardial scar before CRT. Khan et Al., in the randomized TARGET trial, have shown that LV lead positioning in a site far from LV scar and with significant residual contractility (defined as a > 10% amplitude of the corresponding radial strain trace) was associated with a higher percentage of CRT response (70 vs. 55%, $p < 0.031$) and significantly better survival (log-rank $p = 0.002$). However, when compared with scar assessment at cardiac magnetic resonance (CMR), the predictive value of segmental radial strain for the identification of myocardial scar was low (sensitivity 33% and specificity 72%) [35].

This suggests the usefulness of a multimodality imaging approach to plan and ease CRT implantation. Specifically, echocardiography can assess mechanical dyssynchrony, whereas CMR can quantify the extent and localization of myocardial scar. If CMR is not available or contraindicated, SPECT might be applied for the localization of the scar and to assess viability [36].

Clinical Evidence in Cardiac Resynchronization Therapy and Current Guidelines

Randomized multi-center trials have provided solid evidence concerning the benefits of CRT in heart failure treatment.

The initial trials including limited numbers of severe HF failure patients (NYHA III-IV; QRS duration ≥ 150 ms; LVEF ≤ 35%) only showed symptomatic benefit [37, 38]. In 2004, COMPANION was the first randomized trial to show a survival benefit following CRT in HF patients [39]. It included 1520 HF patients, NYHA class III-IV with QRS ≥ 120 ms and LVEF ≤ 35%, that were randomized to either CRT or optimal medical treatment (OMT). Patients with pacemaker CRT (CRT-P) had the risk of the combined end point of death or hospitalization for HF reduced by 34% ($p < 0.002$), while in those with defibrillator CRT (CRT-D), the risk was reduced by 40% ($p < 0.001$). These results were confirmed a year later by the CARE-HF trial [8].

The COMPANION and CARE-HF trials were followed by 3 cornerstone trials addressing less severe HF patients (NYHA class I–II), with low LVEF and wide QRS: the REVERSE [40], RAFT [41] and MADIT-CRT trials [42].

The REVERSE trial demonstrated in 610 patients with NYHA class I or II HF, wide QRS ≥ 120 ms and low LVEF ≤ 40%, that CRT in combination with OMT (±defibrillator) reduces the risk for HF hospitalization and improves ventricular structure (LV end-systolic volume reduction), with no effect however on mortality [40].

The RAFT trial randomized 1798 patients suffering from NYHA class II-III HF with wide or paced QRS and LVEF ≤ 30%, to CRT with defibrillator (CRT-D) versus implantable cardioverter defibrillator alone (ICD). The trial showed a significant mortality reduction of 25% ($p = 0.003$) and a reduction of 32% for HF hospitalization ($p < 0.001$) in the CRT group, at the cost of more peri-procedural adverse events [41].

The MADIT-CRT trial included 1820 patients with NYHA class I-II HF, wide QRS ≥ 130 ms, and reduced LVEF ≤ 30%, that were randomized into CRT-D versus ICD alone. The initial results, published in 2009, showed, after an average follow-up of 2.4 years, a significant 41% reduction in the risk of HF events ($p = 0.001$), a finding primarily evident in a pre-specified subgroup of patients with a QRS ≥ 150 ms. CRT was also associated with a significant reduction in LV volumes and LVEF improvement, with no influence however on mortality [42].

In 2014, the long-term follow-up of the MADIT-CRT trial has been published. At 7 years of follow-up, among the 1818 patients enrolled in the post-trial registries, CRT-D was associated with significant mortality reduction in LBBB patients (hazard ratio (HR): 0.59; 95% confidence interval (CI) 0.43–0.80; $p < 0.001$). In contrast, CRT-D was not associated with any clinical benefit, and proved potentially harmful in patients without LBBB (HR: 1.57; 95% CI 1.03–2.39; $p = 0.04$) (Fig. 13.1) [43].

While all the main randomized trials addressed the issue of mechanical dyssynchrony correction in the presence of electrical dyssynchrony (defined mainly as wide QRS of at least 120 ms), the EchoCRT trial investigated the potential benefit of CRT in HF patients with narrow QRS. The trial enrolled 809 patients suffering from NYHA class III-IV HF, with narrow QRS < 130 ms and low LVEF ≤ 35%, in whom there was echocardiographic evidence of LV dyssynchrony (defined using color-coded tissue Doppler imaging as an opposing-wall delay in the peak systolic velocity of 80 msec or more in apical four-chamber or apical long-axis views, or using speckle-tracking radial strain as a delay in the anteroseptal-to-posterior wall of 130 ms or more in the mid-left ventricular short-axis view). All patients had a CRT device implanted and were randomized to have CRT capability turned on or off. After a mean follow-up of 19 months, the trial was prematurely stopped because of increased mortality in the CRT ON group (11.1% vs. 6.4%; HR: 1.81; 95% CI 1.11–2.93; $p = 0.02$) [44].

The EchoCRT trial demonstrated that in HF patients with narrow QRS < 130 ms, CRT does not reduce the rate of death or HF hospitalization and may increase mortality.

These pivotal trials represent the basis for current HFrEF treatment guidelines, where CRT is recommended in HF patients (NYHA class II–IV) with wide QRS ≥ 130 ms and reduced LVEF ≤ 35% (Table 13.3) [2]. The American Guidelines dating are similar to the European ones, with one significant difference—the inferior cut-off duration for the QRS remained at 120 ms [3].

Right ventricular apical pacing has been shown to have deleterious effects on LV systolic function, as it is associated with a delayed electrical LV activation, with consequences similar (but not identical) to that seen with LBBB (LV dyssynchrony with reduced LVEF and mitral regurgitation). Clinical consequences include increased risk for atrial fibrillation, HF hospitalization, and death [45–47], especially in the setting of pre-existing HF and LV systolic dysfunction (below 40%) [47].

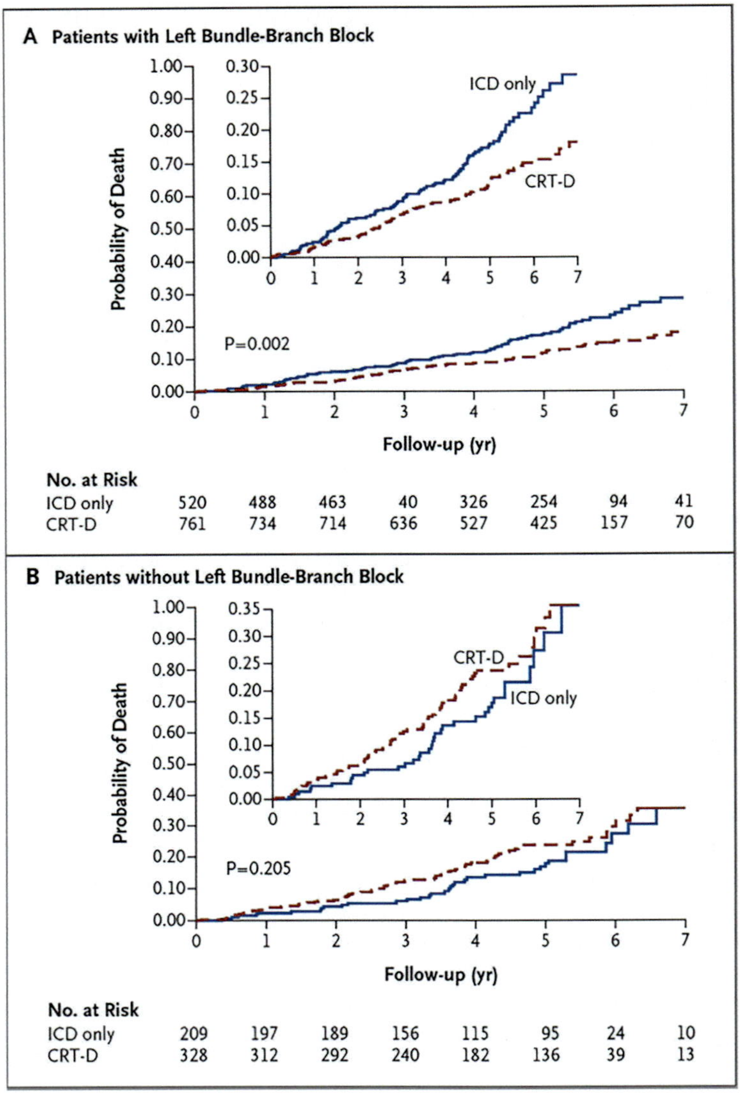

Fig. 13.1 Kaplan–Meier estimates of the cumulative probability of death from any cause among patients with and those without left bundle-branch Block. CRT-D denotes cardiac-resynchronization therapy with defibrillator, and ICD implantable cardioverter–defibrillator. The insets show the same data on an enlarged y-axis. (Goldenberg et Al. from the long-term follow-up of the MADIT-CRT trial [43])

Table 13.3 Indications according to class of recommendation and level of evidence, for cardiac resynchronization therapy (biventricular or conduction system pacing) according to current European (2021) and North American (2023) guidelines

NYHA II–IV heart failure with reduced LV ejection fraction ≤35%, under OMT			If CS leads to implantation failure:
LBBB	≥150 ms	CRT I—A[a, b] CSP IIb—B[b]	CSP IIa—B[a, b]
	130[c]—149 ms	CRT IIa[d]—B[a, b]	Limited data for CSP[a]
Non-LBBB	≥150 ms	CRT IIa[e]—B[a, b]	CSP IIb—C[b]
	130[c]—149 ms	CRT IIb—B[a, b]	CSP IIb—C[b]
QRS < 130[c] ms		No CRT/CSP III—A[a, b]	

CRT cardiac resynchronization therapy, *CSP* conduction system pacing (His bundle or left bundle branch area pacing), *LBBB* left bundle branch block, *OMT* optimal medical therapy

[a]2021 ESC Guidelines on cardiac pacing and CRT

[b]2023 HRS/APHRS/LAHRS Guideline on Cardiac Physiologic Pacing

[c]120 ms for 2023 HRS/APHRS/LAHRS Guideline on Cardiac Physiologic Pacing

[d]For female sex: Class of recommendation I, level of evidence A, for 2023 HRS/APHRS/LAHRS Guideline on Cardiac Physiologic Pacing

[e]For NYHA II: Class of recommendation IIb, for 2023 HRS/APHRS/LAHRS Guideline on Cardiac Physiologic Pacing

The BLOCK-HF trial randomized 691 patients with NYHA class I—III HF, LVEF ≤ 50%, and an indication for bradycardia pacing to standard right ventricular pacing or biventricular pacing. The study has shown that patients receiving biventricular pacing had a lower incidence of primary outcome (urgent care visit for HF; death from any cause; progression of HF, defined as a significant increase of left ventricular end-systolic volume index). The BLOCK-HF trial supports the use of CRT over standard right ventricular pacing in HF patients with LV systolic dysfunction and atrioventricular block requiring ventricular pacing [48].

Therefore, for patients with an indication for bradycardia pacing, in whom the percentage of ventricular pacing is expected to be high, in the presence of reduced LVEF (although debatable—usually below 40%), de novo CRT implantation should be considered. In patients with ventricular pacing who develop HF and left ventricular systolic dysfunction (LVEF < 35%), an upgrade to CRT is indicated, as the benefit has been demonstrated by us and other studies [49].

Most patients included in large CRT randomized trials were in sinus rhythm. In one prospective study for HF patients with permanent AF, reduced LVEF ≤ 35% and wide QRS > 120 ms, the per-protocol analysis including patients with biventricular pacing percentage > 85% showed a slight but significant symptomatic improvement at 6 months and 1-year follow-up [50]. A meta-analysis by Wilton et Al. that included 7495 CRT recipients, 25% with atrial fibrillation, from 23 observational studies, with a mean follow-up of 33 months, demonstrated an attenuated improvement of symptoms and LV end systolic volume, in the presence of AF, but not for the LVEF [51]. Current guidelines recommend CRT for AF patients with ambulatory NYHA class III-IV, wide

QRS ≥ 130 ms and reduced LVEF ≤ 35%, provided a high percentage of biventricular pacing (ideally 100%) can be achieved—a target for which atrioventricular junction ablation should be taken into consideration.

Response to CRT: Patient Selection and Improving CRT Delivery

Response to CRT can be evaluated from a clinical and structural perspective (Table 13.4), using individual or composite parameters (such as "functional response" [52]).

Depending upon the definition of response, the historical rates of non-response to CRT from 10 years ago varied between 20% and 40% [53]. Patient's characteristics (underlying heart disease, comorbidities, and arrhythmias; type and severity of conduction disorder; presence and degree of dyssynchrony; presence and extent of scar tissue; functional myocardial reserve), as well as CRT-related aspects (electrical and anatomical positioning of LV lead; programming mode and percentage of effective bi-ventricular pacing), have been shown to influence the response to CRT [10, 53–56].

Diagnosing dyssynchrony is crucial for patient selection given successful cardiac resynchronization therapy. Despite remarkable cardiac imaging advancements in the evaluation and understanding of mechanical dyssynchrony, electrical dyssynchrony (i.e.: wide QRS) remains the guideline criterion for CRT recommendation.

The role of LV dyssynchrony assessment in predicting response in CRT patients remains controversial to date. The PROSPECT trial investigated the predictive value of several echocardiographic dyssynchrony parameters (Doppler, M-mode, tissue Doppler imaging, and delayed longitudinal contraction) on LV reverse remodeling and a composite clinical score. The conclusion was that given the modest sensitivity and specificity in this multicenter setting despite training and central analysis, no single echocardiographic measure of dyssynchrony may be

Table 13.4 Response to cardiac resynchronization therapy evaluation

Clinical		Structural	
Parameter	Responder	Parameter	Responder
NYHA	Reduction ≥ 1 class	LVEF	Absolute increase ≥ 5–6%
6MWT	Increase ≥ 10–20%	LVESV	Decrease ≥ 10–15%
VO_2 max	Increase ≥ 10–15%	Mitral regurgitation reduction	
Hospitalization rate	Decrease > 25–30%		
QOL	Decrease ≥ 8–10 points		

6MWT 6-minute walk test, *LVEF* left ventricular ejection fraction, *LVESV* left ventricular end-systolic volume, *NYHA* New York Heart Association heart failure class, *QOL* quality of life questionnaire, *VO_2 max* maximal oxygen consumption recommended to improve patient selection for CRT beyond current guidelines [55]. The EchoCRT trial has shown that mechanical dyssynchrony detected by echocardiography is not a good target for CRT correction, in the absence of electrical dyssynchrony (i.e.: QRS < 130 ms) [44]. Still, other trials have shown that the amount of LV dyssynchrony at baseline and the remainder of LV dyssynchrony following CRT are correlated with clinical outcomes and response to CRT [11, 57].

Interestingly, the PREDICT-CRT trial by Stankovic et Al. has shown that the presence of apical rocking and septal flash—two subjectively measured echocardiographic dyssynchrony parameters (Table 13.2), is associated with more favorable long-term survival after CRT. Both apical rocking and septal flash were also indicators of an effective therapy [58].

To conclude, mechanical dyssynchrony documentation by cardiac imaging is not mandatory for CRT patient selection. The presence of echocardiographic dyssynchrony parameters is associated with better CRT response, but their absence does not preclude CRT for that patient. Current guidelines recommend the use of echocardiography only for CRT optimization in case of non-response.

Cardiac imaging remains very important for better understanding the underlying disease—in terms of etiology, global cardiac size and function, myocardial contractility and functional reserve, scar extent and localization, all of which correlate with prognosis and outcome beyond cardiac dyssynchrony in patients undergoing CRT [36]. Despite recent changes in the guideline's definition of HFrEF for LVEF < 40%, the cut-off for biventricular CRT implantation remains 35%, as all major CRT trials have used this specific value (or even lower cut-off ≤ 30% as inclusion criterium) [59].

The type of electric disease is important for CRT response. LBBB morphology and a QRS duration >150 ms are associated with the best response following CRT. The question remains in patients with wide QRS of right bundle branch (RBBB) or intraventricular conduction delay (IVCD) morphology, where the benefit of CRT has not been proven. The long-term MADIT-CRT follow-up has shown the absence of mortality benefit of CRT-D versus ICD alone in mild-to-moderate HF with reduced LVEF ≤ 30%, who presented with RBBB or IVCD at baseline [43] (Fig. 13.1, Section B). Specific subgroup analysis from MADIT-CRT demonstrated that the use of CRT-D in non-LBBB patients with prolonged PR ≥ 230 ms was associated with a significant 73% reduction in the risk of HF/death (HE: 0.27; 95% CI 0.13–0.57; P < 0.001) and 81% reduction in the risk of all-cause mortality (HR: 0.19; 95% CI 0.13–0.57; P < 0.001). At the same time, CRT-D use in non-LBBB patients with normal PR < 230 ms was associated with an increased risk of HF/death [60].

A recent meta-analysis has confirmed that RBBB morphology is not associated with a lower risk for heart failure hospitalization or death following CRT, regardless of QRS duration. Interestingly though, intra-ventricular conduction delay (IVCD) morphology with a QRS duration ≥ 150 ms was still associated with a benefit in terms of reduced heart failure hospitalization and death. This suggests that among IVCD patients, some may still benefit from CRT [61].

Ongoing registry trials (such as FACT-CRT) are currently trying to identify those IVCD candidates for CRT.

The underlying heart condition and co-morbidities influence the overall prognostic and response to CRT. Although LV reverse remodeling after CRT is not affected by the duration of HF, clinical outcomes are better in patients implanted earlier in their disease course [62]. Atrial fibrillation, by comparison to sinus rhythm, is associated with an increased risk of non-response to CRT (34.5% vs 26.7%; pooled relative risk 1.32; 95% CI 1.12–1.55; P = 0.001), as demonstrated by Wilton's meta-analysis [51]. In ischemic heart disease, the benefit of CRT exists but is attenuated by comparison to non-ischemic heart disease, as shown in the MIRACLE trial [63]. Focal scar burden detected by late-Gadolinium enhancement on cardiac magnetic resonance was shown to correlate with poorer CRT response [64] as did lead localization in scar areas. Co-morbidities such as renal failure may also affect CRT. Interestingly, we have demonstrated that functional response to CRT at 1 year did not differ significantly between patients with or without chronic kidney disease and was shown to be an independent predictor of improved long-term survival in patients with renal dysfunction (eGFR < 60 ml/min/1.73m^2) [52]. Although data regarding CRT response in severe renal failure patients is scarce, data shows that dialysis does not significantly modify the adverse outcomes associated with severe renal dysfunction (eGFR < 30 ml/min/1.73m^2) following ICD/CRT-D implantation [65].

To ensure CRT response, *optimal LV lead placement is essential.* Ideally, it should be placed in the utmost late contracting segment of the left ventricle [66]. The area of delayed contraction can be previously detected by using echocardiography (tissue Doppler imaging and two-dimensional speckle tracking are considered the most sensitive) [66, 67]. Cardiac magnetic resonance and SPECT MPI may also detect it, with the advantage of offering supplemental information concerning its viability.

Reaching the target area for the LV lead is largely dependent upon the venous anatomy. Non-invasive pre-procedural visualization of the cardiac venous system can be performed using 64-slice computed tomography, which may offer important information concerning the existence of a potential target vein [68].

Sometimes the target vein is difficult to access due to tortuosity or stenosis. For overcoming anatomical obstacles, the operator has now several tools and techniques, including telescopic delivering systems [69], performing venoplasty, and the use of Lasso snaring techniques [70]. Once the target vein has been reached, electrical problems can arise such as local high pacing thresholds or phrenic capture. The introduction of quadripolar LV leads has significantly reduced these issues (Fig. 13.2) [71, 72]. Furthermore, the possibility to pace from multiple sites from the quadripolar LV lead has improved response to CRT [73]. When the target vein is unreachable or the patient has no target vein, the LV lead can still be implanted either using a transeptal approach [74] or surgically [75], and more recently, by replacing CRT with conduction system pacing

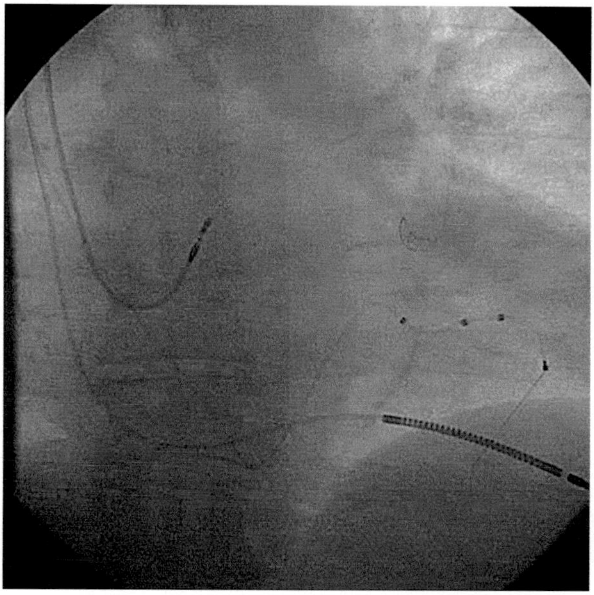

Fig. 13.2 A CRT-D system using a quadripolar LV lead

[76]. Finally, the LV lead should not be placed in an apical position but left in a basal or mid-ventricular segment [77].

Following implantation, to deliver optimal cardiac resynchronization therapy, the device has to be programmed to reach an ideal of 100% biventricular pacing [78]. Further efforts should be performed to maximize the percentage of biventricular pacing (very strict AF rate control—including atrioventricular node ablation if needed; ventricular premature beats elimination [79]).

Thus, preventing non-response should include:

- Prior electro-mechanical dyssynchrony documentation (wide QRS/LBBB) and myocardial scar burden assessment
- Identify the target area (latest contracting LV segments) for optimal LV lead positioning (preferably quadripolar lead)
- Obtaining consistent biventricular pacing (as close to 100% of the time as possible)

In the case of non-response, a protocol-driven approach for CRT optimization involving HF physicians, electrophysiologists, and focused echocardiography has been shown to improve response rates [80].

The focus over the last 10 years has been to improve the CRT response rate—by careful procedure planning (correct patient selection; scar and apical segments avoidance for LV lead implantation), the use of last-generation tools (quadripolar LV lead; special coronary sinus sheaths and catheters) and CRT optimization by the long-term use of validated automated algorithms and multipoint pacing [81].

The latest CRT randomized controlled trial published in August 2023—the AdaptReponse trial enrolled 3797 patients with HFrEF, successfully implanted with CRT systems, and followed up for a median of 59 months. Although negative in terms of the primary endpoint (by failing to demonstrate a significant added clinical benefit of using an optimized LV-only pacing algorithm versus standard biventricular pacing), the AdaptResponse trial has shown that mortality in HFrEF in the era of modern pathogenic treatment combined with CRT has dropped spectacularly (16.5% at 5 years). Furthermore, 93% of all patients either improved or stabilized clinically with CRT—which is the highest response rate yet reported in any randomized CRT trial. Response to CRT was evaluated by using a clinical composite score at 6 months (NYHA class, quality of life, adverse events, health care service utilization, device data). The exceptionally high response rate was explainable mainly by patient selection: NYHA II–III, LVEF ≤ 35%, adjudicated LBBB with a QRS duration ≥140 ms (men) or ≥130 ms (women). These are the patients for which CRT is intended [82].

Cardiac Resynchronization Therapy and Conduction System Pacing

Conduction system pacing has emerged as a new method for ventricular physiological pacing, in patients with an indication of anti-bradycardia therapy. By the ability to intercept and directly pace the ¬His bundle or its branches, conduction system pacing has the potential to correct the intra LV dyssynchrony in a more physiological way and without the need for a coronary sinus catheter. The concept is already supported by published clinical data showing that CSP can successfully replace biventricular CRT [83].

In an initial study, Vijayaraman et Al. have demonstrated that permanent His bundle pacing was achievable in 95/106 (90%) patients eligible for CRT, as a bailout for failed LV lead implantation/non-response, or as or as a primary strategy in patients with AV block, BBB, or high ventricular pacing burden as an alternative to BVP. However, because of the currently recognized electrical limitations of His bundle pacing (low sensing thresholds, atrial far field, high pacing thresholds, associated with high rates of re-interventions), just like for anti-bradycardia pacing, operators are now moving towards left bundle branch area pacing when using CSP as an alternative to biventricular CRT [84].

Some of the most compelling data comes from Vijayaraman et Al., showing that in a large cohort of 325 patients with wide QRS (152 ± 32 ms; LBBB 39%) and an LVEF < 50% (33 ± 10%), left bundle branch area pacing was successfully achieved in 85% of the cases, leading to significant QRS narrowing (137 ± 22 ms) and LVEF increase (44 ± 11%) [85]. Numerous case reports and series of patients with CSP replacing biventricular CRT have been reported since with variable but generally

Table 13.5 Clinical trials using cardiac resynchronization therapy for the treatment of more than 20,000 patients with HFrEF over the last 25 years

Trial	Patients (No.)	NYHA class	LVEF (%)	SR/AF	QRS (ms)	Year of publication
PATH CHF	41	III, IV	≤35%	SR	≥120	1999
MUSTIC-SR	58	III	≤35%	SR	≥150	2002
MIRACLE	453	III, IV	≤35%	SR	≥130	2002
MUSTIC AF	43	III	≤35%	AF	≥200	2002
MIRACLE ICD	369	III, IV	≤35%	SR	≥130	2003
MIRACLE ICD II	186	II	≤35%	SR	≥130	2004
COMPANION	1520	III, IV	≤35%	SR	≥120	2004
CARE HF	814	III, IV	≤35%	SR	≥120 & Dys	2005
CONTAK CD	227	II,IV	≤35%	SR	≥120	2006
RethinQ	172	III, IV	≤35%	SR	≤130 & Dys	2007
REVERSE	610	I, II	≤40%	SR	≥120	2009
BLOCK-HF	691	I–III	≤50%	SR/AF	Any	2013
Echo-CRT	821	III, IV	≤35%	SR	≤130 & Dys	2013
BIOPACE	1810	No	UK	SR/AF	No criteria	2013
MADIT CRT	1800	I, II	≤30%	SR	≥130	2014
RAFT	1800	II,III	≤30%	SR/AF	≥130; ≥200	2014
More CRT MMP	5850	II, III	≤35%	SR	≥130	2019
AdaptResponse	3620	II, III	≤35%	SR	≥130/140	2023

high rates of success. Recently, data from the multicenter European MELOS registry study has shown that across 14 European centers, CSP lead implantation was successfully achieved in 82.2% of cases for heart failure indications. There is a learning curve—steepest for the initial 110 cases, with heart failure, broad baseline QRS, and left ventricular end-diastolic diameter as independent predictors for CSP lead implantation failure. Complication rates were quite high—11.7%, reminding the need for safety improvement [86].

Currently, conduction system pacing can be considered as an alternative to biventricular CRT when biventricular CRT has failed. There are no long-term randomized trials supporting CSP as first-line therapy for HFrREF with LBBB, instead of biventricular CRT. Several small randomized control trials including a total of 125 patients with HFrEF and wide QRS, have shown that CSP versus biventricular CRT can achieve similar degrees of cardiac resynchronization, ventricular reverse remodeling, and clinical outcomes at 6-month follow-up [87–89].

Concerns remain regarding the long-term performance and effect of CSP leads as well as their behavior when the need comes for extraction. Furthermore, there are no dedicated cardiac implantable electronic devices to be used with CSP leads and the tools for CSP lead implantation can suffer improvements. Given the wide acceptance of biventricular CRT based on randomized control trials with long follow up, that have enrolled over 20,000 patients (Table 13.5), it is considered at a higher level of recommendation for use as CRT (Table 13.3).

Another possibility for CRT is to combine biventricular pacing with CSP, leading to a new hybrid technique: the His optimized CRT (HOT-CRT) [90] and the left bundle branch area pacing-optimized CRT (LOT-CRT) [86]. By introducing one lead for CSP (either His or LBBB area) and one LV lead via the coronary sinus, both HOT-CRT, and LOT-CRT were proven to be feasible and safe. It is also worth noting that in the latter study, LOT-CRT reduced QRS duration to a greater extent than biventricular pacing or left bundle branch area pacing alone [89].

Still, these hybrid methods require randomized controlled trials to assess the actual benefits by comparison to standard CRT, as the majority of data on CSP is observational, and long-term data on lead survival is lacking.

Conclusion

Cardiac resynchronization therapy has become part of the standard of care for heart failure patients with reduced left ventricular ejection fraction and wide QRS. Despite its role in evaluating and understanding cardiac dyssynchrony, cardiac imaging—especially echocardiography, was unable to top the classic ECG criteria (QRS morphology and duration) for patient selection.

Biventricular cardiac resynchronization therapy remains the mainstay treatment for HFrEF patients with LVEF $\leq 35\%$ and LBBB. Conduction system pacing is an emerging new technique that can offer an alternative for cases with failed biventricular CRT or can be used complementary when classic CRT is suboptimal or in the case of non-response. Further studies are required to better understand the role of conduction system pacing for CRT, as well as the role of CRT for HFrEF patients with IVCD.

References

1. Cazeau S, et al. Four chamber pacing in dilated cardiomyopathy. Pacing Clin Electrophysiol. 1994;17(11 Pt 2):1974–9.
2. Glikson M, et al. 2021 ESC Guidelines on cardiac pacing and cardiac resynchronization therapy: developed by the Task Force on cardiac pacing and cardiac resynchronization therapy of the European Society of Cardiology (ESC) with the special contribution of the European Heart Rhythm Association (EHRA). Eur Heart J. 2021;42(35):3427–520. https://doi.org/10.1093/eurheartj/ehab364.
3. Chung MK, et al. 2023 HRS/APHRS/LAHRS guideline on cardiac physiologic pacing for the avoidance and mitigation of heart failure. Heart Rhythm. 2023;20(9):e17–91. https://doi.org/10.1016/j.hrthm.2023.03.1538.
4. Nagueh SF. Mechanical dyssynchrony in congestive heart failure: diagnostic and therapeutic implications. J Am Coll Cardiol. 2008;51(1):18–22. https://doi.org/10.1016/j.jacc.2007.08.052.
5. Cazeau S, et al. Echocardiographic modeling of cardiac dyssynchrony before and during multisite stimulation: a prospective study. Pacing Clin Electrophysiol. 2003;26(1 Pt 2):137–43.

6. Ritter P, Silvestre J. AV delay optimisation by peak endocardial acceleration in cardiac resynchronisation therapy: comparison with standard echocardiographic procedure (abstract). Europace. 2004;6(Suppl. 1):209.
7. León AR, et al. Cardiac resynchronization with sequential biventricular pacing for the treatment of moderate-to-severe heart failure. J Am Coll Cardiol. 2005;46(12):2298–304. https://doi.org/10.1016/j.jacc.2005.08.032.
8. Cleland JGF, et al. The effect of cardiac resynchronization on morbidity and mortality in heart failure. N Engl J Med. 2005;352(15):1539–49. https://doi.org/10.1056/NEJMoa050496.
9. Nof E, et al. Mechanism of diastolic mitral regurgitation in candidates for cardiac resynchronization therapy. Am J Cardiol. 2006;97(11):1611–4. https://doi.org/10.1016/j.amjcard.2005.12.064.
10. Delgado V, et al. Relative merits of left ventricular dyssynchrony, left ventricular lead position, and myocardial scar to predict long-term survival of ischemic heart failure patients undergoing cardiac resynchronization therapy. Circulation. 2011;123(1):70–8. https://doi.org/10.1161/CIRCULATIONAHA.110.945345.
11. Pitzalis MV, et al. Cardiac resynchronization therapy tailored by echocardiographic evaluation of ventricular asynchrony. J Am Coll Cardiol. 2002;40(9):1615–22.
12. Khan SG, Klettas D, Kapetanakis S, Monaghan MJ. Clinical utility of speckle-tracking echocardiography in cardiac resynchronisation therapy. Echo Res Pract. 2016;3(1):R1–R11. https://doi.org/10.1530/ERP-15-0032.
13. Bax JJ, et al. Left ventricular dyssynchrony predicts benefit of cardiac resynchronization therapy in patients with end-stage heart failure before pacemaker implantation. Am J Cardiol. 2003;92(10):1238–40.
14. Bax JJ, et al. Left ventricular dyssynchrony predicts response and prognosis after cardiac resynchronization therapy. J Am Coll Cardiol. 2004;44(9):1834–40. https://doi.org/10.1016/j.jacc.2004.08.016.
15. Notabartolo D, et al. Usefulness of the peak velocity difference by tissue Doppler imaging technique as an effective predictor of response to cardiac resynchronization therapy. Am J Cardiol. 2004;94(6):817–20. https://doi.org/10.1016/j.amjcard.2004.05.072.
16. Van de Veire NR, et al. Usefulness of triplane tissue Doppler imaging to predict acute response to cardiac resynchronization therapy. Am J Cardiol. 2007;100(3):476–82. https://doi.org/10.1016/j.amjcard.2007.03.051.
17. Yu C-M, Fung W-H, Lin H, Zhang Q, Sanderson JE, Lau C-P. Predictors of left ventricular reverse remodeling after cardiac resynchronization therapy for heart failure secondary to idiopathic dilated or ischemic cardiomyopathy. Am J Cardiol. 2003;91(6):684–8.
18. Mele D, et al. Left intraventricular myocardial deformation dyssynchrony identifies responders to cardiac resynchronization therapy in patients with heart failure. Eur Heart J. 2006;27(9):1070–8. https://doi.org/10.1093/eurheartj/ehi814.
19. Suffoletto MS, Dohi K, Cannesson M, Saba S, Gorcsan J. Novel speckle-tracking radial strain from routine black-and-white echocardiographic images to quantify dyssynchrony and predict response to cardiac resynchronization therapy. Circulation. 2006;113(7):960–8. https://doi.org/10.1161/CIRCULATIONAHA.105.571455.
20. Marsan NA, et al. Real-time three-dimensional echocardiography permits quantification of left ventricular mechanical dyssynchrony and predicts acute response to cardiac resynchronization therapy. J Cardiovasc Electrophysiol. 2008;19(4):392–9. https://doi.org/10.1111/j.1540-8167.2007.01056.x.
21. Sengupta PP, et al. Left ventricular structure and function: basic science for cardiac imaging. J Am Coll Cardiol. 2006;48(10):1988–2001. https://doi.org/10.1016/j.jacc.2006.08.030.
22. Torrent-Guasp F, et al. Towards new understanding of the heart structure and function. Eur J Cardiothorac Surg. 2005;27(2):191–201. https://doi.org/10.1016/j.ejcts.2004.11.026.
23. Notomi Y, et al. Measurement of ventricular torsion by two-dimensional ultrasound speckle tracking imaging. J Am Coll Cardiol. 2005;45(12):2034–41. https://doi.org/10.1016/j.jacc.2005.02.082.

24. Fuchs E, Müller MF, Oswald H, Thöny H, Mohacsi P, Hess OM. Cardiac rotation and relaxation in patients with chronic heart failure. Eur J Heart Fail. 2004;6(6):715–22. https://doi.org/10.1016/j.ejheart.2003.12.018.
25. Matsuoka K, et al. Right ventricular apical pacing impairs left ventricular twist as well as synchrony: acute effects of right ventricular apical pacing. J Am Soc Echocardiogr. 2009;22(8):914–9. quiz 970–971. https://doi.org/10.1016/j.echo.2009.05.001.
26. Hara M, et al. Chronic effect of right ventricular pacing on left ventricular rotational synchrony in patients with complete atrioventricular block. Echocardiogr Mt Kisco N. 2011;28(1):69–75. https://doi.org/10.1111/j.1540-8175.2010.01257.x.
27. Lee Y, et al. New approach for rotational dyssynchrony using three-dimensional speckle tracking echocardiography. Echocardiogr Mt Kisco N. 2014;31(4):492–8. https://doi.org/10.1111/echo.12406.
28. Norisada K, et al. Myocardial contractile function in the region of the left ventricular pacing lead predicts the response to cardiac resynchronization therapy assessed by two-dimensional speckle tracking echocardiography. J Am Soc Echocardiogr. 2010;23(2):181–9. https://doi.org/10.1016/j.echo.2009.11.017.
29. Hor KN, et al. Presence of mechanical dyssynchrony in Duchenne muscular dystrophy. J Cardiovasc Magn Reson. 2011;13:12. https://doi.org/10.1186/1532-429X-13-12.
30. Petryka J, et al. Magnetic resonance imaging assessment of intraventricular dyssynchrony and delayed enhancement as predictors of response to cardiac resynchronization therapy in patients with heart failure of ischaemic and non-ischaemic etiologies. Eur J Radiol. 2012;81(10):2639–47. https://doi.org/10.1016/j.ejrad.2011.10.003.
31. Chan Y-H, Wang C-L, Kuo C-T, Yeh Y-H, Wu C-T, Wu L-S. Clinical assessment and implication of left ventricular mechanical dyssynchrony in patients with heart failure. Acta Cardiol Sin. 2013;29(6):505–14.
32. Chen J, Garcia EV, Bax JJ, Iskandrian AE, Borges-Neto S, Soman P. SPECT myocardial perfusion imaging for the assessment of left ventricular mechanical dyssynchrony. J Nucl Cardiol. 2011;18(4):685–94. https://doi.org/10.1007/s12350-011-9392-x.
33. Boogers MM, et al. Quantitative gated SPECT-derived phase analysis on gated myocardial perfusion SPECT detects left ventricular dyssynchrony and predicts response to cardiac resynchronization therapy. J Nucl Med. 2009;50(5):718–25. https://doi.org/10.2967/jnumed.108.060657.
34. Koepfli P, et al. Left bundle branch block causes relative but not absolute septal underperfusion during exercise. Eur Heart J. 2009;30(24):2993–9. https://doi.org/10.1093/eurheartj/ehp372.
35. Bakos Z, et al. A comparison between radial strain evaluation by speckle-tracking echocardiography and cardiac magnetic resonance imaging, for assessment of suitable segments for left ventricular lead placement in cardiac resynchronization therapy. Europace. 2014;16(12):1779–86. https://doi.org/10.1093/europace/euu167.
36. Galli E, et al. The saga of dyssynchrony imaging: are we getting to the point. Front Cardiovasc Med. 2023;10. [Online]. Available: https://www.frontiersin.org/articles/10.3389/fcvm.2023.1111538. Accessed 15 Oct 2023.
37. Cazeau S, et al. Effects of multisite biventricular pacing in patients with heart failure and intraventricular conduction delay. N Engl J Med. 2001;344(12):873–80. https://doi.org/10.1056/NEJM200103223441202.
38. Auricchio A, et al. Clinical efficacy of cardiac resynchronization therapy using left ventricular pacing in heart failure patients stratified by severity of ventricular conduction delay. J Am Coll Cardiol. 2003;42(12):2109–16.
39. Bristow MR, et al. Cardiac-resynchronization therapy with or without an implantable defibrillator in advanced chronic heart failure. N Engl J Med. 2004;350(21):2140–50. https://doi.org/10.1056/NEJMoa032423.
40. Linde C, et al. Randomized trial of cardiac resynchronization in mildly symptomatic heart failure patients and in asymptomatic patients with left ventricular dysfunction and previous

heart failure symptoms. J Am Coll Cardiol. 2008;52(23):1834–43. https://doi.org/10.1016/j.jacc.2008.08.027.
41. Tang ASL, et al. Cardiac-resynchronization therapy for mild-to-moderate heart failure. N Engl J Med. 2010;363(25):2385–95. https://doi.org/10.1056/NEJMoa1009540.
42. Moss AJ, et al. Cardiac-resynchronization therapy for the prevention of heart-failure events. N Engl J Med. 2009;361(14):1329–38. https://doi.org/10.1056/NEJMoa0906431.
43. Goldenberg I, et al. Survival with cardiac-resynchronization therapy in mild heart failure. N Engl J Med. 2014;370(18):1694–701. https://doi.org/10.1056/NEJMoa1401426.
44. Ruschitzka F, et al. Cardiac-resynchronization therapy in heart failure with a narrow QRS complex. N Engl J Med. 2013;369(15):1395–405. https://doi.org/10.1056/NEJMoa1306687.
45. Sweeney MO, et al. Adverse effect of ventricular pacing on heart failure and atrial fibrillation among patients with normal baseline QRS duration in a clinical trial of pacemaker therapy for sinus node dysfunction. Circulation. 2003;107(23):2932–7. https://doi.org/10.1161/01.CIR.0000072769.17295.B1.
46. Connolly SJ, et al. Effects of physiologic pacing versus ventricular pacing on the risk of stroke and death due to cardiovascular causes. Canadian Trial of Physiologic Pacing Investigators. N Engl J Med. 2000;342(19):1385–91. https://doi.org/10.1056/NEJM200005113421902.
47. Wilkoff BL, et al. Dual-chamber pacing or ventricular backup pacing in patients with an implantable defibrillator: the Dual Chamber and VVI Implantable Defibrillator (DAVID) Trial. JAMA. 2002;288(24):3115–23.
48. Curtis AB, et al. Biventricular pacing for atrioventricular block and systolic dysfunction. N Engl J Med. 2013;368(17):1585–93. https://doi.org/10.1056/NEJMoa1210356.
49. Marai I, et al. Improvement of congestive heart failure by upgrading of conventional to resynchronization pacemakers. Pacing Clin Electrophysiol. 2006;29(8):880–4. https://doi.org/10.1111/j.1540-8159.2006.00455.x.
50. Linde C, et al. Long-term benefits of biventricular pacing in congestive heart failure: results from the MUltisite STimulation in cardiomyopathy (MUSTIC) study. J Am Coll Cardiol. 2002;40(1):111–8.
51. Wilton SB, Leung AA, Ghali WA, Faris P, Exner DV. Outcomes of cardiac resynchronization therapy in patients with versus those without atrial fibrillation: a systematic review and meta-analysis. Heart Rhythm. 2011;8(7):1088–94. https://doi.org/10.1016/j.hrthm.2011.02.014.
52. Bogdan S, et al. Functional response to cardiac resynchronization therapy in patients with renal dysfunction and subsequent long-term mortality. J Cardiovasc Electrophysiol. 2014;25(11):1188–95. https://doi.org/10.1111/jce.12463.
53. Yu C-M, Sanderson JE, Gorcsan J. Echocardiography, dyssynchrony, and the response to cardiac resynchronization therapy. Eur Heart J. 2010;31(19):2326–37. https://doi.org/10.1093/eurheartj/ehq263.
54. McAlister FA, et al. Cardiac resynchronization therapy for patients with left ventricular systolic dysfunction: a systematic review. JAMA. 2007;297(22):2502–14. https://doi.org/10.1001/jama.297.22.2502.
55. Chung ES, et al. Results of the predictors of response to CRT (PROSPECT) trial. Circulation. 2008;117(20):2608–16. https://doi.org/10.1161/CIRCULATIONAHA.107.743120.
56. Miyazaki C, et al. Dyssynchrony indices to predict response to cardiac resynchronization therapy: a comprehensive prospective single-center study. Circ Heart Fail. 2010;3(5):565–73. https://doi.org/10.1161/CIRCHEARTFAILURE.108.848085.
57. Pitzalis MV, et al. Ventricular asynchrony predicts a better outcome in patients with chronic heart failure receiving cardiac resynchronization therapy. J Am Coll Cardiol. 2005;45(1):65–9. https://doi.org/10.1016/j.jacc.2004.09.058.
58. Stankovic I, et al. Relationship of visually assessed apical rocking and septal flash to response and long-term survival following cardiac resynchronization therapy (PREDICT-CRT). Eur Heart J Cardiovasc Imaging. 2016;17(3):262–9. https://doi.org/10.1093/ehjci/jev288.
59. McDonagh TA, et al. 2021 ESC Guidelines for the diagnosis and treatment of acute and chronic heart failure: developed by the Task Force for the diagnosis and treatment of acute and

chronic heart failure of the European Society of Cardiology (ESC) with the special contribution of the Heart Failure Association (HFA) of the ESC. Eur Heart J. 2021;42(36):3599–726. https://doi.org/10.1093/eurheartj/ehab368.
60. Kutyifa V, et al. PR interval identifies clinical response in patients with non-left bundle branch block: a multicenter automatic defibrillator implantation trial-cardiac resynchronization therapy substudy. Circ Arrhythm Electrophysiol. 2014;7(4):645–51. https://doi.org/10.1161/CIRCEP.113.001299.
61. Friedman DJ, et al. Cardiac resynchronization therapy improves outcomes in patients with intraventricular conduction delay but not right bundle branch block: a patient-level meta-analysis of randomized controlled trials. Circulation. 2023;147(10):812–23. https://doi.org/10.1161/CIRCULATIONAHA.122.062124.
62. Verbrugge FH, et al. Time from emerging heart failure symptoms to cardiac resynchronisation therapy: impact on clinical response. Heart Br Card Soc. 2013;99(5):314–9. https://doi.org/10.1136/heartjnl-2012-302807.
63. Abraham WT, et al. Cardiac resynchronization in chronic heart failure. N Engl J Med. 2002;346(24):1845–53. https://doi.org/10.1056/NEJMoa013168.
64. Chen Z, et al. Focal but not diffuse myocardial fibrosis burden quantification using cardiac magnetic resonance imaging predicts left ventricular reverse modeling following cardiac resynchronization therapy. J Cardiovasc Electrophysiol. 2016;27(2):203–9. https://doi.org/10.1111/jce.12855.
65. Bogdan S, et al. Clinical outcomes in patients with severe renal dysfunction including dialysis following defibrillator implantation. Am J Nephrol. 2015;42(4):295–304. https://doi.org/10.1159/000440772.
66. Khan FZ, et al. Targeted left ventricular lead placement to guide cardiac resynchronization therapy: the TARGET study: a randomized, controlled trial. J Am Coll Cardiol. 2012;59(17):1509–18. https://doi.org/10.1016/j.jacc.2011.12.030.
67. Risum N, et al. Left bundle-branch block: the relationship between electrocardiogram electrical activation and echocardiography mechanical contraction. Am Heart J. 2013;166(2):340–8. https://doi.org/10.1016/j.ahj.2013.04.005.
68. Van de Veire NR, et al. Non-invasive visualization of the cardiac venous system in coronary artery disease patients using 64-slice computed tomography. J Am Coll Cardiol. 2006;48(9):1832–8. https://doi.org/10.1016/j.jacc.2006.07.042.
69. Worley SJ. CRT delivery systems based on guide support for LV lead placement. Heart Rhythm. 2009;6(9):1383–7. https://doi.org/10.1016/j.hrthm.2009.04.038.
70. Soga Y, et al. Efficacy of coronary venoplasty for left ventricular lead implantation. Circ J. 2007;71(9):1442–5.
71. Shetty AK, Duckett SG, Bostock J, Rosenthal E, Rinaldi CA. Use of a quadripolar left ventricular lead to achieve successful implantation in patients with previous failed attempts at cardiac resynchronization therapy. Europace. 2011;13(7):992–6. https://doi.org/10.1093/europace/eur032.
72. Ohlow M-A, Lauer B, Brunelli M, Daralammouri Y, Geller C. The use of a quadripolar left ventricular lead increases successful implantation rates in patients with phrenic nerve stimulation and/or high pacing thresholds undergoing cardiac resynchronisation therapy with conventional bipolar leads. Indian Pacing Electrophysiol J. 2013;13(2):58–65.
73. Pappone C, et al. Abstract 13412: cardiac resynchronization therapy with multisite left ventricular pacing improves acute hemodynamic response in patients. Circulation. 2012;126(21 Suppl):A13412.
74. Bracke FA, van Gelder BM, Dekker LRC, Houthuizen P, ter Woorst JF, Teijink JA. Left ventricular endocardial pacing in cardiac resynchronisation therapy: moving from bench to bedside. Neth Hear J. 2012;20(3):118–24. https://doi.org/10.1007/s12471-011-0210-5.
75. Ailawadi G, et al. Surgically placed left ventricular leads provide similar outcomes to percutaneous leads in patients with failed coronary sinus lead placement. Heart Rhythm. 2010;7(5):619–25. https://doi.org/10.1016/j.hrthm.2010.01.014.

76. Burri H, et al. EHRA clinical consensus statement on conduction system pacing implantation: endorsed by the Asia Pacific Heart Rhythm Society (APHRS), Canadian Heart Rhythm Society (CHRS), and Latin American Heart Rhythm Society (LAHRS). Europace. 2023;25(4):1208–36. https://doi.org/10.1093/europace/euad043.
77. Singh JP, et al. Left ventricular lead position and clinical outcome in the multicenter automatic defibrillator implantation trial–cardiac resynchronization therapy (MADIT-CRT) trial. Circulation. 2011;123(11):1159–66. https://doi.org/10.1161/CIRCULATIONAHA.110.000646.
78. Hayes DL, et al. Cardiac resynchronization therapy and the relationship of percent biventricular pacing to symptoms and survival. Heart Rhythm. 2011;8(9):1469–75. https://doi.org/10.1016/j.hrthm.2011.04.015.
79. Lakkireddy D, et al. Radiofrequency ablation of premature ventricular ectopy improves the efficacy of cardiac resynchronization therapy in nonresponders. J Am Coll Cardiol. 2012;60(16):1531–9. https://doi.org/10.1016/j.jacc.2012.06.035.
80. Mullens W, et al. Insights from a cardiac resynchronization optimization clinic as part of a heart failure disease management program. J Am Coll Cardiol. 2009;53(9):765–73. https://doi.org/10.1016/j.jacc.2008.11.024.
81. Leclercq C, et al. Cardiac resynchronization therapy non-responder to responder conversion rate in the more response to cardiac resynchronization therapy with MultiPoint Pacing (MORE-CRT MPP) study: results from Phase I. Eur Heart J. 2019;40(35):2979–87. https://doi.org/10.1093/eurheartj/ehz109.
82. Wilkoff BL, et al. Adaptive versus conventional cardiac resynchronisation therapy in patients with heart failure (AdaptResponse): a global, prospective, randomised controlled trial. Lancet. 2023;402(10408):1147–57. https://doi.org/10.1016/S0140-6736(23)00912-1.
83. Bogdan S, Ababei A, Glikson M. How to treat cardiac dyssynchrony in heart failure with reduced ejection fraction—a review. Romanian J Cardiol. 2024;34(1):1–6.
84. Sharma PS, et al. Permanent His-bundle pacing as an alternative to biventricular pacing for cardiac resynchronization therapy: a multicenter experience. Heart Rhythm. 2018;15(3):413–20. https://doi.org/10.1016/j.hrthm.2017.10.014.
85. Vijayaraman P, et al. Left bundle branch area pacing for cardiac resynchronization therapy: results from the international LBBAP Collaborative Study Group. JACC Clin Electrophysiol. 2021;7(2):135–47. https://doi.org/10.1016/j.jacep.2020.08.015.
86. Jastrzębski M, et al. Left bundle branch-optimized cardiac resynchronization therapy (LOT-CRT): results from an international LBBAP collaborative study group. Heart Rhythm. 2022;19(1):13–21. https://doi.org/10.1016/j.hrthm.2021.07.057.
87. Vinther M, Risum N, Svendsen JH, Møgelvang R, Philbert BT. A randomized trial of his pacing versus biventricular pacing in symptomatic HF patients with left bundle branch block (his-alternative). JACC Clin Electrophysiol. 2021;7(11):1422–32. https://doi.org/10.1016/j.jacep.2021.04.003.
88. Pujol-Lopez M, et al. Conduction system pacing vs biventricular pacing in heart failure and wide QRS patients: LEVEL-AT trial. JACC Clin Electrophysiol. 2022;8(11):1431–45. https://doi.org/10.1016/j.jacep.2022.08.001.
89. Wang Y, et al. Randomized trial of left bundle branch vs biventricular pacing for cardiac resynchronization therapy. J Am Coll Cardiol. 2022;80(13):1205–16. https://doi.org/10.1016/j.jacc.2022.07.019.
90. Upadhyay GA, et al. On-treatment comparison between corrective His bundle pacing and biventricular pacing for cardiac resynchronization: a secondary analysis of the His-SYNC Pilot Trial. Heart Rhythm. 2019;16(12):1797–807. https://doi.org/10.1016/j.hrthm.2019.05.009.

Chapter 14
Mechanical Circulatory Support

Sylvie Baudart and Liviu Klein

Introduction and Epidemiology

Heart failure incidence and prevalence are increasing due to the success in treating acute myocardial infarction with primary angioplasty and due to the overall increase in life expectancy, with a significant increase in the elderly population. In the United States, 6.5 million patients have heart failure, with a similar number in Western Europe [1]. The incidence in the United States is close to 800,000 new cases annually, with more than 300,000 deaths/year being attributed to heart failure, and with an annual cost to manage these patients estimated at over $30 billion [1]. Close to 40% of the heart failure patients have heart failure with reduced ejection fraction, and approximately 5–10% of these patients have advanced disease, yielding an estimated cohort of 100,000–200,000 patients who have a high 1-year mortality (over 30%) and can benefit of advanced therapies such as heart transplantation or ventricular assist devices [1].

The number of heart transplants performed worldwide is limited due to donor availability. Advances in organ preservation [e.g. temperature control transport such as Paragonix SherpaPak (Paragonix Technologies, Waltham, Massachusetts, United States), or ex-vivo perfusion such as TransMedics OCS Heart System (TransMedics Inc., Andover, Massachusetts, United States) and XVIVO Heart Assist (XVIVO, Gothenburg, Sweden)], utilization of donors after cardiovascular death and donors with hepatitis C, has allowed a marked increase in the number of available organs [2]. In 2023, over 4000 adult heart transplants were performed in the United States, and about 2300 in Europe [3, 4]. However, the number of waitlisted candidates for heart transplant has simultaneously increased (44% increase in the United States in the last 12 years) [5] thus leaving the supply-demand gap unchanged and the need

S. Baudart · L. Klein (✉)
Advanced Heart Failure Comprehensive Care Center, San Francisco, CA, USA
e-mail: Liviu.Klein@ucsf.edu

M. Dorobanţu et al. (eds.), *Current Approach to Heart Failure*, https://doi.org/10.1007/978-3-031-96562-3_14

for mechanical support device alternatives critical. The revision of the donor heart allocation system in 2018 in the United States has transformed the type and utilization of mechanical circulatory support devices with an increase in patients bridged to transplant via acute (temporary) devices such as extracorporeal membrane oxygenation (ECMO), intra-aortic ballon pump (IABP), and microaxial flow pump (Impella) and a simultaneous decrease in durable left ventricular assist device (LVAD) [6, 7]. Simultaneously patients on durable LVAD have seen an increase in wait time to transplant since the new allocation system was implemented and the LVAD prioritization was downgraded [8].

The clinical profile of the advanced heart failure patients includes several of the following characteristics despite optimal medical and electrical therapies: (1) severe symptoms with New York Heart Association (NYHA) functional class III or IV, continuously for at least 2 months; (2) severe impairment of functional capacity demonstrated by either inability to exercise, a 6-min walk distance below 300 m, or a peak oxygen consumption below 12–14 ml/kg/min; (3) recurrent episodes of hospitalization with signs of fluid retention and/or peripheral hypoperfusion; (4) left ventricular ejection fraction below 25–30%; (5) high left and/or right ventricular filling pressures with low cardiac output at cardiac catheterization; and (6) evidence of systemic organ injury, in particular renal and hepatic dysfunctions (hyponatremia, elevated blood urea nitrogen, creatinine and bilirubin levels) [9]. In our center we emphasize to the treating cardiologists that any two or more of these findings should prompt referral to our comprehensive heart failure program for consideration of advanced therapies.

To further refine the prognosis and the risk of surgical intervention in advanced heart failure patients, the Interagency Registry for Mechanically Assisted Circulatory Support (INTERMACS) scale assigns patients into seven levels according to their hemodynamic profile and functional capacity (Table 14.1) [10]. Based on this risk profile, the time frame for intervention should be within hours (profile 1) or days (profile 2), or more elective such as weeks to months (profiles 3–6). During the first decade of modern circulatory support (2000–2010) most patients implanted with durable LVAD were profiles 1 (40–50% of patients) or 2 (25–35% of patients) and, as consequence, the long-term survival was marginal [11]. Mortality occurred during the initial hospitalization for LVAD surgery, closely related to the degree of organ compromise and urgency at the time of implantation, which might have been associated with irreversible organ dysfunction. The current approach to LVAD implantation puts a great emphasis on patient selection and pre-operative optimization. In selected patients, temporary mechanical assist devices such as Impella 5.5 are used to optimize patients' hemodynamics, renal function, nutrition and pre habilitation [12]. Great strides have been made in the last decade to the pump design and long-term post LVAD implant medical management yielding significant improvement in survival (1- and 5-year survival of 83% and 52%, respectively) with a lower rate of adverse events [13].

Table 14.1 Interagency Registry for Mechanically Assisted Circulatory Support (INTERMACS) clinical profiles

Profile 1	Critical Cardiogenic Shock ("crash and burn")	Patients with life-threatening hypotension despite rapidly escalating inotropic support, critical organ hypoperfusion, often confirmed by worsening acidosis and/or lactate levels
Profile 2	Progressive Decline ("sliding on inotropes")	Patient with declining function despite intravenous inotropic support; may be manifested by worsening renal function, nutritional depletion, or inability to restore volume balance. Also describes declining status in patients unable to tolerate inotropic therapy
Profile 3	Stable but Inotrope Dependent ("dependent stability")	Patient with stable blood pressure, organ function, nutrition, and symptoms on continuous intravenous inotropic support (or a temporary circulatory support device or both), but demonstrating repeated failure to wean from support because of recurrent symptomatic hypotension or renal dysfunction
Profile 4	Resting Symptoms ("frequent flyer")	Patient can be stabilized close to normal volume status but experiences daily symptoms of congestion at rest or during activities of daily living. Doses of diuretics generally fluctuate at very high levels. More intensive management and surveillance strategies should be considered, which may in some cases reveal poor compliance that would compromise outcomes with any therapy. Some patients may shuttle between profiles 4 and 5
Profile 5	Exertion Intolerant ("housebound")	Comfortable at rest and with activities of daily living but unable to engage in any other activity, living predominantly within the house. Patients are comfortable at rest without congestive symptoms, but may have underlying refractory elevated volume status, often with renal dysfunction. If underlying nutritional status and organ function are marginal, patient may be more at risk than in profile 4 and require definitive intervention
Profile 6	Exertion Limited ("walking wounded")	Patient without evidence of fluid overload is comfortable at rest, and with activities of daily living and minor activities outside the home, but fatigues after few minutes of any meaningful activity. Attribution to cardiac limitation requires careful measurement of peak VO2, in some cases with hemodynamic monitoring to confirm severity of cardiac impairment
Profile 7	Advanced New York Heart Association functional class III	A placeholder for more precise specification in future, this level includes patients who are without current or recent episodes of unstable fluid balance, living comfortably with meaningful activity limited to mild physical exertion

Adapted from Ref. [10]
Possible profile modifiers are the need for temporary circulatory support (TCS) for profiles 1–3; arrhythmias (A) for profiles 1–7; and frequent flyer (FF) for profiles 3–6

Acute (Temporary) Mechanical Circulatory Support Devices

These devices are used primarily in three patient populations including high-risk percutaneous coronary interventions, post-cardiotomy failure to wean from the cardiopulmonary bypass, and cardiogenic shock. Although the devices used are similar for all these indications, the current chapter will address only the setting of cardiogenic shock.

Cardiogenic shock occurs secondary to acute left or right ventricular systolic dysfunction, acute (on chronic) aortic or mitral valvular disease, and vasodilatory abnormalities in patients with acute myocardial infarction, out of hospital cardiac arrest, and worsening chronic heart failure. In clinical practice, patients with cardiogenic shock represent a spectrum of disease that can be classified via the SCAI shock stages A-E (A: at risk E: extremis) depending on the level of blood pressure, heart rate, intracardiac filling pressures, cardiac output, tissue perfusion (lactate, urine output) and need for vasoactive medications [14, 15]. Potential benefits of temporary mechanical circulatory support devices in this setting include the ability to provide circulatory support (thereby maintaining vital organ perfusion and preventing systemic shock syndrome); provide ventricular unloading (left, right, biventricular) in order to reduce intracardiac filling pressures (thereby reducing congestion and/or pulmonary edema), reduce ventricular volumes, wall stress, and myocardial oxygen consumption; and augment myocardial perfusion by increasing coronary blood flow (theoretically also limiting the infarct size in the setting of myocardial infarction). Each of the currently available devices (Fig. 14.1) is designed to tackle the entire equation (i.e. circulatory support, ventricular unloading, myocardial perfusion) but primarily address specific aspects of that equation [14–16].

The temporary mechanical circulatory support devices can be largely categorized by the amount of cardiac support or flow they provide. The lowest amount of flow device is the IABP that has been in use since the early 1960s. This pulsatile device primarily functions by augmenting the diastolic pressure and, as a result, increasing coronary perfusion. The ventricular unloading aspect of the IABP (counter pulsation) relies on an intact ventricular-vascular coupling and may be diminished in patients with sicker left ventricles. The third part of the equation (i.e. circulatory support) relies on the augmented mean arterial pressure that is driven primarily by the augmented diastolic pressure. While the IABP positively impacts coronary perfusion, it augments the cardiac output by only 0.5 liters per minute (LPM). Its usefulness is therefore limited to patients in the early shock phase, in patients with active coronary ischemia or ischemic ventricular arrhythmias. While the majority of IABP are placed in the femoral artery, they can also be inserted percutaneously via the axillary artery allowing patient mobilization [16, 17].

The Impella left sided micro-axial temporary ventricular assist devices (Abiomed, Danvers, Massachusetts, United States) can provide up to 5.3 LPM of flow. The right sided Impella RP can provide up to 4.3 LPM of flow and is designed to support the right ventricle by draining blood from the inferior vena cava and pumping it into the pulmonary artery. The left sided support Impella pumps (CPs or 5.5) can provide up to 5.3 LPM and work by pulling blood from the left ventricle and directly ejecting it into the ascending aorta, past the aortic valve. These pumps effectively increase mean arterial pressure and directly unload the left ventricle, thereby reducing ventricular pressure. As a result of the increased mean aortic pressure and lower ventricular pressure, the trans myocardial perfusion gradient changes and coronary perfusion will increase [16, 17]. The Impella 5.5 can be placed in the subclavian or

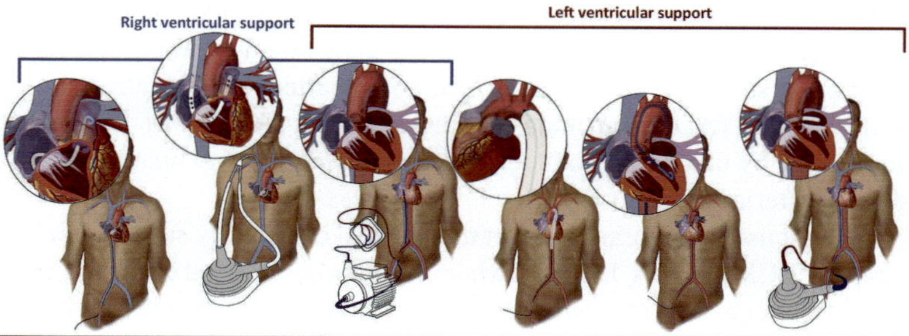

	Impella RP	TandemHeart RA-PA	VA-ECMO	IABP	Impella (2.5, CP, 5.0, 5.5)	TandemHeart LA-FA
Flow	max 4.0 l/min	max 4.0 l/min	max 7.0 l/min	0.5 l/min	2.5 - 5.5 l/min	max 4.0 l/min
Pump Speed	33000 rpm	max 7500 rpm	max 5000 rpm	NA	max 51,000 rpm	max 7500 rpm
Mechanism	Axial flow continuous pump (RA-to-PA)	Centrifugal flow continuous pump (RA-to-PA)	Centrifugal flow continuous pump (RA-to-AO)	Balloon inflation-deflation (AO)	Axial flow continuous pump (LV-to-AO)	Centrifugal flow continuous pump (LA-to-AO)
Cannula Size	22 F venous	29 F venous	14-19 F arterial 17-21 F venous	7-8 F arterial	13-21 F arterial	12-19 F arterial 21 F venous
Insertion/Placement	Femoral vein	Internal jugular vein	Femoral vein Femoral artery	Femoral artery Axillary artery	Femoral artery Axillary artery	Femoral artery Femoral vein
LV Unloading	-	-	-	+	+ to +++	++
RV Unloading	+	+	++	-	-	-
Cardiac Power	-	-	↑↑	↑	↑↑	↑↑
Afterload	-	-	↑↑	↓	↓↓	↑
Coronary Perfusion	-	-	-	↑	↑	-
Considerations	• *RECOVER RIGHT: 73% survival-to-30 days in RVF post LVAD, AMI or cardiotomy* • *May 2019 - FDA post-approval study: 33% survival-to-30 days*	• *IJ access may facilitate early ambulation*	• *Bi-V + oxygenation support for CS following:* *- AMI, ADHF or cardiac arrest* *- Cardiotomy* *- Myocarditis* *- Allograft rejection*	• *Requires stable cardiac rhythm and native heart function* • *May consider in select cases of post-AMI mechanical complications*	• *June 2008 – FDA 510(k) approval for HR-PCI* • *April 2016: Expanded Indication for CS* • *Contraindicated with mechanical aortic valve, LV thrombus*	• *Requires transseptal access* • *Oxygenator may be added to the circuit*

Fig. 14.1 The hemodynamic profiles of the various circulatory support devices available for treatment of cardiogenic shock. *ADHF* acute decompensated heart failure, *AMI* acute myocardial infarction, *AO* aorta, *Bi-V* biventricular, *CS* cardiogenic shock, *FA* femoral artery, *FDA* Food and Drug Administration, *HR-PCI* high risk percutaneous coronary intervention, *IABP* intra-aortic balloon pump, *IJ* internal jugular, *LA* left atrium, *LV* left ventricular, *LVAD* left ventricular assist device, *PA* pulmonary artery, *RA* right atrium, *RPM* revolutions per minute, *RV* right ventricular, *RVF* right ventricular failure, *VA-ECMO* venoarterial extracorporeal membrane oxygenation. (With permission from Ref. [14])

axillary artery thereby facilitating patient's mobility. Its sturdiness and reliability allow patients to remain on support for weeks to allow potential recovery or become optimized for heart transplant or durable LVAD surgical candidacy [12].

Finally, centrifugal flow pumps are extracorporeal, provide the greatest amount of flow and include a wide array of configurations with or without gas exchange (Fig. 14.1). The Tandem Heart (Cardiac Assist, Pittsburgh, Pennsylvania, United States) configuration supports the left ventricle by draining blood from the left atrium (via a trans-septal catheter) and delivering it to the systemic circulation via the femoral artery. The Tandem Heart effectively tackles all three components of the equation on the left side by unloading the left ventricle, by reducing left atrial volume (reducing left ventricular preload), and by increasing mean arterial pressure, which leads to increase in the coronary perfusion pressure [16, 17].

The Centrimag (Abbott Medical, Pleasanton, California, United States) BiVAD system utilizes two separate, independent centrifugal pumps thereby providing biventricular support (right atrium to pulmonary artery and left atrium to ascending aorta). The BiVAD Centrimag addresses each element of the equation biventricularly by unloading both ventricles, reducing preload bilaterally and increasing mean arterial pressure.

The most used temporary support mechanical circulatory support device remains peripheral ECMO (pVA ECMO) whereby blood is drained from the right atrium and inferior vena cava, oxygenated and propelled to the systemic arterial circulation via the femoral artery. The VA ECMO system is distinct from all the other devices by its flow capability (up to 7 LPM), its bypassing of the lung and its gas exchange capability as blood flows through an oxygenator that efficiently adds oxygen and removes carbon dioxide. However, by supporting blood flow in a *retrograde* fashion it increases left ventricular afterload and may lead to worsening left ventricular function, left ventricular dilatation and pulmonary edema. Patients placed on pVA ECMO may need additional interventions to unload the left ventricle such as inotropic agents, mechanical devices such as IABP or Impella or surgical procedures (atrial septostomy, left atrial or ventricular vent).

A clear understanding of each device strengths and weakness [15–21] is crucial to utilize the configuration that will best match the patient's cardiogenic shock pattern while minimizing complications (Table 14.2). Patients are kept on support until end organ function has improved and a decision of weaning for recovery or proceeding to permanent support is achieved, or palliative withdrawal is instituted.

In our center, we use preferentially the Centrimag pVA ECMO system for patients in cardiogenic shock, due to its ease of implantation (percutaneous, surgical), portability ("ECMO to go") and versatility, and we use a combination of pharmacological (i.e. dobutamine or epinephrine) and mechanical (IABP or Impella) unloading to achieve optimal hemodynamics. Our initial approach is to quickly achieve normal perfusion (mean arterial pressure above 65 mmHg, lactate level below 2 mmol/L), while maintaining the acid base equilibrium (pH 7.3–7.4), adequate tissue oxygenation (hematocrit above 30%), and urine output (greater than 1.5–2 mL/kg/h). We anticoagulate all patients with intravenous heparin, targeting unfractionated heparin level of 0.3–0.5 U/mL. When hemodynamics have improved (right atrial pressure < 10–12 mmHg, pulmonary capillary wedge pressures < 20 mmHg), we perform echocardiography guided turndown of the pVA ECMO. If cardiac function has improved, we gradually decrease the amount of support (from full support of 4–5 LPM to minimal support of 1.5 LPM), while paying attention to left ventricular size, severity of mitral regurgitation, right ventricular function (fractional area change, free wall s'), hemodynamics (mean arterial pressure, right atrial pressure and pulmonary capillary wedge pressures) and peripheral oxygen saturation. If the weaning is successful, the ECMO is explanted, and patients are bridged via inotropes to oral heart failure therapies. If the weaning is unsuccessful, the patients can either be implanted with durable ventricular assist devices or undergo heart transplant. The pVA ECMO often requires patients to be on bedrest which increases risks of deconditioning. Our approach is to transition patient off

Table 14.2 Acute (temporary) mechanical circulatory support device contraindications and complications

	IABP	Impella	Tandem heart	VA-ECMO
Contraindications	Moderate to severe AI	Moderate to severe AI	Moderate to severe AI	Moderate to severe AI
	Severe PVD	Severe PVD	Severe PVD	Severe PVD
	Aortic disease (atherosclerosis, dissection)	Contraindication to anticoagulation	Contraindication to anticoagulation	Contraindication to anticoagulation
		LV thrombus	LA thrombus	
		Mechanical AV	HIT or DIC	
		AV area < 0.6 cm^2	VSD	
Complications	Limb ischemia	Limb ischemia	Limb ischemia	Limb ischemia
	Vascular trauma	Vascular trauma	Vascular trauma	Vascular trauma
	Infection	Infection	Infection	Infection
	Stroke	Stroke	Stroke	Stroke
	Acute kidney injury			
	Thrombocytopenia	Hemolysis	Hemolysis	Hemolysis
			Air embolism	Air embolism
			Thromboembolism	Thromboembolism
	IABP rupture	Device migration	Device dislodgement	Bleeding
		Device thrombosis		
	Bowel ischemia		Cardiac tamponade	Compartment syndrome
				Peripheral nerve injury
Bleeding/hemolysis	+	++	++	++
Peripheral vascular complications	+	++	+++	++++

AI aortic insufficiency, *AV* aortic valve, *DIC* disseminated intravascular coagulation, *HIT* heparin-induced thrombocytopenia, *IABP* intra-aortic balloon pump, *LA* left atrium, *LV* left ventricle, *PVD* peripheral vascular disease, *VA-ECMO* veno-arterial extracorporeal membrane oxygenation, *VSD* ventricular septal defect pVA ECMO as soon as possible, often to an axillary Impella 5.5 if their right ventricular function will tolerate it. The device will continue to support the patient's hemodynamics while allowing effective rehabilitation and nutritional enhancement. This strategy is particularly insightful if the patient is too be bridged to a durable LVAD as it allows us to evaluate the response of the patient's right ventricle to single sided left ventricular support.

Durable (Permanent) Ventricular Assist Devices

Durable ventricular assist devices are evolving into an effective and reasonably cost-effective therapy for a growing population of patients with advanced heart failure. They provide significant left ventricular unloading and increased cardiac output and improve end-organ function. Patients supported with ventricular assist device enjoy a 1 and 5-year survival of 83% and 52%, respectively and marked improvement in symptoms and quality of life [13]. While the traditional indications for implantation were divided into bridge to transplantation, bridge to decision and destination therapy, the improved reliability of today's devices, enhanced medical management and lack of available organs for transplantation has led to a paradigm shift where device is used for long term, without a transplant associated label [22–24].

First generation positive displacement pulsatile devices (e.g. Thoratec HeartMate XVE, Novacor LVAS) used a diaphragm and unidirectional valves to mimic the pulsatile cardiac cycle through diastolic filling and systolic emptying of the pump. The use of HeartMate XVE in the Randomized Evaluation of Mechanical Assistance for the Treatment of Congestive Heart Failure (REMATCH) trial [25] opened the door for mechanical circulatory support for long-term use in transplant ineligible patients ("destination therapy"). However, due to their size, adverse events and limited durability (18–24 months), their use was very limited, and these pumps were eventually discontinued in mid to late 2000s.

Second and third generation continuous flow pumps are smaller, enjoy simpler implantation, and have more limited blood contacting area with fewer moving parts and without valves, air vents and compliance chambers, leading to longer durability and reduced risks for thromboembolism, infection, and malfunction. They use a permanent magnetic field designed to rapidly spin a single impeller supported by mechanical, hydrodynamic (using a layer of blood—blood bearing—to lift the rotor) or magnetic bearings (using magnetic bearings to levitate the rotor) [24]. Second-generation axial pumps have the impeller outflow directed parallel to the axis of rotation with the rotor spinning on mechanical (Thoratec HeartMate II, Jarvik 2000) [26, 27] or contact-free bearings (Berlin Heart Incor). Third-generation centrifugal pumps have the impeller outflow perpendicular to the axis of rotation (Medtronic HeartWare Ventricular Assist Device [HVAD] and Abbott HeartMate III) [28, 29]. Additionally, the HeartMate III fully magnetically levitated design allows the impeller to spin without any points of contact thus reducing friction and heat generation. Since the removal from the market of the HeartWare HVAD pump, the HeartMate III is the only durable centrifugal pump available for durable LVAD implantation.

The pump blood flow is directly proportional to the rotor speed and inversely proportional to the pressure differential across the pump (i.e. head pressure, the pressure difference between the left ventricle and aorta). However, the axial and centrifugal pumps differ in their hydrodynamic performance, as characterized by the relation between flow rate and head pressure (Fig. 14.2) [30, 31]. Axial flow pumps have a steep and inverse linear relationship between flow and head pressure, while in centrifugal pumps this relationship is flatter and more susceptible to head pressure changes (i.e., more sensitive to pre-load and afterload). Due to these hydrodynamic characteristics, with the same change in pressure, centrifugal pumps generate larger changes in flow and yield more pulsatile waveforms, more accurate flow estimation, and have a lower risk of suction events (in setting of dehydration, arrhythmias, or right ventricular failure), but are more dependent on the loading conditions when compared with axial flow pumps (Fig. 14.2).

Patient Selection

As previously described in this chapter, the patients most likely to benefit from long-term use of LVAD are patients with advanced heart failure, preferably INTERMACS profiles 3–4, where the surgical risk of implantation is small (in-hospital mortality < 5%). Patients with INTERMACS profiles 1–2 should be bridged with temporary mechanical circulatory support devices and their end-organ function and nutritional status improved significantly or normalized in order to decrease the surgical mortality and morbidity associated with the durable LVAD implant.

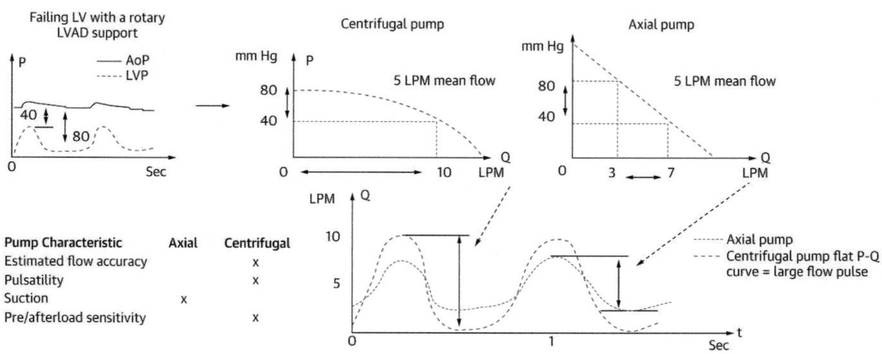

Fig. 14.2 Relationship between head pressure and pump flow in axial and centrifugal pumps and the effect on pulsatility. *AoP* mean aortic pressure, *LPM* liters per minute, *LV* left ventricle, *LVAD* left ventricular assist device, *LVP* left ventricular pressure, *P* pressure, *Q* flow. (With permission from Ref. [30])

Ideal candidates are patients with large left ventricles, relatively preserved right ventricular function, elevated left ventricular filling pressures and low cardiac output, with competent aortic valve, without history of gastrointestinal bleeding, compliant, with adequate social support, and with few extracardiac comorbidities that could limit the long-term benefit of LVAD [32, 33]. Carefully selected patients with restrictive cardiomyopathy [34] or congenital heart disease [35] could also benefit from ventricular assist device implantation.

In our center, the absolute contraindications to implantation include recent stroke (within 3 months), active systemic infection, uncorrectable peripheral vascular disease or aortic disease, severe irreversible lung disease (forced expiratory volume in first second < 1 L or diffusing lung capacity for carbon monoxide < 35% of predicted values), severe cardiac cachexia (body mass index < 19 kg/m^2, serum albumin level < 2.5 g/dL, or serum pre-albumin level < 15 mg/dL), end stage renal disease on dialysis or with high likelihood of needing dialysis post implant (e.g. creatinine > 3 mg/dL, unless the patient is considered as bridge to heart-kidney transplantation), biopsy proven liver cirrhosis, irreversible cognitive dysfunction (as established by formal neurocognitive testing) and marked frailty [33]. Patients are also deemed to not be good candidates for implantation if they lack social support or have a recent or active history of significant alcohol or illicit substance use. Older patients (older than 80 years) or morbidly obese patients (body mass index above 45 kg/m^2) are evaluated on case-by-case basis.

Current Clinical Results with Continuous Flow Pumps

Several modern trials with LVAD have shown a progressive increase in survival. The early trials focused on 1 year survival with the survival ranging from 68% (in the initial Thoratec HeartMate II bridge to transplant and destination therapy trials and HeartWare HVAD destination therapy trial) [36–39] to 86% (HeartWare HVAD bridge to transplant trial, Thoratec HeartMate II post approval studies) [40–42]. Patients with INTERMACS profiles 3–7 had better survival, slightly greater than 90% at 1 year. More recent trials have focused on long term survival with 2-year survival at 81% and surprisingly comparable results for INTERMACS profile 1,2 and 3,4 where 5-year survival reaches 55%. The HeartMate III demonstrated superior survival free of stroke compared to axial pumps with a 55% 5-year survival for the fully magnetically levitated device vs 44% for the axial pumps [22].

Durable LVAD outcomes and survival have increased but the therapy remains hampered by the relatively high probability of device related adverse events. The most common adverse events in the early and late periods after implant are major infection (early, 1.349; late, 0.440 events per patient-year) and major bleeding (early, 1.433; late, 0.347 events per patient-year) [23]. Stroke (early, 0.3 and late, 0.1 events per patient-year) and pump thrombosis (early, 0.18 and late, 0.09 event ser patient-year) have seen a marked decrease in the recent era [23]. In addition, significant right heart failure can occur in up to 30% of patients, and 5–10% require insertion of a temporary or permanent right ventricular assist device [43]. Over time, up to 30% of patients will develop aortic insufficiency, which may be related to the degree of opening allowed by the ongoing assist device settings [4]. The hospitalization rates for device related complications are high, with reportedly up to 65% of patients being hospitalized at least once during the first year on support [44].

In Hospital Management

Once the patient selection process has been completed and the patient has been determined to be a suitable candidate for LVAD implantation, pre-operative optimization using a multi-systems approach prepares the patient for the best chance of a successful outcome. Although several risk scores have been proposed, there are currently no validated risk prediction models to identify patients at highest risk for perioperative complications for ventricular assist device implant. All efforts should be made to ensure that all patients go into surgery with optimal organ functions, irrespective of its baseline state.

Pre-operative Optimization

The use of inotropes, vasopressors and temporary mechanical circulatory support devices can improve renal blood flow, while judicious decongestion with combination of intravenous diuretics, aquaretics or ultrafiltration will reduce the central and renal venous pressures. In our center, all attempts are made to improve renal function to pre-operative creatinine and blood urea nitrogen values of less than 2 mg/dL and 50 mg/dL, respectively. Hepatic dysfunction in heart failure is a result of circulatory shock from acute decompensation and persistently high right atrial pressures in the setting of venous congestion and poor right ventricular function. Hepatic dysfunction can lead to coagulation abnormalities and increased risk of bleeding in patients undergoing LVAD implantation. In our center, those with acute heart failure decompensation and elevations of transaminases or bilirubin receive aggressive therapy with diuresis, inotropes, and temporary mechanical circulatory support devices as necessary to improve hepatic function prior to implantation, to preoperative transaminases and bilirubin values of less than 100 IU/L and 2 mg/dL, respectively.

Right ventricular dysfunction is common in advanced heart failure patients and is consequence of pulmonary venous hypertension from chronically elevated left ventricular filling pressures, valvular pathology, or a combination of these processes. In our center, all patients with right ventricular dysfunction (more than mild) are admitted to the hospital prior the implant surgery and are optimized by receiving inotropes (e.g. dobutamine or milrinone) and/or temporary mechanical circulatory support devices to increase the cardiac index > 2.2 L/min/m^2. In addition, all patients receive intravenous diuretics or ultrafiltration to achieve a preoperative central venous pressure < 10 mmHg. In patients with pulmonary vascular resistance above 5 Wood units and moderate to severe right ventricular dysfunction we use treatment with sildenafil or inhaled nitric oxide to decrease the pulmonary vascular resistance and enhance the right ventricular function preoperatively. Poor nutritional state is associated with a high risk of post-operative complications, including infections, poor healing, poor functional recovery and prolonged length of stay. In our center, for patients with cardiac cachexia we use intensive nutritional optimization with high caloric oral supplements, enteral feedings or parenteral nutrition to boost nutritional status on the short term (e.g. few days pre-op). We attempt to improve nutritional status to a pre-operative albumin and pre-albumin values of above 3 mg/dL and 15 mg/dL, respectively.

Intra-operative Management

The intraoperative period is the most critical time of the implant and proper anesthetic techniques, hemodynamic management and surgical techniques are key to a successful outcome. To ensure a coordinated and successful operation, we conduct a multidisciplinary preoperative meeting the day prior to the operation, where the surgeon, heart failure cardiologist, LVAD coordinator, anesthesiologist and perfusionist are present. We review the medical history, comorbidities, echocardiogram, right heart catheterization, CT scans, and set specific plans for everything from line placement, ventilation strategy, perfusion, to how to treat possible right heart failure, bleeding and vasoplegia. This approach has improved significantly our outcomes and intraoperative errors.

During the LVAD implant surgery, the right ventricle is particularly vulnerable. Right coronary artery hypoperfusion from hypotension or air emboli should be avoided. Vasopressors (or vasodilators as needed) should be used to maintain a mean arterial pressure of 65–75 mmHg during the implant procedure. Inotropes should be used to maintain a good contractile function and intravenous diuretics or ultrafiltration should be used to maintain euvolemia. Judicious blood product and fluid management is key to prevent right ventricular volume overload and dysfunction. During surgical implantation, the LVAD inflow cannula should be placed parallel to the septum directed towards the mitral valve, away from the free wall. This should be verified by transesophageal echocardiography. Correct inflow cannula placement will minimize the chance of suction events. For patients where bilateral thoracotomy is used for implantation, sufficient surgical space should be available for a good visualization of the coring area and inflow cannula implantation. The outflow graft should be positioned to the right of sternal midline and avoid compression of right ventricle. Minimizing total cardiopulmonary bypass time may reduce the unfavorable extracorporeal-induced trauma of blood elements and the chance of bleeding. At the separation from cardio-pulmonary bypass, pulmonary vasodilation therapy with inhaled nitric oxide should be initiated prior to separation from bypass to provide the most favorable conditions for the right heart. Inotropic therapy should be continued or initiated, and volume management should be maintained. Sequential atrio-ventricular pacing can enhance right ventricular function and should be attempted if bradyarrhythmia is present.

Post-operative Management

The primary objective of early post-operative management is to support organ recovery and to avoid multi-system organ failure through optimization of organ perfusion. We use invasive monitoring of the patient for the first 48–72 h to ensure adequate optimization of hemodynamic support. Pump speed should be adjusted to maintain an output that provides the patient with adequate cardiac output while avoiding left ventricular suction and septum deviation to the left. A low pump output should trigger evaluation for hypovolemia (e.g. bleeding), tamponade, right heart failure, and in rare cases, inflow or outflow cannula obstruction. Surgical bleeding that occurs despite correction of coagulopathies will require that the patient be returned promptly to the operating room to identify the source. Uncontrolled bleeding should always be surgically evaluated.

Intravenous heparin is started after 24–48 h post-operatively if the surgical bleeding is controlled. We gradually increase the anticoagulation target to a goal heparin level of 0.3–0.5 U/mL and start warfarin once the patient tolerates oral medications. We no longer use aspirin in patients implanted with HeartMate III, based on recent trial data [45].

The impact of the LVAD on right ventricular function can be both beneficial and detrimental. The beneficial effects are realized through unloading the left ventricle and decreasing filling pressures, thereby reducing right ventricular afterload. The potential detrimental effects include an increase in right ventricular preload from the normalized cardiac support, and the septal shift observed with unloading the left ventricle. With lower left ventricular filling pressures, the septum will tend to shift to the left and decrease the septal contribution to right ventricular output. Pump speed should be maintained to achieve an optimal balance between an adequate cardiac output and avoidance of right ventricular dysfunction. Weaning of inotropic support should be initiated once the patient is euvolemic and is clinically guided by the physical examination with close monitoring of device parameters. As inotropes are weaned, the clinician should evaluate for evidence of right ventricular dysfunction including increasing edema; elevation in jugular venous pressure above 12–15 mmHg; low cardiac output (mean arterial pressure below 60 mmHg, poor urine output, decrease central venous saturation); end organ dysfunction (renal or liver failure); and change in pump parameters (decrease in flows and PI). If needed, intravenous inotropes could be used for an extended period of time. All sustained atrial and ventricular arrhythmias should be treated with anti-arrhythmic agents and synchronized cardioversion should be used in refractory cases.

We obtain a comprehensive transthoracic echocardiogram prior to discharge to evaluate ventricular size and function, cannula position and flow, aortic valve opening, tricuspid valve regurgitation and perform a ramp test to determine the best pump speed that unloads the left ventricle without inducing right ventricular dysfunction.

Long-Term Management

After LVAD implantation and discharge from the index hospitalization, the clinician is faced with the challenge of caring for the patient in the outpatient setting. This phase of care may last years, and the clinical concerns may evolve (e.g. moving from rehabilitation in the early period to preventing or treating comorbid conditions over time). Patients can be followed at the implant center or in coordination with the referring cardiologist ("shared care"). If a shared care approach is used, management guidelines should be distributed to the referring cardiologist to ensure a uniform approach and long-term success [46].

In our center, patients are seen in the outpatient clinic or telehealth weekly or biweekly for the first 30 days post discharge, then at 1 month and every 3 months afterwards. We obtain a panel of laboratory values (basic chemistry, complete blood count, lactate dehydrogenase, plasma free hemoglobin, international normalized ratio [INR], natriuretic peptide) with every clinic visit and monthly after the 1-month clinic visit. All patients receive home monitoring equipment to record daily weights, blood pressure, pump parameters and biweekly INRs. Automatic thresholds are set to alert the clinic staff when patients' parameters deviate from desired values (e.g. weight gain, high pump power, sub- or supra-therapeutic INR, hypo- or hypertension) to promptly intervene and correct them. Using this approach our center has managed to drastically reduce our rehospitalization rates during the first-year post implant to below 40%, compared to the 65% reported in the literature [23].

We maintain all patients on oral anticoagulation with a combination of warfarin (target INR 2–2.5) and aspirin 81 mg daily for older generation LVADs (e.g. HeartMate II and HeartWare HVAD) and warfarin alone for HeartMate III. The INR target is lowered to 1.8–2.2 for patients with evidence of gastrointestinal bleeding or individuals older than age 70 years at high risk for bleeding. All patients check their INRs biweekly using an INR home meter and in case of subtherapeutic values, patients inject enoxaparin 40 mg daily subcutaneously until the INR returns to desired values.

Blood pressure control is key to preventing strokes in patients on ventricular assist devices [47]. In patients with pulsatile hemodynamics (pulse pressure > 20 mmHg), we target a systolic blood pressure below 90–110 mmHg while in patients with non-pulsatile physiology we target mean arterial pressures of 70–90 mmHg. We make every effort to place patients on guideline directed medical therapy using angiotensin receptor/neprilysin inhibitors, mineralocorticoid receptor antagonists, sodium-glucose cotransporter-2 as first line therapy and use beta-blockers only in patients without evidence of significant right ventricular failure [32, 48].

Driveline management is an important part of the long-term care. We use an abdominal driveline exit site and silver containing driveline dressings that are changed every week using a standardized driveline management tray (chlorhexidine wand, silver patch, Tegaderm dressing, anchor). If trauma to driveline exists site occurs (e.g. dropping the controller, pulling the driveline during physical activities), patients remotely send a picture of their exit site, and if erythema or early infection are identified, patients are promptly started on oral antibiotics.

We make every effort to optimize patients on guideline directed medical therapy using angiotensin receptor/ neprilysin inhibitors, mineralocorticoid receptor antagonists, sodium-glucose cotransporter-2 and beta blockers if tolerated. We use transthoracic echocardiography periodically (at 30 days, 3 months, then every 6 months for the first 2 years and yearly thereafter) to optimize the LVAD speed. In setting of recurrent heart failure, we use cardiac catheterization in conjunction with echocardiography to assess and optimize the device function. We perform routine cardiac catheterization at 3 months post LVAD implant to ensure optimal hemodynamics. In patients with difficulty in management, we use implantable hemodynamic sensors (e.g. Abbott CardioMeMS or Endotronix Cordella) to allow for better long-term guidance [49].

Atrial and ventricular arrhythmias should be controlled, using specific antiarrhythmic drugs (e.g. dofetilide, amiodarone, mexiletine) or cardioversion. The cardiac implantable electric devices should be interrogated every 3 months, at the time of the clinic visit, to correlate potential ventricular assist device malfunction with concomitant arrhythmias.

Management of Ventricular Assist Device Long-Term Complications

Management of Gastrointestinal Bleeding

After hospital discharge, the most common cause of bleeding is the gastrointestinal tract. The reasons for this common complication are likely related to the use of antithrombotic therapy, acquired von Willebrand factor deficiency, acquired impaired platelet aggregation, and intestinal angiodysplasia related to continuous flow technology [50]. Our general approach to the first bleeding episode is to explore the gastrointestinal tract in detail (upper endoscopy, colonoscopy, capsule endoscopy and double balloon enteroscopy) and treat the identified lesions. If no lesions are identified or if the bleeding is recurrent, further investigations are not performed and we transfuse patients to a hematocrit above 30%. We use intravenous or oral iron supplements, but do not use erythropoietin-stimulating agents, as they have been associated with thrombotic complications in patients with ventricular assist devices

[51]. In patients with recurrent bleeding or significant need for transfusion, we have used octreotide (monthly injections of long-acting octreotide), oral thalidomide, oral danazole or intravenous bevacizumab with good results [32, 48].

Management of Infections

The most common pathogens in ventricular assist device-related infections are Staphylococcus and Pseudomonas and the most common site of infections if the percutaneous driveline exit site [52]. We have a low threshold for blood culture collection to evaluate for an occult bloodstream infection and are aggressive with empiric antibiotics after blood cultures are obtained. We use empiric therapy with cephalexin 500 mg oral every 6 h for 10–14 days, or doxycycline 100 mg oral every 12 h for 10–14 days in patients with a history of/colonized with methicillin resistant Staphylococcus Aureus. The antibiotics are modified accordingly based on culture data. If the initial treatment has not led to resolution of the superficial driveline infection, we use a 48–72 h course of intravenous antibiotics, followed by longer oral antibiotic course (14–28 days). For recurrent superficial driveline infections, we use lifetime suppressive coverage. Deep driveline infections are treated with intravenous vancomycin 15–20 mg/kg mg every 8–12 h and piperacillin/tazobactam 4.5 g every 6 h for a minimum of 14 days. Consideration for surgical exploration, debridement and vacuum assisted closure system should be given early for deep driveline infections.

Management of Atrial and Ventricular Arrhythmias

In patients who develop symptomatic or sustained ventricular arrhythmias we optimize the hemodynamics with medical therapy and pump optimization. Additional medical therapy consists of beta-blockers (irrespective of the right ventricular function) and antiarrhythmic agents (including amiodarone, mexiletine, and sotalol). For patients with refractory ventricular tachycardia, catheter ablation is an option [53, 54]. Atrial arrhythmias are common in patients on ventricular assist device support and persistent atrial fibrillation has been associated with worse right ventricular function and impaired functional capacity [55]. We attempt rhythm control strategies in these patients and increase the INR goal to 2.5–3 to prevent microembolization. Rarely, if needed, catheter ablation can be used [56].

Management of De Novo Aortic Insufficiency

Aortic valve insufficiency can develop de novo or underlying aortic valve pathology may be exacerbated post LVAD implant. To prevent it, we replace at the time of implant all aortic valves with more than mild regurgitation. De novo occurrence of aortic insufficiency is more common with continuous-flow pumps and occurs due to commissural fusion associated with reduced rates of aortic valve opening [44]. Medical management of aortic insufficiency includes aggressive blood pressure management to reduce the pressure gradient between the aorta and left ventricles. While percutaneous closure of the valve and transcatheter aortic valve replacement have been reported, we believe that the best long-term solution is surgical replacement [32].

Management of Pump Thrombosis and Pump Malfunction

Continuous flow devices are more likely to fail due to pump thrombosis rather than mechanical pump failure. In most cases, pump thrombosis is due to poor surgical pump or outflow graft positioning, and/or suboptimal long-term anticoagulation. Typical presentations for pump thrombosis range from asymptomatic rise in plasma free hemoglobin or lactate dehydrogenase, to hemolysis with hemoglobinuria, or to frank heart failure symptoms, associated with ventricular assist device flow and power elevations [57, 58]. Initial management strategies focus on patient stabilization and consideration of emergent surgical interventions or thrombolytic agents, especially in HeartWare HVAD pumps, which seem to be more amenable to medical management [59]. For these patients, we use tissue plasminogen activator in a dose of 10 mg intravenous as bolus, followed by an infusion of 10 mg over an hour, with high dose unfractionated heparin (heparin level 0.5–0.7 U/mL). If successful (normalization of pump power and a decrease of lactate dehydrogenase levels below 400 U/L), we then use aggressive antithrombotic therapy to prevent further thrombosis (INR 2.5–3) (Fig. 14.3). In patients with hemolysis refractory to intensification of antithrombotic therapy early device exchange should be considered in order to minimize the risk of stroke and death [60].

Management of Neurological Events

Neurological events (strokes) are relatively frequent in patients with ventricular assist devices, with a higher proportion of patients supported by HeartWare HVAD having hemorrhagic strokes compared to patients supported by Thoratec HeartMate II or HeartMate III devices (10% vs. 5%) [23]. Data from recent clinical trials have shown that these events are likely due to uncontrolled blood pressure. Ischemic

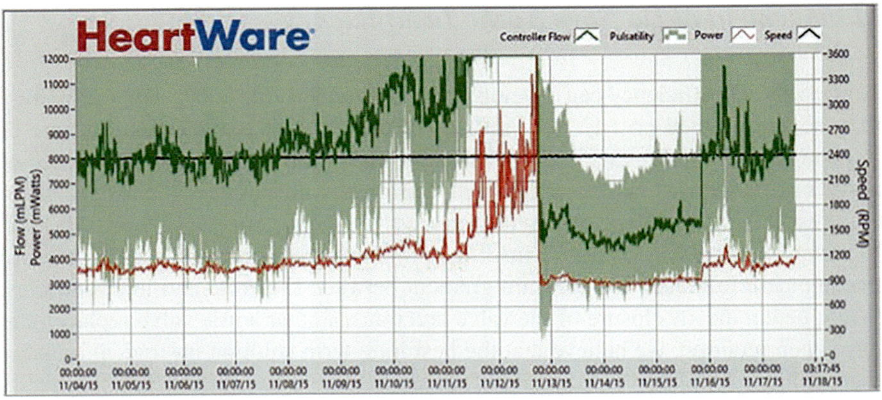

Fig. 14.3 Left ventricular assist device parameters and flow pulsatility in a patient with biochemical evidence of thrombosis. Clear increase in power (*solid red line*) starting in early November 2015, with a marked increase starting November 10, 2015, associated with marked increase in flow (*solid green line*). After administration of intravenous tissue plasminogen activator on November 13, 2015, the power returns to baseline (3 W). There is a subsequent power increase associated with a second episode of thrombosis on November 16, 2015 that responded to a second dose of intravenous tissue plasminogen activator. (Data not shown)

strokes are equally frequently seen in the two devices (5%) and are due to suboptimal anticoagulation [23].

We hospitalize all patients presenting with a neurological event and withhold warfarin and antiplatelet agents in the setting of hemorrhagic stroke, intracranial hemorrhage, and subdural hemorrhage. We reverse anticoagulation immediately with prothrombin factor concentrates followed by intravenous phenytoin, and obtain Neurosurgery and Neurology consultation. Warfarin and antiplatelet agents typically continue to be withheld for 5–7 days until the source of the hemorrhage has been addressed or, if a source has not been identified, until the bleeding subsides, and the affected area is determined to be small enough to not bleed again. In the setting of ischemic stroke, we withhold antihypertensive medications to allow for a higher systemic pressure (mean arterial pressure of 90 mmHg) to improve perfusion to the affected brain areas. In the setting of hemorrhagic stroke, intracranial hemorrhage, and subdural hemorrhage, the blood pressure targets are lower. If the patient recovers, warfarin is reinstituted upon discharge. All patients are provided with intensive inpatient physical and occupational therapy with the goal of discharging the patient to a stroke rehabilitation center to maximize their functional recovery.

Total Artificial Heart

Compared to LVAD, the total artificial heart is implanted in a much smaller proportion of patients, such as patients with severe biventricular failure, fulminant myocarditis or primary heart transplant graft failure.

The Syncardia total artificial heart has a very simple design, delivering pulsatile flow by filling two artificial ventricles lined with polyurethane, and ejecting blood via a four-layer, pneumatically driven, moving diaphragm [61]. Four mechanical valves guarantee the unidirectional flow. The ventricles are connected to patient's circulatory system by cuffs sutured to the atria and vascular grafts sutured to the aorta and pulmonary artery. At maximal stroke volume (70 mL), the device can deliver a cardiac output of more than 9 L per min. The use of Syncardia total artificial heart has been associated with a 70% survival to transplantation in a population of patients ineligible for left ventricular assist devices [62]. Patients are at risk of thrombotic or hemorrhagic stroke, which, alongside the high risk of infection due to the large percutaneous driveline and relatively heavy external power driver, limit the widespread use of this device.

The French Carmat total artificial heart was first implanted in December 2013 and it contains two ventricles, each with a blood compartment and a driving fluid compartment, separated by a flexible hybrid membrane. The hybrid membrane has a polyurethane layer at the fluid-contacting surface and bovine pericardial tissue on the blood-contacting surface. The use of bioprosthetic valves and partial pericardium lining of the blood chambers are the most innovative features of this device [63].

The clinical utility of the total artificial hearts is likely to be expanded once appropriate technological improvements are made.

Conclusions

Mechanical circulatory support devices represent a significant advancement in the field of heart failure. Device technology continues to evolve, patient survival is improving, both for those with cardiogenic shock and for those with chronic advanced heart failure. Better patient selection, surgical techniques and post-operative and long-term management can minimize the device-related complications and allow more patients to benefit from this therapy. It is likely than within the next decade advanced heart failure patients will benefit from a completely implantable assist device. This device will provide full support, including physiologic optimization (i.e. during exercise), will be implanted via a minimally invasive surgery, will enjoy limited complications rate, will be remotely monitored and accessed, and will do so within cost effective parameters.

Future Directions

- Design of hemocompatible surfaces will alleviate the need for anticoagulation and minimize the risk of bleeding, pump thrombosis and stroke.
- Modulation of pulsatility in newer LVADs will likely decrease the complications related to gastrointestinal bleeding.
- In the future, speed modulation algorithms will respond to specific physiological demands, such as those related to exercise and remote monitoring will be able to control the pump (both monitoring data and programming the pump).
- The advent of transcutaneous energy transfer will allow the development of completely implantable devices, with improved quality of life and marked decrease in the risk for infections.
- Newer LVADs will be miniaturized and will allow for smaller surgical or transcatheter implantation.
- LVADs will be used as platforms allowing concomitant administration of full dose neurohormonal blockade, gene therapies, and intramyocardial injections of stem cells that will lead to myocardial recovery.

References

1. Martin SS, Aday AW, Almarzooq ZI, et al. 2024 heart disease and stroke statistics: a report of US and global data from the American Heart Association. Circulation. 2024;149(8):e347–913.
2. DeFilippis EM, Khush KK, Farr MA, Fiedler A, Kilic A, Givertz MM. Evolving characteristics of heart transplantation donors and recipients: JACC focus seminar. J Am Coll Cardiol. 2022;79(11):1108–23.
3. Hsich E, Singh TP, Cherikh WS, International Society for Heart and Lung Transplantation, et al. The International thoracic organ transplant registry of the international society for heart and lung transplantation: thirty-ninth adult heart transplantation report-2022; focus on transplant for restrictive heart disease. J Heart Lung Transplant. 2022;41(10):1366–75.
4. Eurotransplant statistics library. https://statistics.eurotransplant.org/index.php?search_type=transplants&search_organ=heart&search_region=&search_period=&search_characteristic=&search_text=&search_collection=
5. Parker WF, Chung K, Anderson AS, Siegler M, Huang ES, Churpek MM. Practice changes at U.S. transplant centers after the new adult heart allocation policy. J Am Coll Cardiol. 2020;75(23):2906–16.
6. Mastoris I, Tonna JE, Hu J, et al. Use of extracorporeal membrane oxygenation as bridge to replacement therapies in cardiogenic shock: insights from the extracorporeal life support organization. Circ Heart Fail. 2022;15(1):e008777.
7. Cogswell R, John R, Estep JD, et al. An early investigation of outcomes with the new 2018 donor heart allocation system in the United States. J Heart Lung Transplant. 2020;39(1):1–4.
8. Mullan CW, Chouairi F, Sen S, et al. Changes in use of left ventricular assist devices as bridge to transplantation with new heart allocation policy. JACC Heart Fail. 2021;9(6):420–9.
9. Morris AA, Khazanie P, Drazner MH, American Heart Association Heart Failure and Transplantation Committee of the Council on Clinical Cardiology; Council on Arteriosclerosis, Thrombosis and Vascular Biology; Council on Cardiovascular Radiology and Intervention; and Council on Hypertension, et al. Guidance for timely and appropriate referral of patients

with advanced heart failure: a scientific statement from the American Heart Association. Circulation. 2021;144(15):e238–50.
10. Stevenson LW, Pagani FD, Young JB, et al. INTERMACS profiles of advanced heart failure: the current picture. J Heart Lung Transplant. 2009;28:535–41.
11. Goodman D, Stulak J, Rosenbaum AN. Left ventricular assist devices: a historical perspective at the intersection of medicine and engineering. Artif Organs. 2022;46(12):2343–60.
12. Funamoto M, Kunavarapu C, Kwan MD, Matsuzaki Y, Shah M, Ono M. Single center experience and early outcomes of Impella 5.5. Front Cardiovasc Med. 2023;10:1018203.
13. Yuzefpolskaya M, Schroeder SE, Houston BA, et al. The Society of Thoracic Surgeons Intermacs 2022 annual report: focus on the 2018 heart transplant allocation system. Ann Thorac Surg. 2023;115(2):311–27.
14. Tehrani BN, Truesdell AG, Psotka MA, et al. A standardized and comprehensive approach to the management of cardiogenic shock. JACC Heart Fail. 2020;8(11):879–91.
15. Baran DA, Grines CL, Bailey S, et al. SCAI clinical expert consensus statement on the classification of cardiogenic shock: this document was endorsed by the American College of Cardiology (ACC), the American Heart Association (AHA), the Society of Critical Care Medicine (SCCM), and the Society of Thoracic Surgeons (STS). Catheter Cardiovasc Interv. 2019;94(1):29–37.
16. Bernhardt AM, Copeland H, Deswal A, et al. The International Society for Heart and Lung Transplantation/Heart Failure Society of America Guideline on acute mechanical circulatory support. J Heart Lung Transplant. 2023;42(4):e1–e64.
17. Baran DA, Jaiswal A, Hennig F, Potapov E. Temporary mechanical circulatory support: devices, outcomes, and future directions. J Heart Lung Transplant. 2022;41(6):678–91.
18. Thiele H, Zeymer U, Neumann FJ, et al. Intra-aortic balloon support for myocardial infarction with cardiogenic shock. N Engl J Med. 2012;367:1287–96.
19. Møller JE, Engstrøm T, Jensen LO, DanGer Shock Investigators, et al. Microaxial flow pump or standard care in infarct-related cardiogenic shock. N Engl J Med. 2024;390(15):1382–93.
20. Tempelhof MW, Klein L, Cotts WG, et al. Clinical experience and patient outcomes associated with the Tandem Heart percutaneous transseptal assist device among a heterogeneous patient population. ASAIO J. 2011;57:254–61.
21. Eckman PM, Katz JN, El Banayosy A, Bohula EA, Sun B, van Diepen S. Veno-arterial extracorporeal membrane oxygenation for cardiogenic shock: an introduction for the busy clinician. Circulation. 2019;140(24):2019–37.
22. Mehra MR, Goldstein DJ, Cleveland JC, et al. Five-year outcomes in patients with fully magnetically levitated vs axial-flow left ventricular assist devices in the MOMENTUM 3 randomized trial. JAMA. 2022;328(12):1233–42.
23. Jorde UP, Saeed O, Koehl D, et al. The Society of Thoracic Surgeons Intermacs 2023 annual report: focus on magnetically levitated devices. Ann Thorac Surg. 2024;117(1):33–44.
24. Tedford RJ, Leacche M, Lorts A, Drakos SG, Pagani FD, Cowger J. Durable mechanical circulatory support: JACC scientific statement. J Am Coll Cardiol. 2023;82(14):1464–81.
25. Rose EA, Gelijns AC, Moskowitz AJ, For the Randomized Evaluation of Mechanical Assistance for the Treatment of Congestive Heart Failure (REMATCH) Study Group, et al. Long-term use of a left ventricular assist device for end-stage heart failure. N Engl J Med. 2001;345:1435–43.
26. Griffith BP, Kormos RL, Borovetz HS, et al. HeartMate II left ventricular assist system: from concept to first clinical use. Ann Thorac Surg. 2001;71:S116–20.
27. Frazier OH, Myers TJ, Jarvik RK, et al. Research and development of an implantable, axial-flow left ventricular assist device: the Jarvik 2000 Heart. Ann Thorac Surg. 2001;71:S125–32.
28. Larose JA, Tamez D, Ashenuga M, Reyes C. Design concepts and principle of operation of the HeartWare ventricular assist system. ASAIO J. 2010;56:285–9.
29. Farrar DJ, Bourque K, Dague CP, Cotter CJ, Poirier VL. Design features, developmental status, and experimental results with the Heartmate III centrifugal left ventricular assist system with a magnetically levitated rotor. ASAIO J. 2007;53:310–5.

30. Mancini D, Colombo PC. Left ventricular assist devices: a rapidly evolving alternative to transplant. J Am Coll Cardiol. 2015;65(23):2542–55.
31. Giridharan GA, Koenig SC, Soucy KG, et al. Left ventricular volume unloading with axial and centrifugal rotary blood pumps. ASAIO J. 2015;61:292–300.
32. Saeed D, Feldman D, Banayosy AE, et al. The 2023 International Society for Heart and Lung Transplantation guidelines for mechanical circulatory support: a 10-year update. J Heart Lung Transplant. 2023;42(7):e1–e222.
33. Flint KM, Matlock DD, Lindenfeld JA, Allen LA. Frailty and selection of patients for destination therapy left ventricular assist device. Circ Heart Fail. 2012;5:286–93.
34. Topilsky Y, Pereira NL, Shah DK, et al. Left ventricular assist device therapy in patients with restrictive and hypertrophic cardiomyopathy. Circ Heart Fail. 2011;4:266–75.
35. Cedars A, Vanderpluym C, Koehl D, et al. An Interagency Registry for Mechanically Assisted Circulatory Support (INTERMACS) analysis of hospitalization, functional status, and mortality after mechanical circulatory support in adults with congenital heart disease. J Heart Lung Transplant. 2018;37(5):619–30.
36. Miller LW, Pagani FD, Russell SD, For the HeartMate II Clinical Investigators, et al. Use of a continuous flow device in patients awaiting heart transplantation. N Engl J Med. 2007;357:885–96.
37. Slaughter MS, Rogers JG, Milano CA, For the HeartMate II Investigators, et al. Advanced heart failure treated with continuous-flow left ventricular assist device. N Engl J Med. 2009;361:2241–51.
38. Aaronson KD, Slaughter MS, Miller LW, For the HeartWare Ventricular Assist Device (HVAD) Bridge to Transplant ADVANCE Trial Investigators, et al. Use of an intrapericardial, continuous flow, centrifugal pump in patients awaiting heart transplantation. Circulation. 2012;125:3191–200.
39. Rogers JG, Pagani FD, Tatooles AJ, et al. Intrapericardial left ventricular assist device for advanced heart failure. N Engl J Med. 2017;376:451–60.
40. Jorde UP, Kushwaha SS, Tatooles AJ, For the HeartMate II Clinical Investigators, et al. Results of the destination therapy post U.S. Food and Drug Administration approval study with a continuous flow left ventricular assist device: a prospective study using the INTERMACS registry (Interagency Registry for Mechanically Assisted Circulatory Support). J Am Coll Cardiol. 2014;63:1751–7.
41. Milano CA, Rogers JG, Tatooles AJ, ENDURANCE Investigators, et al. HVAD: the ENDURANCE supplemental trial. JACC Heart Fail. 2018;6(9):792–802.
42. McGee E Jr, Danter M, Strueber M, et al. Evaluation of a lateral thoracotomy implant approach for a centrifugal-flow left ventricular assist device: the LATERAL clinical trial. J Heart Lung Transplant. 2019;38(4):344–51.
43. Loghmanpour NA, Kormos RL, Kanwar MK, Teuteberg JJ, Murali S, Antaki JFA. Bayesian model to predict right ventricular failure following left ventricular assist device therapy. JACC Heart Fail. 2016;4(9):711–21.
44. Jorde UP, Uriel N, Nahumi N, et al. Prevalence, significance, and management of aortic insufficiency in continuous flow left ventricular assist device recipients. Circ Heart Fail. 2014;7:310–9.
45. Mehra MR, Netuka I, Uriel N, ARIES-HM3 Investigators, et al. Aspirin and hemocompatibility events with a left ventricular assist device in advanced heart failure: the ARIES-HM3 randomized clinical trial. JAMA. 2023;330(22):2171–81.
46. Kiernan MS, Joseph SM, Katz JN, Evolving Mechanical Support Research Group (EMERG) Investigators, et al. Sharing the care of mechanical circulatory support: collaborative efforts of patients/caregivers, shared-care sites, and left ventricular assist device implanting centers. Circ Heart Fail. 2015;8:629–35.
47. Eisen HJ, Flack JM, Atluri P, American Heart Association Heart Failure and Transplantation Committee of the Council on Clinical Cardiology; Council on Hypertension; and Council on Lifelong Congenital Heart Disease and Heart Health in the Young, et al. Management

of hypertension in patients with ventricular assist devices: a scientific statement from the American Heart Association. Circ Heart Fail. 2022;15(5):e000074.
48. Trachtenberg B, Cowger J, Jennings DL, et al. HFSA expert consensus statement on the medical management of patients on durable mechanical circulatory support. J Card Fail. 2023;29(4):479–502.
49. Thohan V, Abraham J, Burdorf A, INTELLECT 2-HF Investigators, et al. Use of a pulmonary artery pressure sensor to manage patients with left ventricular assist devices. Circ Heart Fail. 2023;16(6):e009960.
50. Suarez J, Patel CB, Felker GM, Becker R, Hernandez AF, Rogers JG. Mechanisms of bleeding and approach to patients with axial-flow left ventricular assist devices. Circ Heart Fail. 2011;4:779–84.
51. Nassif ME, Patel JS, Shuster JE, et al. Clinical outcomes with use of erythropoiesis stimulating agents in patients with the HeartMate II left ventricular assist device. JACC Heart Fail. 2015;3:146–53.
52. Aslam S, Cowger J, Shah P, et al. The International Society for Heart and Lung Transplantation (ISHLT): 2024 infection definitions for durable and acute mechanical circulatory support devices. J Heart Lung Transplant. 2024;43(7):1039–50.
53. Sacher F, Reichlin T, Zado ES, et al. Characteristics of ventricular tachycardia ablation in patients with continuous flow left ventricular assist devices. Circ Arrhythm Electrophysiol. 2015;8:592–7.
54. Moss JD, Oesterle A, Raiman M, et al. Feasibility and utility of intraoperative epicardial scar characterization during left ventricular assist device implantation. J Cardiovasc Electrophysiol. 2019;30(2):183–92.
55. Brisco MA, Sundareswaran KS, Milano CA, et al. The incidence, risk, and consequences of atrial arrhythmias in patients with continuous flow left ventricular assist devices. J Card Surg. 2014;29:572–80.
56. Maury P, Delmas C, Trouillet C, et al. First experience of percutaneous radiofrequency ablation for atrial flutter and atrial fibrillation in a patient with HeartMate II left ventricular assist device. J Interv Card Electrophysiol. 2010;29:63–7.
57. Goldstein DJ, John R, Salerno C, et al. Algorithm for the diagnosis and management of suspected pump thrombus. J Heart Lung Transplant. 2013;32:667–70.
58. Hollis IB, Jennings DL, Krim S, et al. An ISHLT consensus statement on strategies to prevent and manage hemocompatibility related adverse events in patients with a durable, continuous-flow ventricular assist device. J Heart Lung Transplant. 2024;43(8):1199–234.
59. Najjar SS, Slaughter MS, Pagani FD, HVAD Bridge to Transplant ADVANCE Trial Investigators, et al. An analysis of pump thrombus events in patients in the HeartWare ADVANCE bridge to transplant and continued access protocol trial. J Heart Lung Transplant. 2014;33:23–34.
60. Levin AP, Saeed O, Willey JZ, et al. Watchful waiting in continuous-flow left ventricular assist device patients with ongoing hemolysis is associated with an increased risk for cerebrovascular accident or death. Circ Heart Fail. 2016;9:2896–3003.
61. Morris RJ. Total artificial heart—concepts and clinical use. Semin Thorac Cardiovasc Surg. 2008;20:247–54.
62. Copeland JG, Smith RG, Arabia FA, et al. Cardiac replacement with a total artificial heart as a bridge to transplantation. N Engl J Med. 2004;351:859–67.
63. Carpantier A, Latremouille C, Cholley B, et al. First clinical use of a bioprosthetic total artificial heart: report of two cases. Lancet. 2015;386:1556–63.

Chapter 15
Cell and Gene Therapy in Heart Failure

Lina Badimon, Guiomar Mendieta, Gemma Vilahur, and Maria Borrell-Pages

Abstract This chapter analyses existing data on experimental studies testing different gene therapy approaches and stem cell-based therapies to target heart failure (HF) treatment. It also reports on the results of the different clinical trials testing these innovative therapeutic approaches and briefly discusses the current needs and future directions of this research field in order to favour its successful translation into the clinical practice.

Keywords Gene therapy · Stem cells · Non coding RNAs · Cardiac regeneration · Clinical trials

Introduction

The dramatic increase in the prevalence of heart failure (HF) [1] has led to the expansion of studies on the mechanisms triggering the disease. Different molecular signalling pathways involved in the process are under investigation in order to identify new potential therapeutic targets [2]. Gene and cell therapies are under investigation to understand the complex pathophysiology of HF.

L. Badimon (✉)
CIBER-CV, Instituto de Salud Carlos III, Madrid, Spain

School of Medicine UVic-UCC, IRIS-CC and Cardiovascular Research Foundation for Health and Innovation, Barcelona, Spain
e-mail: lbadimon@santpau.cat

G. Mendieta
Department of Cardiology, Hospital de la Santa Creu i Sant Pau, Barcelona, Spain

G. Vilahur · M. Borrell-Pages
Molecular Pathology and Therapeutic of Ischaemic and Atherothrombotic Diseases, Institut de Recerca Sant Pau (IR-Sant Pau), Barcelona, Spain

CIBER-CV, Instituto de Salud Carlos III, Madrid, Spain

M. Dorobanţu et al. (eds.), *Current Approach to Heart Failure*,
https://doi.org/10.1007/978-3-031-96562-3_15

Gene Therapy

The identification of gene variants involved in disease is crucial in order to specifically target gene function. Current gene therapy studies aim to target abnormalities in calcium metabolism, in beta-adrenergic signaling and in the regeneration of cardiac muscle by the regulation of cellular mRNA translation. The main goal of these therapies is to induce cellular protection, improve cardiac muscle contractility and/or enhance stem cell recruitment into the infarcted myocardium after an ischemic event. In this section we will discuss the preclinical work with genes involved in HF that is moving into clinical trials.

Calcium Homeostasis-Related Therapies

Among the different molecules involved in calcium homeostasis, sarcoplasmic reticulum Ca^{2+} ATPase (SERCA2a) plays a critical role. In several studies abnormal calcium handling in the myocardium is observed in patients with end-stage HF [3]. Similar findings have been reported as well in animal models and humans, showing that both mRNA and protein levels of SERCA2a are reduced in the failing myocardium [4, 5]. These reduced SERCA2a levels lead to impaired calcium re-uptake by the sarcoplasmic reticulum during diastole contributing to the HF-related impaired diastolic relaxation, decreasing calcium availability for systolic contraction and further contributing to systolic impairment [6]. These evidences have been proved in experimental animal models in which SERCA2a gene knock-out induces systolic and diastolic dysfunction [7]. Furthermore, pre-clinical studies in small and large animal models have demonstrated, not only improved cardiac contractility after SERCA2a gene transfer, but also enhanced energy utilization, decreased ventricular arrhythmias and improved blood flow [8–10].

Other approaches to target SERCA2a-mediated calcium homeostasis are the manipulation of SERCA2a regulators, such as phospholamban (PLB) and the Small Ubiquitin-like MOdifier type 1 (SUMO1). Because PLB-phosphorylation regulates SERCA2a activity (unphosphorylated-PLB inhibits SERCA2a), adenoassociated virus (AAV)-mediated overexpression of a mutant PLB was investigated showing prevention of cardiomyocyte deterioration and cardiac dysfunction in small animal models of HF [11] and post-MI remodelling [12, 13]. These results have been further validated in a sheep model of HF where treatment with an inhibitory PLB peptide has enhanced SERCA2a activity leading to improved left ventricular (LV) function [14]. These data have been reproduced by the use of RNA interference in a rat model of HF where adenoviral and AAV vectors were used to silence PLB expression [15]. Furthermore, reduced mortality following PLB ablation has been shown in a murine model of HF [15]. Therefore, overexpression of the mutated PLB form or inhibition of PLB improves cardiac function.

PLB phosphorylation is also regulated by protein phosphatase-1 (PP1) and its inhibitor (I-1). PP1-I-1 overexpression in murine models improves cardiac function, preventing HF progression [16, 17]. In fact, transgenic mice expressing constitutively active PP1 inhibitor-1c (I-1c) show PP1 inhibition together with increased levels of phosphorylated PLB [16]. The relevance of a potential PP1 inhibition gene transfer therapeutic approach was validated in a swine model of ischemic HF (IHF) where it improved cardiac function [18]. Furthermore, PP-1 inhibitor gene therapy in swine improved left ventricular and left atrial contractility in the volume-overload HF model [19].

SUMO1 protein regulates SERCA2a levels and activity through a post-translational modification known as SUMOylation. HF has been associated to a reduction in SERCA2a SUMOylation [19]. Gene therapy with an AAV-SUMO1 vector has shown to increase SUMO1 expression and to improve cardiac function in small and large animal models of HF in a comparable way to that obtained with SERCA2a gene therapy suggesting a potential additive effect of both gene-based therapies [20, 21]. Also, a small molecule activator of SUMOylation has been discovered, N106, that significantly improves ventricular function in mice with HF [22].

Another protein involved in SERCA2a regulation in the heart is S100A1. This is a calcium regulated protein that enhances SERCA2a activity promoting cardiac contraction and relaxation. AAV-mediated long-term expression of S100A1 is able to revert LV dysfunction and adverse remodelling in a rat model of HF [23]. Similarly, AAV-mediated expression of S100A1 prevented and reversed these functional and structural changes in a pig model of post-ischemic HF [24]. Indeed, increased S100A1 expression improved systolic and diastolic cardiac function and performance with no evidence of increased arrhythmia [24].

Therapies for the Treatment of Tachy- and Brady-Arrhythmias

HF implies changes in the electrophysiological function that lead to the manifestation of a wide variety of arrhythmic disorders such as tachy- and brady- arrhythmias. This is crucial as, for example, bradyarrhythmias are associated to a worsening of HF and if extreme they can lead to sudden cardiac death. Moreover, the most prevalent tachyarrhythmia associated to HF, atrial fibrillation (AF), dramatically increases the risk for stroke [25].

Because of the clinical relevance of arrhythmias in HF many efforts have been spent in the search for candidate targets for gene therapy [26]. In this context, adenoviral-mediated delivery of a ras-related small G-protein, Gem, in a guinea pig model shortened the action potential duration (APD) which is an electrophysiological hallmark of the failing heart and decreased the L-type calcium current ($I_{Ca\text{-}L}$) [27]. However, this approach severely blunted contractile function limiting its usefulness in the clinical scenario. Interestingly, *in vivo* knockdown of the L-type Ca^{2+} channel β-subunit in a rat model also reduced

$I_{Ca\text{-}L}$ attenuating the hypertrophic response without affecting systolic performance [28]. Another strategy for shortening APD is increasing the activity of repolarizing K channels. Indeed, adenoviral-mediated overexpression of the gene encoding I_{to}, Kv4.3, is able to prevent pressure overload-induced APD prolongation diminishing the hypertrophic response [29]. Also, the restoration of I_{to} in rabbit cardiomyocytes improved cardiac action potential raising the possibility for a new gene-based therapeutic approach to HF [30].

The great importance of cell-to-cell interaction regulatory mechanisms in HF has lead to propose connexin 43(Cx43) as a potential target for gene therapy [31]. Studies performed on cardiac remodelling post-MI in pigs demonstrated that adenoviral-mediated delivery of Cx43 gene improved conduction velocity and reduced the susceptibility to ventricular tachyarrhythmias [32]. Furthermore increased expression of Cx43 in type-1 diabetic rat hearts [33] and in hypothyroid rat hearts [34] induced resistance to inducible ventricular fibrillation indicating a protective role for Cx43 in the heart. These results have to be taken cautiously due to the previously demonstrated positive association between Cx43 levels and infarct size [35].

An important advantage of gene therapy is that it can be locally delivered to the tissue and/or cell type of interest. Sasano et al. demonstrated that local transfer of a gene encoding a dominant-negative version of the KCNH2 potassium channel (KCNH2-G628S) to the scar border, eliminated all ventricular arrhythmias in a porcine model [36].

In rodent, activation of the calcineurin-NFAT signaling pathway induces hypertrophic growth of the myocardium leading to HF [37]. Decoy oligodeoxynucleotides designed to reduce NFAT transcriptional activity seem to preserve cardiac function during stress overload [37]. Finally a recent study demonstrated that gene therapy with the N-terminus of junctophilin-2 into mice myocardium attenuated HF development [38].

Therapies Targeting Adrenergic Signalling

Sympathetic nervous system hyperactivity is known to play a pivotal role in the pathophysiology and progression of HF. A key pathological event is the hyperactivation of the sympathetic system that leads to a hyperadrenergic state of the heart. The chronic stimulation of β-adrenergic receptors (β-ARs) leads to their desensitization. These β-ARs are coupled to stimulatory G proteins (G_s) which regulate intracellular cAMP levels and are counterbalanced by inhibitory G proteins (G_i) [39]. Several groups have targeted G-proteins as a potential approach for gene therapy. In an *ex vivo* pig model, adenovirus carrying the $G\alpha_{i2}$-subunit suppressed baseline atrioventricular conduction and slowed the heart rate during AF [40]. Similarly, silencing $G\alpha_s$ with an adenovirus-small interfering RNA in pigs, reduced heart rates during normal sinus rhythm and prevented inappropriate rate increase after β-adrenergic stimulation [41].

The most abundantly expressed G protein-coupled receptor kinase (GRK) in the heart is GRK2. Several studies have demonstrated that the expression of a peptide inhibitor of GRK2 (βARKct) is able to improve the contractility of the failing heart and the cardiac-specific overexpression of GRK2 showed to delay HF progression in mice [42] and muscular dystrophy [43]. Moreover, βARKct cardiac gene delivery improves LV haemodynamics and preserves cardiac function in rodents [44] and in pigs [45].

Another approach to target β-adrenergic stimulation is the modulation of cAMP expression. Overexpression of adenylyl cyclase type 6 (AC6) in mice reduced PLB phosphorylation and increased SERCA2a activity [46]. Moreover, transgenic AC6 overexpression in mice increases cAMP production and improve cardiac function [47]. This result has been validated in a pacing pig model of HF where adenovirus-mediated AC6 gene transfer also increased cAMP production improving LV function and remodelling [48]. Finally, overexpression of AC6 in rat cardiac fibroblasts facilitates nodal atrioventricular conduction which is a mechanism of cardioprotection [49].

Therapies Targeting Myofilaments

In muscle contractility, myosin uses ATP hydrolysis energy to move along actin filaments. The overexpression of the enzyme ribonucleotide reductase (R1R2) in transgenic mice increases the production of 2-deoxyATP, significantly improving LV systolic function [50]. In small and large animal models of HF, a single dose of this gene leads to sustained inotropic effects with a benign safety profile [51, 52]. However, further studies are needed before this technology can be translated to humans.

Cardiac Regeneration and Proliferation Therapies

Another approach used is to increase the amount of viable myocardium by targeting key signalling pathways in embryonic and fetal cardiomyocyte proliferation [53], with the aim of stimulating the intrinsic potential of cardiac cells to proliferate. In this context, two key molecular pathways have been investigated in cardiomyocyte proliferation, the Notch and Hippo signalling pathways. Indeed, adenovirus or AAV-mediated overexpression of the Notch Intra Cellular Domain (NICD) has shown to protect neonatal rat cardiomyocytes from apoptosis and to promotes their expansion [54, 55]. Similarly, targeting the Hippo pathway by the miR-302/367 cluster induces cardiac regeneration after an MI [56].

An additional strategy has been to induce stem cell (SC) homing into the failing heart. The stem cell-derived factor 1 (SDF-1) is a chemokine that binds to the G protein-coupled CXC chemokine receptor type 4 (CXCR4) to stimulate anti-inflammatory pathways, improve vascular density and promote stem cell homing into the myocardium, facilitating tissue repair after injury [57]. Plasmid-mediated SDF-1 overexpression in a rat model of HF promoted angiogenesis and improved cardiac function inducing a slight scar remodelling with a decreased myocardial fibrosis [57]. Furthermore, in humans, plasma levels of SDF-1 seem to predict the risk of HF and mortality [58].

Non-coding RNA (ncRNAs) are involved in HF by the regulation of different microRNAs (miRNAs). miRNAs are evolutionarily conserved ncRNAs that post-transcriptionally regulate gene expression, playing a critical role in cellular pathways involved in development, homeostasis, and stress response. miRNAs regulate the expression of approximately 60% of all human genes. Approximately 2500 human miRNAs have been identified, cataloged in the miRBase database (http://www.mirbase.org). Noncoding RNAs in the heart play an essential role in cardiac dysfunction, and become new potential targets for treatments, diagnostic and prognostic biomarkers [59]. HF is enhanced by the upregulation of miR-208a, miR-532-3p or the downregulation of miR30e that modulate cardiotoxiciy mediated by doxorubicin in Dahl hypertensive rats [60]. Moreover, quaking (a RNA binding protein) downregulation by doxorubicin promotes atrophy in mice while quaking overexpression strongly attenuates the cardiotoxicity of doxorubicin by regulating a set of circular RNAs [61]. Also, overexpression of microRNA-199a, which is significantly reduced in hypoxia, improves cardiac muscle contractility, increases muscle mass and reduces scar size in infarcted swine hearts [62, 63]. The prognostic value of miRNAs in HF patients has been recently assessed in a meta-analyses showing that *miR-18a-5p*, *miR-18b-5p*, *miR-30d*, *miR-30e-5p*, and *miR-423-5p* are strong biomarkers of prognosis in HF [64]. A recent study in well treated patients with chronic HF has identified seven miRNAs (*let-7a-5p*, *miR-107*, *miR-125a-5p*, *miR-139-5p*, *miR-150-5p*, *miR-30b-5p* and *miR-342-3p*; clusters 1-4 [C:1-4]), that were able to discriminate between HF with preserved ejection fraction (HFpEF) and HF with reduced ejection fraction (HFrEF), and ischaemic and non-ischaemic aetiologies. Furthermore, system biology analysis and pathway enrichment analysis of miRNAs present in C:1-4 (*let-7a-5p*, *miR-125a-5p*, *miR-30b-5p* and *miR-342-3p*) revealed pathways related to HF pathogenesis, identifying a differential signature of down-regulated miRNAs in the plasma of HF patients [65]. However, there are as yet uncertainties on the origins, transport function and mechanisms of action of miRNAs that need to be resolved before clinical applications in HF can be considered.

Cell-Based Therapies

One of the main challenges of cardiac medicine is the need to restore the cellular loss that occurs after a MI, which is the key trigger for adverse ventricular remodelling leading to HF development. In this scenario, cardiac regenerative therapies have emerged as an important tool with potential to overcome such challenge [66].

Since the regenerative concept of cell therapy started several types of cells have been included within the terminology of "stem cells". Each cell type has a different origin and is characterized by differential properties. In the early years, heterogeneous cell populations were used, but with the improvement of the understanding of SC properties, plasticity and paracrine activity these first generation preparations have been replaced by more sophisticated SC-related therapies, the second generation SC [67].

Non-cardiac Origin SCs

In cardiac regeneration the bone marrow-derived mesenchymal stem cells (BMCs) were initially widely used because of their ability to differentiate towards multiple tissue lineages and to secrete a wide range of factors [68]. Several studies on small animal models reported improved heart function after BMCs delivery [69–71]. Similar results were obtained in large animal models. As such, BMCs administration soon after acute MI in swine showed to improve left ventricular ejection fraction (LVEF) and limit wall thickening in the remote non-infarcted myocardium [72]. As well in a pig model of chronic ischemic cardiomyopathy BMCs significantly improved heart function inducing both structural and functional reverse remodelling [73]. Although these pre-clinical evidence point out towards a potential key role of BMCs in the treatment of HF some reports have produced discouraging results [74, 75].

Adipose-derived stem cells (ASCs) are mesenchymal SC that contribute to tissue homeostasis, cell renewal and spontaneous repair. ASCs share many properties with BMCs such as their potential to differentiate towards multiple tissue lineages, their ability to secrete angiogenic and antiapoptotic cytokines, and their immunomodulatory properties. However, ASCs show clear advantages in terms of accessibility and quantity of available sample and their easy *in vitro* expansion [76, 77]. Pre-clinical studies have demonstrated that ASCs administration improves cardiac function, perfusion and remodelling [78, 79]. Indeed, the transendocardial injection of ASCs in swine improved left ventricular LVEF [80] and human ASC implanted into immunocompetent rat hearts with AMI also improved LVEF [81]. However these results have not translated into clinical practice because when tested in human hearts, results have been poor (Table 15.2) [82–84].

The potential autologous cell use in the clinical setting is hampered by the stem cell loss of stemness properties due to the effects of the risk factors that affected the heart [85–89]. However, mesenchymal stem cells (MSCs) are an excellent source for allogeneic therapy due to the possibility of obtaining cells from healthy donors and to the fact that they have a low immunogenicity profile. In fact, preliminary preclinical studies have proven their safety and efficacy by showing their potential to differentiate into the three cardiac cell types and the improvement of cardiac function in large animal models of acute- [90] and chronic-IHD [91].

MSCs transdifferentiate into cardiomyocytes in *in vivo* mice models [92, 93] where transplanted cells have been shown to inhibit cardiac remodelling by reducing collagen deposition, inflammation and cardiomyocyte hypertrophy and to induce normalization of systolic and diastolic cardiac functions as well as the regeneration of the myocardium [93, 94].

The therapeutic efficacy of MSCs can be modified by epigenetic conditioning, i.e. modulating miRNAs levels [95]. Autologous MSC derived from patients with diabetes mellitus and HF exhibited downregulation of miR-126 levels that reduced their proangiogenic abilities [96, 97]. Also, bone marrow-derived MSCs (BM-MSCs) overexpressing miR-126 showed increased secretion of angiogenic factors and transplantation of murine BM-MSCs overexpressing miR-126 enhanced angiogenesis in the ischemic myocardium of mice after AMI [98]. In contrast, inhibition of miRNA-34, results in decreased cardiac fibrosis, improved cardiac function and enhanced angiogenesis in mice subjected to pressure overload by transverse aortic constriction [99]. Much remains to be investigated on the relationship between miRNAs and diseases before we understand the functions and therapeutic applications of miRNA modulation in MSC and in therapies for patients with HF.

Second Generation SCs

Cardiac Origin SCs

The most logical way to target cardiac regeneration would seem to stimulate the self-renewal ability of the tissue. However, it was not until the discovery of mitotic cardiomyocytes and the existence of a multipotent population of cells able to differentiate into cardiomyocytes, smooth muscle cells and endothelial cells, that the idea of a potential turnover of adult cardiomyocytes was plausible [100, 101]. These cardiac stem cells (CSCs) are rapidly activated after certain stimuli such as myocardial injury [102]. Indeed, in a pig model of chronic ischemic cardiomyopathy, CSCs administration showed to improve regional and global LV function and promote cardiac and vascular regeneration [103]. However, the amount of CSCs in adult hearts is too low, diminishing their potential usefulness in the clinical practice for the treatment of HF. In this scenario, the combination of CSCs with a more abundant and accessible SC type such as BMCs, has shown to enhance scar size reduction and restore diastolic and systolic function in a pig model of MI [104] and in a human clinical trial [105]. Indeed, when properly identified and expanded CSC robustly differentiate into cardiomyocytes both *in vitro* and *in vivo* [106]. Furthermore, through paracrine mechanisms, CSC have potent immunomodulatory effects that induce the reduction of apoptosis, fibrosis and inflammation in mice [107].

Another cardiac-related SC, are cardiospheres-derived cells (CDCs) which are a mixed cell population with clonogenic capacity that express SC markers (c-kit$^+$ and CD105$^+$) and show regenerative potential [108]. Importantly, CDCs have shown to afford equivalent effects on LVEF than CSCs in a pig model of ischemic cardiomyopathy but with higher benefits in improving hemodynamics and regional function, and in attenuating ventricular remodelling [109]. Furthermore, CDCs seem to be superior to other SC types providing the greatest functional benefit in a mouse model of MI [110].

Clinical trials with CDCs have been performed in Duchenne muscular dystrophy patients showing improvement in LVEF and LV chamber dimensions reduction; however their efficacy in HF needs to be tested in large randomised trials [111–113].

Pluripotent SCs

The second generation of SC also includes pluripotent SC (PSCs) which include embryonic stem cells (ESCs) and induced pluripotent stem cells (iPSCs). ESCs are isolated from blastocysts and are able to generate functional cardiomyocytes. Indeed small and large experimental animal models have shown their ability to improve cardiac function after MI [114, 115]. iPSCs are generated by the introduction of certain transcription factors into terminally differentiated cells [116].

Cardiac differentiation of PSCs to generate human CMs artificially seems also possible. These cells show the same electrical characteristics demonstrated by human cardiomyocytes [117]. Also 2- and 3-dimensional culture methods are available for cardiac differentiation. 2- dimensional cultures involve differentiation methods that use low-molecular-weight compounds such as CHIR99021 (an inhibitor of glycogen synthase kinase 3β) and/or inhibitors of the WNT signaling pathway (such as IWR-1 and IWP-2). 2-dimensional cultures have enabled the generation of large quantities of PSC-cardiomyocytes required for transplantation [118]. 3-dimensional culture methods generate large quantities of cardiomyocytes by suspension culture using a bioreactor or spinner flask [119] but it is a very expensive technology. 2- or 3-dimensional cultures cannot achieve 100% efficiency in cardiac differentiation, and fluctuations in differentiation efficiency are observed [120, 121]. Therefore, optimization of the cell-differentiation protocols is constantly revised and investigated.

SC-Derived Products

One of the main unresolved issues regarding SC therapy in the context of cardiac regeneration is the fact that grafted cells are not retained in the tissue for long periods while their effects seem to persist over time. This has led to the idea that SC-mediated beneficial effects can be driven by complex paracrine mechanisms that might stimulate endogenous repair signalling pathways [122]. Indeed, intracoronary administration of IGF-1 and hepatocyte growth factor reduced myocardial remodelling and induced regeneration leading to an improved cardiac function in a pig model of MI [123].

However, due to the high complexity of cardiac regeneration it seems implausible that the administration of single growth factors could fully regenerate the mass of the myocardium that is damaged after an MI and that can afterwards evolve into adverse cardiac remodelling and HF. In this scenario, some investigators have proposed that exosomes and microparticles released by SCs could be responsible for their beneficial effects. In line with this hypothesis, a recent study performed in a mouse model of HF has shown that extracellular vesicles derived from human ESCs exert the same beneficial effects on adverse remodelling and cardiac function than their parent cells [124].

Additionally, gene engineering and SC therapy can be combined to improve the properties and enhance the regenerative potential of SC by the up-regulation of specific transcription factors in order to: favour their differentiation into a cardiac phenotype (e.g. TBX5, MEF2C and GATA-4); enhance their pro-survival properties (e.g. Akt, ERK1/2 and HIF-1α); favour their electromechanical integration (e.g. N-cadherin and connexin-43); promote angiogenesis (e.g. VEGF and SDF-1); revert cell senescence (e.g. Pim-1 kinase and Notch-1) or promote cardiomyocyte regeneration (e.g. by regulating the Hippo pathway) [125–129].

Clinical Evidences

The promising results obtained in pre-clinical studies with both gene and SC-based therapies, led to a quick translation into clinical studies in order to test their potential benefit in humans.

Regarding gene therapy (Table 15.1), clinical trials targeting SERCA2a (CUPID) reported encouraging results with a trend towards reduction of clinical events [130] that was further confirmed after follow-up [131]. Unfortunately, the larger CUPID2 study failed to demonstrate efficacy [132]. Due to the key role of SERCA2a in the development of HF, two other clinical trials were initiated to test the effect of AVV1. SERCA2a gene transfer, AGENT-HF (AAV1-CMV-Serca2a GENe Therapy Trial in Heart Failure [133]) and SERCA-LVAD (Safety and Feasibility of AAV1/SERCA2a Gene Transfer in Patients With Chronic Heart Failure [134]) (https://clinicaltrials.gov). However, both studies were prematurely terminated due to the neutral results obtained in the CUPID2 and the trial data reported [133, 134]. The STOP-HF (SafeTy and efficacy Of JVS-100 administered to adults with ischemic heart failure) trial targeting SDF-1 demonstrated a significant improvement in LVEF in those patients who were in the lowest quartile at inclusion but failed to demonstrated other benefits [135]. Instead of direct endomyocardial delivery used in the STOP-HF trial, RETRO-HF studies the safety and efficacy of SDF-1 gene transfer delivered via retrograde delivery through the coronary sinus (NCT01961726). Results are still not available. Finally, the MUSIC-HFrEF1 Trial will explore if a higher AAV dose (3 × 1013 vg) improves vector uptake and leads to higher efficacy.

Intracoronary delivery of adenovirus encoding AC6 appeared to be safe in the AC6 trial. LV function was measured by echocardiography at rest and under

Table 15.1 Gene therapy based clinical trials for HF treatment

Name/clinical trial registration	Gene	Design	Vector administration	Patients	Outcome (or current status)
CUPID [130, 131]	SERCA2a	Randomized, double-blind, placebo-controlled	AAV1 intracoronary	Advanced HF; N = 39	Reduction in CV events including death. No safety concerns
CUPID2 [132]	SERCA2a	Multinational, randomized, double-blind, placebo-controlled	AAV1 intracoronary	HF LVEF ≤ 35%; N = 250	Lack of improvement in recurrence or death. No safety concerns
AGENT-HF [133]	SERCA2a	Randomized, double-blind, placebo-controlled	AAV1-CMV intracoronary	HF LVEF ≤ 35%; N = 9/40	Terminated prematurely at 9 subjects due to neutral results from CUPID2. None of the 9 subjects showed improved ventricular remodelling.
SERCA-LVAD [134]	SERCA2a	Randomized, double-blind, placebo-controlled	AAV1 intracoronary	Chronic HF with LV assistance device; N = 5/24	Terminated prematurely at 5 subjects due to neutral results from CUPID2. None of the 5 subjects showed functional benefits.
MUSIC-HFrEF1	SERCA2a	Randomized, double-blind, placebo-controlled	AAV1 intracoronary	Heart failure with reduced ejection fraction; N = 56	Recruiting
NCT00787059	AC6	Randomized, double-blind, placebo-controlled	Adenovirus intracoronary	Congestive HF; N = 56	Increased LV function beyond standard heart failure therapy

(continued)

Table 15.1 (continued)

Name/clinical trial registration	Gene	Design	Vector administration	Patients	Outcome (or current status)
STOP-HF [135]	SDF-1	Randomized, double-blind, placebo-controlled	Plasmid endomyocardial	IHF LVEF ≤ 40%; N = 93	No safety concerns. However it is only effective in patients with the lowest EF
RETRO-HF	SDF-	Randomized, controlled, Phase I/II, open label	Plasmid Retrograde injection via coronary sinus	IHF; N = 72	Active but not recruiting

AAV1 Adenoassociated virus, *CMV* Cytomegalovirus promoter, *CV* Cardiovascular, *IHF* Ischemic heart failure, *LVEF* Left ventricular ejection fraction, *LVESV* Left ventricular end-systolic volume

dobutamine stress, and improvement was seen in the high dose group. However, no differences between the AC6 treated and placebo-treated patients were seen in treadmill testing [136].

In the stem cell therapy area, the clear advantages and benefits shown in several pre-clinical studies drove a quick translation into clinical studies in order to test their potential usefulness in the context of IHD and HF (Table 15.2). For instance, different cellular populations of BMC were isolated and used for treatment of HF patients. Bone-marrow- derived mononuclear cells (BM- MNCs) are a heterogeneous population that includes hematopoietic stem cells, endothelial progenitor cells, mesenchymal stem cells, lymphocytes and monocytes. Stem cells within the BM-MNCs can differentiate into hepatocytes, neuroectodermal cells, endothelium and epithelium [157]. However, the fraction of stem cells with multipotent differentiation capacity within BM-MNCs is always below 1%. This is probably the reason why BM-MNC have always performed poorly in clinical trials. Indeed, 2 clinical trials were started in 2014 and 2015 had to be terminated early as no improvement was observed in LVEF [74, 75].

BM-MSCs can differentiate into cardiomyocytes, secrete matrix metalloproteinase and proangiogenic factors and have broad immune-modulatory and anti-inflammatory properties. Because they are easy to expand they have been used in several clinical trials in cardiovascular diseases. The POSEIDON trial in 2012 showed the allogenic cells superiority over autologous cells because allogenic BM-MSC treated patients showed a reduction in LV end-diastolic volume [158]. The TRIDENT study in 2017 compared two different doses of allogenic BM-MSCs in patients with ischemic HF, showing that both doses reduced scar size [149]. Finally, the more recent CONCERT- HF trial [159], comparing transendocardial injection of MSCs combined with cardiac stem cells (CSC), MSCs alone, or CSCs alone showed a significant reduction of HF-related major adverse cardiac events only in the CSCs group [105].

Table 15.2 SC therapy based clinical trials for HF treatments

Name/clinical trial registration	SC type	Design	Route of administration	Patients	Outcome (or current status)
REVIVE [137]	Bone marrow aspirate concentrate	Multinational, prospective, randomized, open-label	Retrograde into coronary sinus	IHF and NIHF; N = 60	Safe procedure. LVEF improved. LVESD and BNP improved only in NIHF patients
REGENERATE-IHD [138]	Bone marrow derived-SCs	Randomized, controlled, pilot study	Intramyocardial vs. intracoronary	IHF; N = 58	Safe and feasible procedures. Trend towards improved symptoms
NCT00418418 [139]	Bone marrow derived-SCs	Randomized, double blind	Intramyocardial in the border area	IHF LVEF $\leq$ 45%; N = 39	Reduced scar size. LV systolic function not improved
CARDIO133 [140]	$CD133^+$ bone marrow derived-SCs	Randomized, double blind, placebo-controlled	Intramyocardial	Chronic IHD and LVEF < 35%; N = 60	Scar size and regional perfusion improved. No effect in global LV function
STAR-heart [141]	Bone marrow derived-SCs	Not randomized	Intracoronary	Chronic HF LVEF $\leq$ 35%; N = 191	Safe procedure. Improved ventricular performance, quality of life and survival
FOCUS-HF [142]	Bone marrow mononuclear cells	Prospective	Transendocardial	Chronic HF; N = 30	Safe procedure. Quality of life scores improved
TAC-HFT [143]	MSCs vs. Bone marrow mononuclear cells	Randomized, blinded, placebo-controlled	Transendocardial	Ischemic cardiomyopathy and LVEF < 50%; N = 65	Safe procedures. Regional myocardial function improved only with MSCs
MSC-HF [144, 145]	BMCs	Randomized, double blind, placebo-controlled	Intramyocardial	Chronic IHF and LVEF < 45%; N = 60	Safe procedure. Reduced LVESV. Improved LVEF, stroke volume and myocardial mass
C-CURE [146]	BMCs	Multinational, prospective, randomized	Endomyocardial	IHF; N = 47	Safe and feasible procedure. LVEF improved and LVESV reduced. Improved clinical scoring
POSEIDON [147]	BMCs (allogenic vs. autologous)	Randomized, without placebo-control group	Transendocardial	Ischemic cardiomyopathy with LV dysfunction; N = 37	Low rates of immunologic reactions and clinical complications.

(continued)

Table 15.2 (continued)

Name/clinical trial registration	SC type	Design	Route of administration	Patients	Outcome (or current status)
PERFECT [148]	Autlogous BMCCD133+	Randomized controlled groups	Intramyocardial	Postinfarction patients with chronic ischemia; N = 82	Less adverse events, improved LVEF and quality of life in allogenic group
INTRACELL [74]	Autologous BM-MNC	Randomized controlled groups	Intramyocardial	Non-ischemic dilated cardiomyopathy; N = 30	Safe, no significant improvement in LVEF
MIHeart [75]	Autlogous BM-MNC	Randomized controlled groups	Intracoronary	Non-ischemic dilated cardiomyopathy; N = 30	No improvement in LVEF
TRIDENT [149]	Allogenic BMCs MSC	Randomized controlled groups	Transendocardial	IHD; N = 30	No improvement in LVEF
CONCERT-HF [105]	Autologous BM-MSC and c-kit+ cardiac cells	Double blind, placebo controlled, Phase II trial	Transendocardial	IHF; N = 125	Reduced scar size Improvement in MACE and quality of life
CCTRN SENECA [150]	Allogenic BM-MSC	Randomized controlled groups	Transendocardial	Cancer survivors with chronic dilated cardiomyopathy; N = 37	Safe, no differences in clinical outcomes
NCT01350310 [104]	$CD34^+$ SCs	Randomized, control group without placebo	Intracoronary	Dilated cardiomyopathy; N = 110	Increased LVEF and 6-min walk distance. Decreased NT-proBNP. Lower total mortality and pump failure, but not sudden cardiac death
CHART-1 [151, 152]	Bone marrow-derived and lineage-directed autologous cardiopoietic	Multicenter, randomized, sham-controlled	Intramyocardial	Chronic HF LVEF < 35% at high risk of recurrent events; N = 351	Decreased LV volumes
PRECISE [153]	ASCs	Randomized, double blind, placebo-controlled	Transendocardial	Ischemic cardiomyopathy; N = 27	Safe procedure. Improved ventricular function, myocardial perfusion and exercise capacity

CADUCEUS [154]	CDCs	Prospective, randomized, two centers	Intracoronary	LV dysfunction after MI; N = 25	Safe procedure. Reduced scar mass. Increased viable myocardium, regional contractility and regional systolic wall thickening. No changes in LVEF and LVESV at 6 months
NCT00442806 [82]	ADRC	Randomized controlled groups, double blind	Intramyocardial	CAD patients with ST-elevation AMI; N = 15	Did not increase LVEF
ATHENA ATHENA II [83]	ADRC	Parallel prospective randomized (2:1 active: placebo), double blind, controlled Phase II trials	Intramyocardial	Chronic myocardial ischemia and reduced LV function; N = 12	LVEF did not differ significantly between the ADRC and placebo groups
NCT02387723 [84]	ADRC	Randomized controlled groups	Intramyocardial	IHD and IHF patients; N = 10	Did not increase LVEF after 6 months
RIMECARD [155]	UC-MSC	Randomized controlled groups	Intravenous infusion	Patients with stable IHF; N = 30	At study completion, groups did not differ in mortality, heart failure admissions, arrythmias or incident malignancy.
HUC-HEART [156]	Allogenic UC-MSC or autologous BM-MNCs	Randomized controlled groups	Intramyocardial	Patients with chronic ischemic cardiomyopathy; N = 54	Increased LVEF and stroke volume only in UC-MSC treated patients.

ADRC adipose tissue derived regenerative cells, *BNP* B-type natriuretic peptide, *BM-MNC* Bone Marrow derived mononuclear cells, *BM-MSC* Bone Marrow derived mesenchymal cells, *CSC* Cardiac Stem Cells, *IHD* Ischemic heart disease, *IHF* Ischemic heart failure, *LVEF* Left ventricular ejection fraction, *LVESD* Left ventricular end-systolic diameter, *LVESV* Left ventricular end-systolic volume, *MACE* Major Adverse Cardiovascular Events, *MI* Myocardial infarction, *MSC* Mesenchimal Stem Cells, *NIHF* Non-ischemic heart failure, *NT-proBNP* N-terminal B-type natriuretic peptide, *UC-MSC* Umbilical cord derived mesenchymal cells

However, we still don't know if it is best to stimulate cardiomyocyte regeneration or to improve the function of the surviving cells; we don't know if the cells are the true reparative agent or if their paracrine secretions are; we don't know the appropriate cardiovascular disease to treat nor at which dose or the best route of administration. Therefore extensive basic research is needed to answer all these questions. What is true is that, for most of these SC-based therapies, we still do not know if they are able to induce clinically meaningful reverse cardiac remodelling and have an impact in the clinical evolution of patients.

In summary, the concept that cell-based repair of myocardial injury might be possible was introduced almost two decades ago; however, the field of cardiovascular reparative medicine has been criticized as translation to clinically effective approaches has been slow. The recent retraction of a series of papers has further impacted negatively the perception on this area of research. It is incumbent to critically appraise the current state of cardiac cell repair, determine what can be learned from past mistakes, and formulate best practices for future work. We need to have a critical assessment of what has fallen short, how to prevent similar issues, and how the field might best move forward in the service of science and patients [159].

Future Directions

Despite the encouraging results obtained in pre-clinical models, gene therapy has not yet demonstrated benefits in HF patients in Phase II clinical trials. This fact highlights the need to deeply analyze the optimal genes, cardiac specific vectors, delivery methods, and experimental models to target this complex disease, in order to obtain reproducible results that would warrant their translation into the clinics.

Regarding SC therapy, the discrepancy between promising pre-clinical animal research and the uncertain efficacy of human clinical trials has revealed the need to improve our understanding of the mechanisms of SCs-mediated protection, delineate their paracrine effects, and develop therapies which maximize their effects [160]. Research is needed before this strategy can be translated into standard clinical therapy. Specifically, three main key issues need to be addressed: (1) the search for the ideal cell type and cell-derived product for each specific situation; (2) the standardization of protocols for SC and cell-derived product preparation; and (3) the identification of the correct subsets of patients and control groups to be tested in clinical trials in order to obtain reliable results.

Acknowledgements This work has been possible thanks to the support of the Spanish Ministry of Economy and Competitiveness of Science "Agencia Estatal de Investigación (AEI)" Proj. Ref. AEI/10.13039/501100011033-[PID2019-107160RB-I00]; Project PMP22/00108 to LB cofounded by FEDER "Una Manera de Hacer Europa"; the Institute of Health Carlos III (ISCIII) CIBERCV-CB16/11/00411 and Red RICORS-TERAV to LB and PI23-00589 to MBP.

Conflict of Interest/Disclosures None

References

1. Roger VL. Epidemiology of heart failure. Circ Res. 2013;113:646–59.
2. Raake PW, Tscheschner H, Reinkober J, Ritterhoff J, Katus HA, Koch WJ, et al. Gene therapy targets in heart failure: the path to translation. Clin Pharmacol Ther. 2011;90:542–53.
3. Cadre BM, Qi M, Eble DM, Shannon TR, Bers DM, Samarel AM. Cyclic stretch downregulates calcium transporter gene expression in neonatal rat ventricular myocytes. J Mol Cell Cardiol. 1998;30:2247–59.
4. Hasenfuss G, Reinecke H, Studer R, Meyer M, Pieske B, Holtz J, et al. Relation between myocardial function and expression of sarcoplasmic reticulum Ca(2+)-ATPase in failing and nonfailing human myocardium. Circ Res. 1994;75:434–42.
5. Hayward C, Patel H, Lyon A. Gene therapy in heart failure. SERCA2a as a therapeutic target. Circ J. 2014;78:2577–87.
6. Andersson KB, Birkeland JA, Finsen AV, Louch WE, Sjaastad I, Wang Y, et al. Moderate heart dysfunction in mice with inducible cardiomyocyte-specific excision of the Serca2 gene. J Mol Cell Cardiol. 2009;47:180–7.
7. Kawase Y, Ly HQ, Prunier F, Lebeche D, Shi Y, Jin H, et al. Reversal of cardiac dysfunction after long-term expression of SERCA2a by gene transfer in a pre-clinical model of heart failure. J Am Coll Cardiol. 2008;51:1112–9.
8. Sakata S, Lebeche D, Sakata N, Sakata Y, Chemaly ER, Liang LF, et al. Restoration of mechanical and energetic function in failing aortic-banded rat hearts by gene transfer of calcium cycling proteins. J Mol Cell Cardiol. 2007;42:852–61.
9. Prunier F, Kawase Y, Gianni D, Scapin C, Danik SB, Ellinor PT, et al. Prevention of ventricular arrhythmias with sarcoplasmic reticulum Ca2+ ATPase pump overexpression in a porcine model of ischemia reperfusion. Circulation. 2008;118:614–24.
10. Hoshijima M, Ikeda Y, Iwanaga Y, Minamisawa S, Date MO, Gu Y, et al. Chronic suppression of heart-failure progression by a pseudophosphorylated mutant of phospholamban via in vivo cardiac rAAV gene delivery. Nat Med. 2002;8:864–71.
11. Iwanaga Y, Hoshijima M, Gu Y, Iwatate M, Dieterle T, Ikeda Y, et al. Chronic phospholamban inhibition prevents progressive cardiac dysfunction and pathological remodeling after infarction in rats. J Clin Invest. 2004;113:727–36.
12. Xin W, Li X, Lu X, Niu K, Cai J. Improved cardiac function after sarcoplasmic reticulum Ca(2+)-ATPase gene transfer in a heart failure model induced by chronic myocardial ischaemia. Acta Cardiol. 2011;66:57–64.
13. Kaye DM, Preovolos A, Marshall T, Byrne M, Hoshijima M, Hajjar R, et al. Percutaneous cardiac recirculation-mediated gene transfer of an inhibitory phospholamban peptide reverses advanced heart failure in large animals. J Am Coll Cardiol. 2007;50:253–60.
14. Suckau L, Fechner H, Chemaly E, Krohn S, Hadri L, Kockskamper J, et al. Long-term cardiac-targeted RNA interference for the treatment of heart failure restores cardiac function and reduces pathological hypertrophy. Circulation. 2009;119:1241–52.
15. Kaneko M, Hashikami K, Yamamoto S, Matsumoto H, Nishimoto T. Phospholamban ablation using CRISPR/Cas9 system improves mortality in a murine heart failure model. PLoS One. 2016;11(12):1–16.
16. Pathak A, del Monte F, Zhao W, Schultz JE, Lorenz JN, Bodi I, et al. Enhancement of cardiac function and suppression of heart failure progression by inhibition of protein phosphatase 1. Circ Res. 2005;96:756–66.
17. Nicolaou P, Rodriguez P, Ren X, Zhou X, Qian J, Sadayappan S, et al. Inducible expression of active protein phosphatase-1 inhibitor-1 enhances basal cardiac function and protects against ischemia/reperfusion injury. Circ Res. 2009;104:1012–20.
18. Ishikawa K, Fish KM, Tilemann L, Rapti K, Aguero J, Santos-Gallego CG, et al. Cardiac I-1c overexpression with reengineered AAV improves cardiac function in swine ischemic heart failure. Mol Ther. 2014;22:2038–45.

19. Quispe-Tintaya W. Protein phosphatase inhibitor-1 gene therapy in a swine model of non-ischemic heart failure. Physiol Behav. 2017;176:139–48.
20. Kho C, Lee A, Jeong D, Oh JG, Chaanine AH, Kizana E, et al. SUMO1-dependent modulation of SERCA2a in heart failure. Nature. 2011;477:601–5.
21. Tilemann L, Lee A, Ishikawa K, Aguero J, Rapti K, Santos-Gallego C, et al. SUMO-1 gene transfer improves cardiac function in a large-animal model of heart failure. Sci Transl Med. 2013;5:211ra159.
22. Kho C, Lee A, Jeong D, Oh JG, Gorski PA, Fish K, et al. Small-molecule activation of SERCA2a SUMOylation for the treatment of heart failure. Nat Commun. 2015;6:7229.
23. Pleger ST, Most P, Boucher M, Soltys S, Chuprun JK, Pleger W, et al. Stable myocardial-specific AAV6-S100A1 gene therapy results in chronic functional heart failure rescue. Circulation. 2007;115:2506–15.
24. Pleger ST, Shan C, Ksienzyk J, Bekeredjian R, Boekstegers P, Hinkel R, et al. Cardiac AAV9-S100A1 gene therapy rescues post-ischemic heart failure in a preclinical large animal model. Sci Transl Med. 2011;3:92ra64.
25. Go AS, Mozaffarian D, Roger VL, Benjamin EJ, Berry JD, Blaha MJ, et al. Heart disease and stroke statistics—2014 update: a report from the American Heart Association. Circulation. 2014;129:e28–e292.
26. Motloch LJ, Akar FG. Gene therapy to restore electrophysiological function in heart failure. Exp Opin Biol Ther. 2015;15:803–17.
27. Murata M, Cingolani E, McDonald AD, Donahue JK, Marban E. Creation of a genetic calcium channel blocker by targeted gem gene transfer in the heart. Circ Res. 2004;95:398–405.
28. Cingolani E, Ramirez Correa GA, Kizana E, Murata M, Cho HC, Marban E. Gene therapy to inhibit the calcium channel beta subunit: physiological consequences and pathophysiological effects in models of cardiac hypertrophy. Circ Res. 2007;101:166–75.
29. Lebeche D, Kaprielian R, del Monte F, Tomaselli G, Gwathmey JK, Schwartz A, et al. In vivo cardiac gene transfer of Kv4.3 abrogates the hypertrophic response in rats after aortic stenosis. Circulation. 2004;110:3435–43.
30. Wang N, Dries E, Fowler ED, Harmer SC, Hancox JC, Cannell M. Inducing $I_{to,f}$ and phase 1 repolarization of the cardiac action potential with a Kv4.3/KChIP2.1 bicistronic transgene. Mol Cell Cardiol. 2022;164:29–41.
31. Kim E, Fishman GI. Designer gap junctions that prevent cardiac arrhythmias. Trends Cardiovasc Med. 2013;23:33–8.
32. Greener ID, Sasano T, Wan X, Igarashi T, Strom M, Rosenbaum DS, et al. Connexin43 gene transfer reduces ventricular tachycardia susceptibility after myocardial infarction. J Am Coll Cardiol. 2012;60:1103–10.
33. Lin H, Mitasikova M, Dlugosova K, Okruhlicova L, Imanaga I, Ogawa K, Weismann P, Tribulova N, Republic S. Thyroid hormones suppress ε-pkc signalling, down-regulate connexin-43 and increase lethal arrhythmia susceptibility in non-diabetic and diabetic rat hearts. J Physiol Pharmacol. 2008;59:271–85.
34. Bacová BS, Vinczenzová C, Žurmanová J, Kašparová D, Knezl V, Benová TE, Pavelka S, Soukup T, Tribulová N. Altered thyroid status affects myocardial expression of connexin-43 and susceptibility of rat heart to malignant arrhythmias that can be partially normalized by red palm oil intake. Histochem Cell Biol. 2017;147:63–73.
35. Kanno S, Kovacs A, Yamada KA, Saffitz JE. Connexin43 as a determinant of myocardial infarct size following coronary occlusion in mice. J Am Coll Cardiol. 2003;41:681–6.
36. Sasano T, McDonald AD, Kikuchi K, Donahue JK. Molecular ablation of ventricular tachycardia after myocardial infarction. Nat Med. 2006;12:1256–8.
37. Remes A, Wagner AH, Schmiedel N, Heckmann M, Ruf T, Ding L, et al. AAV-mediated expression of NFAT decoy oligonucleotides protects from cardiac hypertrophy and heart failure. Basic Res Cardiol. 2021;116:38. https://doi.org/10.1007/s00395-021-00880-w.
38. Wang J, Shi Q, Wang Y, Dawson LW, Ciampa G, Zhao W, et al. Gene therapy with the N-terminus of junctophilin-2 improves heart failure in mice. Circ Res. 2022;130:1306–17.

39. Eschenhagen T. G proteins and the heart. Cell Biol Int. 1993;17:723–49.
40. Donahue JK, Heldman AW, Fraser H, McDonald AD, Miller JM, Rade JJ, et al. Focal modification of electrical conduction in the heart by viral gene transfer. Nat Med. 2000;6:1395–8.
41. Lugenbiel P, Bauer A, Kelemen K, Schweizer PA, Becker R, Katus HA, et al. Biological heart rate reduction through genetic suppression of galpha(s) protein in the sinoatrial node. J Am Heart Assoc. 2012;1(2):jah3-e000372.
42. Pfleger J, Gross P, Johnson J, Carter RL, Gao E, Tilley DG, et al. G protein-coupled receptor kinase 2 contributes to impaired fatty acid metabolism in the failing heart. J Mol Cell Cardiol. 2018;123:108–17.
43. Bauer R, Enns H, Jungmann A, Leuchs B, Volz C, Schinkel S, et al. Various effects of AAV9-mediated bARKct gene therapy on the heart in dystrophin-deficient (mdx) mice and d-sarcoglycan-deficient (Sgcd-/-) mice. Neuromuscul Disord. 2019;29(3):231–41. https://doi.org/10.1016/j.nmd.2018.12.006.
44. Harding VB, Jones LR, Lefkowitz RJ, Koch WJ, Rockman HA. Cardiac bARK1 inhibition prolongs survival and augments b blocker therapy in a mouse model of severe heart failure. Proc Natl Acad Sci USA. 2001;98:5809–14.
45. Raake PWJ, Schlegel P, Ksienzyk J, Reinkober J, Barthelmes J, Schinkel S, et al. AAV6. ARKct cardiac gene therapy ameliorates cardiac function and normalizes the catecholaminergic axis in a clinically relevant large animal heart failure model. Eur Heart J. 2013;34(19):1437–47.
46. Phan HM, Gao MH, Lai NC, Tang T, Hammond HK. New signaling pathways associated with increased cardiac adenylyl cyclase 6 expression: implications for possible congestive heart failure therapy. Trends Cardiovasc Med. 2007;17:215–21.
47. Gao MH, Lai NC, Roth DM, Zhou J, Zhu J, Anzai T, et al. Adenylylcyclase increases responsiveness to catecholamine stimulation in transgenic mice. Circulation. 1999;99:1618–22.
48. Lai NC, Roth DM, Gao MH, Tang T, Dalton N, Lai YY, et al. Intracoronary adenovirus encoding adenylyl cyclase VI increases left ventricular function in heart failure. Circulation. 2004;110:330–6.
49. Sastry A, Arnold E, Gurji H, Iwasa A, Bui H, Hassankhani A, Patel HH, Feramisco JR, Roth DM, Lai NC, Hammond HK, Narayan SM. Cardiac-directed expression of adenylyl cyclase VI facilitates atrioventricular nodal conduction. J Am Coll Cardiol. 2006;48:559–65.
50. Nowakowski SG, Kolwicz SC, Korte FS, Luo Z, Robinson-Hamm JN, Page JL, et al. Transgenic overexpression of ribonucleotide reductase improves cardiac performance. Proc Natl Acad Sci USA. 2013;110:6187–92.
51. Kadota S, Carey J, Reinecke H, et al. Ribonucleotide reductase-mediated increase in dATP improves cardiac performance via myosin activation in a large animal model of heart failure. Eur J Heart Fail. 2015;17(8):772–81.
52. Teichman SL, Thomson KS, Regnier M. Cardiac myosin activation with gene therapy produces sustained inotropic effects and may treat heart failure with reduced ejection fraction. Handb Exp Pharmacol. 2017;243:447–64.
53. Collesi C, Giacca M. Gene transfer to promote cardiac regeneration. Crit Rev Clin Lab Sci. 2016;53(6):359–69.
54. Collesi C, Zentilin L, Sinagra G, Giacca M. Notch1 signaling stimulates proliferation of immature cardiomyocytes. J Cell Biol. 2008;183:117–28.
55. Campa VM, Gutierrez-Lanza R, Cerignoli F, Diaz-Trelles R, Nelson B, Tsuji T, et al. Notch activates cell cycle reentry and progression in quiescent cardiomyocytes. J Cell Biol. 2008;183:129–41.
56. Tian Y, Liu Y, Wang T, Zhou N, Kong J, Chen L, et al. A microRNA-Hippo pathway that promotes cardiomyocyte proliferation and cardiac regeneration in mice. Sci Transl Med. 2015;7:279ra38.
57. Sundararaman S, Miller TJ, Pastore JM, Kiedrowski M, Aras R, Penn MS. Plasmid-based transient human stromal cellderived factor-1 gene transfer improves cardiac function in chronic heart failure. Gene Ther. 2011;18:867–73.

58. Subramanian S, Liu C, Aviv A, Ho JE, Courchesne P, Muntendam P, et al. Stromal cell-derived factor 1 as a biomarker of heart failure and mortality risk. Arterioscler Thromb Vasc Biol. 2014;34:2100–5.
59. Rutanen J, Rissanen TT, Markkanen JE, Gruchala M, Silvennoinen P, Kivela A, et al. Adenoviral catheter-mediated intramyocardial gene transfer using the mature form of vascular endothelial growth factor-D induces transmural angiogenesis in porcine heart. Circulation. 2004;109:1029.
60. Chatterjee NA, Singh JP. Autonomic modulation and cardiac arrhythmias: old insights and novel strategies. EP Eur. 2021;23:1708–21.
61. Gupta SK, Garg A, Bär C, Chatterjee S, Foinquinos A, Milting H, Streckfus-Bomeke K, Fiedler J, Thum T. Quaking inhibits doxorubicin-mediated cardiotoxicity through regulation of cardiac circular RNA expression short communication. Circ Res. 2018;122:246–54.
62. Kuang G-M-Q, O'Brien S, Thomas D, Hagop Kantarjian HY. Downregulation of MiR-199a derepresses hypoxia-inducible factor-1a and sirtuin 1 and recapitulates hypoxia preconditioning in cardiac myocytes. Circ Res. 2005;23:1–7.
63. Gabisonia K, Prosdocimo G, Aquaro GD, Carlucci L, Zentilin L, Secco I, et al. MicroRNA therapy stimulates uncontrolled cardiac repair after myocardial infarction in pigs. Nature. 2019;569:418–22. https://doi.org/10.1038/s41586-019-1191-6.
64. Yang J, Yang X, Fan S, Zhao X, Li C, Zhao Z, Pei M, Qiu L, Zhuang X, Yang C. Prognostic value of microRNAs in heart failure. Medicine (Baltimore). 2021;100(46):e27744.
65. Vilella-Figuerola A, Gallinat A, Escate R, Mirabet S, Padró T, Badimon L. Systems biology in chronic heart failure-identification of potential miRNA regulators. Int J Mol Sci. 2022;23(23):15226.
66. Ptaszek LM, Mansour M, Ruskin JN, Chien KR. Towards regenerative therapy for cardiac disease. Lancet. 2012;379:933–42.
67. Nunez Garcia A, Sanz-Ruiz R, Fernandez Santos ME, Fernandez-Aviles F. "Second-generation" stem cells for cardiac repair. World J Stem Cells. 2015;7:352–67.
68. Narita T, Suzuki K. Bone marrow-derived mesenchymal stem cells for the treatment of heart failure. Heart Fail Rev. 2015;20:53–68.
69. Cho J, Zhai P, Maejima Y, Sadoshima J. Myocardial injection with GSK-3beta-overexpressing bone marrow-derived mesenchymal stem cells attenuates cardiac dysfunction after myocardial infarction. Circ Res. 2011;108:478–89.
70. Lopez Y, Lutjemeier B, Seshareddy K, Trevino EM, Hageman KS, Musch TI, et al. Wharton's jelly or bone marrow mesenchymal stromal cells improve cardiac function following myocardial infarction for more than 32 weeks in a rat model: a preliminary report. Curr Stem Cell Res Ther. 2013;8:46–59.
71. Hou M, Yang KM, Zhang H, Zhu WQ, Duan FJ, Wang H, et al. Transplantation of mesenchymal stem cells from human bone marrow improves damaged heart function in rats. Int J Cardiol. 2007;115:220–8.
72. Price MJ, Chou CC, Frantzen M, Miyamoto T, Kar S, Lee S, et al. Intravenous mesenchymal stem cell therapy early after reperfused acute myocardial infarction improves left ventricular function and alters electrophysiologic properties. Int J Cardiol. 2006;111:231–9.
73. Schuleri KH, Feigenbaum GS, Centola M, Weiss ES, Zimmet JM, Turney J, et al. Autologous mesenchymal stem cells produce reverse remodelling in chronic ischaemic cardiomyopathy. Eur Heart J. 2009;30:2722–32.
74. Sant'Anna RT, Fracasso J, Valle FH, et al. Direct intramyocardial transthoracic transplantation of bone marrow mononuclear cells for non-ischemic dilated cardiomyopathy: INTRACELL, a prospective randomized controlled trial. Rev Bras Cir Cardiovasc. 2014;29(3):437–47.
75. Martino H, Brofman P, Greco O, et al. Multicentre, randomized, double-blind trial of intracoronary autologous mononuclear bone marrow cell injection in non-ischaemic dilated cardiomyopathy (the dilated cardiomyopathy arm of the MiHeart study). Eur Heart J. 2015;36(42):2898–904.

76. Zuk PA, Zhu M, Ashjian P, De Ugarte DA, Huang JI, Mizuno H, et al. Human adipose tissue is a source of multipotent stem cells. Mol Biol Cell. 2002;13:4279–95.
77. Badimon L, Onate B, Vilahur G. Adipose-derived mesenchymal stem cells and their reparative potential in ischemic heart disease. Rev Esp Cardiol (Engl Ed). 2015;68:599–611.
78. Wang L, Deng J, Tian W, Xiang B, Yang T, Li G, et al. Adipose-derived stem cells are an effective cell candidate for treatment of heart failure: an MR imaging study of rat hearts. Am J Physiol Heart Circ Physiol. 2009;297:H1020–31.
79. Valina C, Pinkernell K, Song YH, Bai X, Sadat S, Campeau RJ, et al. Intracoronary administration of autologous adipose tissue-derived stem cells improves left ventricular function, perfusion, and remodelling after acute myocardial infarction. Eur Heart J. 2007;28:2667–77.
80. Mazo M, et al. Treatment of reperfused ischemia with adipose-derived stem cells in a preclinical swine model of myocardial infarction. Cell Transplant. 2012;21:2723–33.
81. Paul A, et al. Functional assessment of adipose stem cells for xenotransplantation using myocardial infarction immunocompetent models: comparison with bone marrow stem cells. Cell Biochem Biophys. 2013;67:263–73.
82. Houtgraaf JH, et al. First experience in humans using adipose tissue-derived regenerative cells in the treatment of patients with ST-segment elevation myocardial infarction. J Am Coll Cardiol. 2012;59:539–40.
83. Henry TD, et al. The Athena trials: autologous adipose-derived regenerative cells for refractory chronic myocardial ischemia with left ventricular dysfunction. Catheter Cardiovasc Interv. 2017;89:169–77.
84. Kastrup J, et al. Cryopreserved off-the-shelf allogeneic adipose-derived stromal cells for therapy in patients with ischemic heart disease and heart failure—a safety study. Stem Cells Transl Med. 2017;6:1963–71.
85. Onate B, Vilahur G, Camino-Lopez S, Diez-Caballero A, Ballesta-Lopez C, Ybarra J, et al. Stem cells isolated from adipose tissue of obese patients show changes in their transcriptomic profile that indicate loss in stemcellness and increased commitment to an adipocyte-like phenotype. BMC Genomics. 2013;14:625.
86. Onate B, Vilahur G, Ferrer-Lorente R, Ybarra J, Diez-Caballero A, Ballesta-Lopez C, et al. The subcutaneous adipose tissue reservoir of functionally active stem cells is reduced in obese patients. FASEB J. 2012;26:4327–36.
87. Bejar MT, Ferrer-Lorente R, Pena E, Badimon L. Inhibition of Notch rescues the angiogenic potential impaired by cardiovascular risk factors in epicardial adipose stem cells. FASEB J. 2016;30(8):2849–59.
88. Ferrer-Lorente R, Bejar MT, Badimon L. Notch signaling pathway activation in normal and hyperglycemic rats differs in the stem cells of visceral and subcutaneous adipose tissue. Stem Cells Dev. 2014;23:3034–48.
89. Ferrer-Lorente R, Bejar MT, Tous M, Vilahur G, Badimon L. Systems biology approach to identify alterations in the stem cell reservoir of subcutaneous adipose tissue in a rat model of diabetes: effects on differentiation potential and function. Diabetologia. 2014;57:246–56.
90. Amado LC, Saliaris AP, Schuleri KH, St John M, Xie JS, Cattaneo S, et al. Cardiac repair with intramyocardial injection of allogeneic mesenchymal stem cells after myocardial infarction. Proc Natl Acad Sci USA. 2005;102:11474–9.
91. Quevedo HC, Hatzistergos KE, Oskouei BN, Feigenbaum GS, Rodriguez JE, Valdes D, et al. Allogeneic mesenchymal stem cells restore cardiac function in chronic ischemic cardiomyopathy via trilineage differentiating capacity. Proc Natl Acad Sci USA. 2009;106:14022–7.
92. Toma C, Pittenger MF, Cahill KS, et al. Human mesenchymal stem cells differentiate to a cardiomyocyte phenotype in the adult murine heart. Circulation. 2002;105:93–8.
93. Mangi AA, Noiseux N, Kong D, et al. Mesenchymal stem cells modifiedwith Akt prevent remodeling and restore performance of infarctedhearts. Nat Med. 2003;9:1195–201.
94. Tang J, Xie Q, Pan G, et al. Mesenchymal stem cells participate in angiogenesis and improve heart function in rat model of myocardial ischemia with reperfusion. Eur J Cardiothorac Surg. 2006;30:353–61.

95. Zhu K, et al. Developing miRNA therapeutics for cardiac repair in ischemic heart disease. J Thorac Dis. 2016;8:E918–27.
96. Meng S, et al. Downregulation of microRNA-126 in endothelial progenitor cells from diabetes patients, impairs their functional properties, via target gene Spred-1. J Mol Cell Cardiol. 2012;53:64–72.
97. Jakob P, et al. Loss of angiomiR-126 and 130a in angiogenic early outgrowth cells from patients with chronic heart failure: role for impaired in vivo neovascularization and cardiac repair capacity. Circulation. 2012;126:2962–75.
98. Huang F, et al. Mesenchymal stem cells modified with miR-126 release angiogenic factors and activate Notch ligand Delta-like-4, enhancing ischemic angiogenesis and cell survival. Int J Mol Med. 2013;31:484–92.
99. Bernardo BC, et al. Therapeutic inhibition of the miR-34 family attenuates pathological cardiac remodeling and improves heart function. Proc Natl Acad Sci USA. 2012;109:17615–20.
100. Beltrami AP, Urbanek K, Kajstura J, Yan SM, Finato N, Bussani R, et al. Evidence that human cardiac myocytes divide after myocardial infarction. N Engl J Med. 2001;344:1750–7.
101. Beltrami AP, Barlucchi L, Torella D, Baker M, Limana F, Chimenti S, et al. Adult cardiac stem cells are multipotent and support myocardial regeneration. Cell. 2003;114:763–76.
102. Angert D, Berretta RM, Kubo H, Zhang H, Chen X, Wang W, et al. Repair of the injured adult heart involves new myocytes potentially derived from resident cardiac stem cells. Circ Res. 2011;108:1226–37.
103. Bolli R, Tang XL, Sanganalmath SK, Rimoldi O, Mosna F, Abdel-Latif A, et al. Intracoronary delivery of autologous cardiac stem cells improves cardiac function in a porcine model of chronic ischemic cardiomyopathy. Circulation. 2013;128:122–31.
104. Williams AR, Hatzistergos KE, Addicott B, McCall F, Carvalho D, Suncion V, et al. Enhanced effect of combining human cardiac stem cells and bone marrow mesenchymal stem cells to reduce infarct size and to restore cardiac function after myocardial infarction. Circulation. 2013;127:213–23.
105. Bolli R, Mitrani RD, Hare JM, et al. A phase II study of autologous mesenchymal stromal cells andc-kit positive cardiac cells, alone or in combination, in patients with ischaemic heart failure: the CCTRNCONCERT-HF trial. Eur J Heart Fail. 2021;23(4):661–74.
106. Scalise M, Marino F, Salerno L, et al. In vitro CSC-derived cardiomyocytes exhibit the typical microRNA-mRNA blueprint of endogenous cardiomyocytes. Commun Biol. 2021;4(1):1146.
107. Nadal-Ginard B, Ellison GM, Torella D. The cardiac stem cell compartment is indispensable for myocardial cell homeostasis, repair and regeneration in the adult. Stem Cell Res. 2014;13(3Pt B):615–30.
108. Smith RR, Barile L, Cho HC, Leppo MK, Hare JM, Messina E, et al. Regenerative potential of cardiosphere-derived cells expanded from percutaneous endomyocardial biopsy specimens. Circulation. 2007;115:896–908.
109. Lee ST, White AJ, Matsushita S, Malliaras K, Steenbergen C, Zhang Y, et al. Intramyocardial injection of autologous cardiospheres or cardiosphere-derived cells preserves function and minimizes adverse ventricular remodeling in pigs with heart failure post-myocardial infarction. J Am Coll Cardiol. 2011;57:455–65.
110. Li TS, Cheng K, Malliaras K, Smith RR, Zhang Y, Sun B, et al. Direct comparison of different stem cell types and subpopulations reveals superior paracrine potency and myocardial repair efficacy with cardiosphere-derived cells. J Am Coll Cardiol. 2012;59:942–53.
111. Taylor M, Jefferies J, Byrne B, et al. Cardiac and skeletal muscle effects in the randomized HOPE-Duchenne trial. Neurology. 2019;92(8):e866–e78.
112. Rogers RG, Fournier M, Sanchez L, et al. Disease-modifying bioactivity of intravenous cardiosphere-derived cells and exosomes in mdx mice. JCI Insight. 2019;4(7):e125754.
113. Marban L, Rogy S, McDonald C, et al. Late breaking news e-poster presentation: LBP 5 HOPE-2 one-year results show clinically relevant improvements in upper limb &cardiac function in patients with later stage duchenne muscular dystrophy. Neuromuscul Disord. 2020;30:S168–S9.

114. Menard C, Hagege AA, Agbulut O, Barro M, Morichetti MC, Brasselet C, et al. Transplantation of cardiac-committed mouse embryonic stem cells to infarcted sheep myocardium: a preclinical study. Lancet. 2005;366:1005–12.
115. Caspi O, Huber I, Kehat I, Habib M, Arbel G, Gepstein A, et al. Transplantation of human embryonic stem cell-derived cardiomyocytes improves myocardial performance in infarcted rat hearts. J Am Coll Cardiol. 2007;50:1884–93.
116. Takahashi K, Yamanaka S. Induction of pluripotent stem cells from mouse embryonic and adult fibroblast cultures by defined factors. Cell. 2006;126:663–76.
117. Zhang J, Wilson GF, Soerens AG, Koonce CH, Yu J, Palecek SP, et al. Functional cardiomyocytes derived from human induced pluripotent stem cells. Circ Res. 2009;104:e30–41.
118. Tohyama S, Fujita J, Fujita C, Yamaguchi M, Kanaami S, Ohno R, et al. Efficient large-scale 2D culture system for human-induced pluripotent stem cells and differentiated cardiomyocytes. Stem Cell Rep. 2017;9:1406–14.
119. Hemmi N, Tohyama S, Nakajima K, Kanazawa H, Suzuki T, Hattori F, et al. A massive suspension culture system with metabolic purification for human pluripotent stem cell-derived cardiomyocytes. Stem Cells Transl Med. 2014;3:1473–83.
120. Lian X, Zhang J, Azarin SM, Zhu K, Hazeltine LB, Bao X, et al. Directed cardiomyocyte differentiation from human pluripotent stem cells by modulating Wnt/beta-catenin signaling under fully defined conditions. Nat Protoc. 2013;8:162–75. https://doi.org/10.1038/nprot.2012.150.
121. Burridge PW, Matsa E, Shukla P, Lin ZC, Churko JM, Ebert AD, et al. Chemically defined generation of human cardiomyocytes. Nat Methods. 2014;11:855–60.
122. Gnecchi M, Zhang Z, Ni A, Dzau VJ. Paracrine mechanisms in adult stem cell signaling and therapy. Circ Res. 2008;103:1204–19.
123. Koudstaal S, Bastings MM, Feyen DA, Waring CD, van Slochteren FJ, Dankers PY, et al. Sustained delivery of insulin-like growth factor-1/hepatocyte growth factor stimulates endogenous cardiac repair in the chronic infarcted pig heart. J Cardiovasc Transl Res. 2014;7:232–41.
124. Kervadec A, Bellamy V, El Harane N, Arakelian L, Vanneaux V, Cacciapuoti I, et al. Cardiovascular progenitor-derived extracellular vesicles recapitulate the beneficial effects of their parent cells in the treatment of chronic heart failure. J Heart Lung Transplant. 2016;35(6):795–807.
125. Behfar A, Yamada S, Crespo-Diaz R, Nesbitt JJ, Rowe LA, Perez-Terzic C, et al. Guided cardiopoiesis enhances therapeutic benefit of bone marrow human mesenchymal stem cells in chronic myocardial infarction. J Am Coll Cardiol. 2010;56:721–34.
126. Don CW, Murry CE. Improving survival and efficacy of pluripotent stem cell-derived cardiac grafts. J Cell Mol Med. 2013;17:1355–62.
127. Hahn JY, Cho HJ, Kang HJ, Kim TS, Kim MH, Chung JH, et al. Pre-treatment of mesenchymal stem cells with a combination of growth factors enhances gap junction formation, cytoprotective effect on cardiomyocytes, and therapeutic efficacy for myocardial infarction. J Am Coll Cardiol. 2008;51:933–43.
128. Siddiqi S, Sussman MA. Cell and gene therapy for severe heart failure patients: the time and place for Pim-1 kinase. Expert Rev Cardiovasc Ther. 2013;11:949–57.
129. Morikawa Y, Zhang M, Heallen T, Leach J, Tao G, Xiao Y, et al. Actin cytoskeletal remodeling with protrusion formation is essential for heart regeneration in Hippo-deficient mice. Sci Signal. 2015;8:ra41.
130. Jessup M, Greenberg B, Mancini D, Cappola T, Pauly DF, Jaski B, et al. Calcium upregulation by percutaneous administration of gene therapy in cardiac disease (CUPID): a phase 2 trial of intracoronary gene therapy of sarcoplasmic reticulum Ca2+-ATPase in patients with advanced heart failure. Circulation. 2011;124:304–13.
131. Zsebo K, Yaroshinsky A, Rudy JJ, Wagner K, Greenberg B, Jessup M, et al. Long-term effects of AAV1/SERCA2a gene transfer in patients with severe heart failure: analysis of recurrent cardiovascular events and mortality. Circ Res. 2014;114:101–8.

132. Greenberg B, Butler J, Felker GM, Ponikowski P, Voors AA, Desai AS, et al. Calcium upregulation by percutaneous administration of gene therapy in patients with cardiac disease (CUPID 2): a randomised, multinational, double-blind, placebo-controlled, phase 2b trial. Lancet. 2016;387:1178–86.
133. Hulot JS, Salem JE, Redheuil A, Collet JP, Varnous S, Jourdain P, et al. Effect of intracoronary administration of AAV1/SERCA2a on ventricular remodelling in patients with advanced systolic heart failure: results from the AGENT-HF randomized phase 2 trial. Eur J Heart Fail. 2017;19(11):1534–41.
134. Lyon AR, Babalis D, Morley-Smith AC, Hedger M, Suarez Barrientos A, Foldes G, et al. Investigation of the safety and feasibility of AAV1/SERCA2a gene transfer in patients with chronic heart failure supported with a left ventricular assist device: the SERCALVAD TRIAL. Gene Ther. 2020;27(12):579–90.
135. Chung ES, Miller L, Patel AN, Anderson RD, Mendelsohn FO, Traverse J, et al. Changes in ventricular remodelling and clinical status during the year following a single administration of stromal cell-derived factor-1 non-viral gene therapy in chronic ischaemic heart failure patients: the STOP-HF randomized Phase II trial. Eur Heart J. 2015;36:2228–38.
136. Hammond HK, Penny WF, Traverse JH, Henry TD, Watkins MW, Yancy CW, et al. Intracoronary gene transfer of adenylyl cyclase 6 in patients with heart failure: a randomized clinical trial. JAMA Cardiol. 2016;1:163–71.
137. Patel AN, Mittal S, Turan G, Winters AA, Henry TD, Ince H, et al. REVIVE trial: retrograde delivery of autologous bone marrow in patients with heart failure. Stem Cells Transl Med. 2015;4:1021–7.
138. Mozid A, Yeo C, Arnous S, Ako E, Saunders N, Locca D, et al. Safety and feasibility of intramyocardial versus intracoronary delivery of autologous cell therapy in advanced heart failure: the REGENERATE-IHD pilot study. Regen Med. 2014;9:269–78.
139. Patila T, Lehtinen M, Vento A, Schildt J, Sinisalo J, Laine M, et al. Autologous bone marrow mononuclear cell transplantation in ischemic heart failure: a prospective, controlled, randomized, double-blind study of cell transplantation combined with coronary bypass. J Heart Lung Transplant. 2014;33:567–74.
140. Nasseri BA, Ebell W, Dandel M, Kukucka M, Gebker R, Doltra A, et al. Autologous CD133+ bone marrow cells and bypass grafting for regeneration of ischaemic myocardium: the Cardio133 trial. Eur Heart J. 2014;35:1263–74.
141. Strauer BE, Yousef M, Schannwell CM. The acute and long-term effects of intracoronary stem cell transplantation in 191 patients with chronic heARt failure: the STAR-heart study. Eur J Heart Fail. 2010;12:721–9.
142. Perin EC, Silva GV, Henry TD, Cabreira-Hansen MG, Moore WH, Coulter SA, et al. A randomized study of transendocardial injection of autologous bone marrow mononuclear cells and cell function analysis in ischemic heart failure (FOCUS-HF). Am Heart J. 2011;161(1078-87):e3.
143. Heldman AW, DiFede DL, Fishman JE, Zambrano JP, Trachtenberg BH, Karantalis V, et al. Transendocardial mesenchymal stem cells and mononuclear bone marrow cells for ischemic cardiomyopathy: the TAC-HFT randomized trial. JAMA. 2014;311:62–73.
144. Mathiasen AB, Jorgensen E, Qayyum AA, Haack-Sorensen M, Ekblond A, Kastrup J. Rationale and design of the first randomized, double-blind, placebo-controlled trial of intramyocardial injection of autologous bone-marrow derived mesenchymal stromal cells in chronic ischemic heart failure (MSC-HF trial). Am Heart J. 2012;164:285–91.
145. Mathiasen AB, Qayyum AA, Jorgensen E, Helqvist S, Fischer-Nielsen A, Kofoed KF, et al. Bone marrow-derived mesenchymal stromal cell treatment in patients with severe ischaemic heart failure: a randomized placebo-controlled trial (MSC-HF trial). Eur Heart J. 2015;36:1744–53.
146. Bartunek J, Behfar A, Dolatabadi D, Vanderheyden M, Ostojic M, Dens J, et al. Cardiopoietic stem cell therapy in heart failure: the C-CURE (Cardiopoietic stem Cell therapy in heart

failURE) multicenter randomized trial with lineage-specified biologics. J Am Coll Cardiol. 2013;61:2329–38.
147. Hare JM, DiFede DL, Rieger AC, et al. Randomized comparison of allogeneic versus autologous mesenchymal stem cells for non ischemic dilated cardiomyopathy: POSEIDON-DCM trial. J Am Coll Cardiol. 2017;69(5):526–37.
148. Steinhoff G, Nesteruk J, Wolfien M, et al. Cardiac function improvement and bone marrow response-outcome analysis of the randomized PERFECT phase III clinical trial of intramyocardial CD133 (+) application after myocardial infarction. EBio Med. 2017;22:208–24.
149. Florea V, Rieger AC, DiFede DL, et al. Dose comparison study of allogeneic mesenchymal stem cells in patients with ischemic cardiomyopathy (the TRIDENT study). Circ Res. 2017;121(11):1279–90.
150. Bolli R, Perin EC, Willerson JT, et al. Allogeneic mesenchymal cell therapy in anthracycline-induced cardiomyopathy heart failure patients: the CCTRN SENECA trial. JACC Cardio Oncol. 2020;2(4):581–95.
151. Bartunek J, Davison B, Sherman W, Povsic T, Henry TD, Gersh B, et al. Congestive heart failure cardiopoietic regenerative therapy (CHART-1) trial design. Eur J Heart Fail. 2016;18:160–8.
152. Teerlink JR, Metra M, Filippatos GS, et al. Benefit of cardiopoietic mesenchymal stem cell therapy on left ventricular remodelling: results from the congestive heart failure cardiopoietic regenerative therapy (CHART-1) study. Eur J Heart Fail. 2017;19(11):1520–9.24.
153. Perin EC, Sanz-Ruiz R, Sanchez PL, Lasso J, Perez-Cano R, Alonso-Farto JC, et al. Adipose-derived regenerative cells in patients with ischemic cardiomyopathy: the PRECISE trial. Am Heart J. 2014;168(88-95):e2.
154. Makkar RR, Smith RR, Cheng K, Malliaras K, Thomson LE, Berman D, et al. Intracoronary cardiosphere-derived cells for heart regeneration after myocardial infarction (CADUCEUS): a prospective, randomised phase 1 trial. Lancet. 2012;379:895–904.
155. Bartolucci J, Verdugo FJ, Gonzalez PL, et al. Safety and efficacy of the intravenous infusion of umbilical cord mesenchymal stem cells in patients with heart failure: a phase 1/2 randomized controlled trial (RIMECARD trial [randomized clinical trial of intravenous infusion umbilical cord mesenchymal stem cells on cardiopathy]). Circ Res. 2017;121(10):1192–204.
156. Ulus AT, Mungan C, Kurtoglu M, et al. Intramyocardial transplantation of umbilical cord mesenchymal stromal cells in chronic ischemic cardiomyopathy: a controlled, randomized clinical trial (HUC-HEART trial). Int J Stem Cells. 2020;13(3):364–76.
157. Cuende N, Rico L, Herrera C. Concise review: bone marrow mononuclear cells for the treatment of ischemic syndromes: medicinal product or cell transplantation? Stem Cells Transl Med. 2012;1(5):403–8.
158. Hare JM, Fishman JE, Gerstenblith G, DiFede Velazquez DL, Zambrano JP, Suncion VY, et al. Comparison of allogeneic vs autologous bone marrow-derived mesenchymal stem cells delivered by transendocardial injection in patients with ischemic cardiomyopathy: the POSEIDON randomized trial. JAMA. 2012;308:2369–79.
159. Povsic TJ, Sanz-Ruiz R, Climent AM, Bolli R, Taylor DA, Gersh BJ, Menasché P, Perin EC, Pompilio G, Atsma DE, Badimon L, DeMaria AN, Hare JM, Henry TD, Janssens S, Kastrup J, Torella D, Traverse JH, Willerson JT, Fernández-Avilés F. Reparative cell therapy for the heart: critical internal appraisal of the field in response to recent controversies. ESC Heart Fail. 2021;8(3):2306–9. https://doi.org/10.1002/ehf2.13256.
160. Badimon L, Vilahur G. Experimental cell therapy: the search for the best stem cell continues. J Am Coll Cardiol. 2014;64:1695–7.

Chapter 16
Transcatheter Therapies for Tricuspid Regurgitation

Julio C. Echarte Morales, Tomás Benito-González, and Rodrigo Estévez-Loureiro

Abstract Tricuspid regurgitation is a significant component of congestive heart failure and is associated with adverse outcomes when left untreated. It often results from the enlargement of the tricuspid annulus and right-sided heart chambers due to various underlying conditions. Transcatheter tricuspid interventions (TTVI), such as tricuspid valve replacement and tricuspid valve repair, offer promising alternatives to surgery but face challenges related to anatomy, technical aspects, and patient selection. Future improvements in device design and imaging technology hold the potential to overcome these challenges and make TTVI more widely accessible.

Keywords Tricuspid regurgitation · Heart failure · Transcatheter interventions · Transcatheter edge-to-edge repair · Transcatheter replacement

Introduction

The prevalence of tricuspid regurgitation (TR) increases with age and is associated with an elevated risk of heart failure exacerbation and mortality [1–4]. The most common cause of TR is secondary or functional, resulting from the enlargement of right-sided heart chambers due to conditions like left heart disease, pulmonary hypertension, atrial fibrillation (AF), or intrinsic disorders of the right ventricle (RV) [5]. In contrast, primary TR is linked to structural anomalies in the tricuspid valve leaflets or apparatus [6]. Additionally, TR related to cardiac implantable electronic devices (CIEDs) is a less common but emerging issue, and its prevalence is anticipated to increase [7, 8].

J. C. Echarte Morales · R. Estévez-Loureiro (✉)
Department of Cardiology, University Hospital Alvaro Cunqueiro, Vigo, Spain

Cardiovascular Research Group, Department of Cardiology, University Hospital Alvaro Cunqueiro, Fundación Biomédica Galicia Sur, Servizo Galego de Saude, University of Vigo, Vigo, Spain

T. Benito-González
Interventional Cardiology Unit, Complejo Asistencial Universitario de Leon, Leon, Spain

M. Dorobanţu et al. (eds.), *Current Approach to Heart Failure*,
https://doi.org/10.1007/978-3-031-96562-3_16

Current guidelines recommend surgical intervention for tricuspid valve-related issues in cases requiring left-sided valve procedures with severe TR or mild to moderate TR together with tricuspid annulus (TA) dilation ($\geq$40 mm or >21 mm/m^2). In isolated TR scenarios, surgery is recommended for patients experiencing severe TR accompanied by symptoms or RV dilatation. However, surgery is not recommended in the presence of severe RV dysfunction or severe pulmonary hypertension [1, 9]. Since isolated tricuspid surgery is infrequently performed due to significant risks of morbidity and mortality, transcatheter alternatives, such as tricuspid valve repair (TTVr) and replacement (TTVR), have gained prominence [10]. These therapies have emerged as potential alternatives to surgery, offering promising results in terms of safety and efficacy for patients who are not suitable candidates for conventional surgical procedures.

Tricuspid Regurgitation and Heart Failure: An Interlinked Relationship

For an extended duration, TR had been perceived as a result of left-sided cardiac conditions, and subsequently, erroneously regarded as harmless and primarily treated medically, mainly with diuretics [11]. However, the clinical evidence now firmly establishes that significant TR serves as a predictor of mortality and overall adverse cardiovascular outcomes. In patients with chronic heart failure, Neuhold et al. reported that significant TR was a predictor in individuals with mildly or moderately reduced left ventricular ejection fraction (LVEF) and NT-proBNP levels below 280 fmol/ml [12]. However, this predictive significance was not observed in advanced disease. Similarly, Topilsky et al. demonstrated that moderate or severe TR in patients with reduced LVEF was associated with higher rates of heart failure. Furthermore, those patients with severe TR (effective regurgitant orifice $\geq$ 0.4 cm^2) faced an increased mortality rate [13].

The RV can tolerate volume overload better than pressure overload, and RV remodeling may precede dysfunction until advanced stages of TR. Right heart failure (RHF) is a clinical condition marked by diminished exercise capacity and/or indications of right-sided decompensation, similar to left heart failure, and progresses through stages [14]. In patients with secondary TR, postoperative outcomes are significantly influenced by RV function, although specific RV functional parameters for predicting isolated tricuspid valve intervention outcomes lack established recommendations. Introducing a staging system of RV dysfunction and the signs and symptoms of right RHF could be beneficial for standardizing their assessment in clinical practice and may help to identify who will benefit from earlier transcatheter interventions [15].

Impact of TR Etiology

Characterizing the primary morphological and/or functional abnormalities leading to the onset of TR is a fundamental aspect when considering a percutaneous treatment approach [16–20] (Table 16.1 and Fig. 16.1).

Patients with ventricular secondary TR typically have a bleaker prognosis compared to those with atrial secondary TR [21, 22]. Furthermore, when precapillary pulmonary hypertension serves as the primary mechanism of TR, the prognosis becomes even more unfavorable. Although there are limitations to suggesting this approach as a means of determining the etiology, it could prove valuable in identifying the most suitable candidates for interventions.

Table 16.1 Integral classification of Tricuspid Regurgitation

	Pathophysiology	Etiology	Imaging
Primary	Absence of leaflet coaptation resulting from intrinsic changes leading to restricted or excessive leaflet mobility or leaflet perforation	Congenital Infective endocarditis Rheumatic disease Carcinoid heart disease Tumors Myxomatous degeneration	TV leaflet structural abnormalities Leaflet mobility varies across all etiologies Enlargement of right-heart side in long-standing evolution
Ventricular secondary	Enlargement and/or dysfunction of the right ventricle, resulting in pronounced leaflet tethering and annular dilation	1. Postcapillary PH due to left-side cardiac disease: Left ventricular diseases (HFpEF or HFrEF) Significant left valvular disease 2. Precapillary PH due to intrinsic pulmonary diseases: Primary pulmonary hypertension Parenchymal disease (e.g., CLD, CTEPH) 3. Primary RV dysfunction or remodeling: RV infarct RV cardiomyopathy	Significant tethering and tenting of the TV leaflets (typically ≥10 mm) The right side of the heart is commonly dilated, with particular enlargement of the RV Systolic impairment of both the LV and RV is usually observed The systolic pulmonary artery pressure is often ≥50 mmHg
Atrial secondary	Enlargement and dysfunction of the RA result in substantial isolated annular dilation	Long-standing Atrial Fibrillation Long-standing Atrial Flutter HFpEF	The right side of the heart is commonly dilated, with particular enlargement of the RA Preserved systolic function of both the LV and RV is usually observed The systolic pulmonary artery pressure is often <50 mmHg

(continued)

Table 16.1 (continued)

	Pathophysiology	Etiology	Imaging
CIED-induced	TR caused by interference from the device cable with leaflets or subvalvular apparatus causing: Leaflet impingement Leaflet/chordal entanglement/ chordal rupture Leaflet adherence Leaflet laceration/ perforation Annular dilatation secondary to chronic pacing	Pacemaker Implantable cardiac defibrillator CRT devices	Altered valvular apparatus may be present Leaflet mobility varies across all etiologies The right-side heart is typically dilated

CIED cardiac implantable electronic device, *CLD* chronic lung disease, *CTEPH* chronic thromboembolic pulmonary hypertension, *CRT* cardiac resynchronization therapy, *HFpEF* heart failure with preserved ejection fraction, *HFrEF* heart failure with reduced ejection fraction, *LV* left ventricle, *PH* pulmonary hypertension, *RA* right atrium, *RV* right ventricle, *TV* tricuspid valve, *TR* tricuspid regurgitation

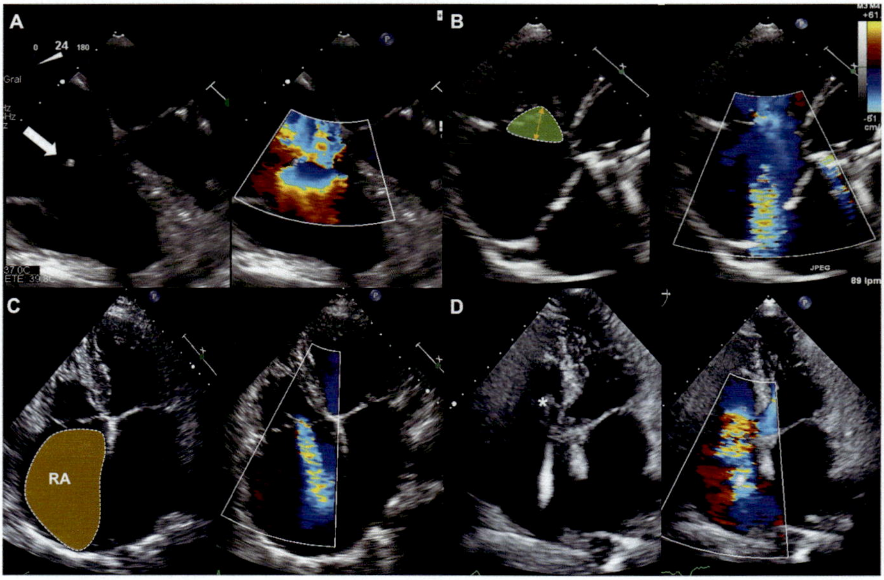

Fig. 16.1 Integral classification of Tricuspid Regurgitation. (**a**) Primary TR due to prolapse of the anterior leaflet. (**b**) Ventricular secondary TR with severe tenting (green area and yellow arrow). (**c**) Atrial secondary TR with severe RA dilatation (yellow area). (**d**) CIED-related TR (* shows impingement of the device over leaflet). *CIED* cardiac implantable electronic device, *RA* right atrium, *TR* tricuspid regurgitation

Patient Selection

TR can be considered a silent killer due to the delayed referral of this population, usually presenting in end-stage of heart failure with concomitant liver dysfunction and chronic kidney disease. Additionally, severe leaflet tethering along with larger tricuspid annulus and dysfunctional RV, leads to a high perioperative mortality and poor outcomes after tricuspid valve surgery [23]. Therefore, a rigorous patient screening is crucial to optimize procedural results and the effectiveness of TTVI. Right heart catheterization is essential to rule out severe pulmonary hypertension, especially when clinical and non-invasive data are inconsistent. Multimodal imaging plays a critical role in identifying patients for whom the intervention may not be beneficial. Additionally, factors like severe RV dysfunction, tethering distance > 0.76 cm or tethering area > 1.63 cm^2, a higher grade of TR, left ventricular disfunction and increase pulmonary pressure are associated with higher risk of TR recurrence following tricuspid valve surgery [24].

Surgery is currently not recommended for patients with severe RV dysfunction/dilatation or severe pulmonary hypertension [1]. The TRI-score was developed with the aim to recognize and characterize better predictors of mortality following isolated tricuspid valve surgery, demonstrating that a TRI-score ≥ 6 is associated with the lower rates of survival and not decrease in heart failure hospitalization rates [25, 26]. In daily clinical practice, TTVI are considered for patients with high surgical risk, considered inoperable, ideally before end-stage of heart disease and severe comorbidities that make the procedure futile (Fig. 16.2).

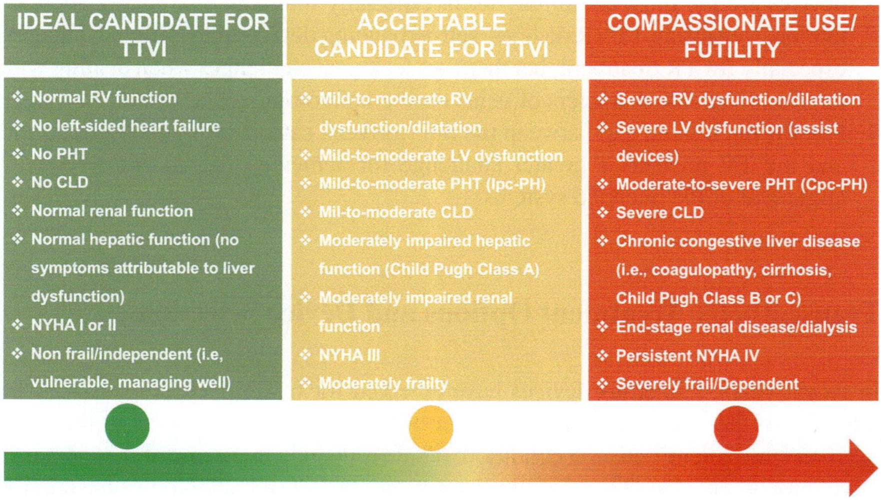

Fig. 16.2 Clinical patient profiles and possible response to intervention. *Cpc-PH* combined post- and pre-capillary pulmonary hypertension, *CLD* chronic lung disease, *Ipc-PH* isolated post-capillary pulmonary hypertension, *LV* left ventricle, *NYHA* New York heart association, *PHT* pulmonary hypertension, *RV* right ventricle, *TTVI* transcatheter tricuspid valve interventions

Considerations for TTVI

The tricuspid valve (TV) is the largest of the heart valves and has a complex structure composed of multiple leaflets (septal, anterior, and posterior) that connect to the fibrous tricuspid annulus, papillary muscles, numerous chordae tendineae, and the associated RV. Importantly, the TV's anatomy can vary significantly among individuals, with some having four or even five leaflets instead of the usual three [27]. The annular size and shape can also change with dilation and during the cardiac cycle based on hemodynamic conditions. Additionally, the TV's proximity to the atrioventricular node (AVN) and the right coronary artery (RCA) running parallel to the TV annulus are crucial considerations for some specific therapies [28, 29].

Performing TTVI requires an understanding of these complex structural elements and several key factors:

1. It features intricate subvalvular components, such as numerous chordae tendineae and papillary muscles, which elevate the risk of entrapment and challenge device maneuverability.
2. Visualizing the TV can be demanding due to its location and acoustic shadowing in echocardiography. Multimodality imaging techniques, including transesophageal, intracardiac echocardiography, and CT imaging, are often necessary to assess TR and RV to achieve a better understanding of etiology and guidance intraprocedure (Fig. 16.3).
3. Selecting the right device is complex due to the TV's mobility, anatomic features that might vary according to the etiology mechanism (primary vs. atrial vs. ventricular vs. CIED), and the need for long-term fixation. As of now, coaptation devices are the most commonly used, especially interventional leaflet approximation. Regarding TTVR devices, self-expanding devices may offer advantages, especially for TR treatment, but there are technical challenges when dealing with large and variable diameters of veins during heterotopic replacement.
4. Finally, the limited gap between the inferior vena cava entering the right atrium and the TV presents a greater challenge for achieving the necessary coaxial alignment of the intended systems.

Transcatheter Treatment Options and Device Selection

In recent years, numerous devices have emerged for treating TR (Fig. 16.4). The selection of these devices should consider both the anatomical aspects of the valve itself and the patient's clinical condition. It's worth noting that some of these devices were initially developed for the mitral valve, but the latest technologies have introduced dedicated devices for TV treatment. These innovations aim to mimic surgical

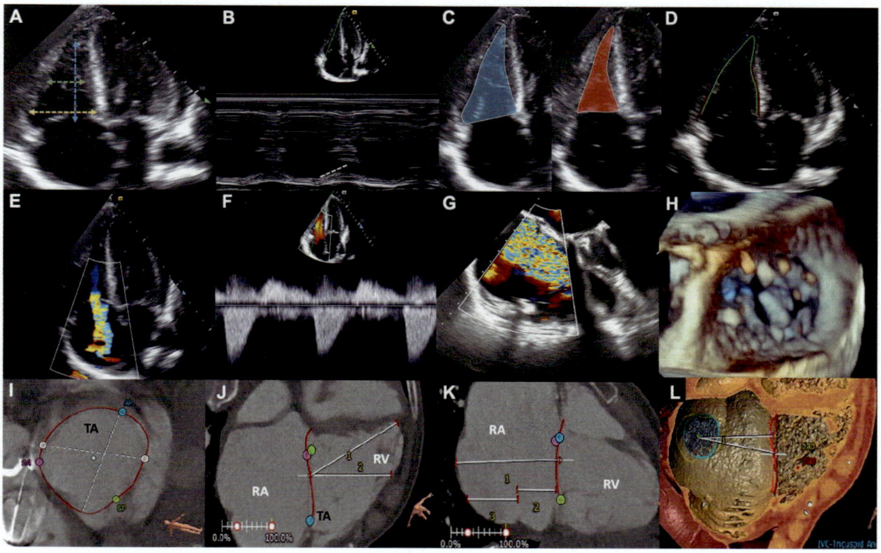

Fig. 16.3 **Multimodality evaluation for TTVI**. (**a**) An apical 4-chamber view with RV dimensions: basal diameter (yellow arrow), mid-diameter (green arrow) and longitudinal diameter (blue arrow). (**b**) The M-mode cursor (white dashed line) aligned with TA, allowing measurement of the tricuspid annular plane systolic excursion. (**c**) The diastolic (blue mask) and systolic (red mask) measurements of the RV area for calculation of fractional area change. (**d**) The measurement of the strain imaging. (**e**) Color doppler showing severe TR. (**f**) Determination of sPAP through TR. (**g**) Mid-esophageal TV 4-chamber view showing severe tricuspid regurgitation. (**h**) Three-dimensional imaging of the TV obtained from TEE as viewed from the RA. (I) TA dimensions in diastole. (**j**) Distance from RV free wall and base to TA. (**k**) Diastolic RA height. (**l**) Assessment of the offset of the IVC and TA. *IVC* inferior vena cava, *RA* right atrium, *RV* right ventricle, *sPAP* systolic pulmonary artery pressure, *TA* tricuspid annulus, *IVC* inferior vein cava, *TR* tricuspid regurgitation, *TTVI* transcatheter tricuspid valve interventions

procedures and offer improved options for patients with TR. Considerable attention has been focused on various trials conducted with both TTVr and TTVR devices. A summary of the characteristics of these patients in main clinical studies and ongoing clinical studies is provided in Tables 16.2 and 16.3, respectively.

Edge-to Edge Repair

Transcatheter tricuspid edge-to-edge repair (T-TEER) devices, designed to enhance leaflet coaptation by implanting a clip, represent the most widely used technique TR treatment. Initially, devices designed for the mitral position, such as the MitraClip (Abbott Vascular, Santa Clara, CA, USA), were proposed for tricuspid use. However,

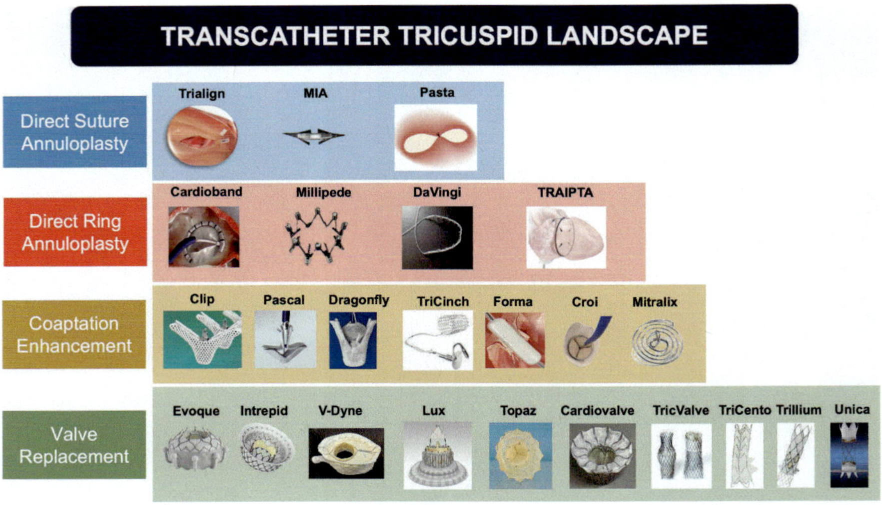

Fig. 16.4 Transcatheter Tricuspid Landscape. In this overview of transcatheter device therapies, the four anchoring methods are presented in the left column, along with device examples in each row

the catheter's curve, originally intended for transseptal puncture into left-sided chambers, makes tricuspid access challenging. Fortunately, a dedicated tricuspid-specific version, the TriClip (Abbott Structural Heart), is now available, offering an increased septal-lateral range of steerability and a shorter curve for improved maneuverability (Fig. 16.5).

The TRILUMINATE Pivotal trial was the first randomized, controlled clinical study to evaluate the safety and efficacy of transcatheter repair using the Triclip system compared to medical therapy in patients with TR [30]. This study included 350 patients and demonstrated lasting reductions in moderate or lesser TR in 89% of cases after 1 year. Although there were no significant differences in mortality or heart failure hospitalization rates between the two groups, the reduction in TR severity was accompanied by symptomatic relief, with 83.9% of patients falling into New York Heart Association [NYHA] Class I or II at 12 months. Similarly, the larger real-world setting of the bRIGHT registry confirmed these findings, highlighting the consistent positive outcomes of the Triclip system [31]. In a cohort of over 500 patients, adverse events were reported rarely, occurring in only 2.5% at 30 days. TR was reduced to ≤ moderate in 77% of patients, accompanied by symptomatic improvement (from 20% to 79% in NYHA Class I/II). It is important to note that the patient population in the bRIGHT study differed from that in the TRILUMINATE trial. These patients had a higher rate of hospitalization, more advanced heart failure symptoms, a higher degree of TR severity, with 88% presenting with massive and torrential TR, lower baseline scores on the Kansas City Cardiomyopathy Questionnaire, and, last but not least, a larger coaptation gap.

Table 16.2 Clinical profile in main transcatheter tricuspid valve interventions

	TRILUMINATE Pivotal RCT [53] n = 350	BRIGHT [31] n = 511	CLASP TR [33] n = 65	TRI-REPAIR [34] n = 30	TRISCEND [54] n = 176	TRICUS EURO [44] n = 35
Management strategy	T-TEER (Triclip)	T-TEER (Triclip)	T-TEER (Pascal)	Annuloplasty (Cardioband)	Orthotopic TTVR (Evoque)	Heterotopic TTVR (TricValve)
Age (years)	78.0 ± 7.4	78.9 ± 7.1	77.4 ± 8.9	75.2 ± 6.6	79.3 ± 7.7	76 ± 6.8
Female (%)	56.0	56.0	55.4	73.3	76.8	82.9
NYHA III/IV (%)	59.4	80.0	70.8	83.3	87.5	100
CIED (%)	16.0	22.5	13.8	13.3	33.9	22.8
Prior HF in the last 12 months (%)	25.1	40.3	37.5	NA	35.7	NA
Massive or torrential TR (%)	72.3	88.0	69.0	NA	45.5	NA
LVEF (%)	59.3 ± 9.3	55.79 ± 10.58	56.5 ± 7.1	57.5 ± 10.8	53.4 ± 10.2	59.2 ± 8.0
TAPSE (cm)	>1.7 cm in 48%	1.70 ± 0.44	1.4 ± 0.4	1.4 ± 0.3	14.9 ± 3.9	18.0 ± 4.0
RVEDD (cm)	50.0 ± 0.8	4.63 ± 0.92	4.0 ± 0.9	3.8 ± 0.6	NA	NA
TA (cm)	4.3 ± 0.7	4.54 ± 0.76	4.5 ± 0.8	43.4 ± 5.0	NA	41.0 ± 9.0

CIED cardiac implantable electronic device, *LVEF* left ventricular ejection fraction, *NA* not available, *NYHA* New York Heart Association, *RCT* randomized clinical trial, *RVEDD* right ventricular end-diastolic diameter, *sPAP* systolic pulmonary artery pressure, *TAPSE* tricuspid annulus plane systolic excursion, *TR* tricuspid regurgitation, *T-TEER* transcatheter tricuspid edge-to-edge repair, *TTVR* transcatheter tricuspid valve replacement

Table 16.3 Ongoing clinical studies evaluating transcatheter tricuspid valve interventions

Type of study	Name of the study	Device	Estimated enrollment (n)	Primary endpoint
RCT (Device vs GDMT)	TRILUMINATE (NCT03904147)	Triclip	700	Hierarchical composite all-cause mortality, TV surgery, HF hospitalizations, QoL with KCCQ
RCT (Device vs GDMT)	TRI-FR (NCR0464811)	Triclip	300	Milton Packer clinical composite score
RCT (Device vs GDMT)	CLASP-TR (NCT04097145)	Pascal	870	Composite of all-cause mortality, RVAD implantation or heart transplant, TV intervention, HF hospitalizations, QoL by KCCQ
RCT (Device vs GDMT)	TRACE-NL (NCT05628779)	Triclip, Pascal	150	Hierarchical composite of all-cause mortality, heart failure hospitalization and QoL
RCT (Device vs GDMT)	TRICI-HF (NCT04634266)	Triclip, Pascal	360	All-cause mortality or HF hospitalization
RCT (Device vs GDMT)	TRISCEND II (NCT04482062)	Evoque	1070	TR grade reduction and composite improvement: KCCQ, NYHA and 6 MWT Rate of MAE Composite: all-cause mortality, RVAD implantation or heart transplant, TV intervention, HF hospitalizations and improvement of KCCQ, NYHA and 6 MWT
Prospective, single-arm	TRAVEL II (NCT05194423)	Lux-Valve Plus	150	All-cause mortality TR reduction
Prospective, single-arm	TRINITY (NCT05436028)	Lux-Valve Plus	135	Composite of MAE
Prospective, single-arm	Early Feasibility Study of the Cardiovalve System for TR (NCT04100720)	Cardiovalve	15	Technical success of Cardiovalve Reduction in TR severity Rate of patients without MAE
Prospective, single arm	TARGET (NCT05486832)	Cardiovalve	100	Freedom for device or procedure-related adverse events Reduction in TR

(continued)

Table 16.3 (continued)

Type of study	Name of the study	Device	Estimated enrollment (n)	Primary endpoint
Prospective, single-arm	TTVR Early Feasibility Study (NCT04433065)	Intrepid	15	Rate of implant or delivery related serious adverse events
Prospective, single arm	TRICURE (NCT05126030)	Topaz (TRiCares)	20	Hierarchical composite endpoint: including all-cause mortality, re-hospitalization for heart failure, re-intervention for failed tricuspid intervention, and KCCQ
Prospective, single arm	Innoventric Trillium Stent Graft First-in-Human Study	Trillium	20	Related rate of device or procedure-related MAEs Freedom from unplanned surgery or re-intervention Technical performance: successful access, delivery and retrieval of the system TR grade as measured on the device valves, or by hepatic vein systolic backflow or reduction in CVP

CVP central venous pressure, *GDMT* guideline-directed medical therapy, *HF* heart failure, *KCCQ* Kansas City Cardiomyopathy Questionnaire, *MAE* major adverse events, *MWT* minute walking test, *NYHA* New York Heart Association, *QoL* quality of life, *RVAD* right ventricular assist device, *RCT* randomized clinical trial, *TR* tricuspid regurgitation, *TV* tricuspid valve

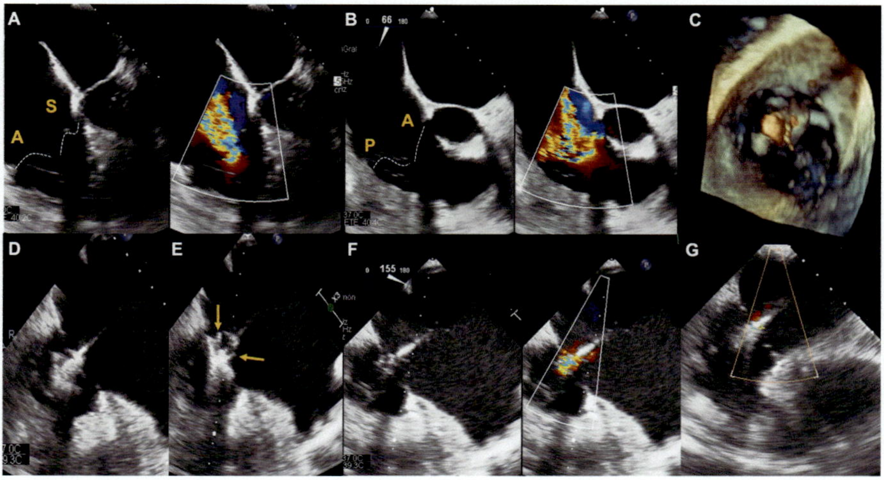

Fig. 16.5 Imaging for T-TEER procedure. (**a**, **b**) Mid-esophageal TV 4-chamber and inflow-outflow views showing severe tricuspid regurgitation. (**c**) Three-dimensional orientation with T-TEER device. (**d**) Leaflets capture. (**e**) Direct view of grasping at the mid-esophageal level showing dropping grippers (yellow arrows). (**f**) Assessment in real time after grasping. (**g**) Immediate result displaying mild TR at the end of the procedure. *A* anterior leaflet, *P* posterior leaflet, *S* septal leaflet, *T-TEER* transcatheter tricuspid edge-to-edge repair, *TV* tricuspid valve

Additionally, the PASCAL system (Edwards Lifesciences) has entered the market, offering versatility for use in both mitral and tricuspid positions, offering greater navigation flexibility, and a central spacer. The early experience with this system demonstrated improvements in RV systolic function, cardiac output, and liver enzyme reduction in patients with documented congestion post T-TEER [32]. Recently, the outcomes of the CLASP TR (Edwards PASCAL TrAnScatheter Valve Repair System in Tricuspid Regurgitation Early Feasibility Study) have highlighted the safety of leaflet approximation using PASCAL and PASCAL Ace devices, demonstrating low complication rates and favorable survival rates [33]. Moreover, at the 1-year follow-up, 86% of patients achieved moderate or less TR, with 100% of patients experiencing a reduction of at least one grade in TR severity. Similar to the TRILUMINATE trial and bRIGHT registry, the CLASP TR revealed enhancements in functional class and overall quality of life.

Annuloplasty

Although there are numerous devices designed to target the TA, the Cardioband Tricuspid Repair System (Edwards Lifesciences) is the only one approved in Europe. This system involves the insertion of a direct, sutureless, and adjustable Dacron band, designed to mimic surgical techniques. It is delivered through a transfemoral 24-F access sheath, deploying up to 17 anchors on the atrial side of the anterior and posterior TA for secure fixation. To fine-tune the sizing, a specialized adjustment tool, capable of bidirectional TA reshaping, is advanced over a wire. This allows for precise cinching of the band, resulting in a controlled reduction of both anteroposterior and septolateral TA diameters.

The 2-year outcomes of TRI-REPAIR (Tricuspid Regurgitation Repair with Cardioband Transcatheter System) demonstrated favorable results in terms of annular reduction and TR severity reduction, along with an associated improvement in quality of life and exercise capacity [34]. Additionally, the recent early feasibility study with the Cardioband reported 1-year outcomes [35]. Among 37 patients with severe TR (76% classified as massive or torrential), of whom 65% had NYHA III/IV symptoms, procedural success was achieved in 92%, accompanied by a significant improvement in the septolateral diameter. Notably, there was a substantial reduction in TR (73% ≤ moderate) and an enhancement in the NYHA functional class (92% classified as I/II) at the 1-year assessment. Follow-up for up to 5 years is planned.

Transcatheter Tricuspid Valve Replacement

TTVR offers the potential for comprehensive TR correction and is relatively unaffected by TV anatomy, in contrast to T-TEER and annuloplasty systems. TTVR encompasses both orthotopic and heterotopic replacement procedures.

Orthotopic Valve Implantation

Evoque

The Evoque valve (Edwards Lifesciences, Irvine, California) is a self-expanding nitinol frame valve with bovine pericardial leaflets. It is inserted via a 28 F transfemoral approach and secured with nine subvalvular arms positioned under the leaflet hinges.

The preliminary compassionate use data for the Evoque TTVR system demonstrated an immediate reduction of TR to ≤1+ in 92% of patients during the procedure, with this improvement maintained in 88% at the 30-day follow-up and 87% at the 1-year follow-up, consistently delivering positive results evaluated over a 2-year follow-up period [36, 37]. The TRISCEND study 1-year results, including 176 patients, were presented at PCR London Valves congress 2022 [38]. The procedure's success rate was reported at 94.4%, with a reduction of 97.6% TR to mild/minimal. Freedom from all-cause mortality was 90.1%, with cardiovascular mortality was reported in 9.4% of patients and 88% of patients free of rehospitalization. Recently, the TRISCEND II outcomes were presented at Transcatheter Cardiac Therapies congress 2023 [39]. At 30 days, the primary composite safety endpoint of major adverse events rate occurred in 27.4% of the 95 patients treated with Evoque, a rate that compared favorably with historic safety data after tricuspid valve surgery (43.8%). At 6 months follow-up 98.8% of patients underwent TTVR had moderate or less TR. TTVR demonstrated a substantial advantage with a win ratio of 4.6 in enhancing both the quality of life and functional status, as evaluated through a hierarchical composite endpoint that quantified alterations in the Kansas City Cardiomyopathy Questionnaire (≥10 points), NYHA functional class (≥1 class), and 6-minute walk test distance (≥30 meters).

LuX-Valve

The LuX-Valve Plus (Ningbo Jenscare Biotechnology Co., Ningbo, China) is a trileaflet bovine pericardium valve with distinctive features. It is delivered through the jugular vein using a 31F steerable system. What sets it apart is its self-adaptive fabric skirt and a ventricular anchor firmly fixed to the interventricular septum, ensuring secure placement. Unlike other valves, it attaches itself to the base of the right atrium and incorporates a specialized three-pronged curved anchoring needle to prevent migration.

In 2022, the first studies of Lux Valve Plus implantation were conducted, involving 10 high-risk patients with severe TR [40]. The procedure was successful in all patients, with no deaths or major complications reported, including significant bleeding, the need for additional surgery, stroke, heart attack, or hospitalization for heart failure within 30 days after the procedure. Furthermore, in the 30-day follow-up with echocardiograms, all patients either did not have tricuspid insufficiency or

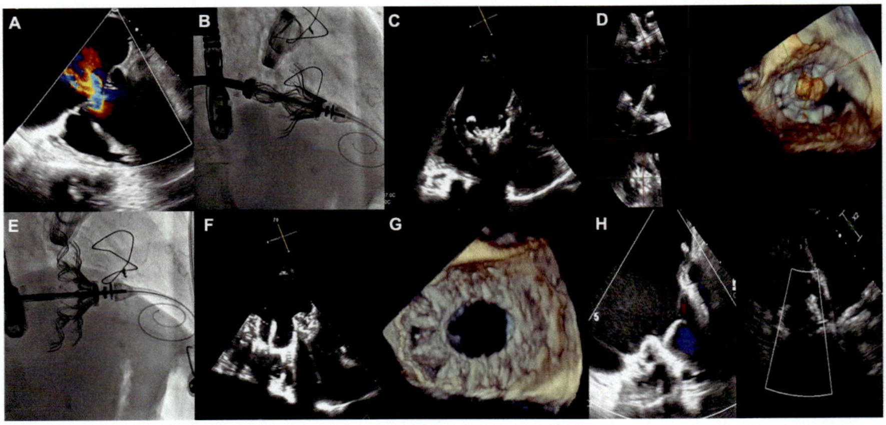

Fig. 16.6 Transcatheter tricuspid valve replacement with Cardiovalve device. (**a**) Severe functional TR with TV annulus dilated. (**b**, **c**) Fluoroscopic and echocardiographic images of the Cardiovalve device with open grasp legs crossing into the RV. (**d**) Multiplanar reconstruction to assess leaflet insertion. (**e**, **f**) Fluoroscopic and echocardiographic images showing the atrial flange and ventricular part deployment. (**g**, **h**) Echocardiographic images showing good expansion and stable position. *RA* right atrium, *RV* right ventricle, *TR* tricuspid regurgitation, *TV* tricuspid valve

had it at a mild level. The patients also experienced significant improvement in their functional class after the procedure.

Cardiovalve

The Cardiovalve (Cardiovalve Ltd., Or Yehuda, Israel), is a self-expanding nitinol frame valve with three bovine pericardial leaflets, designed for secure anchoring on the leaflets (Fig. 16.6). This innovative design incorporates 24 nitinol frames, strategically placed for gentle anchoring and fixation of the device to the native annulus. The system employs a 32 Fr capsule with a 24 Fr shaft. The valve is available in 3 sizes (M, L, XL) for rings of 36–55 mm [41].

Intrepid

The Intrepid TTVR system (Medtronic MN, USA) is a dual stent bovine pericardial valve created for transcatheter delivery via a 35 Fr venous access point. It comes in three outer frame sizes (43 mm, 46 mm, and 50 mm diameter) with a 27 mm inner stent frame. What distinguishes the Intrepid valve is its unique direct annular anchoring mechanism relying on radial force, eliminating the necessity for leaflet anchors. The first cases of compassionate use of the device in the tricuspid position have been successfully presented [42]. The feasibility study of the device in TR is currently underway, and results have not yet been communicated.

Topaz

The Topaz TTVR system, developed by TRiCares, features a distinctive two-stent design comprising an inner and outer stent. The softer outer stent seamlessly aligns with the patient's native annulus, securely anchoring the prosthesis within the TV. Meanwhile, the inner stent independently supports the three-leaflet valve, maintaining its circular shape even in complex anatomies. The atraumatic anchoring system ensures a secure fit without causing harm to native structures. This system is delivered via the femoral vein using a 29 Fr steerable introducer. Currently, the valve is offered in a single size, enabling the treatment of annulus diameters measuring less than 45 mm as determined by diastolic CT scan. The first-in-human experience in compassionate use with the Topaz system demonstrated the feasibility and safety with good outcomes at short-term [43].

Heterotopic Valve Implantation

The goal of heterotopic caval implantation is to alleviate the impact of caval backflow due to TR and reduce systemic venous congestion. The use of specialized devices for cava valve implantation offers a promising option for a significant number of patients who may not have been candidates for edge-to-edge repair, orthotopic valve implantation, or annuloplasty.

Currently, there are four dedicated devices tailored for this patient group: TricValve (P + F Products + Features Vertriebs GmbH, Vienna, Austria), Tricento (MEDIRA, GmbH, Balingen, Germany), Trillium and Unica (Innoventric, Israel), a cross-caval prostheses with radiopaque markers for guidance during fluoroscopy.

TricValve

The TricValve system consists of 2 self-expanding, radiopaque nitinol tubular structures with three bovine pericardial leaflets sutured in place and supplemented with a polyester skirt to prevent paravalvular leaks, for superior and inferior vena cava implantation. The upper vena cava prosthesis is available in sizes ranging from 25 to 33 mm, and for the lower vena cava, it ranges from 31 to 45 mm. The TRICUS EURO study showcased the safety and effectiveness of the TricValve device [44]. All 35 patients began the study in NYHA functional class III/IV. Procedural success was achieved in 94% at 30 days, with no procedural deaths or conversions to surgery. Moreover, it led to an enhanced quality of life and functional class improvement at the 6-month follow-up.

Tricento

The transcatheter cross-caval valved stent graft is constructed with a self-expanding nitinol stent frame, internally lined with delicate porcine pericardium. It is tailor-made to conform to the specific anatomical characteristics of each patient. The screening process takes into account the diameters of the inferior and superior vena cava (ranging from a minimum of 16 mm to a maximum of 35 mm), the length of the right atrium (between 40 and 80 mm), and the distance from the right atrium to the liver veins (a minimum of 10 mm). Wild et al. reported early procedural and clinical outcomes for 21 patients treated with the Tricento system. Technical success was achieved in all 21 patients (100%), which was associated with a significant improvement in functional class (65% in NYHA I/II) during the median 61-day follow-up [45].

Trillium

Trillium (Innoventric, Israel) is a cross-caval device that stands out with its three lateral valves, each capable of accommodating procedures like pacemaker lead placement without interfering with the others. Furthermore, it incorporates a sealing skirt to prevent leaks while ensuring unobstructed suprahepatic veins, an improvement that addresses a common anatomical limitation seen in other devices (Fig. 16.7). Despite being the latest iteration of heterotopic valves, there have been instances of successful cases reported [46].

Unica

Unica (Innoventric, Israel) is a single stent, double valve, cross-caval prosthesis that addresses backflow at both right atrium-inferior vein cava and right atrium-superior vein cava junctions. The core section of the UNICA stent consists of exposed metal,

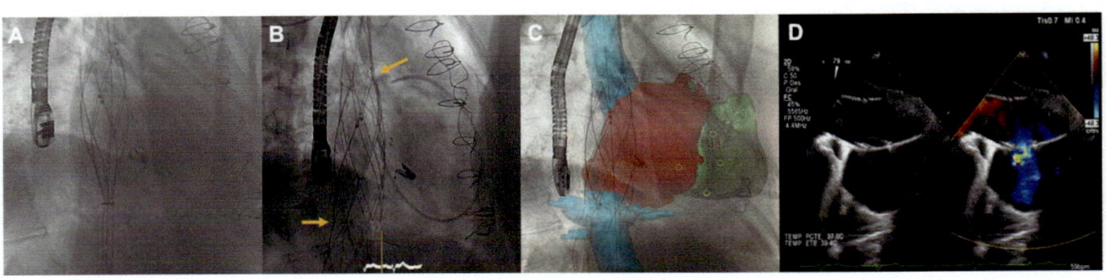

Fig. 16.7 Heterotopic transcatheter tricuspid valve replacement with Trillium device. (**a**) Deployment of the Trillium device from the superior to inferior cava veins. (**b**, **c**) Full deployment of Trillium guided toward the tricuspid valve using radiopaque markers (yellow arrows) and fusion imaging (blue mas: superior and inferior cava veins; red mask: right atrium; green mask: right ventricle). (**d**) Bicaval plane showing proper functioning of the device

complemented by a generous IVC sealing skirt, which enables the possibility of future transseptal punctures and valve-in-valve procedures if required. The first published case involved a successful procedure on an 85-year-old female [47]. After a 60-day evaluation, the patient showed no hospital readmissions, improved quality of life and function, moved from NYHA Class III to Class II, and experienced reduced peripheral swelling while maintaining a consistent diuretic treatment.

Current Unmet Clinical Needs

While TTVI are gaining rapid prominence, there are still significant unresolved clinical questions that need addressing. Addressing these questions is essential to enhance the adoption and utilization of these devices on a larger scale:

- **Screening Failure:** While TTVI systems offer treatment options for a broad spectrum of patients with severe TR, a notable portion of individuals still undergo exclusion during the screening phase. In the case of patients undergoing TTVI, the primary reasons for screening failure are associated with their anatomical and clinical characteristics [48]. In a study conducted by Gercek et al., which examined 547 patients screened for TTVI in Germany and the US, it was observed that among those considered unsuitable for TTVI (42% of the cohort), anatomical factors and clinical futility accounted for 57% and 18% of the exclusions, respectively [49]. A lesser symptom burden, suboptimal imaging quality, and the presence of CIED each contributed to 13% of the screening failures. In the TRILUMINATE randomized trial, it was found that 56% of the screened population, totaling 795 patients, were deemed ineligible to participate in the trial [30]. However, the specific reasons for this exclusion have not been reported as of yet. Data regarding screening failures in patients being evaluated for TTVR are exceedingly limited.
- **Is TV repair on the verge of being replaced?:** TTVr either with Triclip, Pascal or Cardioband has shown to be safe and effective in terms of functional class and quality of life. However, certain patients may not be suitable candidates for TTVr due to various factors, including substantial coaptation gaps, leaflet perforation, significant leaflet tethering, excessively thick chordae, interference from CIED leads resulting in leaflet entrapment, or the intricate geometric complexity of the TV anatomy [50, 51]. The choice between TTVr and TTVR comes with its own set of advantages and disadvantages (Fig. 16.8). TTVR can address a broader range of anatomical variations and can completely abolish TR offering sustained clinical benefits. TTVr tends to be safer, with lower rates of major bleeding, and carries a lower risk of interfering with the conduction system or RCA. However, to date, there have been no studies that directly compare these different approaches.
- **Significance of residual TR:** Assessing residual TR in the native valve is challenging due to reliance on geometric assumptions that may not apply to eccentric

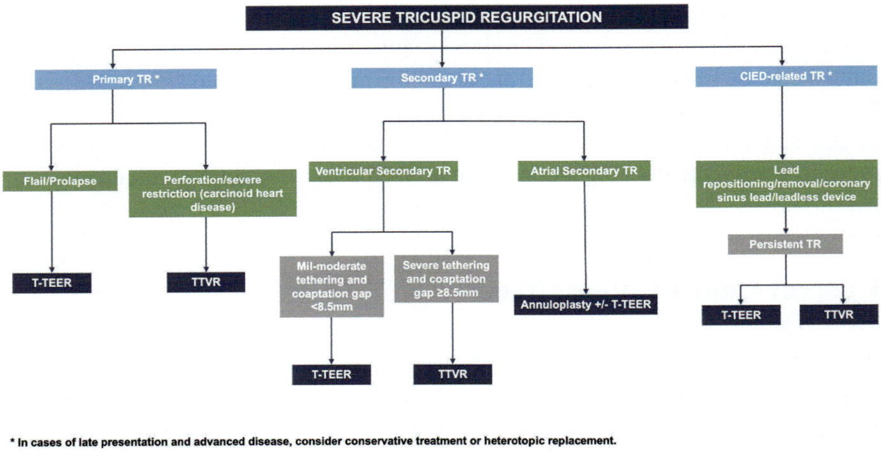

Fig. 16.8 Proposed algorithm to guide transcatheter tricuspid valve intervention device selection. *CIED* cardiac implantable electronic device, *T-TEER* transcatheter tricuspid edge-to-edge repair, *TTVR* transcatheter tricuspid valve replacement, *TR* tricuspid regurgitation

jets. This challenge is even more complex in patients with tricuspid bioprostheses and complex residual TR. Currently, it is unclear whether completely eliminating TR offers better quality of life or improved outcomes compared to reducing its severity based on available evidence. One year after Evoque valve implantation, the majority of patients had mild or less TR (97.6%), and a substantial percentage had no or trace TR (69%) [38]. Similar results were observed with Triclip and Cardioband devices with 89% and 73% having moderate or less TR at 1 year follow up, respectively [30, 35]. All three devices led to comparable improvements in NYHA class and the 6-minute walk test. However, since there are no direct studies comparing these therapies and considering differences in patient populations, the question of whether complete TR elimination is necessary for improved outcomes remains unanswered. Further research is needed to determine if complete TR elimination significantly affects clinically relevant outcomes.

- **Bleeding:** Currently, there is a lack of conclusive evidence regarding the most suitable anticoagulation regimen following TTVI. Nevertheless, due to the relatively reduced flow conditions on the right side of the heart, there is an increased risk of thrombosis, especially post-TTVR. In the TRISCEND study severe bleeding was observed in 25% of patients at the end of the first year, although the majority of these cases occurred around the time of the procedure [38]. In a systematic review and meta-analysis including 991 patients undergoing TTVr, bleeding complications and residual ≥ severe TR were numerically higher in the annuloplasty-like group compared with edge-to-edge repair (13.3% vs. 3.8%, respectively) [52]. Given that all these patients require anticoagulation therapy, either due to AF in the TTVr population or as a mandatory indication in TTVR patients, close monitoring is of utmost importance.

Future Perspectives and Conclusions

In conclusions, the current landscape provides a diverse range of treatment options for patients dealing with TR and heart failure. The pivotal challenge ahead revolves around the meticulous selection and customization of specific devices for individual patients. This task holds paramount significance in the foreseeable future. It is evident that these therapies yield substantial advantages, encompassing symptom alleviation and an enhanced overall quality of life for a patient demographic that, when left untreated, faces elevated mortality and frequent hospitalizations due to heart failure.

As we look ahead, the future prospects of TTVI will necessitate significant advancements in trial design and patient selection. Gaining a deeper understanding of TR, conducting comprehensive assessments of the RV, and pinpointing the optimal timing for intervention will be critical for broadening the scope of patients who can benefit from TTVI. Furthermore, the evolution of TTVI should accommodate diverse anatomical variations, addressing real-world anatomical challenges, and enhancing the feasibility of delivering larger valve sizes through increasingly smaller catheters. Additionally, there must be a shift toward more advanced procedural planning, simulation, and implantation guidance techniques.

References

1. Vahanian A, Beyersdorf F, Praz F, Milojevic M, Baldus S, Bauersachs J, Capodanno D, Conradi L, De Bonis M, De Paulis R, Delgado V, Freemantle N, Gilard M, Haugaa KH, Jeppsson A, Jüni P, Pierard L, Prendergast BD, Sadaba JR, Tribouilloy C, Wojakowski W, Neumann FJ, Myers P, Abdelhamid M, Achenbach S, Asteggiano R, Barili F, Borger MA, Carrel T, Collet JP, Foldager D, Habib G, Hassager C, Irs A, Iung B, Jahangiri M, Katus HA, Koskinas KC, Massberg S, Mueller CE, Nielsen JC, Pibarot P, Rakisheva A, Roffi M, Rubboli A, Shlyakhto E, Siepe M, Sitges M, Sondergaard L, Sousa-Uva M, Tarantini G, Zamorano JL, Benchabi Y, Chilingaryan A, Metzler B, Rustamova Y, Shumavets V, Lancellotti P, Smajic E, Trendafilova-Lazarova D, Samardzic J, Karakyriou M, Palecek T, Dahl JS, Meshaal MS, Palm K, Virtanen M, Bouleti C, Bakhutashvili Z, Boutsikou M, Kertész AB, Danielsen R, Topilsky Y, Golino P, Tuleutayev R, Elezi S, Kerimkulova A, Rudzitis A, Glaveckaite S, Sow R, Demarco DC, Bulatovic N, Aouad A, Van Den Brink R, Antova E, Beitnes JO, Ochala A, Ribeiras R, Vinereanu D, Irtyuga O, Ivanovic B, Simkova I, Gomez AG, Sarno G, Pedrazzini GB, Bsata W, Zakhama L, Korkmaz L, Cherniuk S, Khanji MY, Sharipov I, Baigent C, Aboyans V, Antoniou S, Arbelo E, Baumbach A, Čelutkiene J, Cikes M, Falk V, Fauchier L, Gale CP, Halvorsen S, Jaarsma T, Konradi A, Kotecha D, Landmesser U, Lewis BS, Linhart A, Løchen ML, Neubeck L, Petersen SE, Prescott E, Touyz RM, Galletti L, Hazekamp M, Licht P, Perier P, Prager R, Roessner E, Tsagakis K, Zientara A. ESC/EACTS Guidelines for the management of valvular heart disease. Eur Heart J. 2021;43(2022):561–632. https://doi.org/10.1093/eurheartj/ehab395.
2. Asmarats L, Taramasso M, Rodés-Cabau J. Tricuspid valve disease: diagnosis, prognosis and management of a rapidly evolving field. Nat Rev Cardiol. 2019;16:538–54. https://doi.org/10.1038/s41569-019-0186-1.

3. Nath J, Foster E, Heidenreich PA. Impact of tricuspid regurgitation on long-term survival. J Am Coll Cardiol. 2004;43:405–9. https://doi.org/10.1016/j.jacc.2003.09.036.
4. Topilsky Y, Maltais S, Medina Inojosa J, Oguz D, Michelena H, Maalouf J, Mahoney DW, Enriquez-Sarano M. Burden of tricuspid regurgitation in patients diagnosed in the community setting. JACC Cardiovasc Imaging. 2019;12:433–42. https://doi.org/10.1016/j.jcmg.2018.06.014.
5. Rodés-Cabau J, Taramasso M, O'Gara PT. Diagnosis and treatment of tricuspid valve disease: current and future perspectives. Lancet. 2016;388:2431–42. https://doi.org/10.1016/S0140-6736(16)00740-6.
6. Adler DS. Non-functional tricuspid valve disease. Ann Cardiothorac Surg. 2017;6:204–13. https://doi.org/10.21037/ACS.2017.04.04.
7. Gelves-Meza J, Lang RM, Valderrama-Achury MD, Zamorano JL, Vargas-Acevedo C, Medina HM, Salazar G. Tricuspid regurgitation related to cardiac implantable electronic devices: an integrative review. J Am Soc Echocardiogr. 2022;35:1107–22. https://doi.org/10.1016/j.echo.2022.08.004.
8. Höke U, Auger D, Thijssen J, Wolterbeek R, Van Der Velde ET, Holman ER, Schalij MJ, Bax JJ, Delgado V, Marsan NA. Significant lead-induced tricuspid regurgitation is associated with poor prognosis at long-term follow-up. Heart. 2014;100(12):960–8. https://doi.org/10.1136/heartjnl-2013-304673.
9. Otto CM, Nishimura RA, Bonow RO, Carabello BA, Erwin JP, Gentile F, Jneid H, Krieger EV, Mack M, McLeod C, O'Gara PT, Rigolin VH, Sundt TM, Thompson A, Toly C. ACC/AHA Guideline for the Management of Patients with Valvular Heart Disease: a report of the American College of Cardiology/American Heart Association Joint Committee on Clinical Practice Guidelines. J Am Coll Cardiol. 2020;77(2021):e25–e197. https://doi.org/10.1016/j.jacc.2020.11.018.
10. Scotti A, Sturla M, Granada JF, Kodali SK, Coisne A, Mangieri A, Godino C, Ho E, Goldberg Y, Chau M, Jorde UP, Garcia MJ, Maisano F, Bapat VN, Ailawadi G, Latib A. Outcomes of isolated tricuspid valve replacement: a systematic review and meta-analysis of 5,316 patients from 35 studies. EuroIntervention. 2022;18:840–51. https://doi.org/10.4244/EIJ-D-22-00442.
11. Enriquez-Sarano M, Messika-Zeitoun D, Topilsky Y, Tribouilloy C, Benfari G, Michelena H. Tricuspid regurgitation is a public health crisis. Prog Cardiovasc Dis. 2019;62:447–51. https://doi.org/10.1016/J.PCAD.2019.10.009.
12. Neuhold S, Huelsmann M, Pernicka E, Graf A, Bonderman D, Adlbrecht C, Binder T, Maurer G, Pacher R, Mascherbauer J. Impact of tricuspid regurgitation on survival in patients with chronic heart failure: unexpected findings of a long-term observational study. Eur Heart J. 2013;34:844–52. https://doi.org/10.1093/EURHEARTJ/EHS465.
13. Topilsky Y, Medina Inojosa J, Benfari G, Vaturi O, Maltais S, Michelena H, Mankad S, Enriquez-Sarano M. Clinical presentation and outcome of tricuspid regurgitation in patients with systolic dysfunction. Eur Heart J. 2018;39(39):3584–92. https://doi.org/10.1093/eurheartj/ehy522.
14. Gorter TM, van Veldhuisen DJ, Bauersachs J, Borlaug BA, Celutkiene J, Coats AJS, Crespo-Leiro MG, Guazzi M, Harjola VP, Heymans S, Hill L, Lainscak M, Lam CSP, Lund LH, Lyon AR, Mebazaa A, Mueller C, Paulus WJ, Pieske B, Piepoli MF, Ruschitzka F, Rutten FH, Seferovic PM, Solomon SD, Shah SJ, Triposkiadis F, Wachter R, Tschöpe C, de Boer RA. Right heart dysfunction and failure in heart failure with preserved ejection fraction: mechanisms and management. Position statement on behalf of the Heart Failure Association of the European Society of Cardiology. Eur J Heart Fail. 2018;20:16–37. https://doi.org/10.1002/EJHF.1029.
15. Dietz MF, Prihadi EA, van der Bijl P, Ajmone Marsan N, Delgado V, Bax JJ. Prognostic implications of staging right heart failure in patients with significant secondary tricuspid regurgitation. JACC Heart Fail. 2020;8:627–36. https://doi.org/10.1016/J.JCHF.2020.02.008.
16. Schlotter F, Dietz MF, Stolz L, Kresoja K, Besler C, Sannino A, Rommel K, Unterhuber M, Von Roeder M. Atrial functional tricuspid regurgitation: novel definition and impact

on prognosis. Circ Cardiovasc Interv. 2022;15(9):761–70. https://doi.org/10.1161/CIRCINTERVENTIONS.122.011958.
17. Kwak S, Lim J, Yang S, Rhee TM, Choi YJ, Lee HJ, Hwang IC, Lee H, Yoon YE, Park HE, Lee SP, Kim HK, Choi SY, Kim YJ, Cho GY, Park JB. Atrial functional tricuspid regurgitation: importance of atrial fibrillation and right atrial remodeling and prognostic significance. JACC Cardiovasc Imaging. 2023;16:575–87. https://doi.org/10.1016/j.jcmg.2022.11.014.
18. Hinojar R, Fernández-Golfín C, Gómez AG, García-Martin A, Monteagudo JM, Lunar IG, Sebastian CG, Rivas S, Recalde AS, Zamorano JL. Clinical utility and prognostic value of right atrial function in severe tricuspid regurgitation: one more piece of the puzzle. Eur Heart J Cardiovasc Imaging. 2023; https://doi.org/10.1093/EHJCI/JEAD052.
19. Dietz MF, Prihadi EA, van der Bijl P, Fortuni F, Marques AI, Ajmone Marsan N, Bax JJ, Delgado V. Sex-specific differences in etiology and prognosis in patients with significant tricuspid regurgitation. Am J Cardiol. 2021;147:109–15. https://doi.org/10.1016/j.amjcard.2021.02.016.
20. Hahn RT. Tricuspid regurgitation. N Engl J Med. 2023;388(20):1876–91.
21. Prihadi EA, Delgado V, Leon MB, Enriquez-Sarano M, Topilsky Y, Bax JJ. Morphologic types of tricuspid regurgitation: characteristics and prognostic implications. JACC Cardiovasc Imaging. 2019;12:491–9. https://doi.org/10.1016/J.JCMG.2018.09.027.
22. Topilsky Y, Khanna A, Le Toumeau T, Park S, Michelena H, Suri R, Mahoney DW, Enriquez-Sarano M. Clinical context and mechanism of functional tricuspid regurgitation in patients with and without pulmonary hypertension. Circ Cardiovasc Imaging. 2012;5:314–23. https://doi.org/10.1161/CIRCIMAGING.111.967919.
23. Topilsky Y, Khanna AD, Oh JK, Nishimura RA, Enriquez-Sarano M, Jeon YB, Sundt TM, Schaff HV, Park SJ. Preoperative factors associated with adverse outcome after tricuspid valve replacement. Circulation. 2011;123:1929–39. https://doi.org/10.1161/CIRCULATIONAHA.110.991018.
24. Fukuda S, Song JM, Gillinov AM, McCarthy PM, Daimon M, Kongsaerepong V, Thomas JD, Shiota T. Tricuspid valve tethering predicts residual tricuspid regurgitation after tricuspid annuloplasty. Circulation. 2005;111:975–9. https://doi.org/10.1161/01.CIR.0000156449.49998.51.
25. Dreyfus J, Flagiello M, Bazire B, Eggenspieler F, Viau F, Riant E, Mbaki Y, Bohbot Y, Eyharts D, Senage T, Dubrulle H, Nicol M, Doguet F, Nguyen V, Coisne A, Le Tourneau T, Lavie-Badie Y, Tribouilloy C, Donal E, Tomasi J, Habib G, Selton-Suty C, Raffoul R, Iung B, Obadia JF, Messika-Zeitoun D. Isolated tricuspid valve surgery: impact of aetiology and clinical presentation on outcomes. Eur Heart J. 2020;41:4304–17. https://doi.org/10.1093/eurheartj/ehaa643.
26. Dreyfus J, Galloo X, Taramasso M, Heitzinger G, Benfari G, Kresoja K-P, Juarez-Casso F, Omran H, Bohbot Y, Iliadis C, Russo G, Topilsky Y, Weber M, Nombela-Franco L, Sala A, Eixerés-Esteve A, Iung B, Obadia J-F, Estevez Loureiro R, Riant E, Donal E, Hausleiter J, Badano L, Le Tourneau T, Coisne A, Modine T, Latib A, Praz F, Windecker S, Zamorano JL, von Bardeleben RS, Tang GHL, Hahn R, Webb J, Muraru D, Nejjari M, Chan V, De Bonis M, Carnero-Alcazar M, Nickenig G, Pfister R, Tribouilloy C, Rudolph V, Crestanello J, Lurz P, Bartko P, Maisano F, Bax J, Enriquez-Sarano M, Messika-Zeitoun D, For the T Investigators. TRI-SCORE and benefit of intervention in patients with severe tricuspid regurgitation. Eur Heart J. 2023; https://doi.org/10.1093/EURHEARTJ/EHAD585.
27. Athavale S, Deopujari R, Sinha U, Lalwani R, Kotgirwar S. Is tricuspid valve really tricuspid? Anat Cell Biol. 2017;50:1. https://doi.org/10.5115/ACB.2017.50.1.1.
28. Anderson RH, Yanni J, Boyett MR, Chandler NJ, Dobrzynski H. The anatomy of the cardiac conduction system. Clin Anat. 2009;22:99–113. https://doi.org/10.1002/CA.20700.
29. Van Rosendael PJ, Kamperidis V, Kong WKF, Van Rosendael AR, Van Der Kley F, Marsan NA, Delgado V, Bax JJ. Computed tomography for planning transcatheter tricuspid valve therapy. Eur Heart J. 2017;38(9):665–74. https://doi.org/10.1093/eurheartj/ehw499.
30. Sorajja P, Whisenant B, Hamid N, Naik H, Makkar R, Tadros P, Price MJ, Singh G, Fam N, Kar S, Schwartz JG, Mehta S, Bae R, Sekaran N, Warner T, Makar M, Zorn G, Spinner EM, Trusty PM, Benza R, Jorde U, McCarthy P, Thourani V, Tang GHL, Hahn RT,

Adams DH. Transcatheter repair for patients with tricuspid regurgitation. N Engl J Med. 2023;388:1833–42. https://doi.org/10.1056/nejmoa2300525.

31. Lurz P, Besler C, Schmitz T, Bekeredjian R, Nickenig G, Möllmann H, Stephan von Bardeleben R, Schmeisser A, Atmowihardjo I, Estevez-Loureiro R, Lubos E, Heitkemper M, Huang D, Lapp H, Donal E. Short-term outcomes of tricuspid edge-to-edge repair in clinical practice. J Am Coll Cardiol. 2023; https://doi.org/10.1016/j.jacc.2023.05.008.
32. Kodali S, Hahn RT, Eleid MF, Kipperman R, Smith R, Lim DS, Gray WA, Narang A, Pislaru SV, Koulogiannis K, Grayburn P, Fowler D, Hawthorne K, Dahou A, Deo SH, Vandrangi P, Deuschl F, Mack MJ, Leon MB, Feldman T, Davidson CJ. Feasibility study of the transcatheter valve repair system for severe tricuspid regurgitation. J Am Coll Cardiol. 2021; https://doi.org/10.1016/j.jacc.2020.11.047.
33. Kodali SK, Hahn RT, Davidson CJ, Narang A, Greenbaum A, Gleason P, Kapadia S, Miyasaka R, Zahr F, Chadderdon S, Smith RL, Grayburn P, Kipperman RM, Marcoff L, Whisenant B, Gonzales M, Makkar R, Makar M, O'Neill W, Wang DD, Gray WA, Abramson S, Hermiller J, Mitchel L, Lim DS, Fowler D, Williams M, Pislaru SV, Dahou A, Mack MJ, Leon MB, Eleid MF. 1-year outcomes of transcatheter tricuspid valve repair. J Am Coll Cardiol. 2023;81:1766–76. https://doi.org/10.1016/J.JACC.2023.02.049.
34. Nickenig G, Weber M, Schüler R, Hausleiter J, Näbauer M, Von Bardeleben RS, Sotiriou E, Schäfer U, Deuschl F, Alessandrini H, Kreidel F, Juliard JM, Brochet E, Latib A, Montorfano M, Agricola E, Baldus S, Friedrichs K, Deo SH, Gilmore SY, Feldman T, Hahn RT, Maisano F. Tricuspid valve repair with the cardioband system: two-year outcomes of the multicentre, prospective TRI-REPAIR study: two-year outcomes of the TRI-REPAIR study. EuroIntervention. 2021;16:e1264. https://doi.org/10.4244/EIJ-D-20-01107.
35. Gray WA, Abramson SV, Lim S, Fowler D, Smith RL, Grayburn PA, Kodali SK, Hahn RT, Kipperman RM, Koulogiannis KP, Eleid MF, Pislaru SV, Whisenant BK, McCabe JM, Liu J, Dahou A, Puthumana JJ, Davidson CJ, Feldman T, Gilmore SY, Krzmarzick A, Gerik L, Wang V, Cao A. 1-year outcomes of cardioband tricuspid valve reconstruction system early feasibility study. JACC Cardiovasc Interv. 2022;15:1921–32. https://doi.org/10.1016/J.JCIN.2022.07.006.
36. Webb JG, (Ming yu) Chuang A, Meier D, von Bardeleben RS, Kodali SK, Smith RL, Hausleiter J, Ong G, Boone R, Ruf T, George I, Szerlip M, Näbauer M, Ali FM, Moss R, Kreidel F, Bapat V, Schnitzler K, Ye J, Wild M, Akodad M, Deva DP, Chatfield AG, Mack MJ, Grayburn PA, Peterson MD, Makkar R, Leon MB, Hahn RT, Fam NP. Transcatheter tricuspid valve replacement with the EVOQUE system: 1-year outcomes of a multicenter, first-in-human experience. JACC Cardiovasc Interv. 2022;15:481–91. https://doi.org/10.1016/J.JCIN.2022.01.280.
37. Stolz L, Weckbach LT, Hahn RT, Chatfield AG, Fam NP, von Bardeleben RS, Davidson CJ, Grayburn PA, Zahr F, Hausleiter J. 2-year outcomes following transcatheter tricuspid valve replacement using the EVOQUE system. J Am Coll Cardiol. 2023;81:2374–6. https://doi.org/10.1016/J.JACC.2023.04.014.
38. Windecker S. TRISCEND study one-year outcomes: transfemoral transcatheter tricuspid valve replacement. PCR London Valves, 2022. Available at: https://www.pcronline.com/Cases-resources-images/Resources/Course-videos-slides/2022/TRISCEND-ACURATE-neo2-the-LuX-Valve-Syste
39. Kodali S. TRISCEND II trial: a randomized trial of transcatheter tricuspid valve replacement in patients with severe tricuspid regurgitation; 2023.
40. Zhang Y, Lu F, Li W, Chen S, Li M, Zhang X, Pan C, Qiao F, Zhou D, Pan W, Ge J. A first-in-human study of transjugular transcatheter tricuspid valve replacement with the LuX-Valve Plus system. EuroIntervention. 2023;18:e1088–9. https://doi.org/10.4244/EIJ-D-22-00517.
41. Caneiro-Queija B, Estévez-Loureiro R, Piñón-Esteban M, Barreiro-Pérez M, Baz-Alonso JA, Íñiguez-Romo A. Transfemoral transcatheter tricuspid valve replacement with the Cardiovalve system. Rev Española Cardiol (English Ed). 2023;76:270–2. https://doi.org/10.1016/J.REC.2022.08.011.

42. Bapat VN. The INTREPID valve for severe tricuspid regurgitation: first-inman case experience. In: Presented at CRT. Washington, DC: CRT; 2020.
43. Teiger E, Nejjari M, Lim P, Ruf T, Blanke P, Schäfer U, Treede H, Gallet R, Dreyfus J. First-in-human implantation of the topaz transcatheter tricuspid valve replacement system. EuroIntervention. 2022;18:862–4. https://doi.org/10.4244/EIJ-D-22-00277.
44. Estévez-Loureiro R, Sánchez-Recalde A, Amat-Santos IJ, Cruz-González I, Baz JA, Pascual I, Mascherbauer J, Abdul-Jawad Altisent O, Nombela-Franco L, Pan M, Trillo R, Moreno R, Delle Karth G, Salido-Tahoces L, Santos-Martinez S, Núñez JC, Moris C, Goliasch G, Jimenez-Quevedo P, Ojeda S, Cid-Álvarez B, Santiago-Vacas E, Jimenez-Valero S, Serrador A, Martín-Moreiras J, Strouhal A, Hengstenberg C, Zamorano JL, Puri R, Íñiguez-Romo A. 6-month outcomes of the TricValve system in patients with tricuspid regurgitation: the TRICUS EURO study. JACC Cardiovasc Interv. 2022;15:1366–77. https://doi.org/10.1016/J.JCIN.2022.05.022.
45. Wild MG, Lubos E, Cruz-Gonzalez I, Amat-Santos I, Ancona M, Andreas M, Niklas, Boeder F, Butter C, Carrasco-Chinchilla F, Estevez-Loureiro R, Kempfert J, Köll B, Montorfano M, Nef HM, Toggweiler S, Unbehaun A, Werner P, Windecker S, Praz F. Circulation: cardiovascular interventions early clinical experience with the TRICENTO bicaval valved stent for treatment of symptomatic severe tricuspid regurgitation: a multicenter registry. Circ Cardiovasc Interv. 2022;15(3):e011302. https://doi.org/10.1161/CIRCINTERVENTIONS.121.011302.
46. Cruz-Gonzá Lez I, Martín-Moreiras J, Ló Pez-Tejero S. Trillium: a new treatment for severe tricuspid regurgitation. Rev Esp Cardiol (Engl Ed). 2022;76(9):750. https://doi.org/10.1016/j.rec.2022.12.008.
47. Sherif M, Schmidt A, Path JR, Reinthaler M. Interventions for valvular disease and heart failure cross-caval approach for severe tricuspid insufficiency. EuroIntervention. n.d.:22–3. https://doi.org/10.4244/EIJ-D-23-00503.
48. Latib A, Scotti A. Screen failures for transcatheter tricuspid valve repair: implications for patient management and future innovation. JACC Cardiovasc Interv. 2023;16:1590–3. https://doi.org/10.1016/j.jcin.2023.05.023.
49. Gerçek M, Goncharov A, Narang A, Körber ML, Friedrichs KP, Baldridge AS, Meng Z, Puthumana JJ, Davidson LJ, Malaisrie SC, Thomas JD, Rudolph TK, Pfister R, Rudolph V, Davidson CJ. Characterization of screen failures among patients evaluated for transcatheter tricuspid valve repair (TriSelect-study). JACC Cardiovasc Interv. 2023;16:1579–89. https://doi.org/10.1016/J.JCIN.2023.03.036.
50. Taramasso M, Alessandrini H, Latib A, Asami M, Attinger-Toller A, Biasco L, Braun D, Brochet E, Connelly KA, Denti P, Deuschl F, Englmeier A, Fam N, Frerker C, Hausleiter J, Himbert D, Ho EC, Juliard J-M, Kaple R, Kreidel F, Kuck K-H, Ancona M, Lauten A, Lurz P, Mehr M, Nazif T, Nickening G, Pedrazzini G, Pozzoli A, Praz F, Puri R, Rodés-Cabau J, Schäfer U, Schofer J, Sievert H, Sievert K, Tang GHL, Tanner FC, Vahanian A, Webb JG, Windecker S, Yzeiray E, Zuber M, Maisano F, Leon MB, Hahn RT. Outcomes after current transcatheter tricuspid valve intervention mid-term results from the international TriValve registry. JACC Cardiovasc Interv. 2019; https://doi.org/10.1016/j.jcin.2018.10.022.
51. Fam NP, Braun D, von Bardeleben RS, Nabauer M, Ruf T, Connelly KA, Ho E, Thiele H, Lurz P, Weber M, Nickenig G, Narang A, Davidson CJ, Hausleiter J. Compassionate use of the PASCAL transcatheter valve repair system for severe tricuspid regurgitation: a multicenter, observational, first-in-human experience. JACC Cardiovasc Interv. 2019;12:2488–95. https://doi.org/10.1016/J.JCIN.2019.09.046.
52. Alperi A, Avanzas P, Almendá Rez M, Leó V, Herná Ndez-Vaquero D, Silva I, Ferná Ndez Del Valle D, Lix Ferná Ndez F, Díaz R, Rodes-Cabau J, Sar Morís C, Pascual I. Early and mid-term outcomes of transcatheter tricuspid valve repair: systematic review and meta-analysis of observational studies. Rev Esp Cardiol. 2023;76:322–32. https://doi.org/10.1016/j.rec.2022.06.004.
53. Sorajja P, Whisenant B, Hamid N, Naik H, Makkar R, Tadros P, Price MJ, Singh G, Fam N, Kar S, Schwartz JG, Mehta S, Bae R, Sekaran N, Warner T, Makar M, Zorn G, Spinner EM, Trusty PM, Benza R, Jorde U, McCarthy P, Thourani V, Tang GHL, Hahn RT, Adams

DH. Transcatheter repair for patients with tricuspid regurgitation. N Engl J Med. 2023; https://doi.org/10.1056/NEJMOA2300525/SUPPL_FILE/NEJMOA2300525_DATA-SHARING.PDF.

54. Kodali S, Hahn RT, George I, Davidson CJ, Narang A, Zahr F, Chadderdon S, Smith R, Grayburn PA, O'Neill WW, Wang DD, Herrmann H, Silvestry F, Elmariah S, Inglessis I, Passeri J, Lim DS, Salerno M, Makar M, Mack MJ, Leon MB, Makkar R. Transfemoral tricuspid valve replacement in patients with tricuspid regurgitation: TRISCEND study 30-day results. JACC Cardiovasc Interv. 2022;15:471–80. https://doi.org/10.1016/J.JCIN.2022.01.016.

Chapter 17
20 Years of TAVI—How Can We Get to a Comprehensive Patient Management?

Iliescu Vlad Anton and Parasca Catalina-Andreea

Abstract Twenty years after the first procedure, transcatheter aortic valve implantation (TAVI) has established itself as the most rapidly developing cardiac procedure in the twenty-first century. The road from a lifesaving procedure in inoperable or high-risk patients towards the treatment of choice for most patients with severe aortic stenosis is owed to continuous technological and technique advancements. TAVI surpassed surgery in the treatment of aortic stenosis not only by replacing it in many cases, but also by offering a cure for a whole new cohort of patients, previously constrained only to palliative medical treatment. This chapter aims to provide a comprehensive overview of TAVI in the management of heart failure in the context of aortic stenosis, highlighting past achievements, current practices in the context of established evidence, and possibilities for further development and impending concerns that need to be addressed in the future.

Keywords Aortic stenosis · Transcatheter aortic valve implantation · Transcatheter aortic valve replacement · Heart failure · Durability · Complications · Lifetime management

Abbreviations

AS	aortic stenosis
AI	artificial intelligence
AR	aortic regurgitation
AV	aortic valve

I. V. Anton (✉) · P. Catalina-Andreea
University of Medicine and Pharmacy "Carol Davila", Bucharest, Romania

Emergency Institute for Cardiovascular Diseases "Prof. Dr. C. C. Iliescu", Bucharest, Romania

M. Dorobanţu et al. (eds.), *Current Approach to Heart Failure*,
https://doi.org/10.1007/978-3-031-96562-3_17

AVR	aortic valve replacement
BAV	bicuspid aortic valve
BEV	balloon-expandable valve
CAD	coronary artery disease
CABG	coronary artery bypass grafting
CT	computed tomography
HF	heart failure
LVEF	left ventricular ejection fraction
LVSD	left ventricular systolic dysfunction
SAVR	Surgical aortic valve replacement
SEV	self-expanding valve
SVD	structural valve deterioration
PPM	patient-prosthesis mismatch
STS	Society of Thoracic Surgeons
TVT	Transcatheter Valve Therapy
TAV	tricuspid aortic valve
TAVI	transcatheter aortic valve implantation
TAVR	transcatheter aortic valve replacement
THV	transcatheter heart valves

Aortic Stenosis and Heart Failure—Defining the Landscape

Aortic stenosis (AS) is a relatively high prevalence chronic disease: 3,4% of people aged over 75 years have severe aortic stenosis [1]. The average survival after diagnosis without treatment is 2–3 years [2].

In the natural history of AS, heart failure (HF) is the final stage and is associated with a mortality rate of 67% after 5 years if left untreated [3]. Effective management of heart failure in patients with severe AS requires a thorough understanding of its pathophysiology [4]. This knowledge is essential for making appropriate therapeutic decisions and for avoiding unnecessary or futile interventions. It is important to differentiate between HF in relation to AS, and HF resulting from other coexisting causes, such as severe ischemic cardiomyopathy with significant myocardial infarction sequelae [5]. Effectively reducing the afterload present in AS, by transcatheter aortic valve implantation/replacement (TAVI/TAVR) or surgical aortic valve replacement (SAVR), the intervention significantly improves clinical outcomes but is dependent on the previous extent of cardiac and extracardiac damage [6].

The introduction of TAVI has completely changed AS treatment becoming the mainstay of treatment for patients with AS and concomitant HF [5, 7]. Greater access to TAVI corelates with improved survival rates [8].

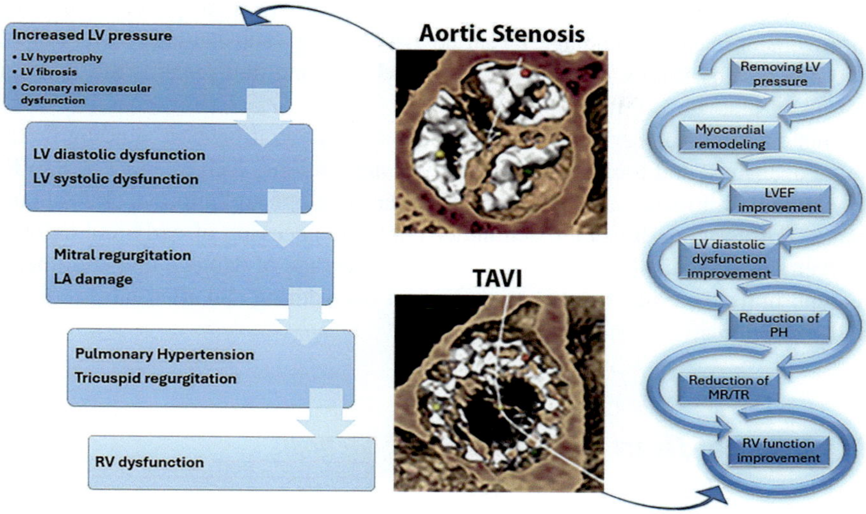

Fig. 17.1 Cardiac damage—pathogenesis in AS and effects of TAVI. Legend: *LA* left atrium, *RV* right ventricle, *PH* pulmonary hypertension, *MR* mitral regurgitation, *TR* tricuspid regurgitation

Stages of Cardiac Damage in Patients with Aortic Stenosis

AS combined with HF represents a progressive condition significantly impacting cardiac structure and function, culminating in various stages of cardiac damage (Fig. 17.1). This progression has been effectively captured through a staged classification that delineates the severity based on extravalvular cardiac damage. The stages of cardiac damage, as they pertain to AS, unfold as follows: Stage 0 indicates no extravalvular damage; Stage 1 involves left ventricular (LV) damage evidenced by measures such as LV hypertrophy, systolic or diastolic dysfunction; Stage 2 encompasses left atrial or mitral valve damage, often marked by conditions such as atrial enlargement, atrial fibrillation or significant mitral regurgitation; Stage 3 includes damage to the pulmonary vasculature or tricuspid valve, including pulmonary hypertension or severe tricuspid regurgitation; and Stage 4 represents right ventricular (RV) damage, which can manifest as moderate to severe RV dysfunction [6].

This stratification not only highlights the incremental risk associated with different stages but also underlines the implications for clinical outcomes after aortic valve replacement (AVR) [6]. Patients exhibiting higher stages of damage generally face poorer prognoses, reflecting a higher mortality risk post-AVR. Moreover, impact assessment of AVR 1-year after procedure offers profound insights. Patients underwent echocardiographic revaluation 1-year after AVR and were reclassified based on the extent of cardiac damage at this point [9]. Data indicate that while some patients experience improvement in cardiac damage 1-year post-AVR (approximately 15%), the majority either show no change (about 60%) or deterioration (around 25%) [9]. The study emphasizes that patients showing improvement in cardiac damage 1-year post-AVR have a substantially lower risk of mortality and morbidity compared to those whose condition remains the same or worsens [9].

This classification serves as a pivotal tool for risk stratification, guiding therapeutic decisions, and timing for aortic valve interventions, such as TAVI or SAVR, to potentially mitigate the progression of cardiac damage and improve clinical outcomes. Furthermore, this approach underscores the necessity of early and tailored interventions in patients with AS to prevent the cascade of damage that culminates in compromised cardiac function and elevated risks during and after valve replacement procedures.

Prevalence of Heart Failure in Aortic Stenosis

In aortic stenosis (AS), the left ventricle (LV) initially adapts through concentric wall hypertrophy to counteract increased pressure and maintain wall stress and LV ejection fraction (LVEF). However, this adaptation impairs diastolic filling and longitudinal shortening, eventually leading to reduced LVEF, heart failure (HF) symptoms, and poor outcomes as the disease progresses. The prevalence of HF in severe AS varies widely, influenced by how HF is defined (e.g., LVEF < 50%, presence of symptoms) and patient demographics. Studies have shown that symptomatic LV systolic dysfunction (LVSD) is common in severe AS, with a prevalence rate of up to 35% for reduced LVEF (<40%). The introduction of TAVI has shifted the management of severe AS, offering an alternative to those previously deemed unsuitable for surgery due to high operative risks.

LVSD is common in patients undergoing TAVI. Initial randomized controlled trials often excluded individuals with severe LVSD, defined as LVEF < 30%. However, real-world registries indicate that mild to moderate LVSD (LVEF 30–50%) occurs in 30% of TAVI patients, and severe LVSD (LVEF < 30%) is observed in approximately 10% of cases [10]. These patients frequently present with multiple comorbidities and an elevated Society of Thoracic Surgeons (STS) mortality risk, positioning them as a high-risk cohort. Prognostic evaluation of LVEF in this group showed mixed outcomes. For example, data from the PARTNER-2 trial and registry suggest that a lower baseline LVEF significantly correlates with increased all-cause and cardiac mortality over two years. Conversely, the Transcatheter Valve Therapy (TVT) registry found that while severe LVSD is associated with higher initial mortality and HF rates, adjusted mortality and HF rates one-year post-TAVI did not significantly differ with changes in LVEF [11].

Several factors have emerged as unfavourable prognostic indicators in patients with LVSD undergoing TAVI. These include low-flow, low-gradient AS, reduced calcification, poor nutritional status, chronic obstructive pulmonary disease, anaemia, atrial fibrillation, significant mitral regurgitation, pulmonary arterial hypertension, and moderate-to-severe paravalvular regurgitation [12, 13].

Identifying the underlying cause (s) of LVSD, such as severe AS, coronary artery disease (CAD), fibrosis, amyloidosis, etc., can be difficult in individuals undergoing TAVI [14]. Differentiating LVSD between afterload mismatch or depressed myocardial contractility is an important aspect in TAVI patients, as the latter is a marker of unfavourable prognosis following intervention. However, data from the TOPAS-TAVI registry and a meta-analysis of five observational studies revealed that while contractile reserve (increase of ≥20% in stroke volume during dobutamine stress echocardiography) is prevalent in approximately half of these patients, it does not significantly impact intermediate-term all-cause or cardiac mortality [12, 15, 16]. Despite notable improvements in stroke volume post-TAVI in patients with contractile reserve, changes in left ventricular ejection fraction (LVEF) and recovery rates are similar regardless of contractile reserve presence [17].

Aortic Stenosis and Concomitant Coronary Artery Disease

In addition to the inability of left ventricular (LV) concentric hypertrophic remodelling to adequately compensate for the increased pressure overload related to aortic stenosis, the coexistence of CAD plays a crucial role in the pathogenesis of HF [18, 19]. This association has significant implications for therapeutic strategies and prognosis [19]. AS and CAD often share pathophysiological pathways, leading to frequent co-occurrence. In the context of SAVR, more than half of the patients over the age of 70 undergo concurrent coronary artery bypass grafting (CABG). Observational studies comparing patients undergoing combined SAVR and CABG with those undergoing isolated SAVR have indicated poorer short- and long-term survival in the combined procedure group, likely due to pre-existing ischemic myocardial damage and other comorbidities [20]. Thus, assessing the presence and impact of significant CAD is crucial for optimizing the timing of intervention.

In randomized clinical trials and registries involving TAVI, the prevalence of CAD varies greatly from 30% to 69% [18, 19]. The management of significant CAD in these patients remains a contentious issue, especially in the elderly, where complete revascularization prior to TAVI may not be deemed critical [21]. However, observational studies suggest that myocardial damage correlates with poorer outcomes [22, 23]. For patients with severe AS undergoing SAVR, significant obstructive CAD often necessitates concurrent revascularization through CABG or a hybrid percutaneous coronary intervention approach [20]. In cases referred for TAVI, significant proximal lesions may warrant revascularization, particularly if they contribute to extensive ischemia or are associated with acute coronary events and hemodynamic instability [19, 20]. Although TAVI is currently playing a centre role, the optimal and comprehensive treatment of AS associated with concomitant CAD and HF is complex and requires additional research.

TAVI: A Paradigm Shift in Interventional Cardiology

TAVI marks a significant milestone in the field of interventional cardiology, emerging as a revolutionary technique that fundamentally changed the management of AS, particularly for patients deemed inoperable or at high surgical risk. After more than 20 years since the first procedure, TAVI highlights not only a scientific and technological leap but also epitomizes the vision and courage of pioneers in the field alongside their first patients. Before the advent of TAVI, the only option for treating severe symptomatic aortic stenosis was open-heart surgery, which many elderly and frail patients were unable to undergo. In 1985, Professor Alain Cribier and his team in Rouen, France performed the first successful percutaneous balloon aortic valvuloplasty, providing immediate clinical improvement for an inoperable patient [24]. After years of research and overcoming challenges, the first successful transcatheter aortic valve implantation was performed in Rouen in 2002 [25]. The introduction of TAVI was met with initial scepticism due to the high restenosis rates seen with balloon aortic valvuloplasty, the precursor to TAVI. However, persistent efforts of developers transformed these challenges into a new, effective treatment paradigm.

The procedural success and widespread adoption of TAVI were propelled forward by enhancements in valve design and procedural approach, driven by a deep understanding of structural heart disease and valve mechanics. Since then, TAVI has undergone extensive scientific evaluation, with numerous randomized trials and international registries demonstrating its safety and efficacy, and continuously expanding its indications from initially being reserved for patients at prohibitive surgical risk to those at low surgical risk [26–29].

Early trials such as PARTNER 1 and the CoreValve US Pivotal Trial focused on patients who were either deemed inoperable or at high surgical risk, demonstrating that TAVI was a viable alternative to surgical aortic valve replacement (SAVR), offering comparable, if not superior, survival benefits with fewer procedural risks [30, 31]. These findings have led to the approval of TAVI for high-risk patients.

Subsequent studies extended to intermediate-risk patients. The PARTNER 2 and SURTAVI trials showed that TAVI was non-inferior to SAVR in terms of survival and stroke rates in this group, further broadening the applicability of TAVI [32]. The most recent paradigm shift came with trials like PARTNER 3 and the Evolut Low Risk trial, which have included low-risk patients [27, 28]. These studies confirmed the non-inferiority of TAVI compared to SAVR and highlighted better post-procedure recovery times and quality-of-life metrics. As a result, guidelines have been updated, and TAVI is now considered a suitable option across all risk categories, revolutionizing the management of severe aortic stenosis and reflecting a significant shift in clinical practice over the last two decades [7, 33]. Currently TAVI is a guideline class I level A indication for patients over 75 years [7].

Continuous advancements in technology, increase in operator experience, broadening of indications, and overall reduction in procedure costs have all played a significant role in the development and rapid growth of TAVI from a novel concept to a widely accepted treatment option. Currently, TAVI is performed worldwide and is supported by extensive clinical trials and robust data that validate its safety and efficacy [34]. TAVI has been a prime example of successful translational research, leading to advancements in cardiac imaging and the Heart Team approach. This procedure has also catalysed further innovations in the treatment of other valvular and structural heart diseases, illustrating the dynamic nature of medical advancement. TAVI has had a significant impact on over 1.5 million patients treated to date, and future stories of TAVI are still being written.

Technological Advancements in TAVI Devices

TAVI technology has expanded its application to a wider range of patient populations with diverse anatomies, owing to its continuous advancement. TAVI volumes consistently increased from 2011 to 2019, surpassing the number of surgical aortic valve replacements in 2019 [35]. Notably, innovations in the design and delivery systems of transcatheter heart valves (THV) have resulted in a decrease in procedural complications and improved clinical outcomes (Fig. 17.2). Improvements in THV sizing and design have led to a reduction in paravalvular leak and conduction disturbances, while the use of lower-profile delivery systems has minimized vascular complications and bleeding [36]. The two main types of THV are balloon-expandable and self-expanding valves, that witness improvements with each iteration [36]. Technological advancements in TAVI devices have focused on addressing several critical issues to enhance procedural success and patient

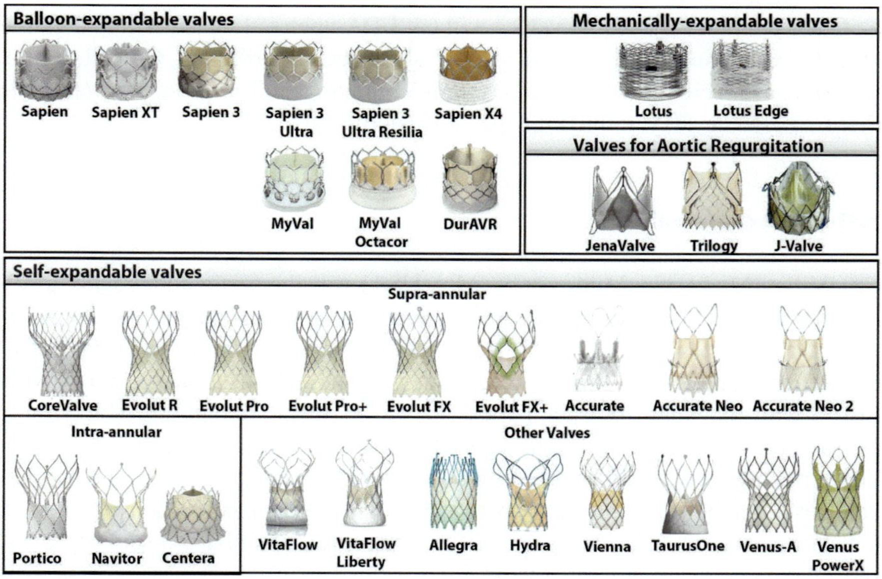

Fig. 17.2 Types of transcatheter aortic valves—past, current, and future devices

outcomes, such as improved sealing mechanisms to minimize paravalvular leak, low-profile devices to decrease the need for pacemaker implantation and facilitate coronary access for future interventions, novel leaflet materials and technologies to extend valve lifespan and prevent degeneration.

THV Technologies—Reiterations and Current Devices

Balloon-Expandable Valves

Since the development of the first transcatheter aortic valve, Cribier-Edwards, the Sapien family of balloon-expandable valves (BEV), has reached five iterations [25, 37]. Sapien 3, Sapien 3 Ultra, and Sapien 3 Ultra Resilia (Edwards Lifesciences, Irvine, CA, USA) are currently the only FDA-approved BEV [38]. Additionally, these valves have CE mark for valve-in-valve procedures. They are characterized by a low-profile cobalt-chromium stent frame with an upper row of large-cell configuration. Developments include a textured polyethylene terephthalate outer cuff instead of the bovine pericardium and increased outer cuff height in the Sapien 3 Ultra; addition of Resilia leaflet tissue with novel anticalcification technology in the Sapien 3 Ultra Resilia.

The latest iteration, Sapien X4, features a new frame design that allows direct adjustable sizing by balloon filling, on-balloon valve preparation, and independent valve rotation control for commissural alignment. Yet not commercially available, Sapien X4 is under assessment for safety and efficacy in all surgical risk categories, in the ongoing ALLIANCE study [NCT05172960].

Other balloon-expandable valves without FDA approval or under investigation include MyVal and the newest valve, MyVal Octacor (Meril, Vapi, Gujarat, India), with nine available sizes; DurAVR (Anteris Technologies, Toowong, Australia), the first single-piece THV, mimicking the native aortic valve [39].

Self-Expandable Valves

CoreValve (Medtronic, Minneapolis, MN, USA) was the first commercially available self-expanding valve (SEV) with a supra-annular design. Further iterations included Evolut R—with a nitinol frame and a completely retrievable and repositionable design, Evolut Pro—with external pericardial tissue wrap, and Evolut Pro+—with extended external pericardial tissue wrap. Evolut FX (Medtronic, Minneapolis, MN, USA) is the latest generation Medtronic valve, featuring improvements in both valve and delivery systems to provide an easier, precise, and predictable result: radiopaque markers on the valve and re-engineered delivery system (smaller nose cone, nitinol capsule, single spine shaft, optimization stability layer) [40]. Going one step further, Evolut FX+ offers enhanced coronary access gaps through a modified stent design. The valve Evolut FX+ received FDA approval since March 2024.

The Acurate Neo (Boston Scientific, Marlborough, MA, USA) features a supra-annular design, porcine pericardial leaflets, stabilization arches above valve leaflets, and a large space between the stabilizers and upper crown for coronary access. Acurate Neo 2 design features taller pericardial sealing skirt, for improved sealing, flexible delivery catheter, and expandable introducer sheet. Acurate Prime XL is a larger copy of Accurate Neo2 and is designed for cases with large native aortic annulus diameters (up to 29 mm) [41]. The ongoing randomized controlled trial Acurate IDE (NCT03735667) aims to compare the results of Acurate Neo 2 with those of other commercially available balloon-expandable or self-expanding valves.

Portico (Abbott, Chicago, IL, USA), the first intra-annular SEV with FDA approval, features a large frame cell design for coronary access, fully resheathable, and partially retrievable mechanism. The latest generation from Abbott, the Navitor valve, features the NaviSealTM active sealing cuff instead of the porcine pericardial cuff. The Navitor Titan valve (35 mm) is the largest available size of Navitor and is used for cases with large native aortic annulus diameter (up to 30 mm) [42].

Other self-expanding valves without FDA approval or under investigation include: Hydra (Sahajanand Medical Technologies Limited, Mumbai, India)—with components to optimize alignment and large open frame cells for coronary access; Venus-A (Venus Medtech Inc., Hangzhou, China), VitaFlow (MicroPort, Shanghai, China) and TaurusOne (Peijia Medical, Suzhou, China)—with high radial force for bicuspid aortic valves; Allegra (New Valve Technology, Hechingen, Germany)—which maintains flow during implantation.

Mechanically Expandable Valves

Lotus and the latest generation Lotus Edge valve system (Boston Scientific, Marlborough, Massachusetts, USA) consists of a bovine pericardial valve embedded in a braided wire Nitinol frame with a very high radial strength and an adaptive seal [43]. Although valve deployment is mechanically controlled, allowing recapturing and repositioning, issues with delivery systems led to their discontinuation in 2020.

THV Technology for Pure Aortic Regurgitation

Although surgery is the recommended treatment option for patients with aortic regurgitation (AR) according to the guidelines, a percutaneous procedure is needed, particularly for patients who are at high or prohibitive surgical risk [16]. TAVI in pure severe AR with common THV devices has been challenging because of valve embolization, significant residual post-procedural AR, and the need for a second valve [44]. To date, only two transcatheter valves are dedicated for AR: the J-Valve (JC Medical) and the JenaValve Trilogy (JenaValve Technology) [45].

J-Valve is a porcine aortic valve set within a self-expandable nitinol stent, featuring three stabilizing anchors, that can be implanted via an 18-Fr steerable delivery system. Although self-expandable, valve recapturing is not possible. The valve is chosen according to annular sizing (5 available sizes) and requires 10% oversizing. The unique features of the J-Valve are addressing the risk of valve embolization: self-expanding valve with self-aligning anchor rings that allow direct capture of aortic valve leaflets. The J-Valve Transfemoral System is currently being evaluated in a clinical trial focused on safety [NCT03876964].

JenaValve is another dedicated valve for treating pure AR. The latest generation, the Trilogy valve, underwent modifications to provide stable annular positioning in the absence of calcified aortic valve and to address previous shortcomings of its predecessor [46, 47]. Trilogy consists of porcine pericardial leaflets mounted in a supra-annular fashion on a self-expanding nitinol support frame available in three different sizes, providing a solution for aortic valves with an annular diameter of 21–27 mm. To ensure proper sealing in pure AR, it is recommended 10–20% oversizing. Refinements brought by the Trilogy valve include large cell design of the stent frame to improve coronary access, diamond-shaped cells in the lower part of the stent frame that provide adequate annular sealing, and integrated radiopaque locators for precise implant depth, sinus, and commissural alignment. The device is essentially clipped to the native leaflets, by grasping forces between locators and nitinol frame. The redesigned introducer system enables transfemoral implantation via an 18F sheet. Since the first in-human transfemoral JenaValve implantation [48], ongoing trials aim to assess safety and efficacy with promising results. In the initial results from the ALIGN-AR clinical trial [NCT02732704] involving 70 patients with pure aortic stenosis who underwent transfemoral TAVI with the Trilogy valve, the device success rate was 94.3% [49].

Patient Selection and Pre-procedural Assessment

Criteria for Selecting Patients for TAVI

Over the past decade, TAVI has become the preferred method for treating symptomatic severe AS [7, 50]. The criteria for patient selection are primarily based on the patient's surgical risk, anatomical considerations, and overall health status (comorbidities). Initially, TAVI was reserved for those at high or prohibitive surgical risk due to factors such as advanced age, presence of multiple comorbidities, or specific conditions that increased the risks associated with open-heart surgery. Over time, as TAVI technology and techniques have advanced, criteria have expanded to include lower-risk patients. This change has been emphasised by results from significant studies such as PARTNER 3 and the Evolut Low-Risk trial [51, 52].

Another important principle involved in patient selection is assessing anatomical suitability for TAVI, requiring detailed and precise analysis of cardiac and vascular anatomy to determine the feasibility and strategy. This assessment is critical for selecting the appropriate prosthetic valve type and size, and for planning the access route. Key anatomical considerations include the type of valve, dimensions, shape, and calcification of the aortic annulus and left ventricle outflow tract, as these factors directly influence the risk of paravalvular leak, conduction abnormalities and post-deployment annular rupture. Vascular access suitability, primarily through the femoral arteries, must be assessed for size, tortuosity, and atheroma burden to determine the feasibility of the transfemoral approach, preferred for its minimally invasive nature and associated rapid recovery. Multidetector computed tomography (MDCT) plays an indispensable role in these evaluations, offering detailed three-dimensional reconstructions of the cardiovascular anatomy [53]. This comprehensive anatomical assessment, conducted by a multidisciplinary Heart Team, ensures that candidates for TAVI are selected with an approach tailored to maximize procedural success and minimize perioperative and long-term complications [54].

As TAVI is increasingly being used for lower-risk and younger patients, it is crucial to employ a shared decision-making process that carefully weighs in life expectancy, valve durability and possibility for reintervention and coronary access [54]. This decision should be grounded in a careful assessment of the patient's preferences, as well as anatomical and procedural considerations, carefully balancing the risks and advantages of each method for the individual patient.

Contraindications and Futility

As its indications continue to expand and more clinical data become available, determining the feasibility of TAVI is a crucial aspect in deciding the appropriate treatment and technique [55, 56]. Absolute contraindications to TAVI include a life expectancy of less than a year secondary to non-cardiac conditions, unlikely improvement in quality of life due to comorbidities, valvular disease other than severe aortic stenosis requiring surgery, active endocarditis, left ventricular thrombus, plaques with mobile trombi in the ascending aorta or arch [57].

The concept of therapeutic futility is characterized by the absence of medical efficacy, particularly in situations where a physician judges that the therapy is unlikely to achieve its intended clinical outcomes or fails to provide meaningful survival based on the patient's personal values (STS score > 15, Life Expectancy < 1 year and/or poor candidate for rehabilitation). Assessment of futility should extend beyond survival and address functional recovery.

Futility in TAVI is influenced by cardiac and extracardiac comorbidities. Cardiac conditions like atrial fibrillation, severe left ventricular dysfunction, right ventricular dysfunction, severe primary mitral regurgitation, and persistent pulmonary hypertension increase mortality and limit symptomatic improvement post-TAVI [58]. Extracardiac factors such as end-stage chronic kidney disease, chronic lung disease, anemia, and active malignancies further elevate the risk of poor prognosis. These comorbidities, particularly when severe, reduce the likelihood of survival and quality of life benefits from TAVI [58]. To minimize the risk of futile interventions, comprehensive pre-procedural evaluation to assess and quantify these comorbidities is required. Consideration must be given to the concept of futility, especially when it comes to transcatheter interventions, which are the primary treatment option for elderly patients. The challenge of assessing the risk/benefit ratios of interventions in elderly patients is amplified by the high prevalence of comorbidity, emphasizing the crucial role of Heart Team in this population.

Although active endocarditis remains an absolute contraindication for TAVI, it appears to be a safe alternative treatment for residual valvular lesion in patients with high surgical risk and healed aortic valve infectious endocarditis [59].

Many of the previously believed relative contraindications of high-risk anatomical features believed to be relative contraindications to TAVI for TAVI have been surmounted. These include inadequate annulus size, bicuspid valve, asymmetric severe valve calcification, low coronary ostia height, small Valsalva sinuses, narrow sinotubular junction, porcelain aorta, and inadequate vascular access (vessel size, calcification, tortuosity, ulcerated plaques, dissection) (Fig. 17.3) [36].

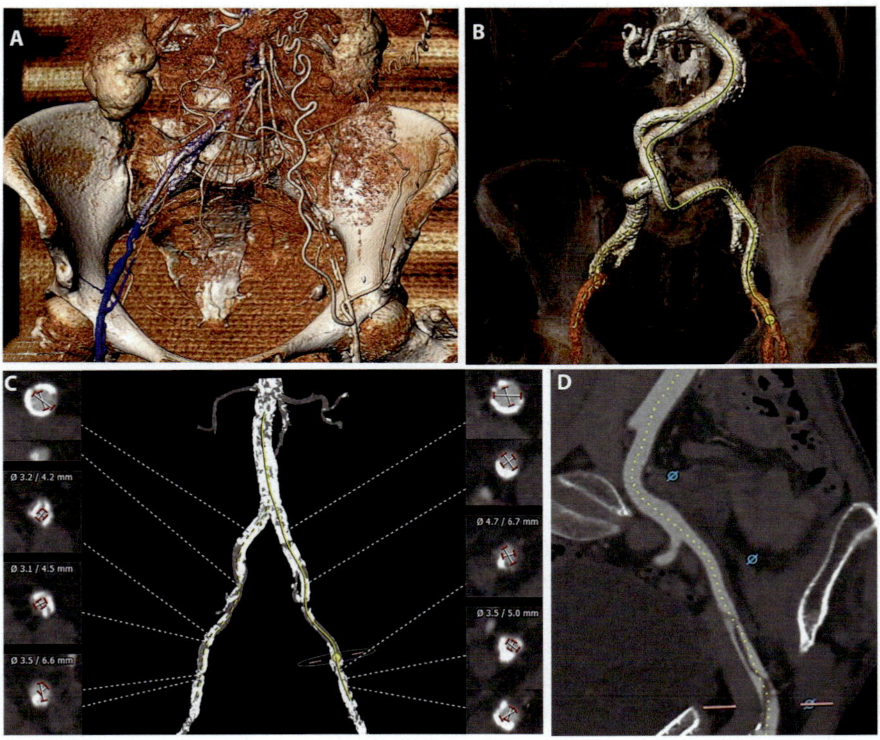

Fig. 17.3 Inadequate vascular access. (**a**) narrow right iliac artery and occluded left iliac artery; (**b**) severe tortuosity; (**c**) severe calcification; (**d**) left external iliac artery dissection

Bicuspid aortic valve (BAV) is one of the most disputed topics when considering TAVI. Anatomical features such as leaflet asymmetry, presence of a calcified raphe, calcifications extending in the left ventricular outflow tract, elliptic or large annular dimensions may impair optimal TAVI positioning and deployment, resulting in an increased risk of paravalvular regurgitation and stroke, but with comparable result in terms of device success and mortality with tricuspid valve [60]. While clinical trials are awaited to provide insights favouring one TAVI device type over another for patients with BAV, procedural planning is essential in achieving good results (morphology, annular and supraanular sizing, implantation height) [61].

For small aortic annuli, a supra-annular valve may be the solution to avoid patient-prosthesis mismatch and achieve superior hemodynamic parameters [62, 63]. Additional tricks include predilatation, high implant depth and balloon post-dilatation to improve frame expansion [62]. In very large aortic annuli, balloon-expandable (with balloon overfilling) have been used beyond manufacturer recommendations with good results [64]. A low-profile with deep implantation depth or a retrievable/repositionable valve may avoid the risk of coronary obstruction, in addition to other strategies to prevent coronary occlusion (prophylactic guidewire, catheter/stent intubation, or leaflet laceration) [65].

With the evolution of technology and improvements in TAVI delivery systems, implying new hydrophilic, thin, expandable, and atraumatic sheaths, together with use of intravascular lithotripsy, transfemoral TAVI is now feasible in more than 95% of cases [66, 67]. For patients without femoral access, alternative access routes may be used: transapical, transaortic, transcarotid, transaxillary, trans-subclavian, and transcaval approaches, posing different adjustments in implantation technique, each with advantages and risks [68].

TAVI and Risk Scores

TAVI has significantly advanced as the main treatment for severe symptomatic aortic stenosis and is applicable across all surgical risk levels assessed by predictive scores, such as the Society of Thoracic Surgeons Predicted Risk of Mortality (STS) or EuroSCORE II. Prediction of postoperative outcomes after valvular surgery using these scores is less accurate in high-risk patients. Moreover, STS and EuroSCORE II, originally designed for surgical cohorts, have limitations when applied to TAVI and often overestimate mortality risk [69]. Assessing the risk of adverse events following TAVI is essential to determine the benefits or futility of the procedure, especially in high-risk patients with AS [43].

In response, TAVI-specific models have been developed to predict outcomes more accurately, such as Transcatheter Valve Therapy (TVT) and FRANCE-2, which are derived from various global registries and studies [69–72]. Comparison of STS and TVT scores in predicting short- and long-term mortality across a large cohort revealed that while TVT scores performed somewhat better in high-risk patients, they did not significantly outperform STS scores in broader patient groups

[73]. Although the TVT risk score has been confirmed in other studies, its usefulness is constrained by its inability to predict long-term results and lack of validation in a population undergoing contemporary TAVI, particularly in younger, lower-risk patients who receive newer-generation THVs [40, 44].

None of the existing risk scores include anatomical factors with impact on the procedure, either surgical or transcatheter, although some attempts have been made with modest results [74]. Moreover, these models do not fully account for factors such as frailty or pre-procedural cognitive status, which have been identified as significant predictors of post-TAVI mortality [75, 76].

Modern advancements in TAVI technology and procedural expertise have notably decreased mortality rates, highlighting the necessity of refining risk prediction models to better reflect current practices and patient profiles [77]. These models must consider a broader range of features, integrating both traditional and emerging risk factors [6, 9, 75]. Machine learning models may provide solutions by analysing large, complex data without the need for constant updates to the models [78]. As the field evolves, assessing extensive real-world data to develop a more robust TAVI risk score is crucial to enhance patient selection and optimize outcomes.

Heart Team Approach in Managing TAVI Patients

The Heart Team ensures that each patient undergoing TAVI receives comprehensive, personalized care that is based on the latest evidence and best practices in the field of cardiology and cardiac surgery. Rapid evolution of TAVI practices has also promoted changes in the architecture and role of the Heat Team in the management of patients with AS [54]. The Heart Team is not only responsible for selection and evaluation of patients, but also procedure planning and risk assessment, intra- and post-procedural care, and remains involved in the long-term management and follow-up. This has led to expansion and diversification in the composition of the Heart Team from its traditional form (consisting of a cardiac surgeon, an interventional cardiologist, and a non-invasive cardiologist) to the contemporary Heart Team (Fig. 17.4) [54].

Risk prediction scores can support the decision-making process of the Heart Team and serve as valuable resources for clinical research, comparing performance standards, and educating patients and their families about the risks associated with the procedure. Nevertheless, these scores should not be utilized as the sole determinant for treatment allocation [79]. The Heart Team's effectiveness lies in its ability to merge diverse expertise towards a unified goal, maximizing patient safety and outcomes while minimizing procedural risks and complications [80].

Decisions concerning treatment and intervention should be made by an active and collaborative Heart Team with expertise in VHD, comprising clinical and interventional cardiologists, cardiac surgeons, imaging specialists, cardiovascular anaesthesiologists, and other specialists if necessary [7]. The Heart Team assessment and decision is especially recommended for the management of high-risk and

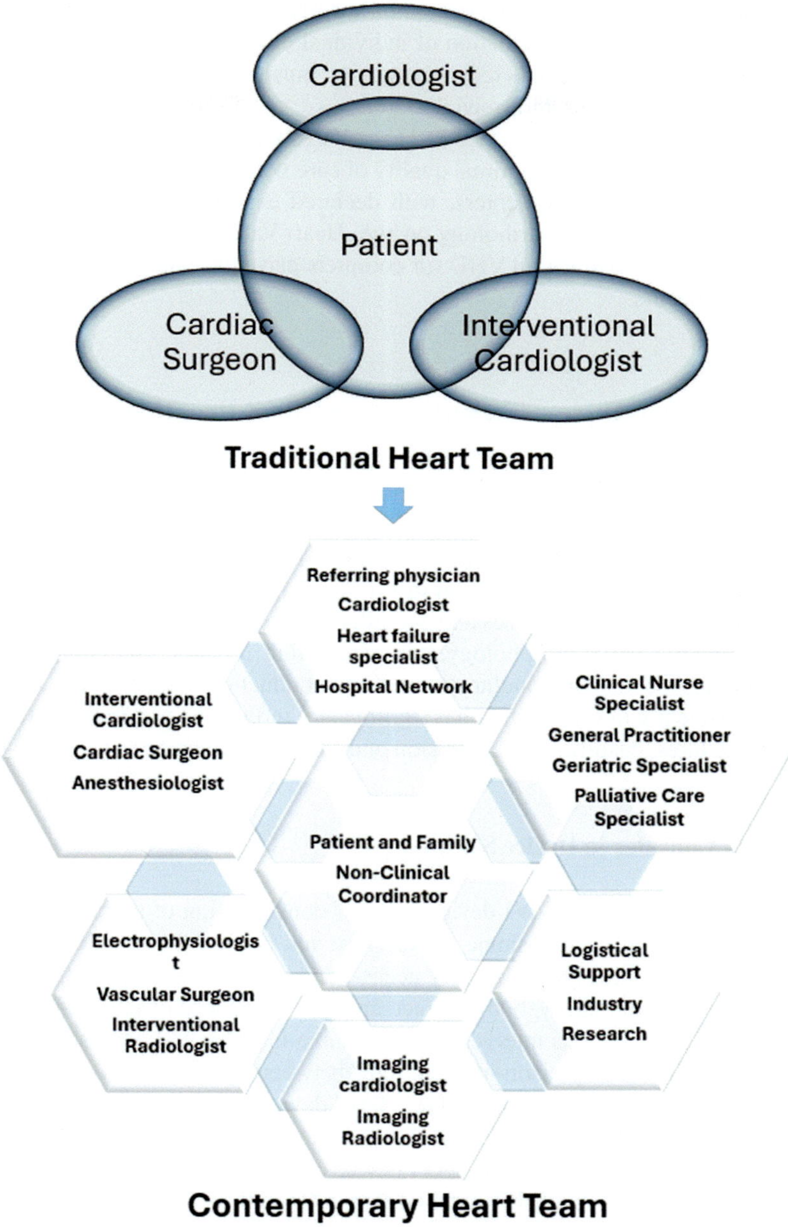

Fig. 17.4 Differences between traditional and contemporary Heart Team composition involved in the management of AS patients

asymptomatic patients, as well as in case of uncertainty or lack of strong evidence. Decision based on careful evaluation of individual clinical, anatomical, and procedural factors. The Heart Team's recommendation must be discussed with the patient to enable them to make an informed decision.

Interventions must be performed in Heart Valve Centres, defined as Centres of Excellence, aimed to deliver optimal quality of care with a patient-centred approach [7]. These are high-volume centers, with declared expertise, and require cardiac surgery and interventional cardiology on site. Heart Valve Centres should promote timely referral of patients with VHD for comprehensive evaluation before irreversible damage occurs.

The TAVI Procedure—Techniques and Best Practices

Procedural Planning

Procedural planning, encompassing valve selection and vascular access, has been enhanced through the standardization of CT imaging, which is now recognized as the definitive modality for assessing vascular access, measuring annular dimensions, examining valve morphology, and forecasting possible complications like acute coronary occlusion, annular rupture, and conduction disturbances [38]. The comprehensive use of CT imaging has significantly refined the preparatory steps for TAVI procedures, ensuring high precision and safe performance.

Factors to Consider in Device Selection

Selecting the appropriate TAVI device requires consideration of several factors: 1. Anatomical—annulus dimensions, aortic valve and aortic root complex calcification, aortic valve phenotype, coronary access, and risk of coronary obstruction; 2. clinical—age and durability, body surface area and avoidance of patient-prosthesis mismatch (PPM); previous interventions and valve-in-valve procedures.

Although direct comparison of event rates between device types is discouraged because of the differences in risk profiles, TAVI devices have unique design characteristics with inherent advantages and disadvantages [81]. Given the lack of large-scale randomized trials on various TAVI devices and the rapid development of new device iterations, there is insufficient evidence to claim the superiority of one device type over another.

Certain patient-related and anatomy-related factors may slightly favour one or several designs [81]. For instance, balloon-expandable valves are particularly suitable for patients with an extremely large annulus that exceeds manufacturer recommendations, a horizontal aorta angled over 70°, a high risk of needing a permanent pacemaker post-procedure, extensive coronary artery disease, or a high probability of requiring future percutaneous coronary interventions. Conversely, self-expanding valves are favoured for cases with dense annular or subannular calcification, patients who are intolerant to rapid pacing such as those with low ejection fraction, or when dealing with small or difficult iliofemoral artery access. Mechanically expandable valves are advantageous for similar reasons as self-expanding valves, particularly in patients who already have a permanent pacemaker. Each valve type is designed to address specific clinical and anatomical challenges, ensuring optimal outcomes for varied patient profiles.

These considerations underscore the importance of a tailored approach in TAVI device selection, integrating detailed anatomical, pathological, and procedural factors to optimize clinical outcomes and ensure device longevity.

Bicuspid Anatomy

As the most prevalent congenital cardiac defect (incidence of 2%), the bicuspid aortic valve (BAV) displays significant morphological diversity, including variations in leaflet geometry, orientation, and the presence or absence of a raphe, with marked differences in the degree of calcification of the valve and surrounding structures. The main concerns regarding TAVI in BAV are related to unfavourable anatomy, choice of appropriate sizing method, optimal device and implantation strategies, and long-term durability of the valve [61].

Specific anatomical features such as severely calcified leaflets, calcified raphe, calcifications protruding in the LVOT, excessively elliptical aortic annuli that exceed THV sizes can lead to suboptimal stent expansion, modified valve hemodynamic parameters with a potential impact on structural valve degeneration, and long-term outcomes [82, 83].

Prosthesis sizing for BAV remains unstandardized, with various approaches being tested, including measurements based on the size of the aortic annuls at different levels (intra-annular, supra-annular, circle method, intercomissural distance, and raphe-based sizing) or direct balloon technique sizing [84]. Alternative innovative sizing algorithms take into consideration the length and calcium load of the raphe and the overall calcium volume in BAV, which could potentially enhance procedural outcomes and THV performance [85]. Furthermore, advanced imaging techniques and CT scan analyses are being utilized to simulate post-TAVI outcomes, providing identification of patients with complex anatomies that might impose challenges [86].

Numerous studies have shown that TAVI is safe and feasible in patients with BAV anatomy, with equivalent results at 30-days and 1-year survival [60, 87]. Moreover, patients with BAV had a significant lower risk of mortality compared to TAV patients, mainly because of lower risk and younger age [87]. However, the follow-up period in these studies is limited beyond one year, requiring further investigation. There are still concerns regarding periprocedural complications such as a higher risk for ischemic cerebrovascular events, moderate to severe paravalvular leak and annular rupture in patients with BAV anatomy [60].

Recent advancements in TAVI technology have significantly improved procedural success and reduced risks like paravalvular leak, annular rupture, and the need for re-implantation. Modern balloon-expandable and self-expanding valves in BAV patients have demonstrated comparable clinical outcomes and device success rates with TAVI in tricuspid aortic valves [60, 88–90].

A recent single centre retrospective study of over 1200 patients undergoing TAVI for severe AS with self-expanding THV (over 90%) shows similar rates of perioperative complications (stroke, pacemaker implantation, PPM) and 1-year survival between different aortic valve morphologies (BAV type 0 vs. BAV type 1 vs. TAV) [91]. Unpublished data from our centre, Emergency Hospital for Cardiovascular Diseases "Prof. Dr, C.C. Iliescu" (Bucharest, Romania), also provide favourable results after TAVI with balloon expandable valves (over 95%) between aortic valve morphologies (Fig. 17.5).

Despite technological advancements, the development of accurate algorithms for transcatheter valve selection in BAV patients requires further research. Currently, there are no comprehensive data supporting one TAVI device type over another for patients with BAV and AS, but procedural planning (morphology, annular and

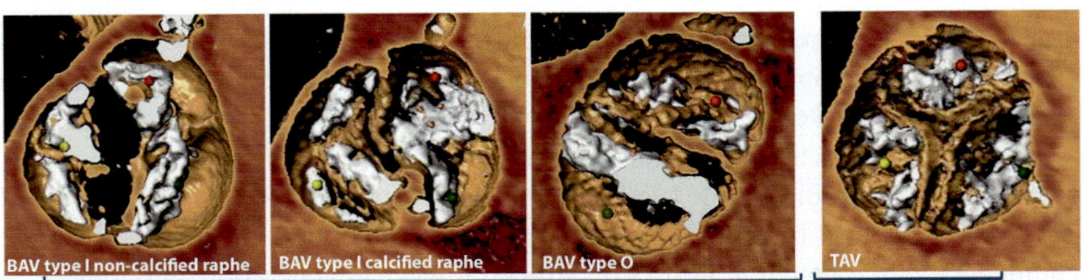

Early follow-up	% (n=1029)	BAV (n=237)	TAV (n=792)	P-value
Periprocedural mortality	1.0%(10)	0.8%(2)	1.0%(8)	1.00
Non-cardiac mortality	1.2%(12)	0.8%(2)	1.3%(10)	0.65
All-cause mortality	2.1%(22)	1.7%(4)	2.3%(18)	1.00
PVL trivial/mild	16.9%(174)	13.5%(32)	17.9%(142)	0.04
moderate	5.6%(58)	7.6%(18)	5.1%(40)	0.22
Annular rupture	1.5%(15)	2.5%(6)	1.1%(9)	0.22
PPI	6.1%(63)	6.3%(15)	5.1%(48)	0.38
Readmission to Hospital	3.9%(40)	3.4%(8)	4.0%(32)	0.25
Late follow-up**	**% (n=1007)**	**BAV (n=233)**	**TAV (n=774)**	**P-value**
All-cause mortality	16.8%(169)	9.4%(22)	19.0(147)	<0.001
Cardiac mortality	2.7%(27)	1.8%(6)	2.9%(21)	0.230

Fig. 17.5 Outcomes of TAVI in BAV vs. TAV morphology. Legend: *PPI* permanent pacemaker implantation, *PVL* paravalvular leak

supraanular sizing, implantation height) is the key to achieving optimal clinical outcomes [61]. As TAVI is expanding to younger patients with longer life expectancy, the initiation of a dedicated prospective RCT on the safety, effectiveness, and limitations of TAVI vs. SAVR on the long-term in different types of bicuspid anatomy in AS is highly needed [92].

Concomitant Coronary Artery Disease

Although SAVR and concomitant myocardial revascularization have already been established for patients with AS and significant CAD, there is a lack of consensus on the percutaneous treatment of CAD in the context of TAVI. Current guidelines and expert consensus statements recommend PCI in patients with left main disease or severe proximal CAD prior to TAVI, but it is unknown whether this translates into improved outcomes [33, 93]. Based on available evidence from randomized controlled trials and large registries, it appears that performing PCI for patients with CAD and planned TAVI does not result in significant improvements in outcomes [94, 95]. The REVASC-TAVI registry revealed comparable outcomes between complete and incomplete revascularization in patients with CAD undergoing TAVI. Furthermore, complete revascularization failed to provide any advantage in patients with impaired LVEF or NYHA class III/IV compared to patients with NYHA class I/II [94]. In a similar fashion, PCI prior to TAVI showed no benefit in terms of rehospitalization and mortality in ACTIVATION, a small randomized clinical trial where over half of patients had NYHA class III/IV [95].

While TAVI is the centrepiece in the treatment of AS, presence of concomitant CAD presents challenges regarding evidence-based protocols for revascularization. Current strategies may include the combined use of TAVI and percutaneous coronary intervention (PCI), especially in high-risk patients. However, the timing, sequence, and choice of the procedures remain the subject of ongoing clinical trials and research.

Bioprosthetic Valve Degeneration and Valve-in-Valve Procedures

The rising prevalence of degenerative bioprosthetic valve disease, largely attributed to an aging population and a preference for bioprostheses over mechanical valves, has led to an increased need for redo interventions [96]. Valve-in-valve (ViV) TAVI has become a favourable alternative to redo SAVR because of its lower risk of periprocedural complications and its suitability for patients with significant comorbidities and frailty [96]. Self-expanding valves are recommended for patients with smaller surgical bioprostheses due to the lower rates of patient-prosthesis mismatch observed with balloon-expandable valves [97].

ViV TAVI has demonstrated lower in-hospital major adverse cardiovascular events (MACE), reduced hospitalizations, and shorter hospital stays than redo SAVR [96]. Long-term outcomes also favour ViV TAVI, with studies such as the PARTNER II—Nested Registry/Valve in Valve indicating better survival rates, improved valve hemodynamic parameters, and enhanced quality of life up to five years post-procedure [98]. The VIVID Registry supports these findings, with a reported five-year survival rate of 38% for high surgical risk patients with TAVI in failed surgical aortic bioprostheses [99]. The study also provides insightful information regarding current practices and their implications, as the size of the initial valve impacts long-term mortality, and the choice of transcatheter valve type affects the need for reintervention after the ViV procedure [99].

Optimal device selection for ViV TAVI requires identification of the mechanism of prosthetic valve failure: structural valve degeneration (SVD), patient-prosthesis mismatch (PPM), or both [100]. While ViV TAVI with a self-expanding valve may be more favorable for small surgical bioprosthesis, balloon fracture of the stent frame of certain prosthetic valves is an option to facilitate ViV TAVI using a larger device for improved hemodinamic parameters [101].

Although less common, TAVI-in-TAVI emerges as a relatively safe and effective procedure for selected patients with structural valve deterioration after TAVI [102]. Recent data show a low rate of redo-TAVI due to probable device failure, only 0.22% out of more than 60,000 TAVI procedures. This low rate of THVs may be attributed to their durability and the competing risk of mortality in high-risk patients undergoing TAVI. The mode of THV failure was balanced (1/3 regurgitation, 1/3 stenosis, 1/3 both) and similar to the mode of surgical valve failure in the TAVI VIVID [103]. Novel concepts emerge in the analysis of redo-TAVI, such as index THV type and mechanism of dysfunction, index THV expansion, neoskirt, leaflet overhang and deflection, valve-to-aorta distances and neosinuses [104]. Before TAVI-in-TAVI becomes a common procedure, additional research is needed to identify the optimal patient and anatomical selection criteria, the ideal type of prosthesis based on the index procedure, and the long-term outcomes for patients undergoing redo-TAVI.

The risks associated with ViV procedures cannot be overlooked, particularly the risk of acute coronary obstruction, primarily due to displacement of the valve-leaflet towards the stent frame and the sinotubular junction during the redo-procedure resulting in sinus sequestration [100]. The risk of acute coronary obstruction in ViV TAVI is high, and careful analysis of the TAVI protocol computed tomography scan should be performed (Fig. 17.6). The BASILICA technique or preemptive coronary protection are adjunctive techniques [100].

Successful ViV procedures, either TAVI-in-SAVR or TAVI-in-TAVI, relies on meticulous pre-procedural planning and precise procedural execution (Fig. 17.7). This involves the accurate identification of the existing valve, selection of an appropriate THV, and optimal placement [100]. Tools like the ViV Aortic application have been developed to assist with the procedural planning process and management for good clinical outcomes [105].

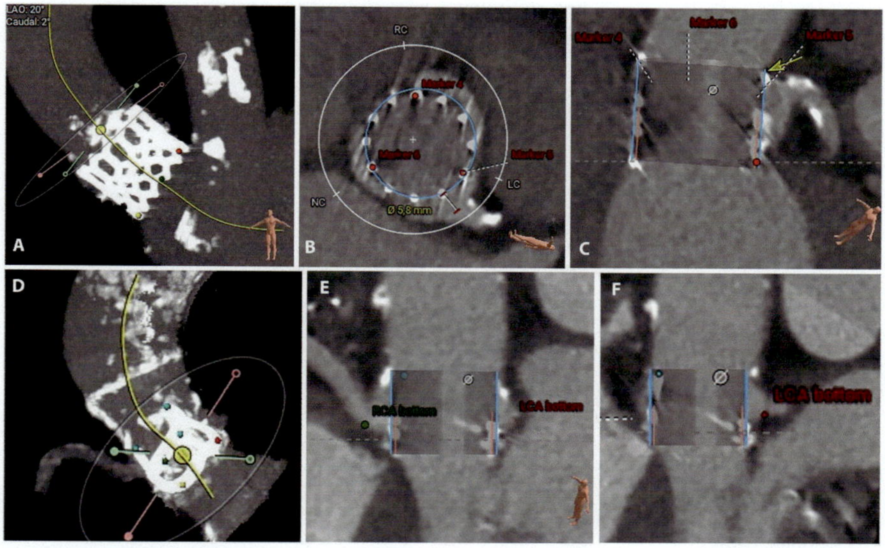

Fig. 17.6 Risk assessment of acute coronary obstruction in ViV TAVI. Upper row: assessment for TAVI-in TAVI: (**a**) Narrow sinuses and small sinotubular junction diameter; (**b**) Valve-to-coronary ostium distance; (**c**) Valve-to-sinotubular junction distance with possible risk of sinus sequestration. Lower row: assessment for TAVI-in-SAVR: (**d**) Supraanular implantation of surgical bioprosthesis in small aortic root; (**e**) Low right coronary artery; (**f**) Low left coronary artery with possible sinus sequestration

Periprocedural Medical Management

Medical Therapy in HF Patients Undergoing TAVI

There is limited information on the current guideline-directed HF therapy in patients with AS and HF undergoing TAVI (Fig. 17.8). While renin–angiotensin system (RAS) inhibitors are present in 40–60% of patients undergoing TAVI at discharge, they have been associated with lower rates of mid-term all-cause mortality, cardiovascular mortality, HF readmission, cerebrovascular events, and new-onset atrial fibrillation [106, 107]. RAS inhibitors following TAVI have also been associated with significant reductions in left ventricular volume and mass, and improved quality of life [108, 109]. The effect on left ventricular remodelling seems to be dose dependent [107]. Discontinuation of RAS inhibitors has been observed in approximately 30% of patients who underwent TAVI and was prompted by post-procedural acute kidney injury or pacemaker requirement [59]. Randomized clinical trials are currently evaluating the effects of RAS and/or SGLT2 inhibition on left ventricular remodelling and post-TAVI outcomes [110, 111].

Although over 30% of patients who undergo TAVI are administered beta-blockers, the association between beta-blockers and post-TAVI outcomes has not been thoroughly investigated [112]. Adequate fluid management with diuretic

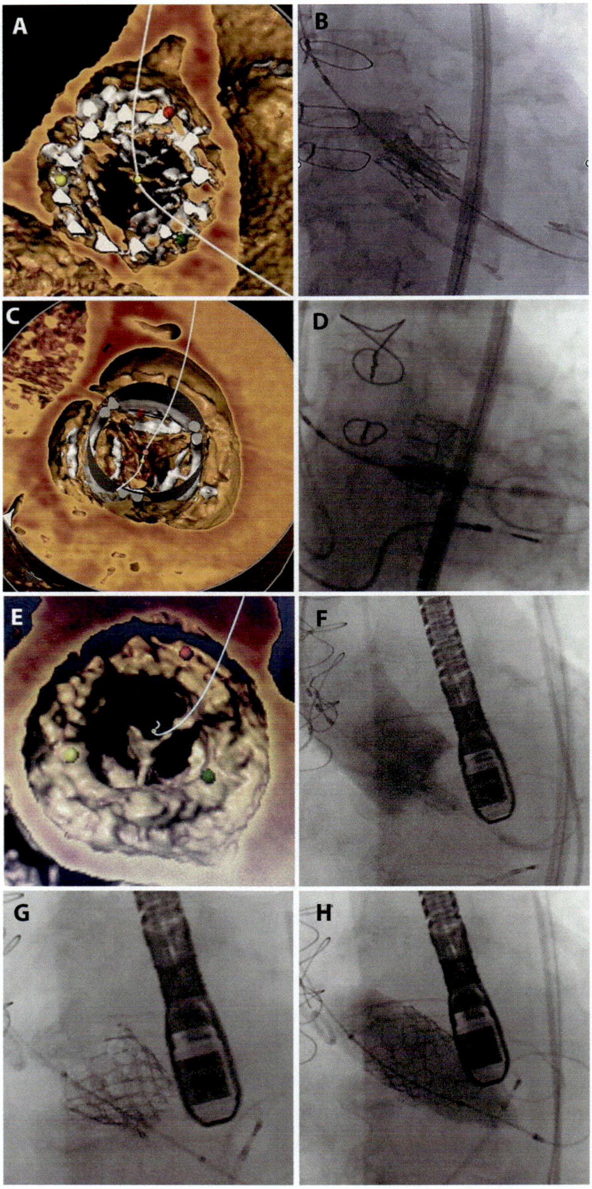

Fig. 17.7 Successful ViV TAVI. First row: TAVI-in-TAVI (Sapien 3). (**a**) Preprocedural reconstruction; (**b**) Intraprocedural aspect of implantation. Second row: TAVI-in-SAVR (CE Perimount no. 21). (**c**) Preprocedural reconstruction; (**d**) Intraprocedural aspect of implantation. Third and fourth row: TAVI-in-SAVR (Epic Supra no. 21). (**e**) Preprocedural reconstruction; (**f**) Intraprocedural aspect of implantation. (**g**) Valve aspect before surgical bioprosthetic valve fracture; (**h**) Balloon fracture

agents prior to intervention is advised, as patients with elevated pulmonary capillary wedge pressure following TAVI have a higher risk of cardiovascular death and hospitalization for HF [113]. While the administration of loop diuretic agents before TAVI has been linked to a trend towards higher mortality rates, it is also considered an indicator of high-risk frail patients with advanced LV remodelling [114]. Approximately half of the patients on chronic beta-blockers undergo

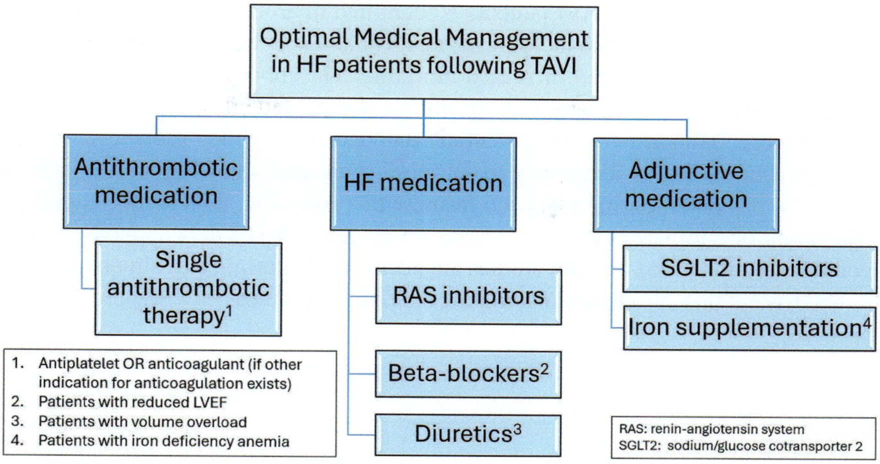

Fig. 17.8 Recommended lines of treatment in patients with AS and HF after TAVI

discontinuation at the time of TAVI due to concerns regarding arrhythmic risk [115]. While pre-procedural beta-blocker administration was not associated with 2-year cardiovascular mortality in the overall TAVI population, it was associated with lower mortality in patients with impaired LVEF, peripheral arterial disease, and prior myocardial revascularization [112]. Whether beta-blockers confer long-term benefits post-TAVI remains to be determined.

Blood Disorders in TAVI Candidates—Anaemia and Thrombocytopenia Management

In patients undergoing TAVI, managing blood disorders such as anaemia and thrombocytopenia is crucial due to their significant impact on outcomes [116].

Anaemia, observed in approximately 45–64% of TAVI candidates prior to the procedure, is commonly related to older age and its associated comorbidities, such as chronic kidney disease and inflammatory conditions, nutritional deficiencies, myelodysplastic syndromes, related to AS such as Heyde syndrome or related to HF (multifactorial) [116]. Anaemia significantly impacts TAVI patient outcomes, increasing the likelihood of requiring blood transfusions due to lower baseline haemoglobin, which can lead to acute kidney injury and higher mortality. Recognizing baseline anaemia is crucial for assessing procedural risks and addressing it pre-operatively is essential. Treatment often involves correcting reversible conditions like iron deficiency. Despite known links between anaemia and poor outcomes, it remains under-treated. Strategies like using erythropoietin and iron supplements are recommended to minimize transfusions and enhance outcomes, though further research is needed to optimize anaemia management in TAVI patients.

Thrombocytopenia in TAVI patients is identified in around 40% of patients pre-procedurally [116]. This rate increases post-TAVI and is linked to clinical complications including bleeding and increased mortality. Thrombocytopenia post-TAVI is primarily due to platelet consumption during the procedure, exacerbated by the inflammatory responses and potential damage from the prosthetic valve. Management strategies focus on careful monitoring and adjusting antithrombotic therapy to balance bleeding risks and thrombotic protection, with some suggesting adjustment of antiplatelet therapy despite no evidence-based data supporting such recommendation [116]. Further studies are necessary to optimize treatment and better understand this complication's impact on TAVI outcomes.

Fast-Track Pathways

Due to the exponential increase in the use of TAVI in the treatment of severe symptomatic AS regardless of the risk profile, there is a need for streamlined patient pathways to improve patient management, both inside and outside the hospital, without compromising patient safety. Several studies have identified specific factors associated with the potential for early and safe discharge after TAVI by examining specific patient characteristics (frailty, favourable anatomy, and left ventricle systolic dysfunction) [117], minimalist procedures (conscious sedation and vascular access) [118], the absence of post-procedural complications (conduction abnormalities, acute kidney injury, and anemia) [119], and the possibility of early mobilization [120]. The multicenter *Vancouver 3M (multidisciplinary, multimodality, but minimalist)* TAVI study in North America, followed by *the Feasibility and Safety of Early Discharge After Transfemoral TAVI (FAST-TAVI)* registry in Europe, demonstrated the feasibility and safety of the clinical pathway of same-day admission, minimalist procedure, and next-day discharge home [121–123].

The latest study on the matter, the BENCHMARK study, evaluated the effect of implementing eight best practices and the use of a TAVI coordinator on efficiency and safety. The study included patients in 28 sites in 7 European countries, including our centre, Emergency Institute for Cardiovascular Diseases "Prof. Dr. C.C. Iliescu", Bucharest, Romania, which occupied 3rd place based on the number of patients included [124]. The BENCHMARK best practices implemented included tailored education of patients and families, determination of an anticipated discharge date at admission based on pre-procedural risk stratification, echocardiographic or angiographic check at the end of the procedure to confirm vascular access closure, nurse-led early mobilization, use of a decision tree to determine the need for new pacemakers, criteria-based discharge, daily visits by implanting physicians, and education and alignment of the internal team (medical, nursing, and paramedical) [124]. The broad implementation of these practices improved the efficiency of the TAVI pathway and reduced the length of hospitalization and costs without compromising patient safety [125].

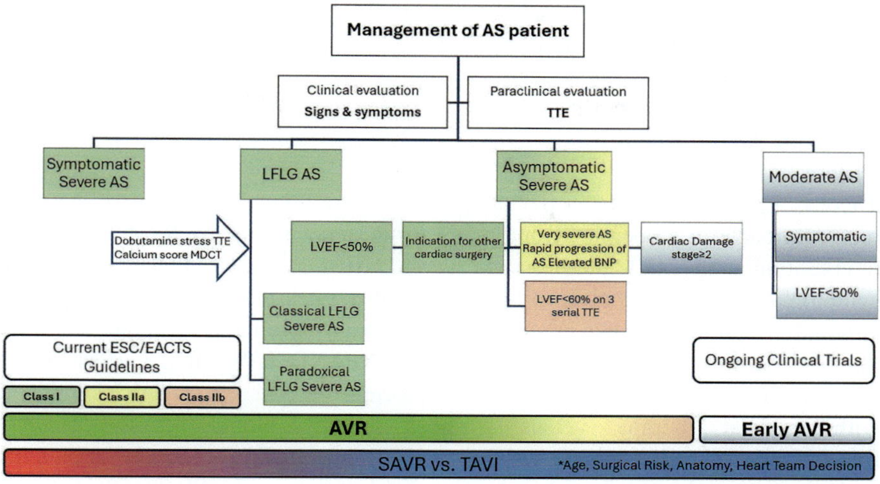

Fig. 17.9 Current and future indications of treatment of AS. Legend: *ESC* European Society of Cardiology, *EACTS* European Society of Cardio-Thoracic Surgery, *LFLG* low flow low gradient

Future Directions and Innovations in TAVI

Expanding Indications

Advancements in imaging, new transcatheter valve designs, and increased operator experience have enhanced the safety and performance of TAVI. Published trials have already shown TAVI's safety and efficacy benefits in low-risk severe aortic stenosis patients, leading to quicker discharges, fewer rehospitalizations and promising mid-term results [27, 28]. Current research extends TAVI applications to various patient groups, including those with asymptomatic or moderate aortic stenosis and isolated aortic regurgitation (Fig. 17.9).

Asymptomatic AS

Current guidelines recommend aortic valve replacement as a possible option for asymptomatic patients under specific conditions (very severe AS, left ventricular systolic dysfunction, or markedly elevated BNP on repeat measures; class IIa, level B) [7]. Recent studies, including the AVATAR and RECOVERY trials, have challenged the conventional approach by demonstrating the benefits of early surgery compared to conservative treatment. The AVATAR trial showed significantly lower rates of adverse events with early SAVR in asymptomatic patients with severe AS, whereas the RECOVERY trial indicated reduced mortality with early intervention over conservative management [126, 127]. The ongoing EARLY TAVR trial

[NCT03042104] aims to evaluate the benefits of TAVI in asymptomatic patients, potentially reshaping treatment paradigms.

Moderate AS

There is a growing interest in deviating from the traditional conservative management approach for moderate symptomatic aortic stenosis (AS) by considering early intervention with TAVI. Studies such as VALVENOR suggest that patients with symptomatic moderate AS have higher mortality rates than those with mild AS, although the mortality rates are similar between asymptomatic moderate and mild AS [128]. Several ongoing trials, including EXPAND TAVR II [NCT05149755] and PROGRESS [NCT04889872], are exploring the efficacy of TAVI combined with medical therapy versus medical therapy alone. TAVR-UNLOAD [NCT02661451] will compare TAVI to optimal heart failure treatment in patients with moderate AS and left ventricular systolic dysfunction (LVEF 20–50%). These studies aim to evaluate whether earlier interventions could improve outcomes, such as functional performance, and reduce risks, such as sudden cardiac death and cardiac remodelling. However, potential benefits must be weighed against procedural and long-term complications [129]. Currently, guidelines do not recommend intervention for moderate AS, reflecting the limited data supporting this approach [7].

Aortic Regurgitation

TAVI is generally not indicated for AR because of the primary indications for surgery and technical anatomical challenges (absence of annular calcification, large and elliptic annulus, concomitant aortopathy), which increase the risk of valve malposition/embolization (lack of valve anchoring) and aortic root injury (oversizing) [44, 45]. Despite this, almost 40% of off-label TAVI cases between 2011 and 2014 targeted AR, driven by the substantial clinical need among patients considered ineligible for SAVR owing to frailty or a high operative risk [45]. Innovations such as Jena Valve's Trilogy Valve and JC Medical's J-Valve are addressing these challenges [45]. These devices feature unique mechanisms to ensure stability and alignment and show promising early outcomes in specialized trials and ongoing studies [44].

Technological Refinements

The main concern of existing THV is the biological tissue used, which is prone to structural valve degeneration, with an impact on long-term durability. SVD is an evolutive physiopathologic process associated with morphological valve changes due to leaflet deterioration that ultimately leads to hemodynamic alteration (stenosis, regurgitation, or both). SVD is related to prosthesis characteristics (stent design, leaflet tissue, and patient-prosthesis mismatch) as well as to patient characteristics (young age, renal failure, subclinical valve thrombosis, dysregulation of calcium metabolism, or anticoagulation cascade) [130]. To address the issue of bioprosthesis durability, especially in younger and lower-risk patients with longer life expectancy, newer bioprosthesis are being developed and tested, focusing on innovations in leaflet materials and designs to improve durability profiles.

Resilia Tissue

After acknowledging the impact of SVD on hemodynamic performance in several registries, Edwards Lifesciences (Irvine, CA, USA) developed the Resilia tissue technology with the attempt to solve the issue of calcification of the bovine pericardium in SVD [98]. Tissue calcification is influenced by various factors, among which the exposure of tissue to free aldehydes during glutaraldehyde fixation and storage stands out [131]. This technology aims to reduce calcification by implementing a stable and irreversible capping technology to eliminate free glutaraldehyde residuals and prevent calcium binding, followed by tissue glycerolization to decrease water content, thus enabling dry, glutaraldehyde-free storage [132].

Resilia tissue was initially used for Edwards' surgical valves, including aortic valve, mitral valve and aortic root conduit. The safety and hemodynamic performance of the Inspiris Edwards Lifesciences (Irvine, CA, USA) with Resilia tissue at 5 years have been shown in the COMMENCE trial, with good hemodynamic performance, no significant regurgitation or SVD [133].

The Resilia tissue has recently been used into latest generation of Edwards` THV. The Sapien 3 Ultra Resilia valve was made available in the US in limited series since late 2022 and only recently in Europe. The clinical performance of Sapien 3 Ultra Resilia compared with Sapien 3 was evaluated in a real-world propensity-matched analysis of data from the TVT Registry [38]. TAVI with the Sapien 3 Ultra Resilia valve was associated with improved hemodynamic parameters in comparison with previous generation Sapien valves, without differences in procedural outcomes, complications, or in 30-day clinical outcomes [38]. The incorporation of the Resilia tissue in the next-generation Sapien X4 THV, which also brings a novel frame and leaflet design for optimal deployment and enhanced outer skirt, may lead to a more durable THV option, potentially tipping the scales in its favor [NCT05172960].

DurAVR

The DurAVR THV System (Anteris Technologies) is a novel BEV specifically designed to address the issues of hemodynamic performance, durability, and possibility for reintervention. In contrast to the existing THV, the novel feature of this valve technology is its unique three-dimensional single-piece leaflet design, built to mimic the native AV anatomy. According to computational fluid modelling, the single-piece leaflet design exhibits a larger coaptation area with improved coaptation height, resulting in a more uniform distribution of leaflet stress, optimal laminar flow, and reduced leaflet strain [134]. The leaflet design also allows for a shorter stent height with a large open-cell geometry, while maintaining a large EOA. In addition, the temporal risk of leaflet calcification and SVD is further mitigated by advancements in leaflet tissue formulation using DNA and glutaraldehyde-free acellular bovine pericardial leaflet tissue that is processed with ADAPT tissue-engineered anticalcification technology [135]. In the initial human study, which was a prospective, nonrandomized, single-arm, single-centre investigation to assess the safety and practicality of DurAVR THV, 13 patients were included [39]. This study found that procedural success was achieved in all patients, with no reported mortality, disabling stroke, or life-threatening bleeding. Additionally, the first five patients who completed follow-up showed excellent native-like 30-day hemodynamic performance. The DurAVR US early feasibility study, which aimed to evaluate the short- and long-term (10-year) safety and feasibility of the DurAVR device, is ongoing [NCT05712161]. The use of DurAVR THV leaflet technology has the potential to significantly impact hemodynamic performance and THV durability, making it a promising candidate for next-generation THV, as TAVI continues to expand and treat younger, lower-risk patients at earlier stages of the disease process.

Foldax TRIA Heart Valve

To address the challenges of SVD with bioprosthetic valves, various synthetic materials have been evaluated as potential candidates for valve leaflet materials. These materials are biocompatible and biostable, can be designed to ensure physiological function and endure high biomechanical strength. Biomedical-grade siloxane-based polyurethane-urea (TRIA LifePolymer) has recently been developed and has undergone extensive in vitro and in vivo testing as a polymer-based valve leaflet material [136]. The TRIA LifePolymer heart valve consists of three flexible polymer leaflets set onto a radiopaque polyether-ether ketone stent with a polytetrafluoroethylene-felt sewing ring. Valve manufacturing relies on automated robotic processes to ensure precise leaflet thickness [136]. Moreover, the valve allows dry storage and does not require preparation prior to implantation. Preliminary clinical results in 15 patients undergoing SAVR have demonstrated promising results [137]. A large-scale clinical trial evaluating the TRIA LifePolymer heart valve is currently underway [NCT03851068]. Further research and development are required to transform this type of technology into a feasible valve for TAVI.

Advancements in Patient Care Strategies—Controversies

One Day Procedure?

Since the COVID-19 pandemic began worldwide in early 2020, healthcare systems have faced challenges in optimizing limited space and personnel resources during hospitalization in compliance with clinical triage recommendations. One study confirmed the safety of same-day discharge (SDD) for carefully selected "minimalist" outpatient TF-TAVI recipients, showing post-discharge safety comparable to that of patients discharged on the day after TAVI [138]. SDD may be suitable for patients without procedural complications or post-TAVI conduction issues. Historically, SDD following TAVI was uncommon before the COVID-19 pandemic, with readmission rates similar to those discharged later (next day or second day discharge). Moreover, SDD TAVI showed significantly lower hospitalization costs compared to non-SDD approaches [139].

Although these studies provide preliminary safety data on SDD in a small cohort of carefully selected patients post-TAVI, larger prospective studies are necessary to further evaluate the safety and feasibility of SDD-TAVI and to establish criteria for identifying suitable candidates. However, it is important to note that the logistical and clinical considerations for TAVI are considerably complex and involve intricate pre-procedural planning, including detailed cardiovascular imaging and assessments to ensure optimum management. While SDD following TAVI is achievable and can be safe for selected patients, it requires a robust framework of patient selection criteria and procedural planning that distinguishes it from the less complex preparations typical of other 1-day procedures (i.e., percutaneous angioplasty).

Lifetime Management

TAVI represents a pivotal shift in managing severe aortic stenosis (AS), particularly for younger, low-risk patients. Traditionally reserved for older, higher-risk populations due to concerns about durability and complications related to repeated interventions, recent expansions in TAVI use necessitate a comprehensive lifetime management approach for these younger patients [140].

In the lifetime management of young, low-risk patients with severe AS multiple scenarios are possible [141]:

1. TAVI-SAVR-TAVI—in this theoretical scenario patients would undergo only one surgical intervention, but later in life. This implies a minimally invasive procedure with presumably low risk at young age, but limited experience with TAVI explantation and need for concomitant aortic root repair with additional risk when first valve degeneration occurs. However, TAV-in-SAV is a feasible procedure, provided that a third valve is required for surgical bioprosthesis degeneration.

2. TAVI-TAVI-TAVI—in this theoretical scenario patients would undergo only transcatheter interventions, however the number of repeat procedures is limited by aortic root anatomy and the choice of device. This approach implies a series of limitations such as risk patient-prosthesis mismatch, paravalvular regurgitation, pacemaker implantation, restricted coronary access, valve thrombosis and uncertainty in long-term durability.
3. SAVR-SAVR-TAVI or SAVR-TAVI-TAVI—most common scenario found in real-life. This promotes surgery at young age, with consideration for aortic root enlargement (Nicks, Manougian, Konno, Yang) to accommodate larger and ViV-friendly surgical bioprosthesis (Carpentier-Edwards Perimount, Inspiris Resilia Edwards Lifesciences) [141].

Main concerns in interpretation of each scenario are defined by durability and valve performance, repeated interventions and valve-in-valve procedures, coronary re-access (Fig. 17.10) and risk of coronary obstruction with repeated procedures, impact of concomitant or occurring disease, and last, but not least, patient preferences and quality of life [142]. Lifetime management should integrate patient-specific factors and robust evidence from trials and registries, to optimize treatment timing and technique for extended functional valve lifespan and improved quality of life.

Role of Artificial Intelligence

The integration of artificial intelligence in the field of cardiology offers a series of advantages, enabled by advanced computational capabilities and efficient data processing, ultimately improving care and reducing costs in medicine [143]. Machine learning comprises techniques that allow high-power computers to analyse large datasets and enhance their performance over time without explicit programming. Deep learning, a specific type of machine-learning technique, focuses on training deep neural networks that process and transform data during learning. Consequently, artificial intelligence can assist in the interpretation of medical imaging such as echocardiography, cardiac CTs, and MRIs [144]. The application of artificial intelligence in TAVI procedures has been explored to improve patient selection (evidence-based risk stratification) [145], aid procedural planning (image analysis) [146], optimize patient outcomes (prediction of specific complications) [147], and assist with post-implantation valve monitoring (through-powered wearable devices and remote monitoring systems) [148]. Artificial intelligence can integrate large amounts of data (preoperative imaging, intraoperative parameters, and postoperative continuously tracked cardiac parameters), providing patient-specific and real-time insights that can result in improved patient care [143].

Artificial intelligence has been shown to detect severe aortic stenosis based on electrocardiograms (EKGs) [149]. Based on echocardiograms, machine learning can provide real-time, automated, and personalized timing for the next

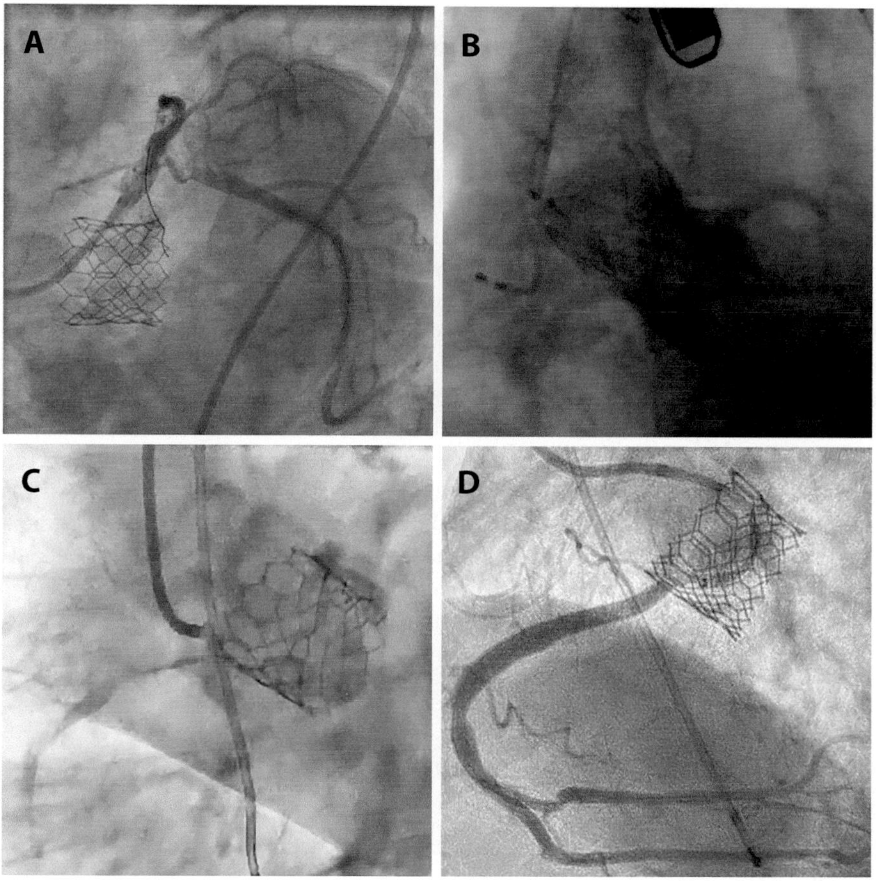

Fig. 17.10 Coronary re-access after TAVI. (**a**) Unstable angina 2-years after TAVI with severe stenosis of proximal circumflex artery (**b**) Coronary access after self-expandable valves; (**c**) Acute coronary obstruction of proximal right coronary artery on preexisting non-significant lesion; (**d**) Percutaneous angioplasty of proximal right coronary artery

echocardiographic follow-up examination in patients with mild-to-moderate aortic stenosis [150]. Another study described an automated assessment of echocardiographic studies that may minimize inter-scan variability, improve the interpretation and diagnosis of AS, and allow for precise and reproducible identification and management of AS patients [151].

Computed tomography (CT) calcium scoring of the aortic valve can be useful in cases with discordant echocardiographic results or low-flow, low-gradient severe aortic stenosis and is predictive of mortality [152]. Deep learning models that use CT scans to automatically segment and score aortic valve calcification have been developed, and some studies have aimed to derive aortic valve calcium scores [153].

Artificial intelligence can make significant contributions to patient selection for TAVI, especially in the context of a paradigm shift from risk assessment to age and durability considerations [154]. Hasimbegovic et al. developed a machine learning-based approach for predicting the decision for TAVI versus surgical aortic valve replacement (AUC 0.91 with 90% accuracy, 92% sensitivity and 90% specificity), demonstrating its usefulness in aiding complex clinical decision-making processes [155].

Recent studies have shown that artificial intelligence can assist in pre-procedural planning, screening for coronary artery disease on coronary CT angiography, non-invasive assessment of the hemodynamic significance of intermediate lesions [156], anatomical analysis for annular sizing, and valve selection [157] and could provide important insights required during the procedure [158]. Artificial intelligence has been shown to aid informed decision-making by assessing mortality risk by outperforming conventional risk scores [159] and predicting specific complications such as readmission due to heart failure [160], cerebrovascular events [161], leaflet thrombosis [162], conduction abnormalities [163], and bleeding events [164].

Despite promising results, artificial intelligence techniques come with inherent limitations such as poor selection of data, outdated data, selection bias, positive publication bias, accuracy, and interpretability of models [143]. Although artificial intelligence possesses great potential and could provide useful tools to enhance TAVI periprocedural management, the clinical judgment of the Heart Team is responsible for ensuring safe and responsible integration of information and providing the gold standard of care.

Conclusion: The Road Ahead for TAVI and Patient Management

Twenty years after the initial procedure, transcatheter aortic valve replacement (TAVI) has radically changed the management of aortic stenosis (AS) across the entire surgical risk range. As TAVI devices have been extended to include lower-risk patients, further efforts should focus on refining valve selection, ensuring device durability, and defining optimal for long-term management of AS.

References

1. Osnabrugge RL, Mylotte D, Head SJ, Van Mieghem NM, Nkomo VT, LeReun CM, et al. Aortic stenosis in the elderly: disease prevalence and number of candidates for transcatheter aortic valve replacement: a meta-analysis and modeling study. J Am Coll Cardiol. 2013;62(11):1002–12.
2. Badran AA, Vohra HA, Livesey SA. Unoperated severe aortic stenosis: decision making in an adult UK-based population. Ann R Coll Surg Engl. 2012;94(6):416–21.
3. Strange G, Stewart S, Celermajer D, Prior D, Scalia GM, Marwick T, et al. Poor long-term survival in patients with moderate aortic stenosis. J Am Coll Cardiol. 2019;74(15):1851–63.

4. McDonagh TA, Metra M, Adamo M, Gardner RS, Baumbach A, Böhm M, et al. 2021 ESC Guidelines for the diagnosis and treatment of acute and chronic heart failure: developed by the Task Force for the diagnosis and treatment of acute and chronic heart failure of the European Society of Cardiology (ESC) With the special contribution of the Heart Failure Association (HFA) of the ESC. Eur Heart J. 2021;42(36):3599–726.
5. Himbert D, Vahanian A. Transcatheter aortic valve replacement for patients with heart failure. Heart Fail Clin. 2015;11(2):231–42.
6. Genereux P, Pibarot P, Redfors B, Mack MJ, Makkar RR, Jaber WA, et al. Staging classification of aortic stenosis based on the extent of cardiac damage. Eur Heart J. 2017;38(45):3351–8.
7. Vahanian A, Beyersdorf F, Praz F, Milojevic M, Baldus S, Bauersachs J, et al. 2021 ESC/EACTS Guidelines for the management of valvular heart disease. Eur Heart J. 2022;43(7):561–632.
8. Hartley A, Hammond-Haley M, Marshall DC, Salciccioli JD, Malik IS, Khamis RY, et al. Trends in mortality from aortic stenosis in Europe: 2000-2017. Front Cardiovasc Med. 2021;8:748137.
9. Genereux P, Pibarot P, Redfors B, Bax JJ, Zhao Y, Makkar RR, et al. Evolution and prognostic impact of cardiac damage after aortic valve replacement. J Am Coll Cardiol. 2022;80(8):783–800.
10. Durand E, Doutriaux M, Bettinger N, Tron C, Fauvel C, Bauer F, et al. Incidence, prognostic impact, and predictive factors of readmission for heart failure after transcatheter aortic valve replacement. JACC Cardiovasc Interv. 2017;10(23):2426–36.
11. Furer A, Chen S, Redfors B, Elmariah S, Pibarot P, Herrmann HC, et al. Effect of baseline left ventricular ejection fraction on 2-year outcomes after transcatheter aortic valve replacement: analysis of the PARTNER 2 trials. Circ Heart Fail. 2019;12(8):e005809.
12. Ribeiro HB, Lerakis S, Gilard M, Cavalcante JL, Makkar R, Herrmann HC, et al. Transcatheter aortic valve replacement in patients with low-flow, low-gradient aortic stenosis: the TOPAS-TAVI registry. J Am Coll Cardiol. 2018;71(12):1297–308.
13. Ludwig S, Gossling A, Seiffert M, Westermann D, Sinning JM, Sugiura A, et al. Risk prediction in patients with low-flow, low-gradient aortic stenosis and reduced ejection fraction undergoing TAVI. Open Heart. 2022;9(1):e001912.
14. Carabello BA. Where do low-gradient, low-ef as patients come from?: maybe they're born that way. J Am Coll Cardiol. 2018;71(12):1322–4.
15. Barbash IM, Minha S, Ben-Dor I, Dvir D, Magalhaes MA, Torguson R, et al. Relation of preprocedural assessment of myocardial contractility reserve on outcomes of aortic stenosis patients with impaired left ventricular function undergoing transcatheter aortic valve implantation. Am J Cardiol. 2014;113(9):1536–42.
16. Bavishi C, Trivedi V, Sellke FW, Gordon PC, Abbott JD. Myocardial contractile reserve and mortality in patients with severe aortic stenosis with impaired left ventricular function who underwent transcatheter aortic valve implantation. Am J Cardiol. 2021;141:150–2.
17. Buchanan KD, Rogers T, Steinvil A, Koifman E, Xu L, Torguson R, et al. Role of contractile reserve as a predictor of mortality in low-flow, low-gradient severe aortic stenosis following transcatheter aortic valve replacement. Catheter Cardiovasc Interv. 2019;93(4):707–12.
18. Kamperidis V, Delgado V, van Mieghem NM, Kappetein AP, Leon MB, Bax JJ. Diagnosis and management of aortic valve stenosis in patients with heart failure. Eur J Heart Fail. 2016;18(5):469–81.
19. Paradis JM, Fried J, Nazif T, Kirtane A, Harjai K, Khalique O, et al. Aortic stenosis and coronary artery disease: what do we know? What don't we know? A comprehensive review of the literature with proposed treatment algorithms. Eur Heart J. 2014;35(31):2069–82.
20. de Azevedo Filho AF, Accorsi TA, Ribeiro HB. Coronary artery disease in patients with aortic stenosis and transcatheter aortic valve implantation: implications for management. Eur Cardiol. 2021;16:e49.

21. Van Mieghem NM, van der Boon RM, Faqiri E, Diletti R, Schultz C, van Geuns RJ, et al. Complete revascularization is not a prerequisite for success in current transcatheter aortic valve implantation practice. JACC Cardiovasc Interv. 2013;6(8):867–75.
22. Barone-Rochette G, Pierard S, Meester D, de Ravenstein C, Seldrum S, Melchior J, Maes F, et al. Prognostic significance of LGE by CMR in aortic stenosis patients undergoing valve replacement. J Am Coll Cardiol. 2014;64(2):144–54.
23. Scully PR, Patel KP, Klotz E, Augusto JB, Thornton GD, Saberwal B, et al. Myocardial fibrosis quantified by cardiac CT predicts outcome in severe aortic stenosis after transcatheter intervention. JACC Cardiovasc Imaging. 2022;15(3):542–4.
24. Cribier A, Saoudi N, Berland J, Savin T, Rocha P, Letac B. Percutaneous transluminal valvuloplasty of acquired aortic stenosis in elderly patients: an alternative to valve replacement? Lancet. 1986;327(8472):63–7.
25. Cribier A, Eltchaninoff H, Bash A, Borenstein N, Tron C, Bauer F, et al. Percutaneous transcatheter implantation of an aortic valve prosthesis for calcific aortic stenosis: first human case description. Circulation. 2002;106(24):3006–8.
26. Nguyen V, Willner N, Eltchaninoff H, Burwash IG, Michel M, Durand E, et al. Trends in aortic valve replacement for aortic stenosis: a French nationwide study. Eur Heart J. 2022;43(7):666–79.
27. Mack MJ, Leon MB, Thourani VH, Pibarot P, Hahn RT, Genereux P, et al. Transcatheter aortic-valve replacement in low-risk patients at five years. N Engl J Med. 2023;389(21):1949–60.
28. Forrest JK, Deeb GM, Yakubov SJ, Gada H, Mumtaz MA, Ramlawi B, et al. 3-year outcomes after transcatheter or surgical aortic valve replacement in low-risk patients with aortic stenosis. J Am Coll Cardiol. 2023;81(17):1663–74.
29. Pibarot P. Transcatheter vs surgical aortic valve replacement in low-risk patients: so far (3 years), so good. J Am Coll Cardiol. 2023;81(17):1675–9.
30. Kapadia SR, Leon MB, Makkar RR, Tuzcu EM, Svensson LG, Kodali S, et al. 5-year outcomes of transcatheter aortic valve replacement compared with standard treatment for patients with inoperable aortic stenosis (PARTNER 1): a randomised controlled trial. Lancet. 2015;385(9986):2485–91.
31. Gleason TG, Reardon MJ, Popma JJ, Deeb GM, Yakubov SJ, Lee JS, et al. 5-year outcomes of self-expanding transcatheter versus surgical aortic valve replacement in high-risk patients. J Am Coll Cardiol. 2018;72(22):2687–96.
32. Van Mieghem NM, Deeb GM, Sondergaard L, Grube E, Windecker S, Gada H, et al. Self-expanding transcatheter vs surgical aortic valve replacement in intermediate-risk patients: 5-year outcomes of the SURTAVI randomized clinical trial. JAMA Cardiol. 2022;7(10):1000–8.
33. Otto CM, Nishimura RA, Bonow RO, Carabello BA, Erwin JP 3rd, Gentile F, et al. 2020 ACC/AHA Guideline for the management of patients with valvular heart disease: executive summary: a report of the American College of Cardiology/American Heart Association Joint Committee on Clinical Practice Guidelines. Circulation. 2021;143(5):e35–71.
34. Makkar RR, Thourani VH, Mack MJ, Kodali SK, Kapadia S, Webb JG, et al. Five-year outcomes of transcatheter or surgical aortic-valve replacement. N Engl J Med. 2020;382(9):799–809.
35. Carroll JD, Mack MJ, Vemulapalli S, Herrmann HC, Gleason TG, Hanzel G, et al. STS-ACC TVT registry of transcatheter aortic valve replacement. Ann Thorac Surg. 2021;111(2):701–22.
36. Rheude T, Pellegrini C, Allali A, Bleiziffer S, Kim WK, Neuser J, et al. Multicenter comparison of latest-generation balloon-expandable versus self-expanding transcatheter heart valves: Ultra versus Evolut. Int J Cardiol. 2022;357:115–20.
37. Eltchaninoff H, Gilard M, Cribier A. TAVI at 20: how a crazy idea led to a clinical revolution. EuroIntervention. 2022;18(1):15–8.
38. Stinis CT, Abbas AE, Teirstein P, Makkar RR, Chung CJ, Iyer V, et al. Real-world outcomes for the fifth-generation balloon expandable transcatheter heart valve in the United States. JACC Cardiovasc Interv. 2024;17(8):1032–44.

39. Meduri C, Bapat V, Kodali S, Sorajja P, Hamid N, Poon K, et al. TCT-471 first-in-human study results with the novel anteris DurAVRTM three-dimensional single-piece TAVR device. J Am Coll Cardiol. 2022;80(12, Suppl):B190.
40. Khera S, Krishnamoorthy P, Sharma SK, Kini AS, Dangas GD, Goel S, et al. Improved commissural alignment in TAVR with the newest evolut FX self-expanding supra-annular valve: first-in-human experience. JACC Cardiovasc Interv. 2023;16(4):498–500.
41. Gooley R, Murdoch D, Ng MK, Modolo R, Allocco DJ. First results from the ACURATE Prime XL human feasibility study. Cardiovasc Revasc Med. 2023;57:1–5.
42. Bajoras V, Nuyens P, Vanhaverbeke M, Wang X, Bieliauskas G, De Backer O, et al. TAVR with the novel navitor titan™ transcatheter heart valve to treat aortic stenosis patients with large aortic annuli. Cardiovasc Revasc Med. 2022;40:120–2.
43. Seigerman ME, Nathan A, Anwaruddin S. The lotus valve system: an in-depth review of the technology. Curr Cardiol Rep. 2019;21(12):157.
44. Yoon SH, Schmidt T, Bleiziffer S, Schofer N, Fiorina C, Munoz-Garcia AJ, et al. Transcatheter aortic valve replacement in pure native aortic valve regurgitation. J Am Coll Cardiol. 2017;70(22):2752–63.
45. Costanzo P, Bamborough P, Peterson M, Deva DJ, Ong G, Fam N. Transcatheter aortic valve implantation for severe pure aortic regurgitation with dedicated devices. Interv Cardiol. 2022;17:e11.
46. Kempfert J, Rastan AJ, Mohr FW, Walther T. A new self-expanding transcatheter aortic valve for transapical implantation—first in man implantation of the JenaValve. Eur J Cardiothorac Surg. 2011;40(3):761–3.
47. Nijenhuis VJ, Swaans MJ, Michiels V, de Kroon T, Heijmen RH, Ten Berg JM. First experience with JenaValve: a single-centre cohort. Neth Hear J. 2015;23(1):35–41.
48. Schafer U, Schirmer J, Niklas S, Harmel E, Deuschl F, Conradi L. First-in-human implantation of a novel transfemoral selfexpanding transcatheter heart valve to treat pure aortic regurgitation. EuroIntervention. 2017;13(11):1296–9.
49. Vahl T, Makkar R, Kodali S, Baldus S, Treede H, Daniels D, et al. 30-day outcomes of transfemoral transcatheter aortic valve replacement for aortic regurgitation with a novel self-expanding prosthesis. J Am Coll Cardiol. 2021;77(18, Suppl 1):919.
50. Otto CM, Nishimura RA, Bonow RO, Carabello BA, Erwin JP, Gentile F, et al. 2020 ACC/AHA Guideline for the management of patients with valvular heart disease: a report of the American College of Cardiology/American Heart Association Joint Committee on Clinical Practice Guidelines. Circulation. 2021;143(5):e35–71.
51. Mack MJ, Leon MB, Thourani VH, Makkar R, Kodali SK, Russo M, et al. Transcatheter aortic-valve replacement with a balloon-expandable valve in low-risk patients. N Engl J Med. 2019;380(18):1695–705.
52. Popma JJ, Deeb GM, Yakubov SJ, Mumtaz M, Gada H, O'Hair D, et al. Transcatheter aortic-valve replacement with a self-expanding valve in low-risk patients. N Engl J Med. 2019;380(18):1706–15.
53. Francone M, Budde RPJ, Bremerich J, Dacher JN, Loewe C, Wolf F, et al. CT and MR imaging prior to transcatheter aortic valve implantation: standardisation of scanning protocols, measurements and reporting-a consensus document by the European Society of Cardiovascular Radiology (ESCR). Eur Radiol. 2020;30(5):2627–50.
54. Archbold A, Akowuah E, Banning AP, Baumbach A, Braidley P, Cooper G, et al. Getting the best from the heart team: guidance for cardiac multidisciplinary meetings. Heart. 2022;108(11):e2.
55. Vahanian A, Beyersdorf F, Praz F, Milojevic M, Baldus S, Bauersachs J, et al. 2021 ESC/EACTS Guidelines for the management of valvular heart disease. EuroIntervention. 2022;17(14):e1126–e96.
56. Bhogal S, Rogers T, Aladin A, Ben-Dor I, Cohen JE, Shults CC, et al. TAVR in 2023: who should not get it? Am J Cardiol. 2023;193:1–18.

57. Joint Task Force on the Management of Valvular Heart Disease of the European Society of C, European Association for Cardio-Thoracic S, Vahanian A, Alfieri O, Andreotti F, Antunes MJ, et al. Guidelines on the management of valvular heart disease (version 2012). Eur Heart J. 2012;33(19):2451–96.
58. Patel KP, Treibel TA, Scully PR, Fertleman M, Searle S, Davis D, et al. Futility in transcatheter aortic valve implantation: a search for clarity. Interv Cardiol. 2022;17:e01.
59. Santos-Martínez S, Alkhodair A, Nombela-Franco L, Saia F, Muñoz-García AJ, Gutiérrez E, et al. Transcatheter aortic valve replacement for residual lesion of the aortic valve following "healed" infective endocarditis. J Am Coll Cardiol Intv. 2020;13(17):1983–96.
60. Montalto C, Sticchi A, Crimi G, Laricchia A, Khokhar AA, Giannini F, et al. Outcomes after transcatheter aortic valve replacement in bicuspid versus tricuspid anatomy: a systematic review and meta-analysis. JACC Cardiovasc Interv. 2021;14(19):2144–55.
61. Tarantini G, Fabris T. Transcatheter aortic valve replacement for bicuspid aortic valve stenosis: a practical operative overview. Circ Cardiovasc Interv. 2021;14(7):e009827.
62. Leone PP, Regazzoli D, Pagnesi M, Sanz-Sanchez J, Chiarito M, Cannata F, et al. Predictors and clinical impact of prosthesis-patient mismatch after self-expandable TAVR in small annuli. JACC Cardiovasc Interv. 2021;14(11):1218–28.
63. Scotti A, Sturla M, Costa G, Saia F, Pilgrim T, Abdel-Wahab M, et al. Evolut PRO and SAPIEN ULTRA performance in small aortic annuli: the OPERA-TAVI registry. J Am Coll Cardiol Intv. 2024;17(5):681–92.
64. Sengupta A, Zaid S, Kamioka N, Terre J, Miyasaka M, Hirji SA, et al. Mid-term outcomes of transcatheter aortic valve replacement in extremely large annuli with edwards SAPIEN 3 valve. J Am Coll Cardiol Intv. 2020;13(2):210–6.
65. Lederman RJ, Babaliaros VC, Rogers T, Khan JM, Kamioka N, Dvir D, et al. Preventing coronary obstruction during transcatheter aortic valve replacement: from computed tomography to BASILICA. JACC Cardiovasc Interv. 2019;12(13):1197–216.
66. Walther T, Hamm CW, Schuler G, Berkowitsch A, Kotting J, Mangner N, et al. Perioperative results and complications in 15,964 transcatheter aortic valve replacements: prospective data from the GARY registry. J Am Coll Cardiol. 2015;65(20):2173–80.
67. Sawaya FJ, Bajoras V, Vanhaverbeke M, Wang C, Bieliauskas G, Sondergaard L, et al. Intravascular lithotripsy-assisted transfemoral TAVI: the Copenhagen experience and literature review. Front Cardiovasc Med. 2021;8:739750.
68. Kalogeropoulos AS, Redwood SR, Allen CJ, Hurrell H, Chehab O, Rajani R, et al. A 20-year journey in transcatheter aortic valve implantation: evolution to current eminence. Front Cardiovasc Med. 2022;9:971762.
69. Khan AA, Murtaza G, Khalid MF, Khattak F. Risk stratification for transcatheter aortic valve replacement. Cardiol Res. 2019;10(6):323–30.
70. Codner P, Malick W, Kouz R, Patel A, Chen CH, Terre J, et al. Mortality risk after transcatheter aortic valve implantation: analysis of the predictive accuracy of the transcatheter valve therapy registry risk assessment model. EuroIntervention. 2018;14(4):e405–e12.
71. Kjonas D, Dahle G, Schirmer H, Malm S, Eidet J, Aaberge L, et al. Risk scores for prediction of 30-day mortality after transcatheter aortic valve implantation: results from a two-center study in Norway. Health Sci Rep. 2021;4(2):e283.
72. Al-Farra H, de Mol B, Ravelli ACJ, Ter Burg W, Houterman S, Henriques JPS, et al. Update and, internal and temporal-validation of the FRANCE-2 and ACC-TAVI early-mortality prediction models for Transcatheter Aortic Valve Implantation (TAVI) using data from the Netherlands heart registration (NHR). Int J Cardiol Heart Vasc. 2021;32:100716.
73. Al-Azizi K, Shih E, DiMaio JM, Squiers JJ, Moubarak G, Kluis A, et al. Assessment of TVT and STS risk score performances in patients undergoing transcatheter aortic valve replacement. J Soc Cardiovasc Angiogr Interv. 2023;2(3):100600.
74. Corcione N, Morello A, Ferraro P, Cimmino M, Albanese M, Pepe M, et al. TAVI-CT score to evaluate the anatomic risk in patients undergoing transcatheter aortic valve implantation. Sci Rep. 2022;12(1):7612.

75. Kiani S, Stebbins A, Thourani VH, Forcillo J, Vemulapalli S, Kosinski AS, et al. The effect and relationship of frailty indices on survival after transcatheter aortic valve replacement. J Am Coll Cardiol Intv. 2020;13(2):219–31.
76. El-Sabawi B, Cloud H, Patel JN, Bell SP, Elmariah S, Fearon WF, et al. Association of depression and cognitive dysfunction with patient-centered outcomes after transcatheter aortic valve replacement. Circ Cardiovasc Interv. 2023;16(8):e012875.
77. Goel SS, Reardon MJ. Is it time to move beyond STS and TVT scores for predicting TAVR mortality? J Soc Cardiovasc Angiogr Interv. 2023;2(3):100633.
78. Alhwiti T, Aldrugh S, Megahed FM. Predicting in-hospital mortality after transcatheter aortic valve replacement using administrative data and machine learning. Sci Rep. 2023;13(1):10252.
79. Mylotte D, Piazza N. Patient selection for transcatheter or surgical intervention: the Heart Team TRUMPS the STS. EuroIntervention. 2016;12(12):1439–40.
80. Trivi M, Castro MF, Trossero R, Henquin R, Botto FO, Lamelas PO, et al. Results of a heart team assessment of aortic stenosis candidates for percutaneous valve replacement in an upper-middle-income country. Eur Heart J. 2023;44(Suppl_2):ehad655.022.
81. Claessen BE, Tang GHL, Kini AS, Sharma SK. Considerations for optimal device selection in transcatheter aortic valve replacement: a review. JAMA Cardiol. 2021;6(1):102–12.
82. Yoon SH, Kim WK, Dhoble A, Milhorini Pio S, Babaliaros V, Jilaihawi H, et al. Bicuspid aortic valve morphology and outcomes after transcatheter aortic valve replacement. J Am Coll Cardiol. 2020;76(9):1018–30.
83. Waksman R, Craig PE, Torguson R, Asch FM, Weissman G, Ruiz D, et al. Transcatheter aortic valve replacement in low-risk patients with symptomatic severe bicuspid aortic valve stenosis. JACC Cardiovasc Interv. 2020;13(9):1019–27.
84. Costa G, Angelillis M, Petronio AS. Bicuspid valve sizing for transcatheter aortic valve implantation: the missing link. Front Cardiovasc Med. 2021;8:770924.
85. Petronio AS, Angelillis M, De Backer O, Giannini C, Costa G, Fiorina C, et al. Bicuspid aortic valve sizing for transcatheter aortic valve implantation: development and validation of an algorithm based on multi-slice computed tomography. J Cardiovasc Comput Tomogr. 2020;14(5):452–61.
86. Dowling C, Firoozi S, Brecker SJ. First-in-human experience with patient-specific computer simulation of TAVR in bicuspid aortic valve morphology. J Am Coll Cardiol Intv. 2020;13(2):184–92.
87. Sá MP, Van den Eynde J, Jacquemyn X, Tasoudis P, Erten O, Dokollari A, et al. Late outcomes of transcatheter aortic valve implantation in bicuspid versus tricuspid valves: meta-analysis of reconstructed time-to-event data. Trends Cardiovasc Med. 2023;33(7):458–67.
88. Vincent F, Ternacle J, Denimal T, Shen M, Redfors B, Delhaye C, et al. Transcatheter aortic valve replacement in bicuspid aortic valve stenosis. Circulation. 2021;143(10):1043–61.
89. Forrest JK, Ramlawi B, Deeb GM, Zahr F, Song HK, Kleiman NS, et al. Transcatheter aortic valve replacement in low-risk patients with bicuspid aortic valve stenosis. JAMA Cardiol. 2021;6(1):50–7.
90. Saeed Al-Asad K, Martinez Salazar A, Radwan Y, Wang E, Salam MF, Sabanci R, et al. Transcatheter aortic valve replacement in bicuspid versus tricuspid aortic valve stenosis: meta-analysis and systemic review. Am J Cardiol. 2023;203:105–12.
91. He J, Xiong TY, Yao YJ, Peng Y, Wei JF, Zhao ZG, et al. Outcomes following transcatheter aortic valve replacement for aortic stenosis in patients with type 0 bicuspid, type 1 bicuspid, and tricuspid aortic valves. Circ Cardiovasc Interv. 2023;16(12):e013083.
92. Nuyens P, De Backer O, Sathananthan J, Højsgaard Jørgensen T, Treede H, Leipsic JA, et al. TAVR in bicuspid aortic stenosis: current evidence and proposal for a randomized controlled trial design. J Am Coll Cardiol Intv. 2023;16(13):1682–7.
93. Tarantini G, Tang G, Nai Fovino L, Blackman D, Van Mieghem NM, Kim WK, et al. Management of coronary artery disease in patients undergoing transcatheter aortic valve implantation. A clinical consensus statement from the European Association of Percutaneous

Cardiovascular Interventions in collaboration with the ESC Working Group on Cardiovascular Surgery. EuroIntervention. 2023;19(1):37–52.

94. Costa G, Pilgrim T, Amat Santos IJ, De Backer O, Kim WK, Barbosa Ribeiro H, et al. Management of myocardial revascularization in patients with stable coronary artery disease undergoing transcatheter aortic valve implantation. Circ Cardiovasc Interv. 2022;15(12):e012417.
95. Patterson T, Clayton T, Dodd M, Khawaja Z, Morice MC, Wilson K, et al. ACTIVATION (PercutAneous Coronary inTervention prIor to transcatheter aortic VAlve implantaTION): a randomized clinical trial. JACC Cardiovasc Interv. 2021;14(18):1965–74.
96. Malik AH, Yandrapalli S, Zaid S, Shetty SS, Aronow WS, Ahmad H, et al. Valve-in-valve transcatheter implantation versus redo surgical aortic valve replacement. Am J Cardiol. 2020;125(9):1378–84.
97. Nuche J, Abbas AE, Serra V, Vilalta V, Nombela-Franco L, Regueiro A, et al. Balloon- vs self-expanding transcatheter valves for failed small surgical aortic bioprostheses: 1-year results of the LYTEN trial. JACC Cardiovasc Interv. 2023;16(24):2999–3012.
98. Hahn RT, Webb J, Pibarot P, Ternacle J, Herrmann HC, Suri RM, et al. 5-year follow-up from the PARTNER 2 aortic valve-in-valve registry for degenerated aortic surgical bioprostheses. JACC Cardiovasc Interv. 2022;15(7):698–708.
99. Bleiziffer S, Simonato M, Webb JG, Rodés-Cabau J, Pibarot P, Kornowski R, et al. Long-term outcomes after transcatheter aortic valve implantation in failed bioprosthetic valves. Eur Heart J. 2020;41(29):2731–42.
100. Hayek A, Prieur C, Durrleman N, Chatelain Q, Ibrahim R, Asgar A, et al. Clinical considerations and challenges in TAV-in-TAV procedures. Front Cardiovasc Med. 2024;11:1334871.
101. Chhatriwalla AK, Allen KB, Saxon JT, Cohen DJ, Aggarwal S, Hart AJ, et al. Bioprosthetic valve fracture improves the hemodynamic results of valve-in-valve transcatheter aortic valve replacement. Circ Cardiovasc Interv. 2017;10(7):e005216.
102. Landes U, Webb JG, De Backer O, Sondergaard L, Abdel-Wahab M, Crusius L, et al. Repeat transcatheter aortic valve replacement for transcatheter prosthesis dysfunction. J Am Coll Cardiol. 2020;75(16):1882–93.
103. Duncan A, Moat N, Simonato M, Weger A, Kempfert J, Eggebrecht H, et al. Outcomes following transcatheter aortic valve replacement for degenerative stentless versus stented bioprostheses. J Am Coll Cardiol Intv. 2019;12(13):1256–63.
104. Tarantini G, Delgado V, de Backer O, Sathananthan J, Treede H, Saia F, et al. Redo-transcatheter aortic valve implantation using the SAPIEN 3/ultra transcatheter heart valves-expert consensus on procedural planning and techniques. Am J Cardiol. 2023;192:228–44.
105. Bapat V. Valve-in-valve apps: why and how they were developed and how to use them. EuroIntervention. 2014;10(Suppl U):U44–51.
106. Sun Y, Li J, Li G, Fan R, Luo J. Impact of renin-angiotensin system inhibitors on outcomes after transcatheter aortic valve replacement: a meta-analysis. Catheter Cardiovasc Interv. 2021;97(1):E88–94.
107. Ledwoch J, Olbrich I, Poch F, Thalmann R, Fellner C, Stundl A, et al. Dose-dependent effect of renin-angiotensin system blockade following transcatheter aortic valve replacement. Can J Cardiol. 2021;37(3):443–9.
108. Rodriguez-Gabella T, Catala P, Munoz-Garcia AJ, Nombela-Franco L, Del Valle R, Gutierrez E, et al. Renin-angiotensin system inhibition following transcatheter aortic valve replacement. J Am Coll Cardiol. 2019;74(5):631–41.
109. Inohara T, Manandhar P, Kosinski AS, Matsouaka RA, Kohsaka S, Mentz RJ, et al. Association of renin-angiotensin inhibitor treatment with mortality and heart failure readmission in patients with transcatheter aortic valve replacement. JAMA. 2018;320(21):2231–41.
110. Liao YB, Xia C, Cheng Y, Li Q, Wei X, Ou Y, et al. Angiotensin-converting enzyme inhibitor for post-transcatheter aortic valve implantation patients: study protocol for a multicenter randomized, open-label blinded endpoint control trial. Trials. 2021;22(1):462.

111. Amat-Santos IJ, Sanchez-Luna JP, Abu-Assi E, Melendo-Viu M, Cruz-Gonzalez I, Nombela-Franco L, et al. Rationale and design of the dapagliflozin after transcatheter aortic valve implantation (DapaTAVI) randomized trial. Eur J Heart Fail. 2022;24(3):581–8.
112. Saito T, Yoshijima N, Hase H, Yashima F, Tsuruta H, Shimizu H, et al. Impact of beta blockers on patients undergoing transcatheter aortic valve replacement: the OCEAN-TAVI registry. Open Heart. 2020;7(2):e001269.
113. Imamura T, Narang N, Sobajima M, Tanaka S, Ushijima R, Fukuda N, et al. Inadequate cardiac unloading following transcatheter aortic valve replacement. Circ Rep. 2021;3(10):615–9.
114. Cantey EP, Chang KY, Blair JEA, Brummel K, Sweis RN, Pham DT, et al. Impact of loop diuretic use on outcomes following transcatheter aortic valve implantation. Am J Cardiol. 2020;131:67–73.
115. Younis A, Orvin K, Nof E, Barabash IM, Segev A, Berkovitch A, et al. The effect of periprocedural beta blocker withdrawal on arrhythmic risk following transcatheter aortic valve replacement. Catheter Cardiovasc Interv. 2019;93(7):1361–6.
116. De Larochellière H, Puri R, Eikelboom John W, Rodés-Cabau J. Blood disorders in patients undergoing transcatheter aortic valve replacement. J Am Coll Cardiol Intv. 2019;12(1):1–11.
117. Kamioka N, Wells J, Keegan P, Lerakis S, Binongo J, Corrigan F, et al. Predictors and clinical outcomes of next-day discharge after minimalist transfemoral transcatheter aortic valve replacement. JACC Cardiovasc Interv. 2018;11(2):107–15.
118. Lauck SB, Wood DA, Baumbusch J, Kwon JY, Stub D, Achtem L, et al. Vancouver transcatheter aortic valve replacement clinical pathway: minimalist approach, standardized care, and discharge criteria to reduce length of stay. Circ Cardiovasc Qual Outcomes. 2016;9(3):312–21.
119. Aldalati O, Keshavarzi F, Kaura A, Byrne J, Eskandari M, Deshpande R, et al. Factors associated with safe early discharge after transcatheter aortic valve implantation. Cardiol J. 2018;25(1):14–23.
120. Vendrik J, Vlastra W, van Mourik MS, Delewi R, Beijk MA, Lemkes J, et al. Early mobilisation after transfemoral transcatheter aortic valve implantation: results of the MobiTAVI trial. Neth Hear J. 2020;28(5):240–8.
121. Wood DA, Lauck SB, Cairns JA, Humphries KH, Cook R, Welsh R, et al. The Vancouver 3M (multidisciplinary, multimodality, but minimalist) clinical pathway facilitates safe next-day discharge home at low-, medium-, and high-volume transfemoral transcatheter aortic valve replacement centers: the 3M TAVR study. JACC Cardiovasc Interv. 2019;12(5):459–69.
122. Lauck SB, Sathananthan J, Park J, Achtem L, Smith A, Keegan P, et al. Post-procedure protocol to facilitate next-day discharge: Results of the multidisciplinary, multimodality but minimalist TAVR study. Catheter Cardiovasc Interv. 2020;96(2):450–8.
123. Barbanti M, van Mourik MS, Spence MS, Iacovelli F, Martinelli GL, Muir DF, et al. Optimising patient discharge management after transfemoral transcatheter aortic valve implantation: the multicentre European FAST-TAVI trial. EuroIntervention. 2019;15(2):147–54.
124. McCalmont G, Durand E, Lauck S, Muir DF, Spence MS, Vasa-Nicotera M, et al. Setting a benchmark for resource utilization and quality of care in patients undergoing transcatheter aortic valve implantation in Europe-Rationale and design of the international BENCHMARK registry. Clin Cardiol. 2021;44(10):1344–53.
125. Frank D, Durand E, Lauck S, Muir DF, Spence M, Vasa-Nicotera M, et al. A streamlined pathway for transcatheter aortic valve implantation: the BENCHMARK study. Eur Heart J. 2024;45(21):1904–16.
126. Banovic M, Putnik S, Penicka M, Doros G, Deja MA, Kockova R, et al. Aortic valve replacement versus conservative treatment in asymptomatic severe aortic stenosis: the AVATAR trial. Circulation. 2022;145(9):648–58.
127. Kang DH, Park SJ, Lee SA, Lee S, Kim DH, Kim HK, et al. Early surgery or conservative care for asymptomatic aortic stenosis. N Engl J Med. 2020;382(2):111–9.
128. Coisne A, Montaigne D, Aghezzaf S, Ridon H, Mouton S, Richardson M, et al. Association of mortality with aortic stenosis severity in outpatients: results from the VALVENOR study. JAMA Cardiol. 2021;6(12):1424–31.

129. Abdelfattah OM, Krishnaswamy A, Kapadia SR. Cautious optimism regarding early transcatheter aortic valve replacement. J Am Heart Assoc. 2022;11(10):e026010.
130. Ochi A, Cheng K, Zhao B, Hardikar AA, Negishi K. Patient risk factors for bioprosthetic aortic valve degeneration: a systematic review and meta-analysis. Heart Lung Circ. 2020;29(5):668–78.
131. Schoen FJ, Levy RJ. Calcification of tissue heart valve substitutes: progress toward understanding and prevention. Ann Thorac Surg. 2005;79(3):1072–80.
132. Tamagnini G, Bourguignon T, Rega F, Verbrugghe P, Lamberigts M, Langenaeken T, et al. Device profile of the Inspiris Resilia valve for aortic valve replacement: overview of its safety and efficacy. Expert Rev Med Devices. 2021;18(3):239–44.
133. Bavaria JE, Griffith B, Heimansohn DA, Rozanski J, Johnston DR, Bartus K, et al. Five-year outcomes of the COMMENCE trial investigating aortic valve replacement with RESILIA tissue. Ann Thorac Surg. 2023;115(6):1429–36.
134. Lim KH, Candra J, Yeo JH, Duran CM. Flat or curved pericardial aortic valve cusps: a finite element study. J Heart Valve Dis. 2004;13(5):792–7.
135. Neethling W, Rea A, Forster G, Bhirangi K. Performance of the ADAPT-treated cardiocel(R) scaffold in pediatric patients with congenital cardiac anomalies: medium to long-term outcomes. Front Pediatr. 2020;8:198.
136. Bezuidenhout D, Williams DF, Zilla P. Polymeric heart valves for surgical implantation, catheter-based technologies and heart assist devices. Biomaterials. 2015;36:6–25.
137. Kereiakes DJ, Answini GA, Yakubov SJ, Rai B, Smith JM, Duff S, et al. Preliminary evaluation of a novel polymeric valve following surgical implantation for symptomatic aortic valve disease. JACC Cardiovasc Interv. 2021;14(24):2754–6.
138. Krishnaswamy A, Isogai T, Agrawal A, Shekhar S, Puri R, Reed GW, et al. Feasibility and safety of same-day discharge following transfemoral transcatheter aortic valve replacement. JACC Cardiovasc Interv. 2022;15(6):575–89.
139. Zahid S, Rai D, Tanveer Ud Din M, Khan MZ, Ullah W, Usman Khan M, et al. Same-day discharge after transcatheter aortic valve implantation: insights from the nationwide readmission database 2015 to 2019. J Am Heart Assoc. 2022;11(11):e024746.
140. Russo G, Tang GHL, Sangiorgi G, Pedicino D, Enriquez-Sarano M, Maisano F, et al. Lifetime management of aortic stenosis: transcatheter versus surgical treatment for young and low-risk patients. Circ Cardiovasc Interv. 2022;15(11):915–27.
141. Mylonas KS, Angouras DC. Bioprosthetic valves for lifetime management of aortic stenosis: pearls and pitfalls. J Clin Med. 2023;12(22):7063.
142. Moumneh MB, Damluji AA, Heslop AW, Sherwood MW. Structural heart disease review of TAVR in low-risk patients: importance of lifetime management. Front Cardiovasc Med. 2024;11:1362791.
143. Benjamin MM, Rabbat MG. Artificial intelligence in transcatheter aortic valve replacement: its current role and ongoing challenges. Diagnostics (Basel). 2024;14(3):261.
144. LeCun Y, Bengio Y, Hinton G. Deep learning. Nature. 2015;521(7553):436–44.
145. Brendel JM, Walterspiel J, Hagen F, Kubler J, Paul JF, Nikolaou K, et al. Coronary artery disease evaluation during transcatheter aortic valve replacement work-up using photon-counting CT and artificial intelligence. Diagn Interv Imaging. 2024;105(7–8):273–80.
146. Toggweiler S, Wyler von Ballmoos MC, Moccetti F, Douverny A, Wolfrum M, Imamoglu Z, et al. A fully automated artificial intelligence-driven software for planning of transcatheter aortic valve replacement. Cardiovasc Revasc Med. 2024;65:25–31.
147. Agasthi P, Ashraf H, Pujari SH, Girardo ME, Tseng A, Mookadam F, et al. Artificial intelligence trumps TAVI(2)-SCORE and corevalve score in predicting 1-year mortality post-transcatheter aortic valve replacement. Cardiovasc Revasc Med. 2021;24:33–41.
148. Boulif A, Ananou B, Ouladsine M, Delliaux S. A literature review: ECG-based models for arrhythmia diagnosis using artificial intelligence techniques. Bioinform Biol Insights. 2023;17:11779322221149600.

149. Kwon JM, Lee SY, Jeon KH, Lee Y, Kim KH, Park J, et al. Deep learning-based algorithm for detecting aortic stenosis using electrocardiography. J Am Heart Assoc. 2020;9(7):e014717.
150. Sanchez-Puente A, Dorado-Diaz PI, Sampedro-Gomez J, Bermejo J, Martinez-Legazpi P, Fernandez-Aviles F, et al. Machine learning to optimize the echocardiographic follow-up of aortic stenosis. JACC Cardiovasc Imaging. 2023;16(6):733–44.
151. Krishna H, Desai K, Slostad B, Bhayani S, Arnold JH, Ouwerkerk W, et al. Fully automated artificial intelligence assessment of aortic stenosis by echocardiography. J Am Soc Echocardiogr. 2023;36(7):769–77.
152. Patel PP, El Sabbagh A, Johnson PW, Suliman R, Salwa N, Morales-Lara AC, et al. Sex differences in the impact of aortic valve calcium score on mortality after transcatheter aortic valve replacement. Circ Cardiovasc Imaging. 2022;15(8):e014034.
153. Chang S, Kim H, Suh YJ, Choi DM, Kim H, Kim DK, et al. Development of a deep learning-based algorithm for the automatic detection and quantification of aortic valve calcium. Eur J Radiol. 2021;137:109582.
154. Kusunose K, Tsuji T, Hirata Y, Takahashi T, Sata M, Sato K, et al. Unsupervised cluster analysis reveals different phenotypes in patients after transcatheter aortic valve replacement. Eur Heart J Open. 2024;4(1):oead136.
155. Hasimbegovic E, Papp L, Grahovac M, Krajnc D, Poschner T, Hasan W, et al. A sneak-peek into the physician's brain: a retrospective machine learning-driven investigation of decision-making in TAVR versus SAVR for young high-risk patients with severe symptomatic aortic stenosis. J Pers Med. 2021;11(11):1062.
156. Rabbat M, Leipsic J, Bax J, Kauh B, Verma R, Doukas D, et al. Fractional flow reserve derived from coronary computed tomography angiography safely defers invasive coronary angiography in patients with stable coronary artery disease. J Clin Med. 2020;9(2):604.
157. Santalo-Corcoy M, Corbin D, Tastet O, Lesage F, Modine T, Asgar A, et al. TAVI-PREP: a deep learning-based tool for automated measurements extraction in TAVI planning. Diagnostics (Basel). 2023;13(20):3181.
158. Samin M, Juthier F, Van Belle C, Agostoni P, Kluin J, Stella PR, et al. Automated 3D analysis of multislice computed tomography to define the line of perpendicularity of the aortic annulus and of the implanted valve: benefit on planning transcatheter aortic valve replacement. Catheter Cardiovasc Interv. 2014;83(1):E119–27.
159. Abdul Ghffar Y, Osman M, Shrestha S, Shaukat F, Kagiyama N, Alkhouli M, et al. Usefulness of semisupervised machine-learning-based phenogrouping to improve risk assessment for patients undergoing transcatheter aortic valve implantation. Am J Cardiol. 2020;136:122–30.
160. Zahid S, Agrawal A, Salman F, Khan MZ, Ullah W, Teebi A, et al. Development and validation of a machine learning risk-prediction model for 30-day readmission for heart failure following transcatheter aortic valve replacement (TAVR-HF score). Curr Probl Cardiol. 2024;49(2):102143.
161. Okuno T, Overtchouk P, Asami M, Tomii D, Stortecky S, Praz F, et al. Deep learning-based prediction of early cerebrovascular events after transcatheter aortic valve replacement. Sci Rep. 2021;11(1):18754.
162. Bailoor S, Seo JH, Dasi L, Schena S, Mittal R. Prosthetic valve monitoring via in situ pressure sensors: in silico concept evaluation using supervised learning. Cardiovasc Eng Technol. 2022;13(1):90–103.
163. Truong VT, Beyerbach D, Mazur W, Wigle M, Bateman E, Pallerla A, et al. Machine learning method for predicting pacemaker implantation following transcatheter aortic valve replacement. Pacing Clin Electrophysiol. 2021;44(2):334–40.
164. Jia Y, Luosang G, Li Y, Wang J, Li P, Xiong T, et al. Deep learning in prediction of late major bleeding after transcatheter aortic valve replacement. Clin Epidemiol. 2022;14:9–20.

Chapter 18
Heart Failure Treatment—The Last Pieces of the Puzzle

Oana Ioniţă and Lucian Florin Dorobanţu

Abstract Heart failure is a major public health problem, associated with significant morbidity and mortality. Over the years several pathophysiological models of heart failure have been proposed, that led to the development of specific therapeutical agents. Hyperactivation of the renin-angiotensin-aldosterone, neurohormonal and adrenergic system are well known pathophysiological pathways involved in heart failure development. Several drugs have been developed to address these changes, resulting in an improvement in life expectancy. Sodium-glucose co-transporter 2 inhibitors completed the heart failure foundational therapy, through mechanisms not fully understood. Nevertheless, the puzzle is not complete and the patients are still exposed to a residual risk of adverse events or worsening heart failure, so that new pathways, new therapeutic targets and development of adjunctive structural interventions are still required.

Keywords Chronic heart failure · ARNI · SGLT-2 inhibitors · Foundation treatment

Treatment of heart failure with reduced ejection fraction (HFrEF) relies on four therapeutical pillars: angiotensin receptor–neprilysin inhibitors, beta-adrenergic receptor blockers, mineralocorticoid receptor antagonists, and sodium–glucose co-transporter 2 (SGLT2) inhibitors [1, 2]. Large scale trials have proven their effects to reduce mortality and morbidity in patients with chronic heart failure and they form the foundational therapy of HFrEF.

Novel drugs developed for the patients already on the optimal guideline-directed medical therapy, with positive data in some clinical trials are soluble guanylate cyclase stimulators [3], and myosin activators [4].

O. Ioniţă (✉)
Nord Hospital—Grupul Medical Provita, Bucharest, Romania

L. F. Dorobanţu
Nord Hospital—Grupul Medical Provita, Bucharest, Romania

Faculty of Medicine, Titu Maiorescu University, Bucharest, Romania

M. Dorobanţu et al. (eds.), *Current Approach to Heart Failure*,
https://doi.org/10.1007/978-3-031-96562-3_18

Development of treatment for heart failure is based on conceptual models of heart failure pathophysiology and verified afterwards in clinical development programs [5]; most frequently clinical effect and success match the conceptual existing models, while sometimes they do not fit in the current paradigm and require further clarification of the mechanism. One of the examples for the latter are the SGLT-2 inhibitors, which reduce heart failure mortality and morbidity independent of the effects on the renal tubular function, leading to new research in the quest of understanding the mechanisms involved in the observed benefits of this medication [6, 7].

Models in Heart Failure with Reduced Ejection Fraction

Heart failure development is a complex interplay between structural and functional modifications which involve the heart, the kidney, the peripheral vasculature, the autonomic nervous system, and skeletal muscle and can be influenced by aging, genetic background, comorbidities, nutrition or nonbiological environmental factors [3].

Several pathophysiological models were developed over the years. Historically the first one was the cardiorenal model, which linked the initial cardiac injury to the reduced ability of the heart to receive the blood from the peripheral organs or to pump it forward, leading to sodium retention and edema in the peripheral or pulmonary territories. While this model led to the use of diuretics in heart failure treatment [8], which are still the cornerstone of symptomatic treatment nowadays, it is known that sodium retention is neurohumoral mediated and not linked to decreased cardiac output per se. The second model was the cardiocirculatory or hemodynamic one, seeing heart failure as a combination of pump failure and peripheral vasoconstriction, which led to the use of oral peripheral vasodilators and inotropic agents. Studies like V-HeFT I [9], comparing two vasodilators, showed survival benefit with the combination hydralazine—isosorbide dinitrate and not with prazosin, despite significant blood pressure decrease, inconsistent with the cardiocirculatory model. Moreover the inotropic agents with vasodilator properties failed to show long term clinical benefits. The cardiocirculatory model still applies to the acute heart failure syndromes, where diuretics, vasodilators and inotropes form the basis of the therapy. In the 1990s, the neurohormonal conceptual model started to prevail [8], based on the observations that excess activation of sympathetic and renin-angiotensin-aldosterone systems was deleterious to the heart and circulation. This model recognized heart failure as a neurohormonal rather than a hemodynamic problem [5] and led to widespread use of beta-adrenergic blockers, angiotensin-converting enzyme inhibitors, angiotensin receptor blockers, and aldosterone antagonists in the treatment of heart failure. These therapeutical classes have been shown in multiple large scale studies to improve cardiovascular mortality and morbidity and form the basis of the nowadays guideline-directed medical therapy [1, 10]. However, this model also cannot completely explain disease progression and does not explain the benefit of device therapies [5]. Moreover, not all neurohormonal antagonists tested over the time were proven successful.

Maladaptive remodeling and molecular changes in heart failure, that include decreased energetic turnover, slower calcium transport in the sarcoplasmic reticulum, increased expression of low ATPase beta-myosin heavy chain isoforms have been described in heart failure [11].

Apoptosis, necrosis and autophagy play an important role in remodeling [12]. Autophagy, an important degradation/recycling system in cellular homeostasis [13], which can be adaptive or maladaptive, has been recently linked to the worsening of the ventricular function.

In recent years knowledge of genetic pathophysiology of heart failure increased, paving the way to identification of new therapeutical targets which might lead to new cardiovascular treatment options in the future.

Foundational Therapy in HFrEF

Angiotensin-Neprilysin Inhibitors

The renin angiotensin aldosterone system (RAAS) plays a key role in the pathophysiology of heart failure according to the neurohumoral model and RAAS blockade has lead to improved mortality and morbidity in landmark cardiovascular trials [14–16].

The natriuretic peptide system counteracts the effects of RAAS upregulation, inhibits vasopressin secretion and modulates the autonomic nervous system [17]. The release of natriuretic peptides, stimulated by increased ventricular preload and afterload and wall stress promotes natriuresis and vasodilation. This neurohormonal pathway has been targeted during the years. Nesiritide, a form of recombinant BNP with vasodilating properties, failed to show effects on mortality and rehospitalization in a large trial of patients hospitalized for acute heart failure [18]. The next target in the natriuretic peptide system was the inhibition of the breakdown of natriuretic peptides, which is done by an endopeptidase neprilysin and through a natriuretic peptide clearance receptor [17]. While initial attempts to inhibit neprilysin were only partially successful, as it was associated also with an increase of angiotensin II levels, the solution came with dual blockade of RAAS and natriuretic peptide system. First attempts of combining neprilysin and an angiotensin converting enzyme (ACE) were stopped due to high rate of angioedema [19]. The success came from combining an angiotensin receptor blocker with neprilysin inhibitor, under the name sacubitril-valsartan. The Prospective comparison of ARNI with ACEI to Determine Impact on Global Mortality and morbidity in Heart Failure trial (PARADIGM-HF trial) [20, 21] showed sacubitril/valsartan superiority to enalapril in reducing the primary end point of cardiovascular (CV) death or HF hospitalization, leading to a major change in guidelines. Data from PARADIGM-HF showed for each 1000 patients switched from enalapril to sacubitril/

valsartan, over a median period of time of 27 months, 47 less CV death or HF hospitalizations, 33 less CV deaths, 28 less first hospitalizations for HF and 32 less deaths from any cause [17, 20].

Considering the ARNI effect on the degradation of several vasoactive peptides beside de natriuretic ones, there is still an open question regarding a possible added clinical benefit through this mechanism.

Sodium-Glucose Cotransporter-2 Inhibitors

SGLT-2 inhibitors as HF medication were not developed by targeting a specific heart failure model, in the same way as the rest of the HFrEF treatment pillars that address neurohormonal activation. As Food and Drug Administration requires that the cardiovascular safety profiles for all new antidiabetic drugs are tested, this new therapeutic class came into attention after showing significant benefits on cardiac and renal function [5]. Two trials in HFrEF (DAPA-HF and EMPEROR-Reduced) [22, 23] showed significant reduction in cardiovascular mortality and worsening of heart failure in patients treated with dapagliflozin or empagliflozin irrespective of the presence or absence of diabetes. Later, positive effects in HF with preserved ejection fraction (HFpEF) were demonstrated [24, 25], gaining a class I guideline recommendation for both molecules also in the treatment of HFpEF and HF with mildly reduced EF [26].

The classical mechanism of action is related to inhibition of glucose transporter SGLT-2, highly expressed in the kidneys [5], where it is responsible for 90% of glucose reabsorption and it is involved in the proximal tubular reabsorption of sodium and the passive absorption of chloride.

However, it seems that SGLT2 inhibitors exhibit several direct citoprotective effects on the heart, independent of the nephron. SGLT-2 inhibitors increase nutrient-deprivation signaling and autophagic flux, leading to a decrease in cellular stress, a decrease in pro-inflammatory signaling and apoptosis and promoting mitochondrial health and renewal [6]. SGLT-2 inhibitors might also lead to reversal of the metabolic changes that appear in heart failure, which include increased uptake with decreased oxidation of long-chain fatty acids. They have also been connected with a decrease in ferritin and hepcidin levels, leading to better hemoglobin production [6, 27].

Several studies suggest that SGLT-2 inhibitors can lead to cardiac reverse remodeling. One study showed a significant lower change in LV mass index assessed by cardiac magnetic resonance imaging versus placebo, even though the precise mechanism is not clear [28].

Other Classes of Medication

Vericiguat

Vericiguat is a soluble guanylate cyclase stimulator that was associated with reduced incidence of cardiovascular death or heart failure hospitalization in patients with HFrEF, already treated with guideline-based medical therapy [3]. It has been included in clinical guidelines, with a IIb indication in selected HFrEF patients already on optimal medical therapy, with recent HF worsening [1, 10].

It targets nitric oxide(NO)-sGC-cyclic guanosine monophosphate (cGMP) cascade, that has a major role in cardiovascular hemeostasis. NO, whose main source is the endothelium, increases the activity of soluble guanylare cyclase (sGC) and the production of cGMP. In HFrEF a degree of endothelial dysfunction and inflammation leads to a deficiency of NO and cGMP synthesis [3]). sGC can be activated directly, but this approach has been abandoned due to significant symptomatic hypotension or indirectly through medications like vericiguat, which increase de sGC sensitivity to endogenous NO.

Cardiac Myosin Activators

Other heart failure medication targeting one of the conceptual heart failure models are cardiac myosin activators. Considering reduced contractility as a major problem in HFrEF in the cardiocirculatory model, improving contractility might prove clinical benefit. Three distinct mechanisms of action for inotropic drugs have been described [30]. In the first group, addressing the upstream pathways of muscle contraction, medication acts through an increase in intracellular calcium level. This group includes β1-agonists, phosphodiesterase 3 inhibitors or inhibitors of Na^{+}/Ca^{2+} exchange. Except digoxin, that still remains utilized in chronic HF in specific situations, the other drug groups are not used as chronic treatment of HF. The second group of medication acts through an increase of the affinity of troponin C for calcium, including for example levosimendan. It also shares phosphodiesterase-3 inhibitors properties. The third class includes medication that affects directly the connection between myosin and actin, without altering the intracellular calcium level, having as example omecamtiv mecarbil. However, after several clinical trials, the drug failed to get FDA approval in 2023.

Structural Interventions

Besides the advances in heart failure medication (Fig. 18.1, Table 18.1) [1, 26, 31], several structural interventions and device therapies are nowadays available, especially for the subset of patients that remain symptomatic. Surgical techniques maintain their specific roles, however the development of percutaneous or hybrid therapies allow a broader structural approach regardless of the ejection fraction [32]. New pacing strategies focusing on cardiac physiological pacing have emerged, having as goal the treatment or prevention of heart failure development [33].

Moreover, there is an increasing availability of therapies for advanced heart failure like cardiac transplantation and mechanical circulatory support, although the gap between the number of available donors and waiting recipients is widening [34].

Most frequently used structural interventions in heart failure are the mitral valve edge-to-edge repair (TEER), while annuloplasty devices or transcatheter mitral valve replacement systems are also available. Optimal patient selection is an important piece of the puzzle in order to get adequate results. Based on discrepancies between two landmark trials assessing edge-to-edge therapy (Mitra-FR and COAPT) [35, 36] and while waiting for the results from the ongoing RESHAPE-HF2 trial [37], some authors have suggested a selection process that should involve mitral regurgitation proportionality, implying better results in patients in which mitral

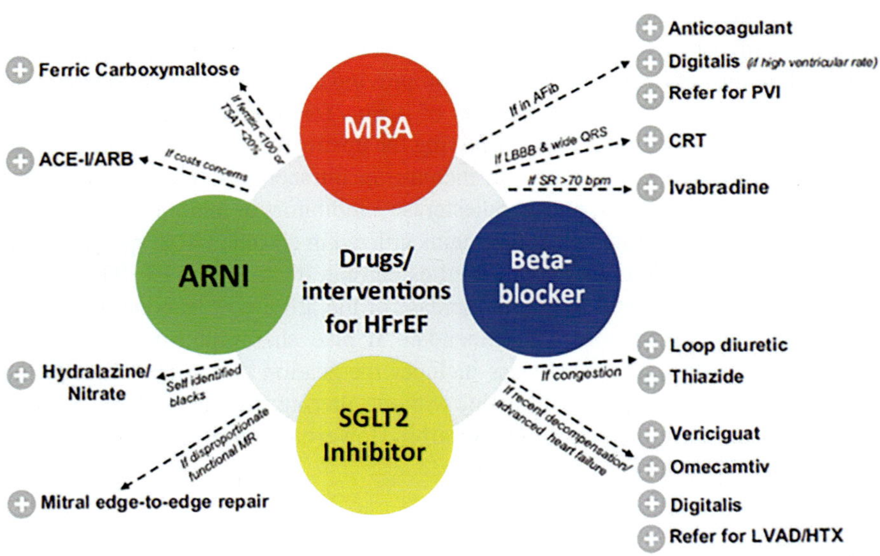

Fig. 18.1 Treatment puzzle of heart failure with reduced ejection fraction (HFrEF). *ARNI* angiotensin receptor/neprilysin inhibitor, *ACE-I* angiotensin-converting enzyme inhibitor, *ARB* angiotensin receptor blocker, *SGLT-2* sodium glucose co-transporter 2, *MRA* mineralocorticoid receptor antagonist, *CRT* cardiac resynchronization therapy, *PVI* pulmonary vein isolation, *HR* heart rate, *SR* sinus rhythm, *LVAD* left ventricular assist device, *TSAT* transferrin saturation

Table 18.1 Interventions in heart failure according to the European Society of Cardiology Guidelines for the diagnosis and treatment of acute and chronic heart failure—2021, updated 2023 (after 1, 26)

Intervention	HF	Evidence class and level
SGLT-2 inhibitors	*HFmrEF* *HFpEF* *HFrEF*	IA IA IA
ARNI/ACEI/ARB	*HFmrEF* *HFrEF*	IIb C IA
MRA	*HFmrEF* *HFrEF*	IIb C IA
Beta-blockers	*HFmrEF* *HFrEF*	IIb C IA
Diuretics	*HFmrEF* *HFpEF* *HFrEF*	For volume overload IC
Rapid uptitration of HF medication with frequent follow up visits in the first 6 weeks after hospitalization		IB
Iron supplementation		IA—improvement of HF symptoms and quality of life IIaA—improvement of HF hospitalizations
ICD	LVEF≤35%, QRS < 130 ms, therapy appropriate	IA—ischemic dysfunction IIaA—nonischemic dysfunction
CRT-D/P	SR and LVEF ≤ 35%, QRS ≥ 130 ms	IIaB—QRS 130–149 ms IA—QRS ≥ 150 ms
Ivabradine	SR, symptomatic HF with LVEF ≤ 35%, HR ≥ 70 bpm despite B-blockers	IIaB
Hidralazine and isosorbide dinitrate	Symptomatic HFrEF when ARNI, ARB, ACE-I are not tolerated or contraindicated	IIbB
Digoxin	Symptomatic patients in HFrEF in sinus rhythm despite optimal treatment	IIbB
Vericiguat	HFrEF with worsening symptoms despite optimal treatment	IIbB

HFrEF heart failure with reduced ejection fraction, *HFmrEF* heart failure with mildly reduced ejection fraction, *HFpEF* heart failure with preserved ejection fraction, *ARNI* angiotensin receptor/neprylisin inhibitor, *ACE-I* angiotensin-converting enzyme inhibitor, *ARB* angiotensin receptor blocker, *SGLT-2* sodium glucose co-transporter 2, *MRA* mineralocorticoid receptor antagonist, *CRT* cardiac resynchronization therapy, *CRT-D* Cardiac resynchronization therapy with Defibrillator, *CRT-P* Cardiac resynchronization therapy pacemaker, *ICD* implantable cardioverter defibrillator, *HR* heart rate, *SR* sinus rhythm, *LVEF* left ventricular ejection fraction regurgitation severity surpassed the degree of regurgitation expected based on left ventricular remodeling [38].

However, there are more factors involved in obtaining TEER benefits, like timing and optimal up-titration of medical therapy, degree of LV fibrosis/scar, presence of severe pulmonary hypertension, tricuspid regurgitation, or RV dysfunction [39]. Optimal medical therapy maintained before, during and after TEER is of utmost importance in these patients, as shown in the European Registry of Transcatheter Repair for Secondary Mitral Regurgitation international registry, in a subgroup of patients with TEER and right ventricular dysfunction.

Transcatheter repair techniques are also increasingly used for the tricuspid valve, improving the prognosis of these patients who were traditionally managed conservatively due to the high or prohibitive surgical risk [40].

Conclusions

Significant advances in heart failure treatment were registered in the last decades. The foundation therapy of heart failure with reduced ejection fraction is based on four classes of medication in three pills that counteract the neurohormonal activation and the newer sodium-glucose co-transporter 2 inhibitors, with complex, not fully understood mechanisms of action. The puzzle is completed by several other therapeutical medical or structural interventions, that can improve the prognosis of patients that were traditionally managed conservatively.

References

1. McDonagh TA, Metra M, Adamo M, ESC Scientific Document Group, et al. 2021 ESC Guidelines for the diagnosis and treatment of acute and chronic heart failure: developed by the Task Force for the diagnosis and treatment of acute and chronic heart failure of the European Society of Cardiology (ESC). With the special contribution of the Heart Failure Association (HFA) of the ESC. Eur J Heart Fail. 2022;24(1):4–131.
2. Packer M, McMurray JJV. Rapid evidence-based sequencing of foundational drugs for heart failure and a reduced ejection fraction. Eur J Heart Fail. 2021;23(6):882–94.
3. Armstrong PW, Pieske B, Anstrom KJ, VICTORIA Study Group, et al. Vericiguat in patients with heart failure and reduced ejection fraction. N Engl J Med. 2020;382(20):1883–93.
4. Teerlink JR, Diaz R, Felker GM, GALACTIC-HF Investigators, et al. Cardiac myosin activation with omecamtiv mecarbil in systolic heart failure. N Engl J Med. 2021;384(2):105–16.
5. Mann DL, Felker GM. Mechanisms and models in heart failure: a translational approach. Circ Res. 2021;128(10):1435–50.
6. Packer M. SGLT2 inhibitors: role in protective reprogramming of cardiac nutrient transport and metabolism. Nat Rev Cardiol. 2023;20:443–62.
7. Joshi SS, Singh T, Newby DE, et al. Sodium-glucose co-transporter 2 inhibitor therapy: mechanisms of action in heart failure. Heart. 2021;107(13):1032–8.
8. Packer M. How should physicians view heart failure? The philosophical and physiological evolution of three conceptual models of the disease. Am J Cardiol. 1993;71(9):3C–11C.

9. Cohn JN, Archibald DG, Ziesche S, et al. Effect of vasodilator therapy on mortality in chronic congestive heart failure: results of a Veterans Administration Cooperative Study. N Engl J Med. 1986;314:1547–52.
10. Maddox T, Januzzi J, Allen L, et al. 2024 ACC expert consensus decision pathway for treatment of heart failure with reduced ejection fraction: a report of the American College of Cardiology Solution Set Oversight Committee. J Am Coll Cardiol. 2024;83(15):1444–88.
11. Katz AM. The "modern" view of heart failure: how did we get here? Circ Heart Fail. 2008;1(1):63–71.
12. Boulet J, Mehra M. Left ventricular reverse remodeling in heart failure: remission to recovery. Struct Heart. 2021;5:466–81.
13. Miyamoto S. Autophagy and cardiac aging. Cell Death Differ. 2019;26:653–64.
14. The SOLVD investigators. Effect of enalapril on survival in patients with reduced left ventricular ejection fractions and congestive heart failure. The SOLVD Investigators. N Engl J Med. 1991;325:293–302.
15. The CONSENSUS investigators. Effects of enalapril on mortality in severe congestive heart failure. Results of the Cooperative North Scandinavian Enalapril Survival Study (CONSENSUS). The CONSENSUS Trial Study Group. N Engl J Med. 1987;316:1429–35.
16. Cohn JN, Tognoni G. A randomized trial of the angiotensin-receptor blocker valsartan in chronic heart failure. N Engl J Med. 2001;345:1667–75.
17. Jhund PS, McMurray JJ. The neprilysin pathway in heart failure: a review and guide on the use of sacubitril/valsartan. Heart. 2016;102(17):1342–7.
18. O'Connor CM, Starling RC, Hernandez AF, et al. Effect of nesiritide in patients with acute decompensated heart failure. N Engl J Med. 2011;365:32–43. 10.1056.
19. Packer M, Califf RM, Konstam MA, et al. Comparison of omapatrilat and enalapril in patients with chronic heart failure: the Omapatrilat Versus Enalapril Randomized Trial of Utility in Reducing Events (OVERTURE). Circulation. 2002;106:920–6.
20. McMurray JJV, Packer M, Desai AS, et al. Angiotensin-neprilysin inhibition versus enalapril in heart failure. N Engl J Med. 2014;371:993–1004.
21. Packer M, McMurray JJV, Desai AS, et al. Angiotensin receptor neprilysin inhibition compared with enalapril on the risk of clinical progression in surviving patients with heart failure. Circulation. 2015;131:54–61.
22. McMurray JJV, Solomon SD, Inzucchi SE, DAPA-HF Trial Committees and Investigators, et al. Dapagliflozin in patients with heart failure and reduced ejection fraction. N Engl J Med. 2019;381(21):1995–2008.
23. Packer M, Anker SD, Butler J, EMPEROR-Preserved Trial Investigators, et al. Cardiovascular and renal outcomes with empagliflozin in heart failure. N Engl J Med. 2020;383(15):1413–24.
24. Anker SD, Butler J, Filippatos G, EMPEROR-Preserved Trial Investigators, et al. Empagliflozin in heart failure with a preserved ejection fraction. N Engl J Med. 2021;385(16):1451–61.
25. Solomon SD, McMurray JJV, Claggett B, DELIVER Trial Committees and Investigators, et al. Dapagliflozin in heart failure with mildly reduced or preserved ejection fraction. N Engl J Med. 2022;387(12):1089–98.
26. McDonagh TA, Metra M, Adamo M, ESC Scientific Document Group, et al. 2023 focused update of the 2021 ESC Guidelines for the diagnosis and treatment of acute and chronic heart failure: developed by the task force for the diagnosis and treatment of acute and chronic heart failure of the European Society of Cardiology (ESC) with the special contribution of the Heart Failure Association (HFA) of the ESC. Eur J Heart Fail. 2024;26(1):5–17.
27. Lam CSP, Chandramouli C, Ahooja V, et al. SGLT-2 inhibitors in heart failure: current management, unmet needs, and therapeutic prospects. J Am Heart Assoc. 2019;8(20):e013389.
28. Verma S, Mazer CD, Yan AT, et al. Effect of empagliflozin on left ventricular mass in patients with type 2 diabetes mellitus and coronary artery disease: the EMPA-HEART CardioLink-6 randomized clinical trial. Circulation. 2019;140(21):1693–702.
29. Falco L, Brescia B, Catapano D, et al. Vericiguat: the fifth harmony of heart failure with reduced ejection fraction. J Cardiovasc Dev Dis. 2023;10(9):388.

30. Zhou S, Liu Y, Huang X, et al. Omecamtiv Mecarbil in the treatment of heart failure: the past, the present, and the future. Front Cardiovasc Med. 2024;11:1337154.
31. Bauersachs J. Heart failure drug treatment: the fantastic four. Eur Heart J. 2021;42:681–3.
32. Katzianer D, Albert C. Structural interventions in heart failure: mending a broken heart. J Clin Med. 2023;12(9):3243.
33. Chung MK, Patton KK, Lau CP, et al. 2023 HRS/APHRS/LAHRS guideline on cardiac physiologic pacing for the avoidance and mitigation of heart failure. J Arrhythm. 2023;39(5):681–756.
34. Kobashigawa JA. The future of heart transplantation. Am J Transplant. 2012;12(11):2875–91.
35. Obadia JF, Messika-Zeitoun D, Leurent G, Iung B, Bonnet G, Piriou N, MITRA-FR Investigators, et al. Percutaneous repair or medical treatment for secondary mitral regurgitation. N Engl J Med. 2018;379:2297–306.
36. Stone GW, Lindenfeld J, Abraham WT, Kar S, Lim DS, Mishell JM, COAPT Investigators, et al. Transcatheter mitral-valve repair in patients with heart failure. N Engl J Med. 2018;379:2307–18.
37. Anker SD, Friede T, von Bardeleben RS, et al. Percutaneous repair of moderate-to-severe or severe functional mitral regurgitation in patients with symptomatic heart failure: baseline characteristics of patients in the RESHAPE-HF2 trial and comparison to COAPT and MITRA-FR trials. Eur J Heart Fail. 2024;26(7):1608–15.
38. Grayburn PA, Sannino A, Packer M. Proportionate and disproportionate functional mitral regurgitation: a new conceptual framework that reconciles the results of the MITRA-FR and COAPT trials. JACC Cardiovasc Imaging. 2019;12(2):353–62.
39. Grayburn PA, Chandrashekhar YS. Functional mitral regurgitation: more questions than answers. JACC Cardiovasc Imaging. 2021;14(4):711–4.
40. Taramasso M, Vanermen H, Maisano F, et al. The growing clinical importance of secondary tricuspid regurgitation. J Am Coll Cardiol. 2012;59:703–10.

Chapter 19
Heart Transplantation—What Is New?

Horatiu Moldovan and Maria Sabina Safta

Nothing can take the place of a well supported and well planned research effort for solving the most difficult of medical problems.

Branislav Radovancevic

Abstract Heart transplantation is a surgical procedure that represents the replacement of a diseased heart with end-stage heart failure, with a healthy heart from a brain-dead donor organism.

Today, heart transplantation, due to its results, represents an unanimously accepted clinical treatment option for patients with end-stage heart failure, where all other therapeutic options have been exhausted. However, the availability of donor hearts limits the number of heart transplant operations performed worldwide.

Keywords Heart transplant · End-stage heart failure · Available donor heart · Cardiectomy · Biatrial technique · Bicaval technique · Immunosuppression · Complications · Follow-up

Historic Note

First experimental surgeries of the cardiac transplantation were performed on dogs in 1905, by Alexis Carrel and Charles Guthrie, at University of Chicago in the US [1].

However, the people who described the technical details of the heart transplant, initially on dogs and then in humans, were Norman Shumway and Richard Lower, also from the US, at Stanford University in California [2].

H. Moldovan (✉)
Department of Cardiovascular Surgery, Bucharest Clinical Emergency Hospital, Bucharest, Romania

M. S. Safta
Faculty of Medicine, Iuliu Hateganu University of Medicine and Pharmacy, Cluj-Napoca, Romania

M. Dorobanţu et al. (eds.), *Current Approach to Heart Failure*,
https://doi.org/10.1007/978-3-031-96562-3_19

The first orthotopic heart transplant in humans was performed by Christian Barnard in the 1967 at Cape Town City, South Africa. Although the first patient died after a short period of time from a mixed cause of atypical pneumonia and an acute rejection reaction, the surgery had an overwhelming worldwide promotion and it immediately won a worldwide trend [3].

The initial results were not what the public expected and the method entered in a shadow period, thus decreasing the worldwide number of such operations performed.

The improvement of the diagnostic procedures and therapeutic control of the acute rejection reaction lead to the return of the heart transplant surgery on the first lines of the hospitals worldwide.

The decisive steps were on the one hand monitoring the rejection reaction by myocardial biopsy and histological examination, and on the other hand the adjustment if the immunosuppression treatment using ciclosporin A.

Ciclosporin A was discovered by JF Borel in 1976 and introduced in the transplantation protocol by Shumway and Lower starting with the 1980s [4–6].

Following these improvements, the results improved significantly, obtaining a postoperative mortality below 10% and a 1-year survival over 80%. Currently surviving after cardiac transplantation may be enough for the patients to further live decades of years [7].

In Romania, experimental research on cardiac transplantation started at Fundeni Hospital in Bucharest by Prof. Dr. Voinea Marinescu, Prof. Dr. Dan Setlacek and Dr. Marian Ionescu, and in Cluj by Prof. Ioan Pop de Popa, at the beginning of the 1960s.

The first human orthotopic cardiac transplant was performed at the Clinical Emergency Hospital of Bucharest—Floreasca by Dr. Serban Bradisteanu and Prof. Dr. Radu Deac in 1999.

Cardiac transplant programs have continued at the Institute of Cardiovascular Diseases from Targu Mures under the supervision of Prof. Radu Deac and today Prof. Horatiu Suciu, as well as at the Clinical Hospital of Urgenta Bucharest under the management of Dr. Serban Bradisteanu and in present under the leadership Prof. Horatiu Moldovan.

Epidemiologic Data

It was considered that congestive heart failure (CHF) affects more than 23 million people from all over the world, prevalence in the population with age of over 20 of years being of 2.6% in the developed countries [8].

Cardiac transplantation represents the optimum therapeutic solution for symptomatic patients with terminal heart failure who do not respond to conventional therapy [9].

Candidates for such an operation are put on a waiting list. This is because the number of donors is relatively low.

The death rate on the waiting list in 2001 in the USA was of 17%. It fell to 13.7% in 2009, most likely due to the therapeutic progress registered by the large-scale application of resynchronization therapy and implantable cardiac defibrillators [10, 11].

Long-term outcomes after cardiac transplant have improved with the progress of candidates' selection, perfected surgical techniques, improved postoperative care and optimized immunosuppressive treatment [12, 13].

According to the statistics from the Register of the International Society for Heart and Lung Transplantation (ISHLT), annually approximately 5000 hearts are transplanted worldwide.

In total, from 1983 until now, more than 90,000 such operations were performed, and the survival rate is approximately 50% at 12 years [14].

Because the number of available organs is much smaller compared to the number of candidates on the waiting lists, a rigorous assessment for the patients more in need that would benefit best from the available donor is crucial [15].

Indications, Contraindications and Criteria of Acceptance in the Heart Registry

Heart Transplant Indications

All patients with severe heart failure should be considered for a possible heart transplant, if the medical therapy and cardiac resynchronization therapy failed to improve the symptomatology and/or failed to slow down the progression of the disease [16].

Primary indications for cardiac transplant are represented by:

- Non-ischemic dilated cardiomyopathy (53%).
- Idiopathic cardiomyopathy (38%).
- Heart valvular disease (3%).
- The dysfunction of heart graft and re-transplant (3%).
- Other (<1%) [15].

Of course that before the necessity of cardiac transplantation, all other conventional methods should be exhausted. This includes surgical or conventional interventions such as: myocardial revascularization, the correction of the valvular lesion, etc.

Patients with heart failure in NYHA class IV require an additional assessment to check if there is a multi-organ involvement. These patients have a mortality of 50% in 1 year [14].

Indications recommended by ACC/AHA for cardiac transplantation are: [17].

- Refractory cardiogenic shock requiring intra-aortic counter-pulsation balloon assistance or left ventricular assistance mechanical devices (LVAD);
- Cardiogenic shock with requirement of positive inotropic support, intravenous need of dobutamine or milrinone.
- Consumption of oxygen ("peak V02") under 10 ml/kg.

- Heart failure in functional class III–IV NYHA, unresponsive to maximal medical therapy and interventional support.
- Malignant ventricular arrhythmias despite an implanted cardiac defibrillator or ablative antiarrhythmic therapy.
- Heart failure due to terminal stage congenital malformations or primary pulmonary hypertension;
- Refractory unstable angina without other medical, interventional or surgical therapeutic options [17].

The indications advisable by the European Society of Cardiology are:

Class function III or IV NYHA with:

- Repetitive episodes of pulmonary or systemic congestion or reduced cardiac output (peripheral hypoperfusion) in conditions of rest.
- Severe cardiac dysfunction
- Ejection fraction lower than 30%
- Pseudo-normal or restrictive mitral flow on doppler echocardiography severely impaired functional capacity demonstrated by one of the following parameters: reduced exercise capacity, decreased walking test for 300 m in 6 min or consumption maximum of oxygen (Peak V02) for 12–14 ml/kg/min;
- Repeated hospitalizations for cardiac failure in the last 6 months [18].

Contraindications for Cardiac Transplantation

The following clinical situations are considered to be ABSOLUTE contraindications for cardiac transplantation: [19].

1. Advanced irreversible renal failure with Creatinine >2 mg/dl or clearance of creatinine <30–50 ml/min without the possibility of concomitant renal transplantation;
2. Advanced irreversible liver disease;
3. Advanced irreversible pulmonary parenchyma disease or (FEB 1 < 1 L/min);
4. Advanced irreversible pulmonary arterial hypertension (pulmonary artery systolic pressure > 60 mmHg, pulmonary vascular resistance >4–5 unity wood, which does not decrease with administration of vasodilators).
5. History of neoplastic disease in the last 5 years [19].

RELATIVE contraindications for cardiac transplantation:

1. Severe peripheral vascular disease;
2. Severe cerebrovascular disease;
3. Severe osteoporosis;
4. Obesity (BMI > 35 kg/m^2) or cachexia;
5. Acute pulmonary embolism;
6. Active Infection (excluding infections related to LVAD);

7. Age (>70 of years);
8. Psychological instability (of example, PTSD);
9. Addiction to psychotropic substances in the last 6 months.
10. Diabetes mellitus with target organ involvement.
11. Lack of social support or insufficient resources to offer medical compliance to permanent immunosuppression medication [19].

Steps of Cardiac Transplant Surgery

The Management of DONOR Patient

Until the brain death declaration, the patient—future potential donor, is fully monitored and evaluated for the status of the possible transplantable organs.

Clinical assessment must contain:

1. Age/weight/height/body surface area and blood group. (these parameters have a primary importance in the selection of the receiving patient).
2. Clinical history:
   - Mechanism of brain death.
   - Any pre-hospital events (cardiac stop, resuscitation, electrical shock, hypotension, hypoxemia, vasoactive and inotrope drug administration, ischemic duration, etc.).
   - Personal history and family history.
   - Any presence of thoracic/cardiac injuries.

Basic patient monitoring includes:

1. Invasive average blood tension.
2. Central venous pressure/pulmonary artery pressure/ pressure in the capillary pulmonary via Swan Gonzalez catheter.
3. Urinary flow on urine probe.
4. Peripheral pulse oximetry,
5. EKG.
6. Temperature: rectal/vesical.
7. Echocardiography: transthoracic/transesophageal.
8. Standard Hematology (hemoglobin, leucocytes, platelet count).
9. Standard acid base and electrolytes balance.
10. Kidney function monitoring.
11. Bacteriological and virology screening:
    - HBsAg
    - Antibodies anti HBs
    - Antibodies anti HBc
    - Antibodies anti HCV

- Antibodies anti HIV (excluding the donor)
- CMV titre

12. For donor patients 35 years or older we need coronarographic screening of possible ischemic cardiac disease.

The diagnosis of brain death is made according to the following criteria:

- absence of cortical activity, known cause of deep coma.
- absence of respiratory movements (apnea).
- fixed bilateral mydriasis.
- abolished brainstem reflexes (corneal reflex, oculocephalic reflex, oculovestibular reflex, reflex of cough, etc.).
- two flat successive EEG recording in a 6 h interval.
- absence of action potentials evoked by the cerebral cortex.

Of course, all these elements must be judged in absence of any humoral or pharmacological agents that influence the cerebral function.

After the patient is officially declared brain dead, he becomes a potential donor. Family consent is required for organ donation. After family consent, the potential donor becomes a real donor, and he/she is officially declared at the national transplant agency.

In the general, Criteria of acceptance for a DONOR HEART are:

1. Absence of a pathology or a traumatic injury of the heart.
2. Age between new born to 60 of years old (with caution over 40 years old).
3. The physical distance between donor and receiver, including technical conditions of transport must be for an ischemia time of less than 4–5 h. (for newborn—infants, ischemic time may expand to 6–8 h).
4. Acceptable doses of positive inotropic and/or vasopressor drugs [21].

Assignment of Cardiac Graft for Transplantation

All the criteria stated by international norms and national regulations that regulate organ transplantation, for the heart the most important is the geographical criteria, because the duration of ischemia is limited to 4–5 h.

Thus, from the data available in the Register National of receivers, the heart available for transplantation is directed to the closest center that has a compatible receiver.

According to updated regulations, clinical priority is done as follows:

- Class I: patient who require:
  - Mechanic circulatory support with an intra-aortic contra-pulsation balloon or LVAD.
  - Positive inotropic support and/or iv vasopressor.
- Class II: all other outpatients on the list of waiting.

Criteria of Compatibility Between Donor and Receiver

1. Same blood group.
2. Same body size. (at receivers with normal pulmonary vascular resistance can be transplanted with hearts from donors weighing up to 20% less; at receptors with pulmonary vascular resistance at its limit or increased can be transplanted with hearts from donors of same weight or higher).
3. Acceptable distance, ischemia time under the 4–5 h.
4. Cross-Matching (all transplant candidates are evaluated for compatibility with a panel of 50 types of lymphocytes, only 10% are positive and they must be analyzed directly).

The HLA compatibility, intensively used in the transplantation of others organs, for heart transplant is less used due to the lower number of available donor hearts and the efficient postoperative immunosuppressive therapy [20].

Surgical Technique

Cardiac Graft Excision from the Donor

After confirming the existence of a real organ donor, the transplant coordinator notifies the coordinators of the accredited units for heart transplant. The assignment complies with the criteria presented above up.

Because most of the time it is a multiple organ/tissues harvest, thus a synchronized multidisciplinary surgical team is required for efficient organ harvest [21]. The aim is to avoid iatrogenic damage to the organs taken, as well as to minimize ischemia time for each organ taken. It should be mentioned that the shortest time is for the heart, of approximate 4–5 h.

The order of harvesting is: heart, liver, pancreas, lung, kidney, other tissues (excepting only the relatively rare situation in which a heart—lung assembly is harvested, which is done first).

Surgical steps include:

1. Full median sternotomy.
2. Longitudinal pericardiotomy.
3. Aortic dissection until the emerging arterial brachiocephalic trunk.
4. Dissection of pulmonary artery until its main branches.
5. Dissection of superior vena cava with the ligature of azygos vein.
6. Dissection of inferior vena cava until the diaphragm.
7. Administration of systemic unfractioned heparin 200 IU/kg.
8. A needle is mounted on the ascending aorta through a purse string suture for administration of cold cardioplegia.

9. Sectioning of the inferior vena cava close to the diaphragm and right pulmonary veins at the edge of the pericardium. The heart will start to decompress through free bleeding in the pericardium.
10. Ascending aorta is clamped at the emergence of the arterial brachiocephalic trunk. (aortic cross clamping).
11. Cold cardioplegic Bretschneider solution is infused and cold serum is applied to the pericardium for cooling topic.

After stopping the heart and finishing the administration of cardioplegia, the left pulmonary veins, superior vena cava, the aorta at the level of the clamp are sectioned. The inferior vena cava and pulmonary arteries sectioning is completed and the heart is released totally from the donor pericardium.

The sampled heart is prepared on a special attached sterile table. After a quick inspection, the heart is inserted in a sterile plastic bag in air-sealed cold physiological serum. This bag is inserted in a second sterile bag with air-sealed sterile cold serum; and then into a third final air-sealed plastic bag. This whole assembly is placed in an isotherm transportation box filled with sterile ice. Transport to receiver must be done in the fastest and safest way available [21].

Preserving the Donor Heart

Preserving the donor heart is based on performing cardioplegia with a cold crystalloid solution whose main functions are: blocking the sodium/potassium membrane pump and easing myocardial in the diastole, the cooling of myocardium to 4 degrees and reduction to minimum myocardial metabolism.

The most used cardioplegia is the Bretshneider solution, which ensures the protection for the myocardium in conditions of hypothermia for 4–5 h.

The extension time of ischemia over this one limit, may be chosen in the conditions of pre-existent pathology of the donor patient—such as left ventricular hypertrophy.

An alternative method of conservation is for the collected heart to be placed in an artificial blood perfusion circuit and maintaining it in mechanical and electrical activity, from the desire to grow the time period between sampling and implantation in the absence of myocardial ischemia.

Next is the heart excision (cardiectomy) from receiver patient and anastomoses of the new graft [21].

Cardiectomy of the Receiver Patient

The receiving patient is admitted to the hospital as soon as a real donor is confirmed and the criteria are considered fulfilled for compatibility (matching).

From the moment the patient is announced, the receiver is questioned about any new arising conditions, especially infections or exacerbations of heart failure.

After the receiver is admitted reassessment from cardiological and anesthesiologic point of view is performed and the receiver is prepared for surgery.

Of great importance is the signing of the informed consent for the general anesthesia, blood transfusion and surgical intervention.

Patient is taken to operating theatre and anesthetized during the time in which the sampling team confirms the quality of the graft after the inspection.

Median sternotomy with central cannulation for extracorporeal circulation is performed.

After the start of extracorporeal circulation in normothermia, the main operative steps are:

- Clamping the ascending aorta.
- Sectioning the superior vena cava at the junction with the right atrium, section of ascending aorta and pulmonary artery just before the valves.
- The left atrium is incised on the upper wall and the incision is continued to the left before the left pulmonary veins, then the lateral and inferior wall until close to inferior vena cava.
- The incision of the left atrium is now continued to the right, before the drainage of right pulmonary veins into the superior vena cava. The section of the lower inferior vena cava is performed at a 1 cm distance from the right atrium (Fig. 19.1).
- Now, the heart can be excised from the receiver, in order to implant the heart graft (Fig. 19.2).

Anastomoses of the Cardiac Graft to the Receiver

The cardiac graft is prepared carefully yet quickly. The holes of the 4 pulmonary veins join through 4 incisions and the edges of the left atrial orifice are adjusted. The ascending aorta, the pulmonary artery and the 2 vena cava were prepared for the harvest.

The graft is placed in the pericardial cavity of the receiver and the anastomoses of the right atrium to the right atrial orifice starts.

It is important to create one orientation for no confusion to survive later during surgery. The left ear of the graft is positioned in the right ostium of the left upper pulmonary vein.

A continuous suture is performed with 4–0 polypropylene thread to the left, circularly, to a point located between the inferior vena cava of the receiver and the ostium of the coronary sinus of the graft.

Then we continue to practice the suture with same thread to right, circular until in the same point.

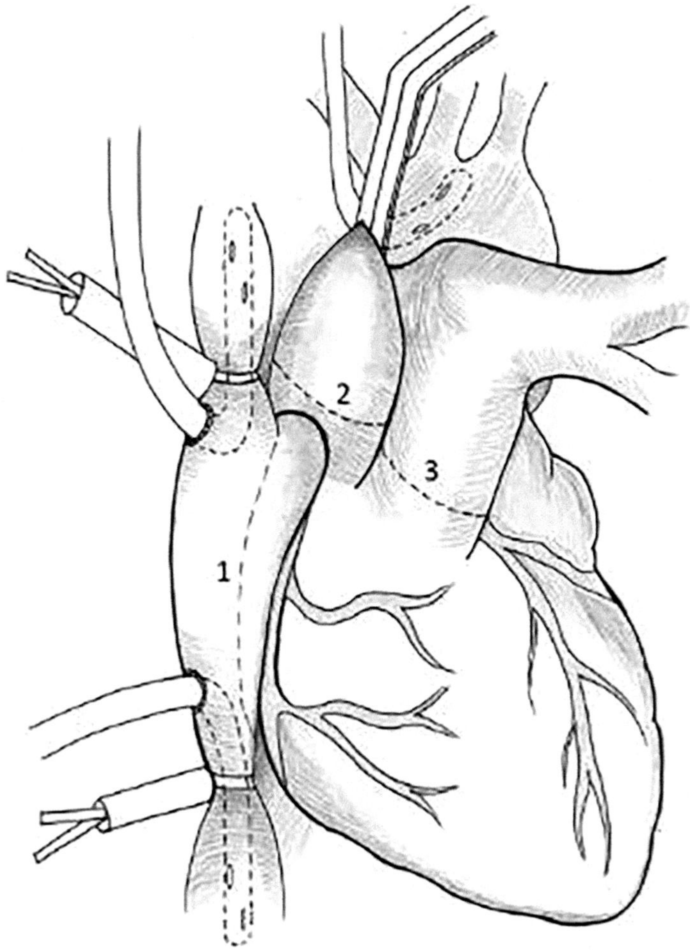

Fig. 19.1 lines of incision for cardiectomy at the receiver

Next, the end-to-end anastomosis of the superior cava is performed between the end of the receiver and that of the graft, a continuous suture with 5–0 polypropylene thread is used. As a rule, the graft being a normal heart and is a lot smaller than the remaining space from the pericardium after cardiectomy, thus using the length of both portions of the superior vena cava is necessary.

Next, the anastomoses of the inferior vena cava is performed with a continuous(surge) suture with a 5–0 polypropylene thread.

The aortic anastomosis follows, through a continuous suture with a 4–0 polypropylene thread. It is important to adjust the two heads of the aorta, so that at the end of the anastomosis it respects as much as possible the natural curvature of the ascending aorta.

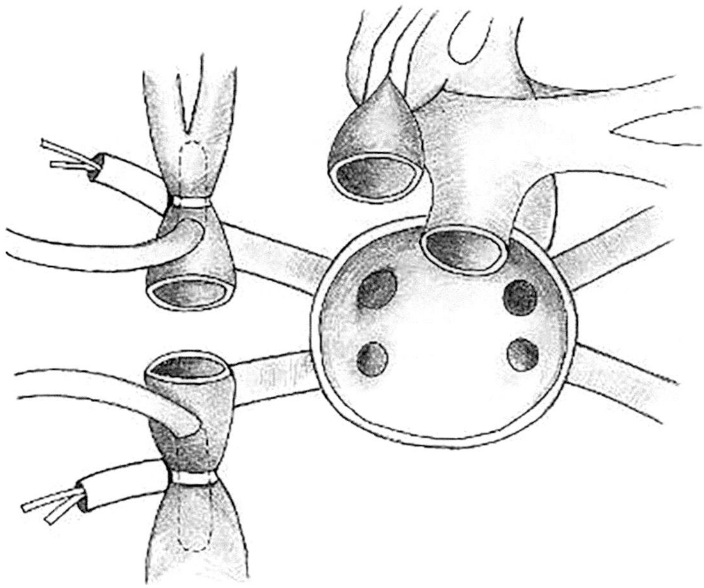

Fig. 19.2 Remaining structures after the cardiectomy of the receiver patient

Finally, the pulmonary artery is anastomosed end to end, via a continuous(surge) suture with 5–0 polypropylene thread.

Some authors have published other technical variants in which the order of the anastomoses differ. You start with the aorta, which is declamped earlier and thus, the ischemia time is shortened considerably, but to technically practice suture is more difficult [22] (Fig. 19.3).

After all anastomoses are performed, the vena cava are relished and the heart is recirculated in a classical way.

The aorta is unclamped and in most cases the cardiac graft resumes spontaneous activity with sinus rhythm.

A generous circulatory assistance time of approximately 30 min for the implanted graft to reach temperature of 37 degrees Celsius, in order to power the mitochondrial myocytes to recover fast and atrioventricular conduction to return to physiological speed.

Finally, the extracorporeal circulation is reduced progressively until it is stopped. Central cannulation is withdrawn and all ligatures are closed.

Control hemostasis is performed and reversion of anticoagulation with sulfate of protamine is infused to the patient.

It is important to place temporary epicardium stimulation at the level of the right ventricle and the right atrium for any temporary perioperative pacemaker stimulation (Figs. 19.4 and 19.5).

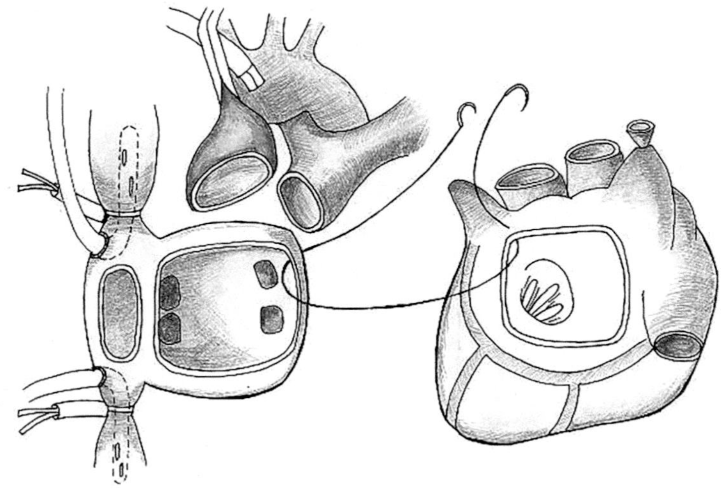

Fig. 19.3 The first step of anastomosis of the right atrium

Fig. 19.4 Suture of the two vena cava

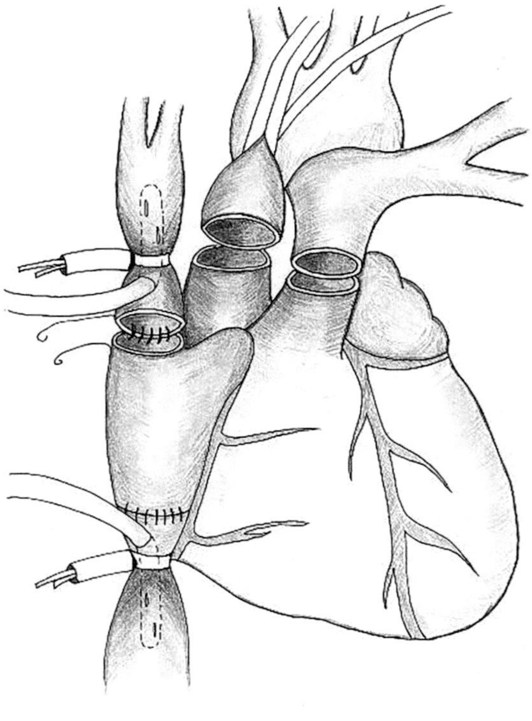

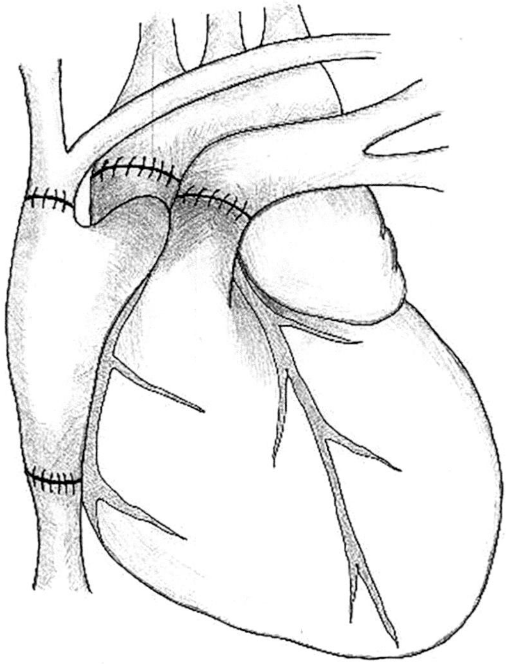

Fig. 19.5 Final anastomosis aspect

This “Bicaval” technique was introduced by Wythenshawe, Jacob and Dreyfus starting in the 90s [22].

Benefits of this surgical technique are:

- It maintains the architecture of the right atrium and preserves the circuits of atrial conduction. Supraventricular rhythm disorders are rare.
- Functionality of atrioventricular valves are well preserved. Incidence of tricuspid regurgitation is rare.
- Better aesthesis aspect.
- It adapts more easily to particular anatomical situations, especially when there is an important discrepancy between graft and the pericardial cavity of the receiver.
- Anastomosis time slightly prolonged, but the suture of the left atrium is simpler and more safer.

There is a “total biatrial” technique described by Trenton in the which independent anastomosis are performed for pulmonary veins as well.

The Classical Biatrial Process

Described initially by Shumway and Lower in the 1961 [23, 24].

Cardiectomy is different at the level of the right atrium whose wall posteriorly, it remains in place together with the ostia of the superior vena cava and the interatrial septum. If there is patent foramen ovale, this is closed.

The graft is prepared differently in the sense that the superior vena cava is ligated and the ostium of the inferior vena cava is joined through an incision with right atrium.

The anastomosis begins similarly to the bicaval technique, through apposition of the left ear to the upper left pulmonary vein. The suture is continuous with 4–0 polypropylene thread. It anastomoses the circular left slope to a point located between the vena cava lower part of the receptor and the ostium of the coronary sinus of the graft. Then, with the same thread, the atrium is circularly anastomosed to the right of the graft with that of the receiver and at the level of the septum interatrial remaining (Fig. 19.6).

Then the two right atria are anastomosed with a continuous thread of polypropylene 5–0, starting at the level interatrial septum (Fig. 19.7).

After finishing the atrial anastomoses, the anastomosis of the ascending aorta is done and that of the pulmonary artery in a similar manner as the bicaval technique (Fig. 19.8).

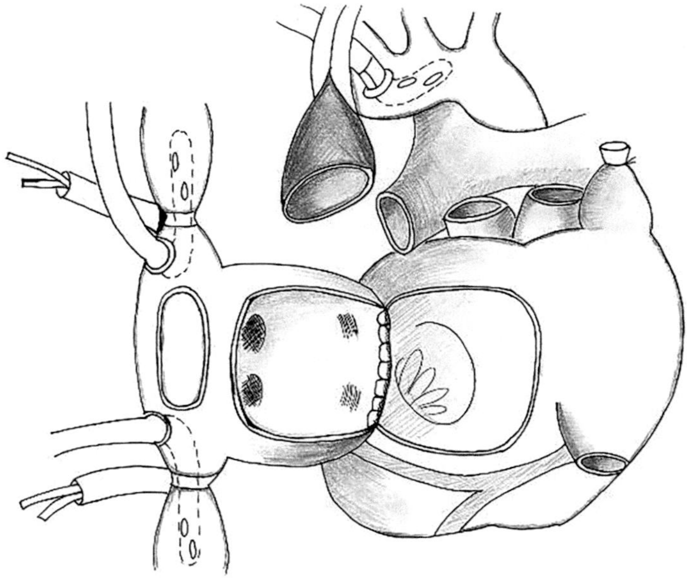

Fig. 19.6 Suture of the atrium in the biatrial procedure

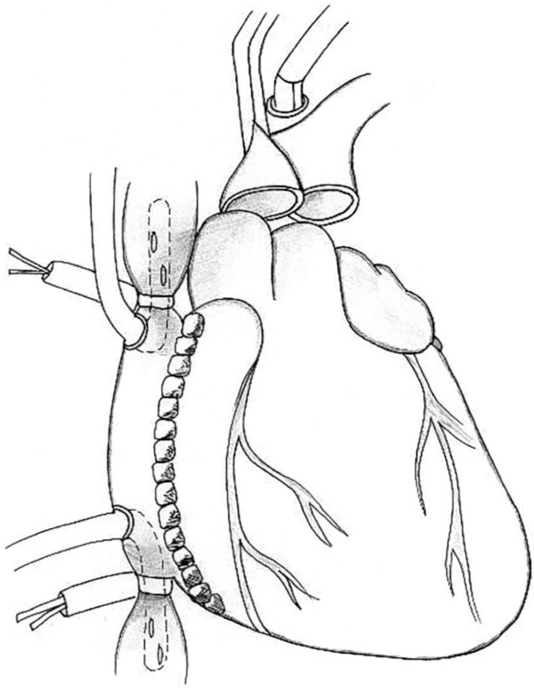

Fig. 19.7 Suture the right atrium

Benefits of this technique are:

1. The experience very big (>40,000 de transplants done).
2. Time of anastomoses can be shorter.

The disadvantages of this technique are:

1. Distortion of the atrias.
2. The interruption the atrial conduction system.
3. Altered intracardiac hemodynamics, frequency of regurgitation is greater for tricuspid valve, the frequency of rhythm troubles with supraventricular arrythmias is bigger.
4. Asynchrony of interatrial contraction.

Heterotopic Intrathoracic Technique

It is an exceptional process in the which the receiver heart remain in the position and it add in the parallel the graft from the donor.

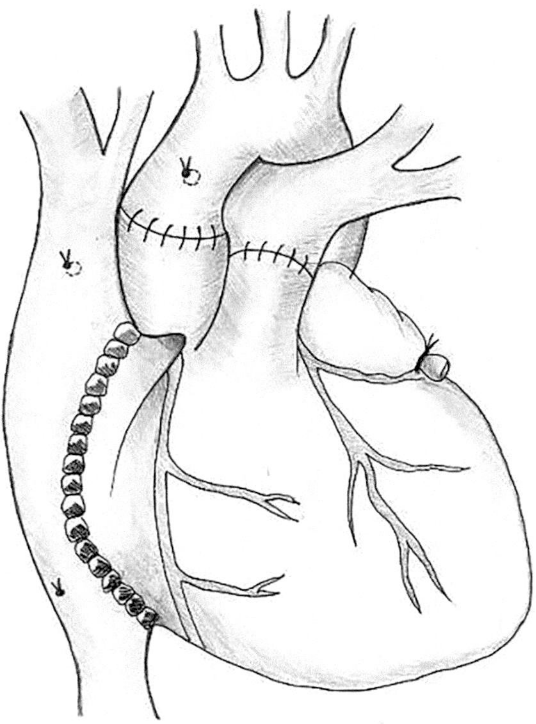

Fig. 19.8 Sutures in the biatrial technique

The atria are anastomosed in the same way as in the biatrial technique, the aorta and the pulmonary artery can be directly anastomosed with the heart of the receiver or through some intermediate synthetic grafts.

Utility of this technique is limited. It remains a last resort technique, if there is an important discrepancy in size between donor and receiver in the conditions of maxim expedite. Bicaval technique, through its actual benefits, is most commonly practiced in the last 20 years.

Making the anastomosis between the graft and the cardiac structures remaining from the receiver take approximate 1 h. This time must taken into account when calculating the global ischemia time, making the amount with the time required for the transport. Global ischemia time of for the cardiac graft is good not to exceed 4–5 h for recovery to be optimal.

Immediate Postoperative Care of the Transplanted Patient

In general, the team caring for a transplant patient must have the usual cardiac intensive care training, but specific experience for these kind of patients is needed.

As a rule, post-transplant patients are isolated in designated intensive care units. The team taking care of these patients are provided with special equipment when entering in contact with the patient.

Before admitting the patient from the operating room, it is necessary to clean and sanitize once more the assigned unit.

The entire staff that is assigned to supervise the patient is careful prepared through hand sanitizing, wear surgical masks permanently and use sterile equipment.

It is also important that the access to patient is limited to when is strictly necessary, so that infectious risk is minimum.

The SPECIFICATIONS for a patient operated on heart open remain the same, in the addition being the need of pulmonary pressure monitoring and the pulmonary capillary pressure using the Swan—Ganz catheter.

Protocol of SURVEILLANCE FOR PATIENTS with HEART TRANSPLANT Includes: In the First 10 Days Postoperative:
Clinical, electrocardiographic, echocardiographic monitoring, radiological, metabolic, invasive hemodynamics, biochemistry, bacteriological and serology screening (1 time in this interval).

A myocardial biopsy is indicated weekly. Some teams have reduced frequency of myocardial biopsy at 3 months. In this interval, other consultations may be necessary (ophthalmological, ENT and gynecological).

In the next 20 days the patient is moved from the intensive care unit to the department ward, where continuous monitoring of clinical aspects, electrocardiography, non-invasive hemodynamics, transthoracic echocardiography and radiological parameters are followed.

Cyclosporinemia continues to be dosed 2 times a week. Some teams practice angiographic exam of coronary arteries before hospital discharge.

In the months following the hospital discharge, the patient must be followed up by monthly consultation. Within it, the following must be practiced: clinical examination, electrocardiogram, transthoracic echocardiography, thoracic x-ray, biochemical, hematological, coagulation and bacteriological examinations, depending on the clinical condition. Angiographic exam of coronary arteries is indicated annually.

Also, the cyclosporine dosage is required at each consultation, follow-up for adjusting the doses remains permanent.

PROTOCOL OF SUPERVISION FOR HEART TRANSPLANT
PERFORMS TO EVERY DAY CONSULT until hospital discharge:

1. Exam clinical completely with mention weights loss/gain.
2. EKG with Shumway index.
3. Full blood count with full biochemistry and inflammatory markers.
4. PH determination.
5. Urine sample with proteinuria determination/24 h.
6. Cyclosporinemia.

IT IS PERFORMED QUARTERLY; in January, April, July, October, of every year:

1. Thorax X-ray.
2. Transthoracic echocardiography/Scintigraphy.
3. Myocardium Biopsy.
4. Coagulation cascade monitoring.
5. Cholesterol. Triglycerides. Lipid profile.
6. Serological screening for CMV, herpes simplex, hepatitis B and C, toxoplasma, candida, aspergillus, legionella, EBV, HIV.

It is PERFORMED ANNUALLY; in the month October of EACH year:

1. coronary angiography—possibly with catheterization of Right Heart if there is indication.
2. Bone x-ray.
3. Ophthalmological, ENT, dental, +/− gynecological check-ups.
4. Bacteriological screening [25].

Immunosuppression

Posttransplant immunosuppression must achieve a balance between rejection reaction control and possible infection control.

If the immunosuppression is very aggressive, the patient can develop severe infections; if but immunosuppression is not enough, there is risk of reject reaction increases.

Happily, once Ciclosporin is introduced in the treatment of heart transplant patients, control of this balance becomes easier.

The principle uses at its basis the following therapeutic scheme:

Intraoperative: Methylprednisolone 500–1000 mg at Aortic declamp.

In the 1st and 2nd postoperative day: Methylprednisolone 125 mg × 3/day associated with Ciclosporin 250 mg × 3/day (for a plasma level of 250–350 ng/ml) and MYCOPHENOLATE of mofetil (Cellcept) 1.5 g × 2/day.

On the 3rd day: Methylprednisolone 125 mg × 3/day associated with Ciclosporin 250 mg × 2/day (for a plasma level of 250–350 ng/ml) and MYCOPHENOLATE of mofetil (Cellcept) 1.5 g × 2/day.

In the 4th day until hospital discharge: prednisone initial 1 mg/kg/day then it decrease with 5 mg/day up to a dose of 0.3 mg/kg/day in the first month. If rejection reaction does not appear it may be reduced a lot after 6 months. This is paired with Cyclosporine 250 mg × 2/day po (for plasma level 250–350 ng/ml) and MYCOPHENOLATE of mofetil (Cellcept) 1.5 g × 2/day [25].

Other Medications Used

Systemic antibiotics used are based on 2nd generation cephalosporin associated with anticytomegalovirus (CMV) from class Vanciclovir and with a antifungals of type Diflucan. Additionally Biseptol 1 thb/day for a year is given.

The scheme used at Bucharest Clinical Emergency Hospital is:

1. CYCLOSPORINE A
   - 200 mg (4 tablets) Morning at 11.00
   - 150 mg (3 tablets) in the evening at 23.00
2. MYCOPHENOLATE MOFETIL MMF (CELL-CEPT)
   - 1.5 mg (3 tablets) Morning at 10.00
   - 1.5 mg (3 tablets) Evening at 22.00
3. PREDNISONE:
   - Month 1: 8 tablets/day Morning at 8.00—until hospital discharge.
   - Month 2–3: 6 tablets /day in the morning at 8.00
   - Month 4: 4 tablets/day in the morning at 8.00
   - Month 5: 3 tablets/day in the morning at 8.00
   - Rest of life: 2 tablets/day in the morning at 8.00
4. BISEPTOL 1tablet/day in the evening for 1 year
5. VALCYTE 2 tablets/day for 6 months after transplantation [27]

Complications

The immediate complications, the most significant are the acute rejection and acute cardiac failure. The right ventricle is the most sensitive and can easily become ineffective under some raised vascular resistance situations.

The acute rejection is responsible of approximate 10% of deaths in the first 3 years after transplantation. Subsequently the incidence and impact on rate of death decreases significantly [26].

There is evidence that the acute rejection favors progression of vasculopathy for the allograft (CAV) [26].

Another serious immediate complication is early infection, favoured by the immunosuppressive treatment. This can cause up to 30% of deaths in the first year after transplantation [26].

High incidence for deaths related to infection in the first year could be explained by the higher dose of immunosuppression, which is necessary to control the more intense immune response immediately after transplantation.

After reduction immunosupression in the next years, the risk of death determined by infection is with 10% less, annually.

Chronic Vasculopathy of Allograft (CAV)

This illness affects the coronary arteries, known also under the name of coronary disease of the transplanted heart, affects up to 10% of patients in 3 years and 30% in 5 years from the operation.

At 10 years, CAV affects over 50% of patients. It has an important impact on rate of survival [26].

The incidence of CAV has decreased minimally in recent years, despite considerably good improvement of the immunosuppressant treatment.

The percentage of patients who do not develop CAV 5 years after transplantation in the last 10 years grew by only 3%, from 67% to 70% [26].

Possible cause of this is the presence of the treatment supported with statins [29] and early detection of the disease is done through coronary angiography [28].

Neoplasia

5 years after the transplant surgery, approximately 15% of patient develop a malignant disease. In 10 years, this percentage grows to 35% [26].

The most common malignant tumor described is skin melanoma.

Globally, it is considered that approximately 20% of deaths at 5 years in a transplant patient is due to cancer [26].

Several studies have confirmed a mortality rate of approximately 25% at 10 years, due to neoplasia. This decreased by 10% in this time frame due to frequent checks in by the doctors [26, 28].

Kidney Failure

Systemic administration of immunosuppressants, especially calcineurin inhibitors—such as Ciclosporin, affect the function of the kidney.

Often this effect overlaps with preexisting kidney failure and favors the evolution of heart transplanted patients towards chronic kidney failure [26].

Five years after the transplant, about 16% of patients have renal failure with creatinine >2.5 mg/dL, or requires dialysis and are candidates for kidney transplant.

Conclusion

At the current stage of heart transplant development, the major goals remain the long-term survival, patient morbidity and the quality life.

Heart Transplantation amends radical evolution of the natural heart disease, especially those that evolve with end-stage heart failure.

This operation, along with the implant of left ventricular assisted devices, may be the difference between the loss of the patient on short term or its survival on term long.

Implantation of modern left ventricular assisted devices (LVAD) represent an alternative potential to transplantation, to some categories of patients.

To achieve this goal, additional data is needed regarding medium and long-term survival, such as and the functional outcome and quality of life of patients with LVAD. These data must to be compared with data obtained from the patients with heart transplant .

References

1. Carl A, Guthrie CC. The transplantation of veins and organs. Am Med. 1905;10:1101–2.
2. Lower RR, Shumway US. Studies on orthotopic homotransplantation of the canine heart. Surge Forum. 1960;11:18–9.
3. Barnard CN. The operation. A human cardiac transplant: an interim report of a successful operation performed at Groote Schur hospital, Cape Town. S Afr Med J. 1967;41:1271–4.
4. Borel JF. Comparative study of in vitro and in vivo drug effects on cell-mediated cytotoxicity. Immunology. 1976;31:631–41.
5. Greene CJ, Allison AC. Extensive prolongation of rabbit kidney allograft survival after short-term cyclosporin—a treatment. Lancet. 1978;1:1182–3.
6. Calne RY, White DJ, Rolles K, Smith DP, Herbertson BM. Prolonged survival of orthotopic pig heart grafts treated with cyclosporin A. Lancet. 1978;1(1):183–5.
7. Bahnson HT. Transplantation of the heart: reminiscences of the past and inklings of the future. Ann Thorac Surg. 1997;64:1561–3.
8. Roger VL, Go AS, Lloyd-Jones DM, Adams RJ, Berry JD, Brown TM, Carnethon MR, Dai S, De Simone G, Ford ES, Fox CS, Fullerton HJ, Gillespie C, Greenlund KJ, Hailpern SM, Heit JA, Michael Ho P, Howard VJ, Kissela BM, Kittner SJ, 21 Others. Heart disease and stroke statistics-2011 update: a report from the American Heart Association. Circulation. 2011;123:e18–e209.
9. Metra M, Ponikowski P, Dickstein K, et al. Advanced chronic heart failure: a position statement from the Study Group on Advanced Heart Failure of the Heart Failure Association of the European Society of Cardiology. Eur J Heart Fail. 2007;9:684–94.
10. 2009 annual report of the American Network for Organ Procurement and Transplantation and REGISTER scientific of recipients of transplantation: DATA about transplantation 1999–2008. US Department of Health and Human Services, Resource Management and a services of health, the desk systems of health, divided of transplantation, Rockville, M.D. Available online: http://www.ustransplant.org/annual_reports/current/
11. Hunt SA, Abraham WT, Chin MH, et al. Focused update in 2009, included in the 2005 ACC/AHA guidelines for the diagnosis and management of heart failure at adults: a report of the American Heart Foundation/American Heart Association panel work on practice guidelines: developed in collaboration with the International Society for transplantation cardiac and pulmonary. Circulation. 2009;119:e391–479.
12. Butler J, Khadim G, Paul KM, et al. Selection of patients for heart transplantation in the current era of heart failure therapy. J Am Coll Cardiol. 2004;43:787–93.
13. Lietz K, Miller LW. Survival improved A PATIENT with insufficiency HEART in the stage terminal LEARN on list for transplantation of heart: analyze the network of organ procurement and transplantation/United States network of organ exchange data, 1990 until in 2005. J Am Coll Cardiol. 2007;50:1282–90.

14. Stehlik J, Edwards LB, Kucheryavaya AY, et al. The registry of the International Society for Heart and Lung Transplantation: twenty-eighth adult heart transplant report—2011. J Heart Lung Transplant. 2011;30:1078–94.
15. Starling RC. Advanced heart failure: transplant, LVAD, and beyond. Cleve Clin J Med. 2013;80:33–40.
16. Yancy CW, Jessup M, Bozkurt B, et al. Guide ACCF/AHA 2013 for the management failure cardiac: a report of Foundation American of Cardiology/Association American A heart—the group of WORK looking GUIDELINES of practice. J Am Coll Cardiol. 2013;62:e147–239.
17. Jessup M, Abraham WT, Casey DE, et al. Focused update in 2009: ACCF/AHA Guidelines for the Diagnosis and Management of Heart Failure in Adults: a report of the foundation US of Cardiology/Association American A heart—group of work on practice guidelines, developed in collaboration with the International Society for Transplantation Cardiac and Pulmonary. Circulation. 2009;119:1977–2016.
18. McMurray JJ, Adamopoulos S, Anker SD, Co Guidelines. ESC for diagnosis and treatment of acute and chronic heart failure 2012: group of work for diagnosis and treatment of heart failure acute and chronic 2012 of company Europeans of Cardiology, developed in the collaboration with Association of Insufficiency HEART (HFA) a ESC. Eur J Heart Fail. 2012;14:803–69.
19. Mancini D, Lietz K. Selection of cardiac transplant candidates in 2010. Circulation. 2010;122:173–83.
20. Hunt SA, Haddad F. The changing face of heart transplantation. J Am Coll Cardiol. 2008;52(8):587–98.
21. Aziz TM, Burgess MI, El-Gamel A, Campbell CS, Rahman AN, Deiraniya AK, et al. Orthotopic cardiac transplantation technique: a survey of current practice. Ann Thorac Surg. 1999;68:1242–6.
22. Dreyfus G, Mihaileanu S, Carpenter A. Total orthotopic heart transplantation: an alternative to the standard technique. Ann Thorac Surg. 1991;52:1181.
23. Lower RR, Stofer RC, Shumway NE. Homovital transplantation of the heart. J Thorac Cardiovasc Surg. 1961;41:196–204.
24. Shumway KE, Lower RR, Stofer RC. Transplantation of the heart. Adv Surg. 1966;2:265–84.
25. McCartney SL, Patel C, Del Rio JM. Long-term outcomes and management of the heart transplant recipient. Best Pract Res Clin Anaesthesiol. 2017;31(2):237–48.
26. Lund LH, Edwards LB, Kucheryavaya AY, et al. The registry of the International Society for Heart and Lung Transplantation: thirty-first official adult heart transplant report—2014; focus theme: retransplantation. J Heart Lung Transplant. 2014;33:996–1008.
27. Deuse T, Haddad F, Pham M, et al. Twenty-year survivors of heart transplantation at Stanford University. Am J Transplant. 2008;8:1769–74.
28. Rodriguez Cetina Biefer H, Sündermann SH, Emmert MY, et al. Surviving 20 years after heart transplantation: a success story. Ann Thorac Surg. 2014;97:499–504.
29. Fröhlich GM, Rufibach K, Enseleit F, et al. Statins and the risk of cancer after heart transplantation. Circulation. 2012;126:440–7.

Further Reading

ANZOD Registry. Annual report, section 7: deceased donor heart donation. Adelaide: Australia and New Zealand Dialysis and Transplant Registry; 2017.

Roussel JC, Baron O, Périgaud C, et al. Outcome of heart transplants 15 to 20 years ago: graft survival, post-transplant morbidity, and risk factors for mortality. J Heart Lung Transplant. 2008;27:486–93.

Dall CH, Snore M, Christensen S, et al. Effect of high-intensity training versus moderate training on peak oxygen uptake and chronotropic response in heart transplant recipients: a randomized crossover trial. Am J Transplant. 2014;14:2391–9.

Chapter 20
Chronic Heart Failure: Multidisciplinary Interventions

Izabella Uchmanowicz

Abstract Chronic heart failure (CHF) presents complex challenges that demand a multidisciplinary approach for effective management. This chapter investigates into the collaborative efforts of cardiovascular professionals, including cardiologists, cardiac nurses, rehabilitation specialists, dietitians, and psychologists, in delivering comprehensive care for CHF patients. Drawing upon European and American guidelines, it explores the integration of patient-centered care, contemporary healthcare trends, and evidence-based interventions within a multidisciplinary framework. Effective management of heart failure patients requires a comprehensive and coordinated approach, involving a multidisciplinary team of healthcare professionals. This chapter explores the pivotal role of a multidisciplinary team in the care of heart failure patients and outlines the key components of heart failure management. It emphasizes the importance of collaboration, communication, and the integration of various healthcare disciplines to optimize patient outcomes.

Keywords Chronic heart failure · Multidisciplinary interventions · Cardiovascular professionals · Patient-centered care · Evidence-based management · Holistic support · Quality of life

Introduction

Heart failure (HF) is a multifaceted, recurring, and severe chronic condition, leading to multisystem dysfunction and imposing a substantial load of illness, fatalities, and healthcare expenditures. It is widespread, impacting more than 10% of individuals aged 70 and above [31]. Despite advancements in treatment, chronic heart failure remains associated with significant morbidity and mortality. The 1-year mortality

I. Uchmanowicz (✉)
Faculty of Health Sciences, Department of Nursing and Obstetrics, Wroclaw Medical University, Wroclaw, Poland
e-mail: izabella.uchmanowicz@umed.wroc.pl

M. Dorobanţu et al. (eds.), *Current Approach to Heart Failure*,
https://doi.org/10.1007/978-3-031-96562-3_20

rate following hospitalization for heart failure is approximately 30%, and the 5-year survival rate is only around 50%. These statistics underscore the critical need for improved therapeutic interventions and collaborative management approaches [8].

Multidyscyplinary Approach

The optimal approach to heart failure (HF) management involves a multidisciplinary team comprising health and social care professionals with diverse expertise, ideally under the guidance of a specialized HF practitioner. This approach is essential for addressing the frequently diverse and evolving requirements of individuals living with HF and their families or caregivers. It plays a vital role in facilitating a continuous care pathway across various healthcare environments [31]. The concept of a multidisciplinary team (MDT) revolves around a group of healthcare professionals united in their mission to enhance the quality of life for heart failure (HF) patients (Fig. 20.1).

Simultaneously, their efforts aim to reduce mortality rates, lower hospital admissions, and ultimately bring down healthcare costs. MDTs have become integral in

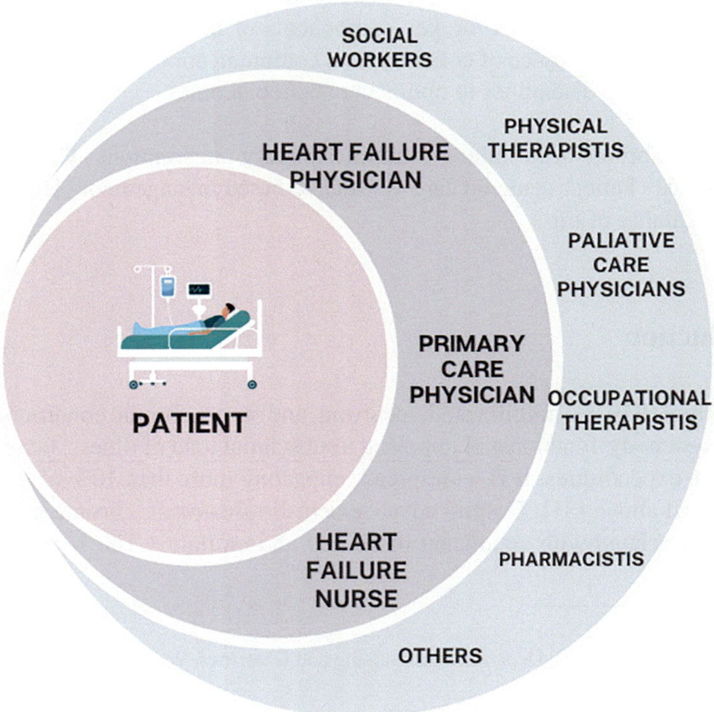

Fig. 20.1 Multidyscyplinary team approach in heart failure care

healthcare systems for delivering optimal care to individuals living with HF, with a focus on improving overall outcomes. Morton and colleagues have categorized MDT interventions into various segments, such as education, self-monitoring and self-management, telemonitoring, medication management and cardiac rehabilitation [26]. Education, self-monitoring, and self-management typically entail instructing patients on adhering to low-sodium diets, regularly checking vital signs, and daily weight monitoring. Telemonitoring of these parameters enhances patient care by involving the expertise of healthcare professionals, often led by an HF nurse. This allows for timely advice and quicker follow-up scheduling to prevent emergency room visits. Medication management involves educating patients on the purpose and potential side effects of each medication, ultimately promoting better adherence. Cardiac rehabilitation integrates evidence-based exercise interventions, which can be conducted either individually or in group settings. In addition to these elements, a multidisciplinary approach may encompass additional services such as psychological support and palliative care [29]. The core team members of this model typically consist of a heart failure physician, a heart failure nurse, and a primary care physician. Complementing this core are other essential team members, including pharmacists, physical therapists, occupational therapists, social workers, and palliative care physicians [29]. The emergency department (ED) serves as the initial point of contact for approximately 80% of individuals suspected of having heart failure (HF). It is often the place where diagnostic assessments and early medical management determinations are made [14]. The early engagement of a multidisciplinary team (MDT) in the ED, comprising cardiologists, HF nurses, geriatricians, and clinical pharmacists, in a patient's care paves the way for a seamless transition to outpatient care upon discharge. To streamline the process, it is advisable to implement a standardized heart failure protocol within the ED. Many hospitals have introduced special heart Failure pathways which encompass standardized orders for acute diuretic therapy, the initiation of guideline-directed medical therapy (GDMT), and consultations with MDT members. Moreover, an efficient triage strategy that involves admitting high-risk patients while discharging low-risk patients with prompt outpatient follow-up has proven effective in reducing the 30-day risk of mortality and hospitalizations related to cardiovascular issues [21]. Considering the robust evidence supporting various heart failure (HF) interventions, particularly guideline-directed medical therapy (GDMT), it becomes imperative to implement quality improvement strategies that maximize evidence-based care. Notably, the wealth of data regarding the initiation of GDMT during hospitalization is compelling, indicating the safety and efficacy of commencing beta-blockers [13], angiotensin receptor/neprilysin [38], and mineralocorticoid receptor antagonists in HF patients admitted to hospitals [9]. Proactive initiatives aimed at initiating and optimizing neurohormonal blockade before hospital follow-up may help mitigate therapeutic hesitancy in the context of GDMT. In addition to therapeutic measures, comprehensive patient education delivered collaboratively by the medical team, nursing staff, and pharmacy plays a pivotal role. An educational approach that encompasses lifestyle modifications, medication guidance, and the development of a post-discharge plan inclusive of cardiac rehabilitation can significantly enhance patient compliance with both pharmacological and non-pharmacological therapies [39]. Due to the persistent issue of high readmission rates among heart failure (HF) patients, it's imperative to initiate discharge planning early in their hospital stay. A significant number of patients experience severe deconditioning upon discharge, and some may rapidly deteriorate during prolonged hospitalizations.

In stark contrast to the steady stream of international clinical guideline recommendations, [3, 17, 24] cardiac rehabilitation still appears to occupy the role of the 'Cinderella' in heart failure management, with fewer than 20% of patients in both Europe and the USA [6, 27, 35]. Perhaps even more concerning is the fact that recent authoritative editorials and commentaries have conspicuously omitted any mention of the necessity, significance, and availability of cardiac rehabilitation for heart failure patients, despite its proven advantages and merits [2]. This disconnect between established guidance and real-world implementation underscores the urgent need for a paradigm shift in the approach to heart failure care and the integration of cardiac rehabilitation as a fundamental component of patient management.

Cardiac rehabilitation represents a comprehensive therapeutic approach encompassing exercise training, dietary education, and psychosocial support. The HF-ACTION trial, a groundbreaking investigation into the safety and effectiveness of cardiac rehabilitation, underscored its positive impact. The trial demonstrated improvements in patients' quality of life (QOL) and suggested a favorable trend toward reduced mortality and rehospitalization, particularly in patients with HF and reduced ejection fraction (HFrEF) [28]. Moreover, cardiac rehabilitation likely extends its benefits to patients with HF and preserved ejection fraction (HFpEF). An in-depth review and meta-analysis unveiled that exercise therapy enhances oxygen consumption, the 6-minute walk distance, and QOL in patients with HFpEF [15]. Despite the compelling evidence supporting its advantages and cost-effectiveness, cardiac rehabilitation remains underutilized [7].

Considering that many patients return home following HF hospitalization, home health services assume a pivotal role in their continued care. These services often involve medication management, monitoring vital signs and weights, and early recognition of signs and symptoms of decompensation. Nevertheless, the landscape of these services is remarkably diverse, posing challenges when it comes to assessing their effectiveness. Transition care services, which encompass nurse home visits and disease management clinics, exhibit considerable potential in reducing all-cause mortality and rehospitalizations, all while contributing to cost savings [37]. Therefore, their role in ensuring smoother post-hospitalization transitions is invaluable. Due to the inherent diversity of multidisciplinary teams (MDT) within various healthcare systems, conducting comprehensive studies to ascertain their efficacy can be a formidable task. The majority of individual studies, often constrained by limited sample sizes, do suggest a tendency towards reducing both mortality and heart failure hospitalizations, albeit frequently failing to reach the threshold of statistical significance. Yet, when aggregated in systematic reviews and meta-analyses, the collective body of evidence for MDT interventions reveals a more consistent and robust benefit. Numerous systematic reviews conducted over the past two decades have strived to standardize MDT interventions to enhance the reliability of comparisons. As an example, McAlister and colleagues conducted a review revealing that strategies involving specialized multidisciplinary follow-up were associated with significant reductions in both mortality rates and overall hospitalizations [23]. Interestingly, patient education in self-care activities and telephone follow-ups exhibited positive trends in reducing these parameters, although the statistical significance was not achieved. Moreover, a Cochrane review by Takeda et al. [34]

The endorsement of MDT in heart failure management is unequivocally reinforced by the 2021 European Society of Cardiology (ESC) Guidelines and the 2022 American Heart Association (AHA)/American College of Cardiology (ACC) Guidelines, which confer Class IA and IB recommendations, respectively [17, 24]. This substantiates the pivotal role of MDTs in optimizing heart failure care, emphasizing their vital contribution to improved patient outcomes and the imperative need for their consistent and widespread implementation. The seamless transition from inpatient to outpatient care assumes paramount significance, particularly for heart failure (HF) patients who face their highest risk of decompensation and readmission during the initial weeks post-discharge [17]. The importance of early and aggressive titration of guideline-directed medical therapy (GDMT) to reach recommended doses immediately after discharge cannot be overstated. This approach has demonstrated its potential to significantly reduce the risk of 180-day all-cause mortality or heart failure-related readmissions [25].

The hallmark of an exemplary outpatient multidisciplinary team (MDT) model is its unwavering patient-centric orientation and comprehensive approach to managing not only HF but also its co-morbid conditions, which may include arrhythmias, hypertension, diabetes, renal dysfunction, and psychological issues Guidelines detail aspects of self-care and patient education [24, 25]. Beyond the core team members, such as primary care physicians, geriatricians, advanced practice providers, and clinical pharmacists, the MDT is further enriched by the contributions of dieticians, social workers, and community healthcare workers, all of whom play indispensable roles in the holistic management of heart failure [17]. The continuity of care from the inpatient to outpatient settings, coupled with the prompt and judicious use of GDMT, represents a pivotal junction where a patient's journey towards improved heart failure management and enhanced quality of life can be decisively influenced. Furthermore, the expanded roles of various healthcare professionals within the MDT demonstrate a holistic approach that addresses the multifaceted nature of heart failure and its associated complexities. This underscores the collective effort required to provide comprehensive, patient-centered, and effective care for individuals living with heart failure.

In community-based healthcare, the delivery of a substantial portion of both cardiac and non-cardiac care to patients with heart failure (HF) heavily relies on primary care physicians (PCPs). These PCPs are responsible for offering rapid outpatient follow-up post-hospitalization, assessing signs and symptoms of congestion, making medication adjustments, and closely monitoring renal function and electrolyte levels. Nonetheless, the effect of directly incorporating PCPs into the multidisciplinary team (MDT) on critical factors like mortality, hospitalization rates, and patient-reported outcome measures (PROMs) remains unclear. To address this question, Raat et al. conducted a systematic review and meta-analysis [32]. Their study investigated how the direct involvement of PCPs in the MDT influenced clinical outcomes, encompassing all-cause readmissions, HF-specific readmissions, all-cause mortality, and PROMs. While their analysis demonstrated that MDT involvement reduced HF readmissions and enhanced PROMs, it could not draw definitive conclusions. Thus, despite the critical role of PCPs in caring for HF patients, the specific impact of their direct integration into the MDT remains unclear, necessitating further research to elucidate this potential benefit. With the ongoing physician shortage, advanced practice providers, including nurse practitioners and physician's assistants, have become indispensable in bridging the gap in patient care. Their responsibilities are expanding, particularly among nurse practitioners, where 70.3% are engaged in primary care. This implies they might be the first healthcare providers patients encounter post-HF hospitalization. Their contributions extend to pivotal roles in cardiology-specific care and multidisciplinary team (MDT) collaboration, rendering them invaluable collaborators for cardiologists. In a noteworthy quality improvement initiative led by Charteris et al., the establishment and utilization of a specialized multidisciplinary HF clinic within the Veterans Administration system, staffed by cardiology nurse practitioners, clinical pharmacists, and a dietitian, led to more veterans receiving care within 2 weeks of HF hospitalization. It also reduced the time between discharge and cardiology follow-up [10]. Apart from the care delivered by healthcare providers, it is imperative that patients take an active role as advocates for their own health. The multidisciplinary team (MDT) should play a pivotal role in promoting patient self-care. Furthermore, the integration of telehealth, device monitoring, electronic health records, and machine learning may open new avenues for enhancing multidisciplinary heart failure care [29].

As self-care management constitutes a critical component of HF treatment, healthcare practitioners working with HF patients acknowledge the necessity for more precise and tailored lifestyle advice recommendations. Self-care encompasses a set of health behaviors crucial for managing chronic illnesses [19, 33]. In the case of individuals with heart failure, this entails health maintenance activities such as medication adherence, dietary management, and exercise, along with the ability to recognize symptoms and respond promptly. Despite the advancements in heart failure treatments over the past decades, individuals with limited self-care capabilities are less likely to fully benefit from these therapeutic measures. This group faces a heightened risk of decompensation, recurrent hospitalizations, and increased mortality, primarily due to higher rates of medication non-adherence, missed medical appointments, and a reduced capacity to detect and respond to early warning signs of decompensation [18].

Assessing self-care capacity can be intricate, given the interplay of personal, family, and community factors. This complexity makes it challenging to identify individuals with a high risk of poor self-care. Nevertheless, the early identification of high-risk individuals can facilitate the implementation of corrective measures during the early stages of the disease. A comprehensive meta-analysis of 20 studies involving 5624 patients revealed that self-management interventions had a favorable impact on reducing heart failure-related hospitalizations and all-cause mortality. Notably, the duration of self-management showed a positive correlation with improved outcomes [18]. Skill training interventions have demonstrated substantial success, whereas interventions focused solely on education have shown mixed results [33]. Furthermore, there is an emerging body of evidence suggesting that personal technologies, such as electronic reminders, telemonitoring, and access to telemedicine, are poised to play a significant role in supporting self-care in the future [30].

Telehealth is a versatile approach that encompasses various methods, such as virtual patient visits, non-traditional multidisciplinary care, telehealth-driven cardiac rehabilitation, remote monitoring, mobile health (m-health) initiatives, and teleconsultations among healthcare professionals [12]. Heart failure's unique features, characterized by periods of stability punctuated by symptomatic phases requiring immediate attention, render it particularly well-suited for telehealth applications. One intriguing aspect of telehealth is its potential to enhance the initiation and optimization of guideline-directed medical therapy (GDMT) through remote interventions led by specialized heart failure teams. Desai et al. demonstrated that predefined algorithms executed by a remote centralized heart failure team improved rates of GDMT optimization while maintaining similar adverse event rates compared to the control group [11]. Similarly, the IMPLEMENT-HF trial, which evaluated the remote optimization of GDMT by a physician-pharmacist heart failure team during non-cardiovascular hospitalizations, reported enhanced GDMT optimization rates without significant safety concerns [5]. Additionally, the AMULET Study, a randomized controlled trial, showed that nurse-led non-invasive assessments combined with remote review and intervention by a cardiologist reduced the incidence of heart failure hospitalization and cardiovascular mortality in individuals with heart failure with reduced ejection fraction [20]. A meta-analysis of smaller studies that investigated telemonitoring of vital signs and weight, coupled with physician intervention, indicated reduced all-cause and cardiovascular mortality and hospitalization when compared to standard care [36]. However, the EMPOWER trial, which examined the benefits of remote monitoring for weight changes and diuretic adherence in individuals discharged after a heart failure admission, did not find a significant difference in all-cause mortality or readmission rates [4].

Considering the limitations of weight-based volume status monitoring, innovative devices for hemodynamic assessment have become an integral component of multidisciplinary team (MDT) care. One such device is the CardioMEMS, an implantable, wireless system designed for pulmonary artery (PA) pressure monitoring. This device, surgically placed in the pulmonary artery during right heart catheterization, continually tracks pulmonary artery pressure, offering insights into a patient's intracardiac filling pressures. These filling pressures tend to rise before visible clinical signs of congestion appear. By closely monitoring these readings, healthcare providers can proactively adjust diuretic doses or intensify the use of neurohormonal blockade agents to prevent decompensation, hospitalization, and potentially even mortality [40]. Clinical trials have shown the CardioMEMS device to be effective in reducing heart failure (HF) hospitalizations among patients with

HF, regardless of their ejection fraction and NYHA class. Studies conducted over 6 and 18 months demonstrated promising outcomes [1, 16]. However, a larger randomized trial that included patients with NYHA class II-IV symptoms yielded inconclusive results regarding the device's benefits, possibly due to the influence of the COVID-19 pandemic [22]. As these devices undergo further enhancements and their usage becomes more widespread, continued assessment of prospective and retrospective data is essential to establish conclusive findings regarding the efficacy of PA pressure sensors.

Summary

The scope of the heart failure epidemic necessitates a concerted effort from a diverse range of healthcare disciplines, extending beyond the realm of cardiology. The adoption of multidisciplinary heart failure care is paramount in mitigating the morbidity, mortality, and economic consequences associated with heart failure. As we navigate the evolving landscape of heart failure management, it is evident that the responsibility for heart failure patient care will increasingly extend beyond the purview of cardiologists. To best address the complex demands of heart failure, a multidisciplinary approach should be instituted at the time of diagnosis, and its implementation should span the entire continuum of the disease course. While there isn't a one-size-fits-all solution, a well-rounded model encompassing clinic-based care, home-based programs, and efficient case management may hold the potential to yield the most significant impact on patient outcomes. Clinical trials have yielded diverse results with respect to specific MDT interventions, but education and empowering patients for self-care play pivotal roles in achieving favorable outcomes.

Furthermore, exploring the integration of novel technologies as complementary tools in heart failure care deserves closer examination. These emerging technologies may offer innovative solutions for enhancing patient management and support, especially in remote or underserved areas. As the quest to provide equitable healthcare continues, concerted efforts should be made to address and mitigate healthcare disparities while simultaneously maintaining cost-effective practices. In the grand scheme of heart failure management, a paradigm shift toward prevention at the primary care level is essential to preempt the onset of heart failure. An emphasis on comprehensive preventive strategies, along with early detection and management of risk factors, will be pivotal in alleviating the burden of heart failure and steering us toward a healthier future.

The multidisciplinary team (MDT) approach is widely regarded as the most effective model for providing care to heart failure (HF) patients. Nevertheless, to establish efficient multidisciplinary HF services, it is essential to comprehend the pertinent evidence base, the fundamental elements of an MDT approach, and how these services may develop over time.

References

1. Abraham WT, Adamson PB, Bourge RC, Aaron MF, Costanzo MR, Stevenson LW, Strickland W, Neelagaru S, Raval N, Krueger S, Weiner S, Shavelle D, Jeffries B, Yadav JS, CHAMPION Trial Study Group. Wireless pulmonary artery haemodynamic monitoring in chronic heart failure: a randomised controlled trial. Lancet (London, England). 2011;377(9766):658–66. https://doi.org/10.1016/S0140-6736(11)60101-3.
2. Adamo M, Gardner RS, McDonagh TA, Metra M. The 'Ten Commandments' of the 2021 ESC Guidelines for the diagnosis and treatment of acute and chronic heart failure. Eur Heart J. 2022;43(6):440–1. https://doi.org/10.1093/eurheartj/ehab853.
3. Ambrosetti M, Abreu A, Corrà U, Davos CH, Hansen D, Frederix I, Iliou MC, Pedretti RFE, Schmid J-P, Vigorito C, Voller H, Wilhelm M, Piepoli MF, Bjarnason-Wehrens B, Berger T, Cohen-Solal A, Cornelissen V, Dendale P, Doehner W, et al. Secondary prevention through comprehensive cardiovascular rehabilitation: from knowledge to implementation. 2020 update. A position paper from the Secondary Prevention and Rehabilitation Section of the European Association of Preventive Cardiology. Eur J Prev Cardiol. 2021;28(5):460–95. https://doi.org/10.1177/2047487320913379.
4. Asch DA, Troxel AB, Goldberg LR, Tanna MS, Mehta SJ, Norton LA, Zhu J, Iannotte LG, Klaiman T, Lin Y, Russell LB, Volpp KG. Remote monitoring and behavioral economics in managing heart failure in patients discharged from the hospital: a randomized clinical trial. JAMA Intern Med. 2022;182(6):643–9. https://doi.org/10.1001/jamainternmed.2022.1383.
5. Bhatt AS, Varshney AS, Nekoui M, Moscone A, Cunningham JW, Jering KS, Patel PN, Sinnenberg LE, Bernier TD, Buckley LF, Cook BM, Dempsey J, Kelly J, Knowles DM, Lupi K, Malloy R, Matta LS, Rhoten MN, Sharma K, …, Vaduganathan M. Virtual optimization of guideline-directed medical therapy in hospitalized patients with heart failure with reduced ejection fraction: the IMPLEMENT-HF pilot study. Eur J Heart Fail. 2021;23(7):1191–201. https://doi.org/10.1002/ejhf.2163.
6. Bjarnason-Wehrens B, McGee H, Zwisler A-D, Piepoli MF, Benzer W, Schmid J-P, Dendale P, Pogosova N-GV, Zdrenghea D, Niebauer J, Mendes M, Cardiac Rehabilitation Section European Association of Cardiovascular Prevention and Rehabilitation. Cardiac rehabilitation in Europe: results from the European Cardiac Rehabilitation Inventory Survey. Eur J Cardiovasc Prev Rehabil. 2010;17(4):410–8. https://doi.org/10.1097/HJR.0b013e328334f42d.
7. Bozkurt B, Fonarow GC, Goldberg LR, Guglin M, Josephson RA, Forman DE, Lin G, Lindenfeld J, O'Connor C, Panjrath G, Piña IL, Shah T, Sinha SS, Wolfel E. Cardiac rehabilitation for patients with heart failure: JACC expert panel. J Am Coll Cardiol. 2021;77(11):1454–69. https://doi.org/10.1016/j.jacc.2021.01.030.
8. Bragazzi NL, Zhong W, Shu J, Abu Much A, Lotan D, Grupper A, Younis A, Dai H. Burden of heart failure and underlying causes in 195 countries and territories from 1990 to 2017. Eur J Prev Cardiol. 2021;28(15):1682–90. https://doi.org/10.1093/eurjpc/zwaa147.
9. Butler J, Anstrom KJ, Felker GM, Givertz MM, Kalogeropoulos AP, Konstam MA, Mann DL, Margulies KB, McNulty SE, Mentz RJ, Redfield MM, Tang WHW, Whellan DJ, Shah M, Desvigne-Nickens P, Hernandez AF, Braunwald E, For the National Heart Lung and Blood Institute Heart Failure Clinical Research Network. Efficacy and safety of spironolactone in acute heart failure: the ATHENA-HF randomized clinical trial. JAMA Cardiol. 2017;2(9):950–8. https://doi.org/10.1001/jamacardio.2017.2198.
10. Charteris EJ, Pounds B. A nurse practitioner-led effort to reduce 30-day heart failure readmissions. J Am Assoc Nurse Pract. 2020;32(11):738–44. https://doi.org/10.1097/JXX.0000000000000470.
11. Desai AS, Maclean T, Blood AJ, Bosque-Hamilton J, Dunning J, Fischer C, Fera L, Smith KV, Wagholikar K, Zelle D, Gaziano T, Plutzky J, Scirica B, MacRae CA. Remote optimization of guideline-directed medical therapy in patients with heart failure with reduced ejection fraction. JAMA Cardiol. 2020;5(12):1430–4. https://doi.org/10.1001/jamacardio.2020.3757.

12. Fedson S, Bozkurt B. Telehealth in heart failure. Heart Fail Clin. 2022;18(2):213–21. https://doi.org/10.1016/j.hfc.2021.12.001.
13. Fonarow GC, Abraham WT, Albert NM, Stough WG, Gheorghiade M, Greenberg BH, O'Connor CM, Sun JL, Yancy CW, Young JB. Influence of beta-blocker continuation or withdrawal on outcomes in patients hospitalized with heart failure: findings from the OPTIMIZE-HF program. J Am Coll Cardiol. 2008;52(3):190–9. https://doi.org/10.1016/j.jacc.2008.03.048.
14. Fonarow GC, ADHERE Scientific Advisory Committee. The Acute Decompensated Heart Failure National Registry (ADHERE): opportunities to improve care of patients hospitalized with acute decompensated heart failure. Rev Cardiovasc Med. 2003;4(Suppl 7):S21–30.
15. Fukuta H, Goto T, Wakami K, Kamiya T, Ohte N. Effects of exercise training on cardiac function, exercise capacity, and quality of life in heart failure with preserved ejection fraction: a meta-analysis of randomized controlled trials. Heart Fail Rev. 2019;24(4):535–47. https://doi.org/10.1007/s10741-019-09774-5.
16. Givertz MM, Stevenson LW, Costanzo MR, Bourge RC, Bauman JG, Ginn G, Abraham WT, CHAMPION Trial Investigators. Pulmonary artery pressure-guided management of patients with heart failure and reduced ejection fraction. J Am Coll Cardiol. 2017;70(15):1875–86. https://doi.org/10.1016/j.jacc.2017.08.010.
17. Heidenreich PA, Bozkurt B, Aguilar D, Allen LA, Byun JJ, Colvin MM, Deswal A, Drazner MH, Dunlay SM, Evers LR, Fang JC, Fedson SE, Fonarow GC, Hayek SS, Hernandez AF, Khazanie P, Kittleson MM, Lee CS, Link MS, et al. 2022 AHA/ACC/HFSA Guideline for the Management of Heart Failure: a report of the American College of Cardiology/American Heart Association Joint Committee on Clinical Practice Guidelines. Circulation. 2022;145(18):e895–e1032. https://doi.org/10.1161/CIR.0000000000001063.
18. Jonkman NH, Westland H, Groenwold RHH, Ågren S, Atienza F, Blue L, Bruggink-André de la Porte PWF, DeWalt DA, Hebert PL, Heisler M, Jaarsma T, Kempen GIJM, Leventhal ME, Lok DJA, Mårtensson J, Muñiz J, Otsu H, Peters-Klimm F, Rich MW, et al. Do self-management interventions work in patients with heart failure? An individual patient data meta-analysis. Circulation. 2016;133(12):1189–98. https://doi.org/10.1161/CIRCULATIONAHA.115.018006.
19. Kent B, Cull E, Phillips NM. A systematic review of the effectiveness of current interventions to assist adults with heart failure to comply with therapy and enhance self-care behaviours. JBI Libr Syst Rev. 2011;9(59):2572–626. https://doi.org/10.11124/01938924-201109590-00001.
20. Krzesiński P, Jankowska EA, Siebert J, Galas A, Piotrowicz K, Stańczyk A, Siwołowski P, Gutknecht P, Chrom P, Murawski P, Walczak A, Szalewska D, Banasiak W, Ponikowski P, Gielerak G. Effects of an outpatient intervention comprising nurse-led non-invasive assessments, telemedicine support and remote cardiologists' decisions in patients with heart failure (AMULET study): a randomised controlled trial. Eur J Heart Fail. 2022;24(3):565–77. https://doi.org/10.1002/ejhf.2358.
21. Lee DS, Straus SE, Farkouh ME, Austin PC, Taljaard M, Chong A, Fahim C, Poon S, Cram P, Smith S, McKelvie RS, Porepa L, Hartleib M, Mitoff P, Iwanochko RM, MacDougall A, Shadowitz S, Abrams H, Elbarasi E, et al. Trial of an intervention to improve acute heart failure outcomes. N Engl J Med. 2023;388(1):22–32. https://doi.org/10.1056/NEJMoa2211680.
22. Lindenfeld J, Zile MR, Desai AS, Bhatt K, Ducharme A, Horstmanshof D, Krim SR, Maisel A, Mehra MR, Paul S, Sears SF, Sauer AJ, Smart F, Zughaib M, Castaneda P, Kelly J, Johnson N, Sood P, Ginn G, et al. Haemodynamic-guided management of heart failure (GUIDE-HF): a randomised controlled trial. Lancet (London, England). 2021;398(10304):991–1001. https://doi.org/10.1016/S0140-6736(21)01754-2.
23. McAlister FA, Stewart S, Ferrua S, McMurray JJJV. Multidisciplinary strategies for the management of heart failure patients at high risk for admission: a systematic review of randomized trials. J Am Coll Cardiol. 2004;44(4):810–9. https://doi.org/10.1016/j.jacc.2004.05.055.
24. McDonagh TA, Metra M, Adamo M, Gardner RS, Baumbach A, Böhm M, Burri H, Butler J, Čelutkienė J, Chioncel O, Cleland JGF, Coats AJS, Crespo-Leiro MG, Farmakis D, Gilard M, Heymans S, Hoes AW, Jaarsma T, Jankowska EA, …, ESC Scientific Document Group.

2021 ESC Guidelines for the diagnosis and treatment of acute and chronic heart failure: developed by the Task Force for the diagnosis and treatment of acute and chronic heart failure of the European Society of Cardiology (ESC) with the special contribution of the Heart Failure Association (HFA) of the ESC. Eur Heart J. 2021;42(36):3599–726. https://doi.org/10.1093/eurheartj/ehab368.

25. Mebazaa A, Davison B, Chioncel O, Cohen-Solal A, Diaz R, Filippatos G, Metra M, Ponikowski P, Sliwa K, Voors AA, Edwards C, Novosadova M, Takagi K, Damasceno A, Saidu H, Gayat E, Pang PS, Celutkiene J, Cotter G. Safety, tolerability and efficacy of up-titration of guideline-directed medical therapies for acute heart failure (STRONG-HF): a multinational, open-label, randomised, trial. Lancet (London, England). 2022;400(10367):1938–52. https://doi.org/10.1016/S0140-6736(22)02076-1.
26. Morton G, Masters J, Cowburn PJ. Multidisciplinary team approach to heart failure management. Heart. 2018;104(16):1376–82. https://doi.org/10.1136/heartjnl-2016-310598.
27. *National Heart Failure Audit (NHFA), 2021 summary report*. 2021, October 14. HQIP. https://www.hqip.org.uk/resource/national-heart-failure-audit-nhfa-2021-summary-report/
28. O'Connor CM, Whellan DJ, Lee KL, Keteyian SJ, Cooper LS, Ellis SJ, Leifer ES, Kraus WE, Kitzman DW, Blumenthal JA, Rendall DS, Miller NH, Fleg JL, Schulman KA, McKelvie RS, Zannad F, Piña IL, For the HF-ACTION Investigators. Efficacy and safety of exercise training in patients with chronic heart failure: HF-ACTION randomized controlled trial. JAMA. 2009;301(14):1439–50. https://doi.org/10.1001/jama.2009.454.
29. Olson M, Thompson Z, Xie L, Nair A. Broadening heart failure care beyond cardiology: challenges and successes within the landscape of multidisciplinary heart failure care. Curr Cardiol Rep. 2023;25(8):851–61. https://doi.org/10.1007/s11886-023-01907-5.
30. Park LG, Beatty A, Stafford Z, Whooley MA. Mobile phone interventions for the secondary prevention of cardiovascular disease. Prog Cardiovasc Dis. 2016;58(6):639–50. https://doi.org/10.1016/j.pcad.2016.03.002.
31. Ponikowski P, Voors AA, Anker SD, Bueno H, Cleland JGF, Coats AJS, Falk V, González-Juanatey JR, Harjola V-P, Jankowska EA, Jessup M, Linde C, Nihoyannopoulos P, Parissis JT, Pieske B, Riley JP, Rosano GMC, Ruilope LM, Ruschitzka F, et al. 2016 ESC Guidelines for the diagnosis and treatment of acute and chronic heart failure: the Task Force for the diagnosis and treatment of acute and chronic heart failure of the European Society of Cardiology (ESC). Developed with the special contribution of the Heart Failure Association (HFA) of the ESC. Eur J Heart Fail. 2016;18(8):891–975. https://doi.org/10.1002/ejhf.592.
32. Raat W, Smeets M, Janssens S, Vaes B. Impact of primary care involvement and setting on multidisciplinary heart failure management: a systematic review and meta-analysis. ESC Heart Fail. 2021;8(2):802–18. https://doi.org/10.1002/ehf2.13152.
33. Riegel B, Moser DK, Buck HG, Dickson VV, Dunbar SB, Lee CS, Lennie TA, Lindenfeld J, Mitchell JE, Treat-Jacobson DJ, Webber DE, American Heart Association Council on Cardiovascular and Stroke Nursing; Council on Peripheral Vascular Disease; and Council on Quality of Care and Outcomes Research. Self-care for the prevention and management of cardiovascular disease and stroke: a scientific statement for healthcare professionals from the American Heart Association. J Am Heart Assoc. 2017;6(9):e006997. https://doi.org/10.1161/JAHA.117.006997.
34. Takeda A, Martin N, Taylor RS, Taylor SJ. Disease management interventions for heart failure. Cochrane Database Syst Rev. 2019;1(1):CD002752. https://doi.org/10.1002/14651858.CD002752.pub4.
35. Taylor RS, Dalal HM, Zwisler A-D. Cardiac rehabilitation for heart failure: 'Cinderella' or evidence-based pillar of care? Eur Heart J. 2023;44(17):1511–8. https://doi.org/10.1093/eurheartj/ehad118.
36. Umeh CA, Torbela A, Saigal S, Kaur H, Kazourra S, Gupta R, Shah S. Telemonitoring in heart failure patients: systematic review and meta-analysis of randomized controlled trials. World J Cardiol. 2022;14(12):640–56. https://doi.org/10.4330/wjc.v14.i12.640.

37. Van Spall HGC, Rahman T, Mytton O, Ramasundarahettige C, Ibrahim Q, Kabali C, Coppens M, Brian Haynes R, Connolly S. Comparative effectiveness of transitional care services in patients discharged from the hospital with heart failure: a systematic review and network meta-analysis. Eur J Heart Fail. 2017;19(11):1427–43. https://doi.org/10.1002/ejhf.765.
38. Velazquez EJ, Morrow DA, DeVore AD, Duffy CI, Ambrosy AP, McCague K, Rocha R, Braunwald E. Angiotensin–neprilysin inhibition in acute decompensated heart failure. N Engl J Med. 2019;380(6):539–48. https://doi.org/10.1056/NEJMoa1812851.
39. Wahbi-Izzettin O, Hopper I, Ritchie E, Nagalingam V, Aung AK. United we stand, divided we conquer: pilot study of multidisciplinary general medicine heart failure care program. Intern Med J. 2018;48(2):178–83. https://doi.org/10.1111/imj.13647.
40. Zile MR, Bennett TD, St John Sutton M, Cho YK, Adamson PB, Aaron MF, Aranda JM, Abraham WT, Smart FW, Stevenson LW, Kueffer FJ, Bourge RC. Transition from chronic compensated to acute decompensated heart failure: pathophysiological insights obtained from continuous monitoring of intracardiac pressures. Circulation. 2008;118(14):1433–41. https://doi.org/10.1161/CIRCULATIONAHA.108.783910.

Part IV
Particular Forms of Heart Failure

Chapter 21
Heart Failure and Hypertension

Roxana Oana Darabont and Maria Dorobanţu

Abstract In developed countries, arterial hypertension carries the greatest population-attributable risk of heart failure. Overall, it is expected that almost 30% of hypertensive patients will develop heart failure over time. High blood pressure has a strong impact on the heart. The morphological and functional transformations induced by hypertension can promote not only left ventricular hypertrophy but also myocardial ischemia or rhythm disorders, each of them representing a potential contributor to the occurrence of heart failure. Left ventricular remodeling mediated by hypertension implies not only an increased size of myocytes but also the process of fibrogenesis. Myocardial ischemia has as its substrate an imbalance between demand and intake, and the appearance of microvascular dysfunction or atherosclerotic lesions in the epicardial coronary arteries, as well. Hypertensive patients usually develop heart failure with preserved ejection fraction. Although diastolic dysfunction can precede left ventricular hypertrophy, it is usually associated with it. The risk of heart failure increases greatly after the appearance of left ventricular hypertrophy. According to the complexity of hypertensive heart disease the diagnostic workup of hypertensive patients starts with electrocardiography and rest transthoracic echocardiography, but must be extended in specific cases with the imagistic evaluation of coronary arteries (angio-CT or conventional angiography), stress tests for myocardial ischemia or even evaluation of microvascular function and cardiac magnetic resonance imaging. Left ventricular hypertrophy, especially left ventricle fibrosis and left atrium dilatation are the main prognostic parameters that augment the risk of heart failure. With each 10 mmHg decrease in systolic blood pressure, the risk of HF falls by 12% making it possible to achieve a global reduction in the occurrence of HF by 50% or even more with antihypertensive treatment. Reducing the risk of heart failure involves the effects of antihypertensive

R. O. Darabont (✉)
Department of Cardiology and Cardiac Surgery—University Emergency Hospital, University of Medicine and Pharmacy "Carol Davila", Bucharest, Romania

M. Dorobanţu
University of Medicine and Pharmacy "Carol Davila", Bucharest, Romania

Romanian Academy, Bucharest, Romania

M. Dorobanţu et al. (eds.), *Current Approach to Heart Failure*,
https://doi.org/10.1007/978-3-031-96562-3_21

treatment on left ventricular hypertrophy, coronary artery disease, mostly acute events, and the occurrence of atrial fibrillation. Thiazides and thiazide-like diuretics are likely the ideal agent for heart failure prevention followed by ACEi/ARBs.

Keywords Arterial hypertension · Heart failure · Left ventricular hypertrophy · Myocardial ischemia

Abbreviations

ACEIs	angiotensin-converting enzyme inhibitors
ARBs	angiotensin-receptor blockers
BBs	beta-blockers
BMI	body mass index
BP	blood pressure
CCBs	calcium-channel blockers
CV	cardiovascular
EDV	end-diastolic volume of left ventricle
EF	ejection fraction
ESV	end-systolic volume of left ventricle
GLS	global longitudinal strain
HF	heart failure
HFpEF	heart failure with preserved ejection fraction
HFrEF	heart failure with preserved ejection fraction
HHD	hypertensive heart disease
HTN	hypertension
IVSd	thickness of interventricular septum at the end of diastole;
LA	left atrium
LVIDd	left ventricular internal diameter at the end of diastole
LVH	left ventricular hypertrophy
LVM	left ventricular mass
LVPWd	thickness of the posterior wall at the end of the diastole
MRI	magnetic resonance imaging

Introduction

In developed countries, arterial hypertension (HTN), along with ischemic heart disease, is the main contributor to the occurrence of heart failure (HF) [1]. The risk of myocardial damage is much higher after a heart attack than that due to prolonged exposure to increased blood pressure (BP) values, but due to its prevalence, HTN carries, in fact, the greatest population-attributable risk of HF [2]. The Framingham Heart Study highlighted the relationship between HTN and HF, confirmed by a large body of evidence since then [2]. This proved to be valid even for slight increases in BP, as long as patients with no history of HTN or cardiovascular (CV) diseases have a 3 times higher risk of CV complications if BP is ≥130/85 mmHg compared with BP values <120/75 mmHg [3]. Overall, we can expect about 30% of hypertensive patients to develop HF [4] within approximately 14 years of the diagnosis of HTN [5].

High BP has a strong impact on the heart. The morphological and functional transformations induced by HTN can promote not only HF but also myocardial ischemia or rhythm disorders. The first definition of hypertensive heart disease (HHD) was proposed by the New York Heart Association in 1970: "anatomofunctional alterations characterized by left ventricular hypertrophy and cardiac failure in patients with systemic hypertension" [6]. In recent years the concept of heart damage mediated by HTN has very much evolved and integrates myocardial fibrosis in the development of left ventricular hypertrophy, the remodeling of the left atrium, and the dysfunction of coronary microcirculation. Thus, a more appropriate definition of HHD could be: "A constellation of changes in the left ventricle, left atrium, and coronary arteries as a result of a chronic blood pressure elevation, which increases the workload on the heart inducing structural and functional changes" [7].

In this chapter we will present the consequences of HTN on the morphology and function of the heart, the clinical manifestations and the diagnostic work-up of patients with HHD, and the current therapeutic options for this pathological condition.

Structural Modifications in Hypertensive Heart Disease

Left Ventricular Remodeling

Left ventricular remodeling represents the main effect of HTN on the heart. The term is attributed to Gibbons and Dzau [8] and consists of the attempt of the left ventricle to reduce the wall stress induced by persistent elevated blood pressures according to Laplace's law:

$$T = \frac{P \times R}{2h},$$

where T is the intraparietal tension, P is the intraventricular pressure induced by the systolic BP, R is the cavity radius and h is the thickness of the left ventricle walls.

As long as wall stress is indirectly proportional to 2 times the thickness of left ventricular walls, an intraparietal pressure increased by the systolic BP promotes the augmentation of left ventricle walls. This pressure overload leads to concentric hypertrophy—in certain cases with a higher thickening of the basal interventricular septum, to increased left ventricular mass, and the reduction of the left ventricular cavity, as well [9]. The high BP load triggers gene expression configured to mediate myocyte hypertrophy and alterations in the extracellular matrix structure [10].

The main morphological modifications in left ventricular hypertrophy (LVH) are presented in Fig. 21.1. Not only do the myocytes increase in size with the multiplication of microtubule density, but they also lose their ability to relax due to the disarray of microtubules, abnormal calcium handling, and hyperphosphorylation of titin protein [11]. Another major contributor to the development of LVH is the process of fibrogenesis which affects the extracellular matrix. It is triggered by the transformation of fibroblasts into myofibroblasts and consists of an increased synthesis of collagen, especially of type I, at this level [12, 13]. It is currently considered that fibrosis is more relevant in HHD than in other causes of heart failure and is characterized by a diffuse and perivascular pattern of distribution [14]. It should be mentioned that myocardial fibrosis develops concomitantly with vascular fibrosis which is known to lead to arterial stiffness in the large arteries and narrowing of the small arteries with secondary hypoperfusion in different territories [15].

The hypertrophic response to pressure overload is highly variable because it is influenced not only by BP values but also by many other determinants like genetic factors [16], demographic factors (advanced age, black race, and female gender) [17–19], and comorbidities, of which obesity and diabetes mellitus are the most important [20, 21]. The development of LVH is strongly mediated by neuro-humoral systems such as the sympathetic nervous system or the renin-angiotensin-aldosterone system, which can be configurated differently from one individual to another [22].

BP values measured at the brachial level have been the most widely studied in correlation with LVH, but we must take into account that central BP values—influenced by the aortic stiffening process [23] or night-time BP levels—recorded during ambulatory blood pressure measurement [24] might contribute independently to left ventricular remodeling.

The prevalence of LVH among hypertensive patients varies with the studied population and the method applied for identification. Based on echocardiography its prevalence is estimated at 20% among hypertensive patients [25].

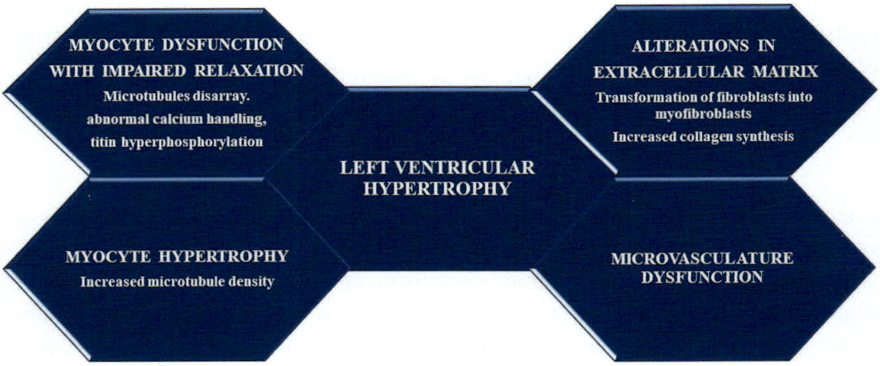

Fig. 21.1 Main histopathological modifications mediated by systemic hypertension in the heart

Other Structural Changes in the Heart Related to Systemic Hypertension

High BP is associated with increased left atrial (LA) size. LA changes are mostly related to left atrium-left ventricle coupling with high filling pressures of the ventricle transmitted to the atrium. As in the case of left ventricular remodeling, this process evolves with the activation of profibrotic cascades [26].

Few studies addressed the relationship between high BP and the right heart chambers. Nonetheless, convergent data are sustaining an association of HTN with right ventricular wall thickening and mass increase, as with the enlargement of the right atrium [27, 28].

It has been emphasized that systemic HTN represents a risk factor for the development of degenerative aortic valve disease [29] or mitral regurgitation [30] which, from the moment they appear and depending on the severity, can contribute to the promotion of heart failure.

Arterial Stiffening

High BP is one of the most important accelerators of the age-related stiffening process in the great arteries [31]. Aortic stiffness can have an important contribution to the development of HF in hypertensives: it increases the risk of LVH [32] and reduces the coronary flow due to the lowering of diastolic pressures in the aorta [33].

Functional and Clinical Consequences of Hypertension-Mediated Cardiac Involvement

The structural modifications that occur in the heart as a result of exposure to high BP have functional effects that lead to myocardial ischemia, arrhythmias, and especially heart failure (Fig. 21.2).

Myocardial Ischemia

Three different mechanisms can induce myocardial ischemia in hypertensive heart disease. The first mechanism is represented by the imbalance between oxygen and nutrient intake and the increased demand for a hypertrophied ventricle. An impaired diffusibility secondary to fibrosis developed in the extracellular matrix may further

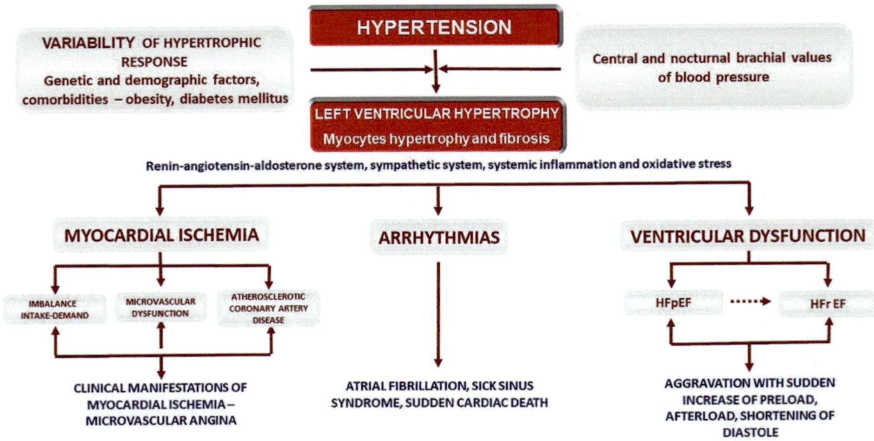

Fig. 21.2 Functional and clinical consequences of hypertension-mediated cardiac involvement. *HFpEF* heart failure with preserved ejection fraction, *HFrEF* heart failure with reduced ejection fraction

limit the blood gas exchange. The second contributor to myocardial ischemia is the microvascular dysfunction. The microvascular vessels constitute more than 70% of the coronary artery circulation: 60% arterioles and 15% capillaries [34]. In the context of HTN microcirculation undergoes systemical morphological and functional transformations. It was shown that microvascular changes in the periphery evolve in parallel with those in the coronary territory [35]. The remodeling process consists of intimal and smooth muscle cell thickening, smooth muscle cell proliferation, and perivascular fibrosis in arterioles, associated with rarefaction and obstruction in capillaries. The endothelium of these vessels becomes progressively dysfunctional manifesting impaired relaxation and in some cases vasospasm [36]. Systemic inflammation and oxidative stress can act as promotors of this phenomenon [37]. Impaired relaxation is responsible for the decrease in coronary flow reserve—an inability of the microvasculature to increase the myocardial flow in stress conditions, like exercise or tachycardia. It has been found that coronary flow reserve can be decreased in hypertensive patients even in the absence of left ventricular hypertrophy [38]. Moreover, microvascular dysfunction objectified by PET-CT along with a decreased global longitudinal strain proved to increase the risk of HF occurrence in patients with adaptative left ventricular remodeling [39]. The most typical manifestation of microvascular dysfunction is represented by angina which occurs in the absence of significant stenosis in the epicardial coronary arteries and is more frequent in women.

It is well known that HTN increases the risk of coronary artery disease [40]. It seems that the risk of incident atherosclerotic cardiovascular disease starts a stepwise increase even from systolic BP values of 90 mmHg [41]. For this reason, myocardial ischemia can also be induced in HHD by atherothrombotic lesions in the epicardial coronary arteries.

Arrythmias

Arterial hypertension is one of the main risk factors for incident atrial fibrillation [42]. The most important substrate for this rhythm disturbance is represented by the left atrial stretching leading to atrial dilatation and dysfunction. The fibrogenesis that characterizes the left ventricle hypertrophy is equally manifested in the left atrium and contributes to the arrhythmogenic process [43].

Along with aging, heart failure, or a history of CV disease, high BP is also recognized as a risk factor for sick sinus syndrome [44].

Not least, hypertensive patients carry the burden of an augmented risk of sudden death. Areas of electrical inhomogeneity may appear in the left ventricle with the progression of fibrosis and the architectural disarrangement of myocardial cells creating conditions for fatal arrhythmias [45].

Heart Failure

Hypertensive patients usually develop heart failure with preserved ejection fraction (HFpEF). Although diastolic dysfunction can precede LVH, it is usually associated with it. The risk of HF occurrence increases greatly after the appearance of left ventricular hypertrophy. Incidence of HF augments with 1% for every 1% increase in LV mass above the normal range on echocardiogram [46]. For many years, it was considered that heart failure with preserved EF mediated by HTN involves only diastolic mechanisms. All phases of diastole are indeed affected in a pathologically hypertrophied ventricle. The active relaxation that characterizes the rapid filling in diastole is impaired, on the one hand, by a decrease in the relaxation capacity of remodeled myocytes and, on the other hand, by the factors that maintain myocardial ischemia in the hypertrophied ventricle. The slow filling in diastole is a passive process strongly influenced by the fibrosis-induced stiffening of the left ventricle. In these conditions, the ventricular filling depends more than usual (20%) on the left atrial systole, which in turn, can be suppressed by the occurrence of atrial fibrillation. Nowadays, much evidence supports the development of an early systolic dysfunction along with the diastolic one, despite a well-preserved ejection fraction. The echocardiographic applications of tissue Doppler, strain, and speckle tracking have contributed to the understanding of this concept [47].

Although it is presumed that heart failure with reduced ejection fraction (HFrEF) evolves from HFpEF the evidence is scarce. Almost three decades ago the occurrence of a myocardial infarction represented a necessary event in the evolution from HFpEF to HFrEF for patients with HHD. However, large populational studies have emphasized that nearly half of the patients with HHD appeared to progress to systolic dysfunction in the absence of coronary artery disease [36]. A disproportionate myocyte loss [48] or an accelerated collagen breakdown could be involved in this deterioration of left ventricular function [49]. Regardless of the pathogenic substrate of the evolution towards HFrEF, it is important to consider, from a practical point of view, that patients with LVH and increased levels of markers reflecting myocardial injury such as NT-pro-BNP and troponin, may be considered at particularly high risk of developing symptomatic HFrEF [50]. Finally, even less explainable, but accepted by some authors, is the direct development of HFrEF without passing through the stage of LVH [5].

HFpEF mediated by HTN has specific etiopathogenic determinants. Small changes in preload or afterload, as well as shortening of diastole, can lead to severe aggravations of HF [51], even harder to endure by older patients with arterial stiffening and impaired natriuresis. In these patients, an altered coupling between the heart and vessels importantly affects cardiovascular reserve function [52].

Other contributors to the development of HF in hypertensive patients might be the dysfunction of the left atrium, right ventricle, or right atrium and, eventually, the association of degenerative aortic valve disease or mitral regurgitation [29, 30, 53, 54].

Diagnostic Workup of Hypertensive Heart Disease

Electrocardiography

Electrocardiography (ECG) is recommended for the routine evaluation of hypertensive patients [55]. It can reveal rhythm disturbances, like atrial fibrillation, or signs of left ventricular hypertrophy. The ECG criteria for LVH are presented in Table 21.1 [56]. The ECG specificity for LVH detection is high, but the sensitivity is low—in the range of 40–50%, even less in patients younger than 50 years old. The presence of strain—ST-T depression in lateral anterior leads—is the most important sign of LVH [57].

Echocardiography

Transthoracic echocardiography is the most useful investigation of the diagnostic workup in HHD. It offers the possibility to evaluate structural, but also functional modifications in the heart, like left ventricular abnormal relaxation or increased filling pressures.

The main hypertension-mediated structural modifications in the heart investigated with 2-D transthoracic echocardiography are listed in Table 21.2 [58]. Figure 21.3 shows a parasternal long-axis view which allows the measurement of the left ventricle walls and end-diastolic diameter of its cavity.

Table 21.1 Electrocardiographic criteria for left ventricular hypertrophy detection [56]

Sokolow-Lyon voltage criteria	$S_{V1} + R_{V5/V6} \geq 35$ mm (3.5 mV) or $R_{aVL} \geq 11$ mm (1.1 mV) $R_{aVL} \geq 1.3$ mm (1.3 mV) if left fascicular block	
Cornell criteria		
Cornell voltage	S_{V3} + RavL ≥ 20 mm—in women S_{V3} + RavL ≥ 28 mm—in men	
Cornell product Criteria for left ventricular hypertrophy	(Cornell voltage + 8 mm) × ORS duration—in women Cornell voltage × ORS duration—in men	Cornell product ≥ 2440 mm × ms
Romhilt-Estes criteria 4 points—probable left ventricular hypertrophy 5 points—definite left ventricular hypertrophy	R or S in any limb lead ≥ 20 mm or $S_{V1/V2}$, $R_{V5/V6} \geq 30$ mm	3 points
	ST-T strain	
	Taking digitalis Not taking digitalis	1 point 3 points
	P terminal force in V1 ≥ 1 mm in depth and ≥40 msec in duration	3 points
	Left axis deviation ≥ -30^0	1 point
	QRS duration ≥ 90 msec	1 point
	Intrinsecoid deflection in V5 or V6 ≥ 50 msec	

Table 21.2 Hypertension-mediated structural modifications in the heart in 2-D transthoracic echocardiography [58]

Left ventricular hypertrophy	Left ventricular mass calculated by Devereux cube formula based on interventricular septal thickness, posterior wall thickness, and left ventricular internal diameter at the end of diastole measured in parasternal long axis view either by M-mode, either directly in 2D	Diagnosis of LVH based on indexed left ventricular mass (LVM/BMI): >95 g/m^2—women >115 g/m^2—men
Left ventricular geometry	Relative wall thickness (RWTd = 2 × posterior wall thickness/left ventricular end-diastolic diameter)	≤0.42—concentric remodeling >0.42—eccentric remodeling
Left atrial volume	Measured by biplane method of disks or area-length technique	Indexed left atrial volume >34 mL/m^2

BMI body mass index, *LVH* left ventricular hypertrophy, *LVM* left ventricular mass

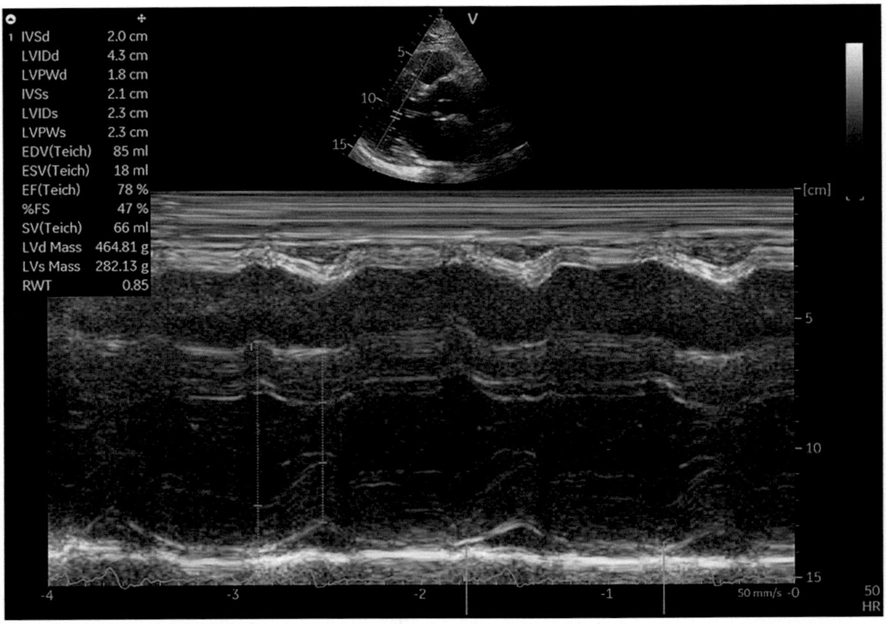

Fig. 21.3 Parasternal long axis view in 2D echocardiography. Calculation of left ventricular mass based on the measurement of left ventricular wall thickness and left ventricular internal diameter at the end of diastole in M-mode. For a male with a body mass index of 2.05, the indexed left ventricular mass is 464.81 g devised by 2.15, which is 226.73 g/m^2. An indexed left ventricular mass ≥ 149 g/m^2 in men indicates severe left ventricular hypertrophy. *IVSd* thickness of interventricular septum at the end of diastole, *LVPWd* thickness of the posterior wall at the end of diastole, *LVIDd* left ventricular internal diameter at the end of diastole

In recent years 3-D echocardiography has proven more accurate than 2-D echocardiography for the evaluation of left ventricle and left atrial volumes [58], as illustrated in Figs. 21.4 and 21.5.

The parameters of the diastolic function are identified based on:

- 2-D echocardiography—for indexed left atrial volume detection;
- Spectral Doppler—for the measurement of the ratio between peak velocity flow in early diastole (E wave) and peak velocity flow in late diastole caused by atrial contraction (A wave) and evaluation of tricuspid regurgitation velocity;
- Tissue Doppler imaging for the interrogation of septal and lateral early diastolic reversal wave (e') [59].

Figure 21.6 exemplifies the case of left ventricle diastolic dysfunction in a patient with HHD.

Finally, based on speckle tracking echocardiography it was emphasized that, despite a preserved ejection fraction, patients with hypertension-mediated heart

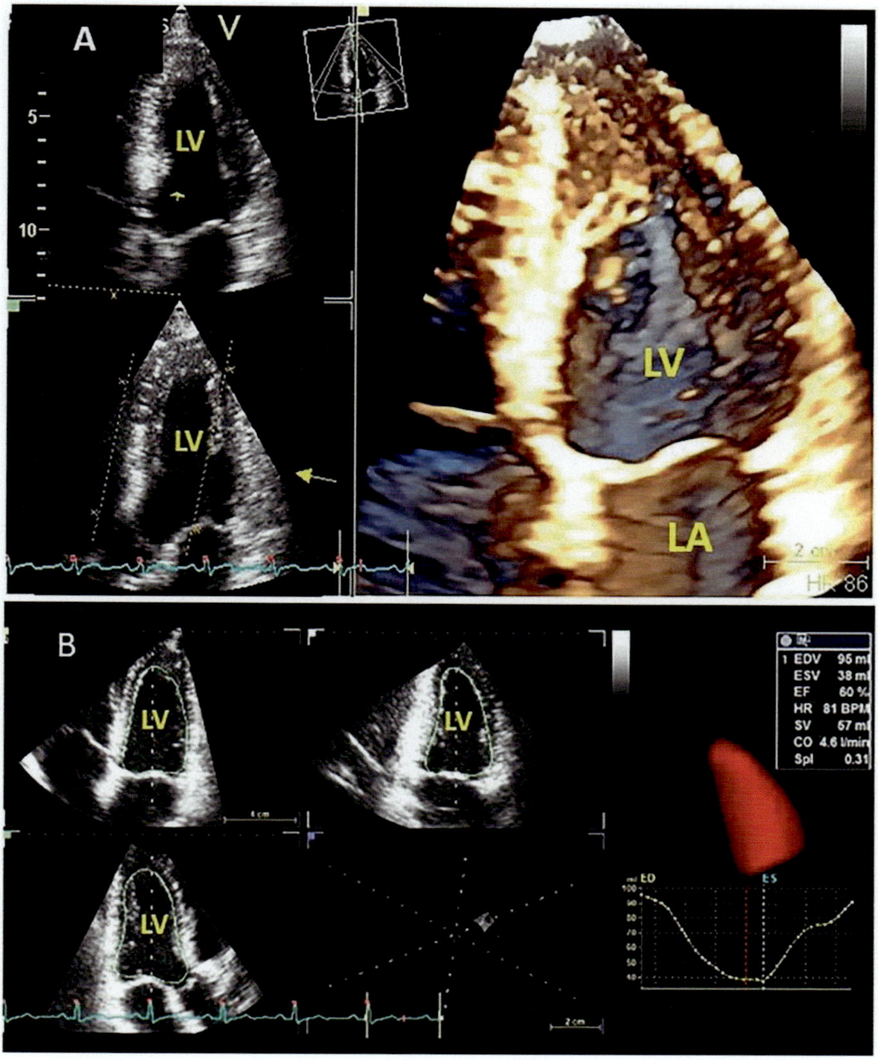

Fig. 21.4 Three-dimensional echocardiography for the assessment of left ventricle volumes and ejection fraction in a patient with left ventricular hypertrophy and preserved ejection fraction. (**Panel A**) Full volume of the left ventricle obtained by multi-beat acquisition; (**Panel B**) Measurements of the left ventricular volumes and ejection fraction by dedicated software. *EDV* end-diastolic volume is 95 ml, *ESV* end-systolic volume is 38 ml, *EF* ejection fraction is 60%

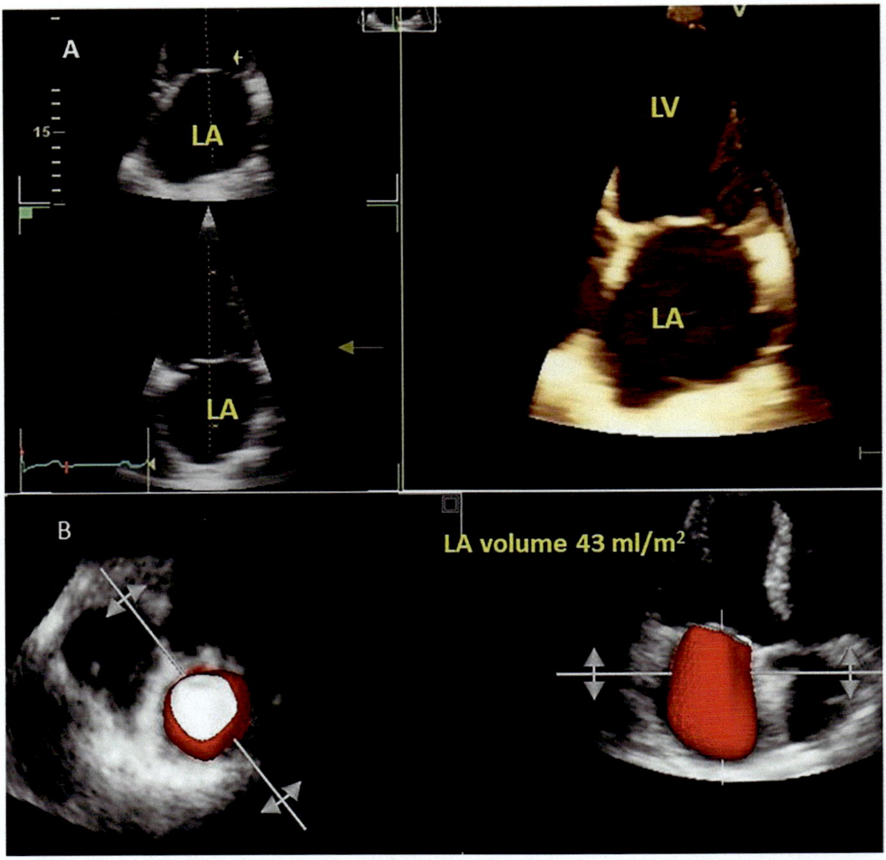

Fig. 21.5 Three-dimensional echocardiography for the assessment of left atrial volumes in a severely hypertensive patient with heart failure with preserved ejection fraction. (**Panel A**) Full volume of the left atrium; (**Panel B**) Measurements of the left atrial maximal volume by dedicated software. An indexed left atrium volume of 43 ml/m^2 indicates a severe enlargement. *LA* left atrium

determinations can be identified with subclinical impairment of systolic function that is assumed when global longitudinal strain is lower than 16% [60], as figured in Fig. 21.7.

Cardiac MRI

Due to its high accuracy for LVH diagnosis and the applications that allow the evaluation of fibrosis cardiac magnetic resonance imaging (MRI) is currently considered the gold standard for cardiac evaluation in HHD. However, it still has

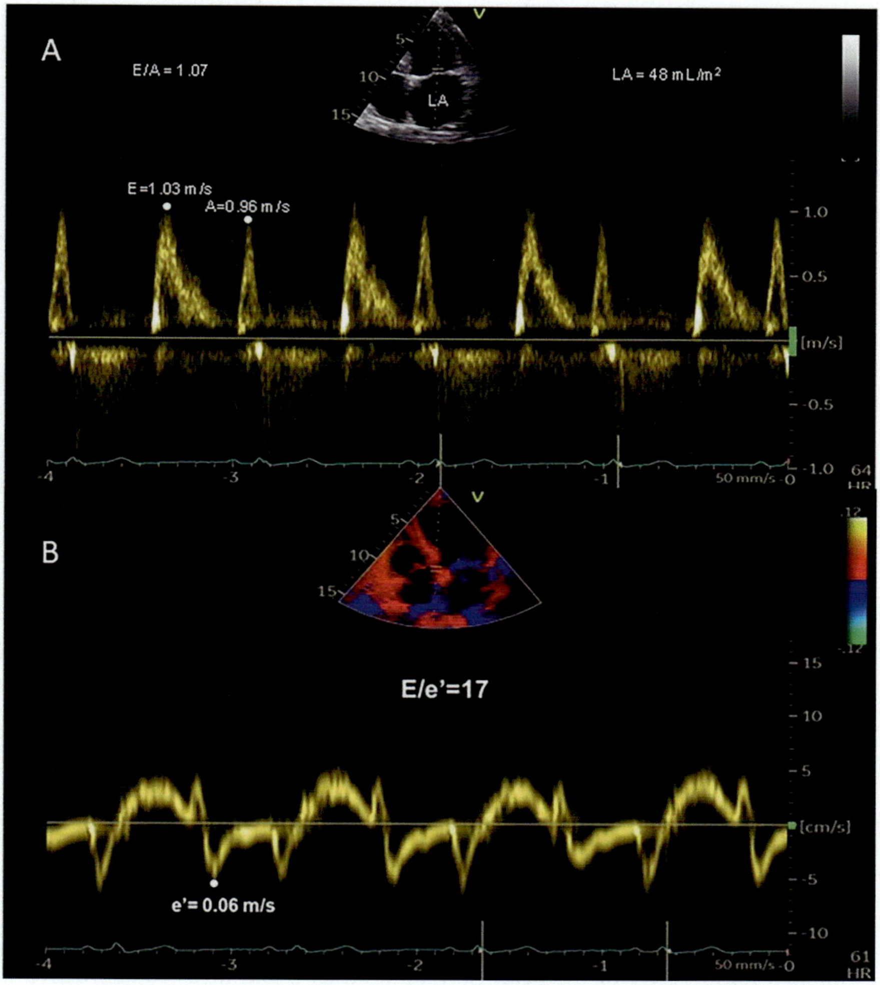

Fig. 21.6 Evaluation of left ventricular diastolic dysfunction. (**Panel A**) E/A ratio is 1.07 with a severely increased left atrial volume of 48 ml/m^2 (>34 ml/m^2); (**Panel B**) A septal E/e' is calculated to be 17 from the ratio between the peak flow velocity of left ventricular filling in early diastole (103 cm/sec) and the septal early diastolic reversal wave (6 cm/sec). In a patient with an E/A ratio of 1.07 (>0.8 and <2) an increased left atrial volume of 48 ml/m^2 (>34 ml/m^2) and an average of septal and lateral E/e' ratio of 17 (>14) supports high filling pressures in the context of a grade II diastolic dysfunction [59]

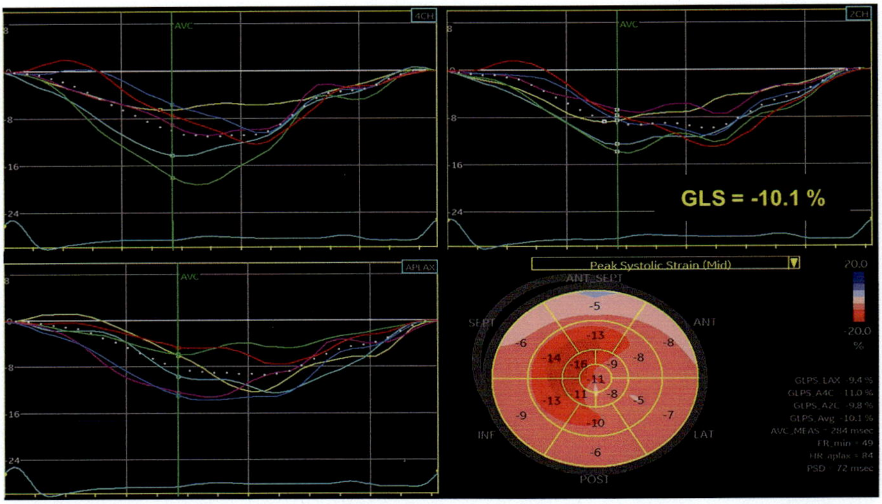

Fig. 21.7 Speckle tracking echocardiography detecting a low global longitudinal strain. A global longitudinal strain of 10.1% is decreased regarding the reference values higher than 18%. *GLS* global longitudinal strain

important limitations imposed by costs and accessibility. The main contributions of cardiac MRI to the evaluation of HHD are tissue characterization—using the late gadolinium enhancement [61], and T1 mapping for extracellular volume [62]. Figure 21.8 displays the morphological evaluation of a hypertrophied left ventricle by cardiac MRI.

Computed Tomography of the Heart

Computed tomography of the heart may be used as a non-invasive alternative to standard coronary angiography. It becomes very valuable for the diagnosis of cardiac microvascular dysfunction which implies, as a first step, the exclusion of significant atherosclerotic disease in epicardial arteries.

Evaluation of Microvascular Dysfunction

Hypertensive patients may develop microvascular dysfunction which must be suspected in patients with manifestations of myocardial ischemia but without hemodynamically significant atherosclerotic disease of the epicardial arteries. Hence, after the evaluation of coronary arteries, the diagnosis of microvascular disease must include:

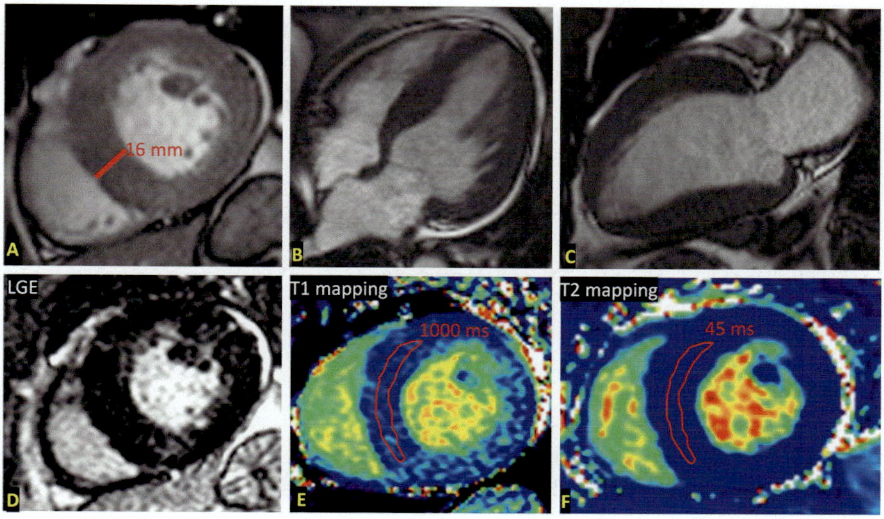

Fig. 21.8 Contrast-enhanced cardiovascular magnetic resonance imaging in a patient with hypertensive heart disease. End-diastolic cine images in short axis, 4 chambers, and 2 chambers views respectively (**a**, **b**, and **c**), showing left ventricular hypertrophy. The late Gadolinium enhancement imaging (**d**) shows patchy areas of myocardial fibrosis at the inferior insertion point. T1 mapping (**e**) identifies a discrete increase in native T1 values. T2 mapping (**f**) shows normal T2 values, excluding myocardial edema. (By courtesy of Dr. Sebastian Onciul from his archive)

- Presence of reversible defect, abnormality, or flow reserve on a functional imaging test like PET-scan, cardiac MRI, transthoracic Doppler echocardiography of left descendent artery;
- Invasive functional coronary angiography for measurement of coronary flow reserve and microvascular resistance with adenosine test [63].

Clinical Forms of Hypertensive Heart Disease

Of all the classifications of HHD we consider that the most practical is the one proposed by Gonzales-Maqueda and his colleagues which integrates the clinical manifestations of HHD with the subclinical effects of HTN on the heart [64] (Table 21.3).

Prognostic Implications of Hypertensive Heart Disease

Regardless of which diagnostic method is used, LVH is associated with a worse cardiovascular prognosis. ECG-based LVH predicts arrhythmias, including sudden cardiac death and atrial fibrillation, myocardial infarction, heart failure, and stroke,

Table 21.3 VIA classification of hypertensive heart disease [64]

Ventricle	0: Normal 1: LVH 2: Diastolic dysfunction/failure 3: Systolic failure
Ischemia	0: Not clinically manifest 1: Microvascular angina/ischemia 2: Macrovascular angina/ischemia 3: Myocardial infarction
Atrial fibrillation	0: None 1: Paroxistical 2: Permanent 3: Embolic

LVH left ventricular hypertrophy

with ECG strain being one of the strongest determinants. Among the morphological parameters related to LVH, indexed left ventricular mass influences mostly the cardiovascular prognosis [65].

Other cardiac parameters that have proven a significant influence on prognosis in hypertensive patients are: myocardial fibrosis [66], left atrial enlargement [67], and left atrioventricular coupling index defined by the ratio between left atrial end-diastolic volume and end-diastolic left ventricle diastolic volume [68].

Treatment of Patients with Hypertensive Heart Disease

With each 10 mmHg decrease in systolic BP, the risk of HF falls by 12% making it possible to achieve a global reduction in the occurrence of HF by 50% or even more with antihypertensive treatment [69]. Reducing the risk of HF involves the effects of antihypertensive treatment on LVH, coronary artery disease—mostly acute events—and the occurrence of atrial fibrillation.

Regression of Left Ventricular Hypertrophy

LVH can regress under antihypertensive treatment but this process is slow and of small amplitude. However, the reduction of left ventricular mass can lead to a reduction in risk events [70]. According to a meta-analysis angiotensin-converting enzyme inhibitors (ACEIs), angiotensin-receptors blockers (ARBs), and calcium-channel blockers (CCBs) appeared to be most effective at reducing LVH [71].

Innovative therapies are currently targeting the process of fibrogenesis and have promising results, as was also proven for sacubitril/valsartan [72–74]. Still, we have to bear in mind that an aggressive attempt to interfere with the extracellular matrix might have harmful effects on myocardial architecture as long as the loss of collagen from the interstitium has been noticed as a critical step in the development of cardiac dilatation [49].

Antihypertensive Treatment and Prevention of Heart Failure

Regarding the class effects of antihypertensives, beta-blockers (BBs) seem to similarly protect against HF as any other class, but due to an increased risk of stroke should be avoided, at least in monotherapy. This adverse impact is attributed to an increase in central BP secondary to heart rate reduction [75].

According to ALLHAT trial doxazosin might increase the risk of CV adverse events compared to chlortalidone, but in ASCOT trial, doxazosin gastrointestinal therapeutic system as a third-line add-on drug did not increase the risk of HF and was well tolerated [76, 77].

Contradictory data also governs the implication of CCBs with the risk of HF. In a Cochrane meta-analysis, CCBs increased the risk of HF events as compared with ACEi, and ARBs. A subsequent evaluation of these data showed that the comparator arm included a larger amount of drugs known to reduce HF symptoms like diuretics, RAA-blockers, and BBs [78, 79].

A network meta-analysis found that diuretics, ACEIs, and ARBs represented the most efficient classes of drugs to reduce HF onset compared with placebo and relegated CCB among the least effective first-line agents in heart failure prevention, together with BBs and α-blockers [80].

SHEP and HYVETT trials revealed a highly protective effect of diuretics—chlortalidone and indapamide, respectively—against HF [81]. In addition, in a meta-analysis of 10 randomized trials, it has been highlighted the superiority of diuretics as a group compared to any other class of antihypertensives [79].

To resume, Thiazides and Thiazide-like diuretics are likely the ideal agents for heart failure prevention followed by ACEi/ARBs.

The 2023 ESH guidelines, also emphasize that antihypertensive treatment is effective in preventing HF and specifies that "all major antihypertensive drug classes, including ACEis, ARBs, BBs, CCBs and Thiazide/Thiazide-like diuretics, can be used for the prevention of heart failure". In addition, these guidelines mention as an I (general agreement) B (moderate evidence) class recommendation that "alpha-1 blockers (e.g. doxazosin) can be used for the prevention of heart failure in hypertension, preferably in combination with Thiazide/Thiazide-like diuretics and BBs to avoid fluid retention and tachycardia". Patients with type-2 diabetes should also be included also the SGLT inhibitors [54].

Once HF occurs, the treatment will be instituted according to the protocols for HFpEF or HFrEF that are described in other chapters of this volume.

Conclusions

In conclusion, cardiac complications mediated by hypertension have complex implications including left ventricular hypertrophy, myocardial ischemia, and predisposition to arrhythmias. The most important clinical expression of hypertensive heart disease is heart failure, although we must not neglect the increased risk for atherosclerotic coronary artery disease, microvascular angina, or atrial fibrillation. Consequently, the diagnostic workup of a hypertensive patient must integrate the investigations that address all the possible consequences of high blood pressure on the heart. Antihypertensive treatment is effective in reducing the occurrence of heart failure and data accumulated up to now pleads for a higher efficiency of Thiazidic or Thiazid-like diuretics and ACEi/ARBs. Studies are underway to evaluate the benefits of new classes of drugs aimed at reducing myocardial fibrosis or improving the determinants of progression from left ventricular hypertrophy to heart failure.

References

1. GBD 2017 Disease and Injury Incidence and Prevalence Collaborators. Global, regional, and national incidence, prevalence, and years lived with disability for 354 diseases and injuries for 195 countries and territories, 1990-2017: a systematic analysis for the Global Burden of Disease Study 2017. Lancet. 2018;392:17891858. https://doi.org/10.1016/S0140-6736(18)32279-7.
2. Levy D, Larson MG, Vasan RS, et al. The progression from hypertension to congestive heart failure. JAMA. 1996;275:1557–62.
3. Vasan RS, Larson MG, Leip EP, et al. Impact of high-normal blood pressure on the risk of cardiovascular disease. N Engl J Med. 2001;345:1291–7. https://doi.org/10.1056/NEJMoa003417.
4. Tocci G, SciaretTa S, Volpe M. Development of heart failure in recent hypertension trials. J Hypertens. 2008;26:1477–86. https://doi.org/10.1097/HJH.0b013e3282fe1d3d.
5. Messerli FH, Rimoldi SF, Bangalore S. The transition from hypertension to heart failure: a contemporary update (2017). JACC Heart Fail. 2017;5:543–51. https://doi.org/10.1016/j.jchf.2017.04.012.
6. New York Heart Association. Nomenclature and criteria for diagnosis of diseases of the heart and vessels. 8th ed. Boston: Little, Brown; 1979. p. 12.
7. Tackling G, Borhade MB. Hypertensive heart disease. In: StatPearls [Internet]. Treasure Island: StatPearls Publishing; 2024.
8. Gibbons GH, Dzau VJ. The emerging concept of vascular remodeling. N Engl J Med. 1994;330:1431–8. https://doi.org/10.1056/NEJM199405193302008.
9. Xie M, Burchfield JS, Hill JA. Pathological ventricular remodeling: therapies: part 2 of 2. Circulation. 2013;128:388–400. https://doi.org/10.1161/CIRCULATIONAHA.113.001879.
10. Lip GY, Felmeden DC, Lee-Saw-Hee FL, et al. Hypertensive heart disease. A complex syndrome or a hypertensive 'cardiomyopathy'? Eur Heart J. 2000;21:1653–65. https://doi.org/10.1053/euhj.2000.2339.
11. Shah SJ, Aistrup GL, Gupta DK, et al. Ultrastructural and cellular basis for the development of abnormal myocardial mechanics during the transition from hypertension to heart failure. Am J Physiol Heart Circ Physiol. 2014;306(1):H88–100. https://doi.org/10.1152/ajpheart.00642.2013.

12. Frangogiannis NG. Cardiac fibrosis: cell biological mechanisms, molecular pathways and therapeutic opportunities. Mol Asp Med. 2019;65:70–99. https://doi.org/10.1016/j.mam.2018.07.001.
13. Wang J, Chen H, Seth A, et al. Mechanical force regulation of myofibroblast differentiation in cardiac fibroblasts. Am J Physiol Heart Circ Physiol. 2003;285(5):H1871–81. https://doi.org/10.1152/ajpheart.00387.2003.
14. Ferrer-Curriu G, Redondo-Angulo I, Guitart-Mampel M, et al. Fibroblast growth factor-21 protects against fibrosis in hypertensive heart disease. J Pathol. 2019;248(1):30–40. https://doi.org/10.1002/path.5226.
15. Harvey A, Montezano AC, Lopes RA, et al. Vascular fibrosis in aging and hypertension: molecular mechanisms and clinical implications. Can J Cardiol. 2016;32(5):659–68. https://doi.org/10.1016/j.cjca.2016.02.070.
16. Post WS, Larson MG, Myers RH, et al. Heritability of left ventricular mass: the Framingham Heart Study. Hypertension. 1997;30(5):1025–8. https://doi.org/10.1161/01.hyp.30.5.1025.
17. Gardin JM, Arnold A, Gottdiener JS, et al. Left ventricular mass in the elderly. The Cardiovascular Health Study. Hypertension. 1997;29(5):1095–103. https://doi.org/10.1161/01.hyp.29.5.1095.
18. Kizer JR, Arnett DK, Bella JN, et al. Differences in left ventricular structure between black and white hypertensive adults: the Hypertension Genetic Epidemiology Network study. Hypertension. 2004;43(6):1182–8. https://doi.org/10.1161/01.HYP.0000128738.94190.9f.
19. Krumholz HM, Larson M, Levy D. Sex differences in cardiac adaptation to isolated systolic hypertension. Am J Cardiol. 1993;72(3):310–3. https://doi.org/10.1016/0002-9149(93)90678-6.
20. Savage DD, Levy D, Dannenberg AL, et al. Association of echocardiographic left ventricular mass with body size, blood pressure and physical activity (the Framingham Study). Am J Cardiol. 1990;65(5):371–6. https://doi.org/10.1016/0002-9149(90)90304-j.
21. Palmieri V, Bella JN, Arnett DK, et al. Effect of type 2 diabetes mellitus on left ventricular geometry and systolic function in hypertensive subjects: Hypertension Genetic Epidemiology Network (HyperGEN) study. Circulation. 2001;103(1):102–7. https://doi.org/10.1161/01.cir.103.1.102.
22. Vasan RS, Short MI, Niiranen TJ, et al. Interrelations between arterial stiffness, target organ damage, and cardiovascular disease outcomes. J Am Heart Assoc. 2019;8(14):e012141. https://doi.org/10.1161/JAHA.119.012141.
23. Cuspidi C, Facchetti R, Bombelli M, et al. Nighttime blood pressure and new-onset left ventricular hypertrophy: findings from the Pamela population. Hypertension. 2013;62(1):78–84. https://doi.org/10.1161/HYPERTENSIONAHA.111.00682.
24. Cuspidi C, Sala C, Negri F, et al. Italian Society of Hypertension. Prevalence of left-ventricular hypertrophy in hypertension: an updated review of echocardiographic studies. J Hum Hypertens. 2012;26(6):343–9. https://doi.org/10.1038/jhh.2011.104.
25. Sardana M, Nah G, Tsao CW, et al. Clinical and echocardiographic correlates of left atrial function index: the Framingham Offspring Study. J Am Soc Echocardiogr. 2017;30(9):904–912.e2. https://doi.org/10.1016/j.echo.2017.05.013.
26. Todiere G, Neglia D, Ghione S, et al. Right ventricular remodelling in systemic hypertension: a cardiac MRI study. Heart. 2011;97(15):1257–61. https://doi.org/10.1136/hrt.2010.221259.
27. Tadic M, Cuspidi C, Suzic-Lazic J, et al. Is there a relationship between right-ventricular and right atrial mechanics and functional capacity in hypertensive patients? J Hypertens. 2014;32(4):929–37. https://doi.org/10.1097/HJH.0000000000000102.
28. Stewart BF, Siscovick D, Lind BK, et al. Clinical factors associated with calcific aortic valve disease. Cardiovascular Health Study. J Am Coll Cardiol. 1997;29(3):630–4. https://doi.org/10.1016/s0735-1097(96)00563-3.
29. Singh JP, Evans JC, Levy D, et al. Prevalence and clinical determinants of mitral, tricuspid, and aortic regurgitation (the Framingham Heart Study). Am J Cardiol. 1999;83(6):897–902. https://doi.org/10.1016/s0002-9149(98)01064-9.

30. Benetos A, Adamopoulos C, Bureau JM, et al. Determinants of accelerated progression of arterial stiffness in normotensive subjects and in treated hypertensive subjects over a 6-year period. Circulation. 2002;105:1202–120. https://doi.org/10.1161/hc1002.105135.
31. Wohlfahrt P, Wichterle D, Seidlerová J, et al. Relation of central and brachial blood pressure to left ventricular hypertrophy. The Czech Post-MONICA Study. J Hum Hypertens. 2011;26(1):14–9. https://doi.org/10.1038/jhh.2011.78.
32. Weber T, Wassertheurer S, O'Rourke MF, et al. Pulsatile hemodynamics in patients with exertional dyspnea: potentially of value in the diagnostic evaluation of suspected heart failure with preserved ejection fraction. J Am Coll Cardiol. 2013;61(18):1874–83. https://doi.org/10.1016/j.jacc.2013.02.013.
33. Ford TJ, Ong P, Sechtem U, et al. Assessment of vascular dysfunction in patients without obstructive coronary artery disease: why, how, and when. JACC Cardiovasc Interv. 2020;13(16):1847–64. https://doi.org/10.1016/j.jcin.2020.05.052.
34. Ford TJ, Rocchiccioli P, Good R, et al. Systemic microvascular dysfunction in microvascular and vasospastic angina. Eur Heart J. 2018;39(46):4086–97. https://doi.org/10.1093/eurheartj/ehy529.
35. Taqueti VR, Di Carli MF. Coronary microvascular disease pathogenic mechanisms and therapeutic options: JACC state-of-the-art review. J Am Coll Cardiol. 2018;72(21):2625–41. https://doi.org/10.1016/j.jacc.2018.09.042.
36. Paulus WJ, Tschöpe C. A novel paradigm for heart failure with preserved ejection fraction: comorbidities drive myocardial dysfunction and remodeling through coronary microvascular endothelial inflammation. J Am Coll Cardiol. 2013;62(4):263–71. https://doi.org/10.1016/j.jacc.2013.02.092.
37. Antony I, Nitenberg A, Foult JM, et al. Coronary vasodilator reserve in untreated and treated hypertensive patients with and without left ventricular hypertrophy. J Am Coll Cardiol. 1993;22(2):514–20. https://doi.org/10.1016/0735-1097(93)90058-9.
38. Zhou W, Brown JM, Bajaj NS, et al. Hypertensive coronary microvascular dysfunction: a subclinical marker of end organ damage and heart failure. Eur Heart J. 2020;41(25):2366–75. https://doi.org/10.1093/eurheartj/ehaa191.
39. Lewington S, Clarke R, Qizilbash N, et al. Prospective Studies Collaboration. Age-specific relevance of usual BP to vascular mortality: a meta-analysis of individual data for one million adults in 61 prospective studies. Lancet. 2002;360:1903–13. https://doi.org/10.1016/s0140-6736(02)11911-8.
40. Whelton SP, McEvoy JW, Shaw L, et al. Association of normal systolic blood pressure level with cardiovascular disease in the absence of risk factors. JAMA Cardiol. 2020;5(9):1011–8. https://doi.org/10.1001/jamacardio.2020.1731.
41. Hindricks G, Potpara T, Dagres N, et al. ESC Guidelines for the diagnosis and management of atrial fibrillation developed in collaboration with the European Association for Cardio-Thoracic Surgery (EACTS): the Task Force for the diagnosis and management of atrial fibrillation of the European Society of Cardiology (ESC) developed with the special contribution of the European Heart Rhythm Association (EHRA) of the ESC. Eur Heart J. 2021;42(5):373–498. https://doi.org/10.1093/eurheartj/ehaa612.
42. Medi C, Kalman JM, Spence SJ, et al. Atrial electrical and structural changes associated with longstanding hypertension in humans: implications for the substrate for atrial fibrillation. J Cardiovasc Electrophysiol. 2011;22(12):1317–24. https://doi.org/10.1111/j.1540-8167.2011.02125.x.
43. Sanders P, Morton JB, Kistler PM, et al. Electrophysiological and electroanatomic characterization of the atria in sinus node disease: evidence of diffuse atrial remodeling. Circulation. 2004;109(12):1514–22. https://doi.org/10.1161/01.CIR.0000121734.47409.AA.
44. Albert CM, Chae CU, Grodstein F, et al. Prospective study of sudden cardiac death among women in the United States. Circulation. 2003;107(16):2096–101. https://doi.org/10.1161/01.CIR.0000065223.21530.11.

45. de Simone G, Gottdiener JS, Chinali M, et al. Left ventricular mass predicts heart failure not related to previous myocardial infarction: the Cardiovascular Health Study. Eur Heart J. 2008;29(6):741–7. https://doi.org/10.1093/eurheartj/ehm605.
46. Marwick TH, Gillebert TC, Aurigemma G, et al. Recommendations on the use of echocardiography in adult hypertension: a report from the European Association of Cardiovascular Imaging (EACVI) and the American Society of Echocardiography (ASE). Eur Heart J Cardiovasc Imaging. 2015;16(6):577–605. https://doi.org/10.1093/ehjci/jev076.
47. Slivnick J, Lampert BC. Hypertension and heart failure. Heart Fail Clin. 2019;15(4):531–41. https://doi.org/10.1016/j.hfc.2019.06.007.
48. Nakahara T, Takata Y, Hirayama Y, et al. Left ventricular hypertrophy and geometry in untreated essential hypertension is associated with blood levels of aldosterone and procollagen type III amino-terminal peptide. Circ J. 2007;71(5):716–21. https://doi.org/10.1253/circj.71.716.
49. Seliger SL, de Lemos J, Neeland IJ, et al. Older adults, "malignant" left ventricular hypertrophy, and associated cardiac-specific biomarker phenotypes to identify the differential risk of new-onset reduced versus preserved ejection fraction heart failure: CHS (Cardiovascular Health Study). JACC Heart Fail. 2015;3(6):445–55. https://doi.org/10.1016/j.jchf.2014.12.018.
50. Drazner MH. The progression of hypertensive heart disease. Circulation. 2011;123(3):327–34. https://doi.org/10.1161/CIRCULATIONAHA.108.845792.
51. Kass DA. Ventricular arterial stiffening: integrating the pathophysiology. Hypertension. 2005;46(1):185–93. https://doi.org/10.1161/01.HYP.0000168053.34306.d4.
52. Tadic M, Cuspidi C, Celic V, et al. Nocturnal hypertension and right heart remodeling. J Hypertens. 2018;36(1):136–42. https://doi.org/10.1097/HJH.0000000000001506.
53. Mauger C, Gilbert K, Lee AM, et al. Right ventricular shape and function: cardiovascular magnetic resonance reference morphology and biventricular risk factor morphometrics in UK Biobank. J Cardiovasc Magn Reson. 2019;21(1):41. https://doi.org/10.1186/s12968-019-0551-6.
54. Mancia G, Kreutz R, Brunström M, et al. ESH Guidelines for the management of arterial hypertension the Task Force for the management of arterial hypertension of the European Society of Hypertension: endorsed by the International Society of Hypertension (ISH) and the European Renal Association (ERA). J Hypertens. 2023;41(12):1874–2071. https://doi.org/10.1097/HJH.0000000000003480.
55. Goldberger AL. Left ventricular hypertrophy: clinical findings and ECG diagnosis. UpToDate. Last updated: 2022, Nov 3. https://www.uptodate.com/contents/left-ventricular-hypertrophy-clinical-findings-and-ecg-diagnosis#H9
56. Hancock EW, Deal BJ, Mirvis DM, et al. AHA/ACCF/HRS recommendations for the standardization and interpretation of the electrocardiogram: part V: electrocardiogram changes associated with cardiac chamber hypertrophy: a scientific statement from the American Heart Association Electrocardiography and Arrhythmias Committee. Council on Clinical Cardiology the American College of Cardiology Foundation, and the Heart Rhythm Society. Endorsed by the International Society for Computerized Electrocardiology. J Am Coll Cardiol. 2009;53:992–1002.
57. Lang RM, Badano LP, Mor-Avi V, et al. Recommendations for cardiac chamber quantification by echocardiography in adults: an update from the American Society of Echocardiography and the European Association of Cardiovascular Imaging. Eur Heart J Cardiovasc Imaging. 2015;16(3):233–70. https://doi.org/10.1093/ehjci/jev014.
58. Nagueh SF, Smiseth OA, Appleton CP, et al. Recommendations for the evaluation of left ventricular diastolic function by echocardiography: an update from the American Society of Echocardiography and the European Association of Cardiovascular Imaging. Eur Heart J Cardiovasc Imaging. 2016;17:1321–60. https://doi.org/10.1093/ehjci/jew082.
59. Mor-Avi V, Lang RM, Badano LP, et al. Current and evolving echocardiographic techniques for the quantitative evaluation of cardiac mechanics: ASE/EAE consensus statement on methodology and indications endorsed by the Japanese Society of Echocardiography. Eur J Echocardiogr. 2011;12:167–205. https://doi.org/10.1093/ejechocard/jer021.

60. Heckbert SR, Post W, Pearson GD, et al. Traditional cardiovascular risk factors in relation to left ventricular mass, volume, and systolic function by cardiac magnetic resonance imaging: the Multiethnic Study of Atherosclerosis. J Am Coll Cardiol. 2006;48(11):2285–92. https://doi.org/10.1016/j.jacc.2006.03.072.
61. Rodrigues JC, Amadu AM, Ghosh Dastidar A, et al. ECG strain pattern in hypertension is associated with myocardial cellular expansion and diffuse interstitial fibrosis: a multi-parametric cardiac magnetic resonance study. Eur Heart J Cardiovasc Imaging. 2017;18(4):441–50. https://doi.org/10.1093/ehjci/jew117.
62. Kunadian V, Chieffo A, Camici PG, et al. An EAPCI Expert Consensus Document on Ischaemia with Non-Obstructive Coronary Arteries in Collaboration with European Society of Cardiology Working Group on Coronary Pathophysiology & Microcirculation Endorsed by Coronary Vasomotor Disorders International Study Group. Eur Heart J. 2020;41(37):3504–20. https://doi.org/10.1093/eurheartj/ehaa503.
63. Gonzales-Maqueda I, Alegria-Ezquerra E, Gonzales-Juanatey JR. Hypertensive heart disease: a new clinical classification. E-J ESC Council Cardiol Pract. 2009;7(20):12.
64. Rautaharju PM, Soliman EZ. Electrocardiographic left ventricular hypertrophy and the risk of adverse cardiovascular events: a critical appraisal. J Electrocardiol. 2014;47(5):649–54. https://doi.org/10.1016/j.jelectrocard.2014.06.002.
65. González A, Schelbert EB, Díez J, et al. Myocardial interstitial fibrosis in heart failure: biological and translational perspectives. J Am Coll Cardiol. 2018;71(15):1696–706. https://doi.org/10.1016/j.jacc.2018.02.021.
66. Armstrong AC, Liu K, Lewis CE. Left atrial dimension and traditional cardiovascular risk factors predict 20-year clinical cardiovascular events in young healthy adults: the CARDIA study. Eur Heart J Cardiovasc Imaging. 2014;15(8):893–9. https://doi.org/10.1093/ehjci/jeu018.
67. Pezel T, Venkatesh BA, De Vasconcellos HD, et al. Left atrioventricular coupling index as a prognostic marker of cardiovascular events: the MESA study. Hypertension. 2021;78(3):661–71. https://doi.org/10.1161/HYPERTENSIONAHA.121.17339.
68. Devereux RB, Dahlöf B, Gerdts E, et al. Regression of hypertensive left ventricular hypertrophy by losartan compared with atenolol: the Losartan Intervention for Endpoint Reduction in Hypertension (LIFE) trial. Circulation. 2004;110(11):1456–62. https://doi.org/10.1161/01.CIR.0000141573.44737.5A.
69. Bangalore S, Wild D, Parkar S, et al. Beta-blockers for primary prevention of heart failure in patients with hypertension insights from a meta-analysis. J Am Coll Cardiol. 2008;52(13):1062–72. https://doi.org/10.1016/j.jacc.2008.05.057.
70. Klingbeil AU, Schneider M, Martus P, et al. A meta-analysis of the effects of treatment on left ventricular mass in essential hypertension. Am J Med. 2003;115(1):41–6. https://doi.org/10.1016/s0002-9343(03)00158-x.
71. Zile MR, O'Meara E, Claggett B, et al. Effects of sacubitril/valsartan on biomarkers of extracellular matrix regulation in patients with HFrEF. J Am Coll Cardiol. 2019;73(7):795–806. https://doi.org/10.1016/j.jacc.2018.11.042.
72. Morfino P, Aimo A, Castiglione V, et al. Treatment of cardiac fibrosis: from neuro-hormonal inhibitors to CAR-T cell therapy. Heart Fail Rev. 2023;2:555–69. https://doi.org/10.1007/s10741-022-10279-x.
73. Lewis GA, Dodd S, Clayton D, et al. Pirfenidone in heart failure with preserved ejection fraction: a randomized phase 2 trial. Nat Med. 2021;27(8):1477–82. https://doi.org/10.1038/s41591-021-01452-0.
74. Lee HY, Shin J, Kim GH, et al. 2018 Korean Society of Hypertension Guidelines for the management of hypertension: part II-diagnosis and treatment of hypertension. Clin Hypertens. 2019;25:20. https://doi.org/10.1186/s40885-019-0124-x.
75. ALLHAT Collaborative Research Group. Major cardiovascular events in hypertensive patients randomized to doxazosin vs chlorthalidone: the antihypertensive and lipid-lowering treatment to prevent heart attack trial (ALLHAT). JAMA. 2000;283(15):1967–75.

76. Chapman N, Chang CL, Dahlöf B, et al. Effect of doxazosin gastrointestinal therapeutic system as third-line antihypertensive therapy on blood pressure and lipids in the Anglo-Scandinavian Cardiac Outcomes Trial. Circulation. 2008;118(1):42–8. https://doi.org/10.1161/CIRCULATIONAHA.107.737957.
77. Chen N, Zhou M, Yang M, et al. Calcium channel blockers versus other classes of drugs for hypertension. Cochrane Database Syst Rev. 2010;10(8):CD003654. https://doi.org/10.1002/14651858.CD003654.pub4. Update in: Cochrane Database Syst Rev. 2021;10:CD003654.
78. Thomopoulos C, Parati G, Zanchetti A. Effects of blood pressure-lowering treatment. 6. Prevention of heart failure and new-onset heart failure—meta-analyses of randomized trials. J Hypertens. 2016;34(3):373–84.; discussion 384. https://doi.org/10.1097/HJH.0000000000000848.
79. Sciarretta S, Palano F, Tocci G, et al. Antihypertensive treatment and development of heart failure in hypertension: a Bayesian network meta-analysis of studies in patients with hypertension and high cardiovascular risk. Arch Intern Med. 2011;171(5):384–94. https://doi.org/10.1001/archinternmed.2010.427.
80. SHEP Cooperative Research Group. Prevention of stroke by antihypertensive drug treatment in older persons with isolated systolic hypertension. Final results of Systolic Hypertension in the Elderly Program (SHEP). JAMA. 1991;265:3255–64.
81. Beckett NS, Peters R, Fletcher AE, et al. Treatment of hypertension in patients 80 years of age or older. N Engl J Med. 2008;358(18):1887–98. https://doi.org/10.1056/NEJMoa0801369.

Chapter 22
Heart Failure and Genetic Cardiomyopathies

Bogdana Ionescu, Pablo Garcia-Pavia, and Ruxandra Jurcut

Abstract Cardiomyopathies, characterized by structural and functional abnormalities of the myocardium, present a diverse spectrum of etiologies, including genetic predispositions, environmental factors, and acquired diseases. This chapter systematically discusses the distinct pathways through which cardiomyopathies contribute to heart failure, considering both systolic and diastolic dysfunction, taking into consideration unique challenges in managing heart failure, necessitating a multifaceted approach that addresses both the underlying cause and the resultant myocardial dysfunction. Consolidation of current knowledge on the particularities of heart failure in cardiomyopathies is of utmost importance. A synthesized perspective on the diverse etiologies, molecular underpinnings, diagnostic advancements, and therapeutic considerations of hypertrophic cardiomyopathy (HCM), dilated and non-dilated left ventricle cardiomyopathy (DCM/NDLVC), arrhythmogenic cardiomyopathy (ARVC), restrictive cardiomyopathy (RCM) and syndromic and metabolic cardiomyopathies is provided.

Keywords Cardiomyopathy · Genetic · Heart failure · Mindset

B. Ionescu · R. Jurcut (✉)
Expert Center for Rare Cardiac Genetic Diseases, Emergency Institute for Cardiovascular Diseases "Prof. Dr. C. C. Iliescu", Bucharest, Romania

Department of Cardiology, University of Medicine and Pharmacy "Carol Davila", Bucharest, Romania

P. Garcia-Pavia
Heart Failure and Inherited Cardiac Diseases Unit, Department of Cardiology, Hospital Universitario Puerta de Hierro Majadahonda, IDIPHISA, CIBERCV, Madrid, Spain

Centro Nacional de Investigaciones Cardiovasculares (CNIC), Madrid, Spain

M. Dorobanţu et al. (eds.), *Current Approach to Heart Failure*,
https://doi.org/10.1007/978-3-031-96562-3_22

Introduction

Cardiomyopathy related heart failure can have distinctive features that shape the clinical landscape of these intricate cardiac disorders. The exploration of genetic cardiomyopathies reveals a complex interplay of molecular mechanisms that impact myocardial contractility, offering insights into tailored therapeutic interventions. The importance of precision medicine in discerning subtle variations in disease presentation is emphasized by the evolving landscape of diagnostic modalities for cardiomyopathies. The role of advanced imaging techniques, biomarkers, and genetic testing in refining diagnosis and risk stratification is detailed to underscore their significance in guiding therapeutic decisions and aiding the development of targeted therapies to mitigate the burden of heart failure in patients with cardiomyopathies.

Definition and Classification

According to the European Society of Cardiology Working Group on Myocardial and Pericardial Diseases, cardiomyopathies are defined as myocardial disorders in which the heart muscle is structurally and functionally abnormal, in the absence of coronary artery disease (CAD), hypertension, valvular disease, and congenital heart disease (CHD) sufficient to cause the observed myocardial abnormality [1].

The broad spectrum of cardiomyopathies is influenced by their underlying causes, which mostly include genetic or inherited factors. However, there are instances when acquired factors such as inflammation, toxicity, or multi-systemic disorders may contribute to the development of cardiomyopathies. Additionally, some cases may have a combination of both hereditary and acquired causes [2].

The latest classification of cardiomyopathies encompasses phenotypic profiles which include hypertrophic cardiomyopathy (HCM), dilated cardiomyopathy (DCM), non-dilated left ventricular cardiomyopathy (NDLVC), arrhythmogenic right ventricular cardiomyopathy (ARVC) and restrictive cardiomyopathy (RCM) [3].

The phenotypic description of the cardiomyopathies at presentation and refinement of their morphological and functional characteristics will lead to more systematic approach of the diagnosis. The most recently published guideline on cardiomyopathies incorporates features that characterize cardiac tissue such as non-ischaemic ventricular fibrosis or fatty replacement, which can occur with or without ventricular dilatation, wall motion abnormalities, or global systolic or diastolic dysfunction, since it may serve as the only indicator for diagnosing a cardiomyopathy and possesses prognostic implications that differ depending on the underlying cause [3].

The continuum of heart failure (HF) in cardiomyopathies is characterized by a wide range of clinical presentations. Cardiovascular manifestations may occur at any stage of disease, leading to sudden cardiac death in individuals who often do not exhibit symptoms. Additionally, these individuals may have a gradual decline in ventricular function, eventually progressing to end-stage heart failure, which can be the leading cause of death in these patients.

Although there have been advancements regarding our knowledge of the precise pathophysiological mechanisms of cardiomyopathies, the treatment is still predominantly following a one-size-fits-all regimen, using non-specific drugs such as beta-blockers, renin-angiotensin-aldosterone axis therapies and sodium–glucose cotransporter 2 inhibitors (SGLT2i) being widely employed currently for all cases of heart failure with reduced ejection fraction (HFrEF), irrespective of aetiology. In the 2021 ESC Guidelines for the diagnosis and treatment of acute and chronic heart failure, the recommendations are not centred around the heart failure aetiology and include the latest medical treatments, devices, interventions and LV assist device (LVAD)/transplantation options [4]. Therefore, we advocate a shift from managing cardiomyopathy related heart failure from a heart failure mindset to a cardiomyopathy mindset.

Also, cardiomyopathies are a setting where preventive therapies are of significant importance, particularly in those with high susceptibility to severe arrhythmias and sudden cardiac death (SCD), even prior to the onset of heart failure.

Improving comprehension of the genotype and its correlation with the phenotype has the potential to enhance the prognosis of individuals with cardiomyopathy. This may be attained through the development of genetic risk scores and the optimization of personalized patient care strategies, including both arrhythmic and heart failure particularities.

Hypertrophic Cardiomyopathy

Hypertrophic cardiomyopathy is characterized by the presence of increased left ventricular (LV) wall thickness or mass, with or without right ventricular (RV) hypertrophy that cannot be explained by abnormal loading conditions [1]. It is typically asymmetric, with the most pronounced hypertrophy affecting the interventricular septum at its base [5].

As far as phenotypic description is concerned, two main forms of HCM can be identified. A diagnosis of obstructive HCM is made when the peak instantaneous Doppler LV outflow tract (LVOT) gradient is greater than 30 mmHg at rest or with provocation (Valsalva maneuver or exercise) [6–8]. Collectively, it has been reported that two thirds of patients with HCM exhibit obstructive physiology at rest or with provocation, at least in patients evaluated at reference centers.

Variants in genes encoding cardiac sarcomere proteins are the most prevalent cause of HCM. Pathogenic variants in beta myosin heavy chain 7 (MYH7) and myosin-binding protein C3 (MYBPC3) are identified in 70% of variant-positive patients. Other genes (TNNI3, TNNT2, TPM1, MYL2, MYL3, ACTC1) account for 1–5% of variant-positive patients [9].

The clinical picture of HCM is usually defined by a phenotype of HF with preserved ejection fraction (HFpEF), explained in general terms by the fact that the LV myocardium becomes abnormally thick, restricting the heart's ability to relax, leading the way towards impaired filling and subsequently, to the development of diastolic dysfunction. Left atrial dilation represents a predictor for the development of atrial fibrillation (AFib) and HF, being an indirect sign of an increased LV diastolic pressure. Distinctive attributes in regard to LVOT obstruction and the degree of HF in patients with HOCM (hypertrophic obstructive cardiomyopathy) are primarily related by the pressure overload caused by a dynamic restriction of left ventricular outflow during systole. The presence of intracavitary obstruction primarily affects the outflow tract and is caused by a combination of factors, including physical obstruction of the hypertrophied septum, abnormal systolic anterior motion (SAM) of the mitral valve, and impairments in diastolic and contractile function. In a subset of individuals, the gradient is generated through mid-cavity obstruction only, resulting from an anomalous alignment between the hypertrophied septum and the anterolateral papillary muscle. The temporal variability and poor consistency of HF symptoms in HCM may be attributed to the dynamic changes in gradients that occur in response to alterations in myocardial contractility and loading circumstances, such as exercise and hydration [10, 11].

Although only a minority of HCM patients can present with end-stage/burn-out clinical phenotype (5%), this group of patients is associated with high mortality due to progressive heart failure (15%), with one fourth of patients requiring advanced HF therapies, including heart transplantation [12]. The distribution of mortality rates associated with heart failure (HF) varies throughout different stages of the illness. Specifically, the "classic" stage is associated with a 14% HF mortality rate, the "adverse remodelling" stage is associated with a 38% mortality rate, and the "overt dysfunction" stage is associated with a 74% mortality rate according to a recent study [13].

Significant predictors for progression towards a dilated phenotype were shown to be atrial fibrillation (AF), nonsustained ventricular tachycardia (NSVT), and left ventricular diameter at end-systole (LVDs) >25.4 mm [14] (Fig. 22.1).

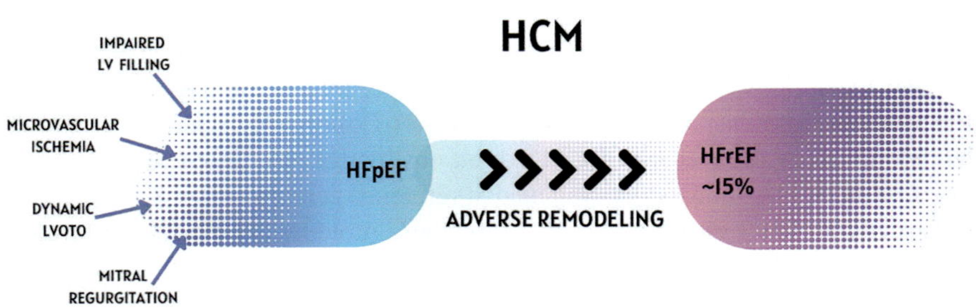

Fig. 22.1 Heart failure spectrum in HCM. *HCM* hypertrophic cardiomyopathy, *HFpEF* heart failure with preserved ejection fraction, *HFrEF* heart failure with reduced ejection fraction, *LV* left ventricle, *LVOTO* left ventricular outflow obstruction

Due to the limited availability of randomized studies, the medical treatment choices are mostly based on direct experience with the aim of improving functional status and alleviating symptoms [15–17].

The basic algorithm for the treatment of symptomatic (NYHA class II-IV) patients with non-obstructive HCM encompasses the management of arrhythmia, reduction of LV filling pressures, and treatment of angina.

Atrial fibrillation has the potential to cause haemodynamic and clinical decompensation due to the reduction in diastolic filling time caused by rapid heart rates and the reliance on atrial contraction for LV filling. Hence, it is particularly important to maintain sinus rhythm, and a strategy focused on rhythm control is preferred, especially when symptoms are present [18]. Pharmacological options for rhythm control include amiodarone, dofetilide and disopyramide [3]. Catheter ablation is a crucial component in the management of AFib. While there is a lack of randomized controlled trials (RCTs) in this specific field, several meta-analyses have been published regarding patients with HCM who undergo catheter ablation for atrial fibrillation that is unresponsive to medication [19–21]. It is generally considered a safe and effective option for HCM patients [22]. Nevertheless, the outcomes seem to be less favourable in HCM, as shown by an increased risk of relapse, a greater need for repeat procedures, and a higher concurrent use of antiarrhythmic medications [23–25]. This can be attributed to the observation that patients with cardiomyopathies exhibit a higher level of structural atrial remodeling [20].

Prompt rhythm/rate control should be considered in patients with LVOT obstruction and new-onset or poorly tolerated AFib (class IIa indication) [3, 18, 26, 27].

The first treatment approach for individuals diagnosed with HCM and resting/provocable LVOTO should consist of non-vasodilating beta-blockers, titrated to maximum tolerated doses [28–33]. This therapeutic strategy aims to decrease myocardial contractility and mitigate the adverse effects of left ventricular diastolic dysfunction by reducing heart rate. Additionally, low-dose loop diuretics should be used to manage symptoms of HF, while concurrently avoiding hypovolemia. Patients should be counselled against dehydration and excessive alcohol consumption. Furthermore, clinicians should be aware of the potential negative impact of arterial/venous dilators drugs on LVOT obstruction [3, 34].Verapamil or diltiazem may serve as viable alternatives in cases when individuals exhibit intolerance or contraindications to beta-blockers [7, 11]. In addition, disopyramide is a class I add-on therapy for patients already on beta-blockers or verapamil for symptoms improvement. Precautions should be taken when using disopyramide due its anticholinergic side effects and risk for QT prolongation during up-titration [3, 28, 29, 35, 36].

Moreover, in patients with progressive systolic dysfunction (LVEF < 50%—entering the burnout phase), the therapeutic armamentarium should include the classical pillars for HFrEF: ACEi (angiotensin-converting enzyme inhibitor), ARB (angiotensin receptor blocker), ARNI (angiotensin receptor neprilysin inhibitor), MRA and SGLT2i [3].

The use of cardiac myosin ATPase inhibitors is supported by recent studies as second-line therapy in addition to optimal medical therapy (beta-blocker or calcium channel blockers) for improving functional capacity and symptoms in patients with resting or provoked LVOT obstruction. Moreover, the use of cardiac myosin ATPase inhibitors in monotherapy should also be considered in patients intolerant or with contraindications to beta-blockers, verapamil/diltiazem or disopyramide. Mavacamten is the first one studied in HCM, acting by reducing actin–myosin cross-bridge formation, thereby reducing contractility and improving myocardial energetics [3] but aficamten has recently communicated beneficial results too.

Patients with HCM and symptomatic LVOT obstruction (NYHA II-III and EF > 55%) benefited from mavacamten's effect on lowering the LVOT gradient and increasing exercise capacity compared to placebo in the EXPLORER-HCM trial [16].

Moreover, in VALOR-HCM (A Study to Evaluate Mavacamten in Adults With Symptomatic Obstructive HCM Who Are Eligible for Septal Reduction Therapy), mavacamten substantially decreased the proportion of adult patients with obstructive HCM referred for septal reduction therapy (SRT) due to refractory symptoms at 16 and 32 weeks [37, 38].

The consideration of an invasive treatment of septal reduction therapy (SRT) is warranted for patients exhibiting a left ventricular outflow tract obstruction (LVOTO) gradient equal to or greater than 50 mmHg. This treatment option is particularly relevant for patients experiencing severe symptoms classified as NYHA functional class III-IV, as well as for those who have exertional or unexplained recurrent syncope despite receiving the highest tolerated dosage of medical therapy. In patients exhibiting mild symptoms (NYHA class II) that are unresponsive to pharmacological treatment, invasive therapy may be deemed appropriate. This is particularly applicable to patients who display a resting or maximum provoked gradient of ≥50 mmHg (during exercise or Valsalva maneuver), along with moderate-to-severe systolic anterior motion-related mitral regurgitation, atrial fibrillation (AF), or moderate-to-severe left atrial dilatation [3, 39] or those with high pulmonary pressures.

The options for invasive treatment include surgical septal myectomy and alcohol septal ablation. The choice between surgical or alcohol septal reduction should be discussed in experienced multidisciplinary teams, as both procedures show improvement of functional status with a similar procedural mortality [40–46]. Moreover, septal reduction therapy (both surgical and interventional) proved significant reduction in rates of HF readmission [47].

One recent study provided evidence that ASA did not accelerate the development of burn-out clinical phase of HCM, while causing a temporary and slight decrease in left ventricular systolic performance immediately after the treatment [14].

A thorough evaluation including the assessment of the obstruction mechanism (SAM related, mid-cavity obstruction, accessory mitral tissue, anomalous papillary muscle insertion etc.), evaluation of mitral valve morphology and function and the distribution and severity of hypertrophy is mandatory before addressing patients to an invasive strategy [3].

Ventricular septal myectomy is highly effective, abolishing or substantially reducing LV outflow tract gradients in over 90% of cases. It also improves systolic anterior motion-related mitral regurgitation, exercise capacity, and symptoms. Preoperative determinants of a good long-term outcome include age under 50 years, left atrial size under 46 mm, absence of atrial fibrillation (AF), and male sex. Surgical complications, such as AV nodal block, left bundle branch block (LBBB), ventricular septal defect, and aortic regurgitation, are uncommon in experienced centers using intra-operative transoesophageal echocardiography guidance.

For patients with intrinsic/primary mitral valve disease or marked mitral leaflet elongation and/or moderate-to-severe mitral regurgitation, septal myectomy can be combined with mitral valve repair or replacement. In patients with AF, concomitant ablation using the Cox–Maze procedure can also be performed.

Alcohol septal ablation (ASA) is discussed as an alternative to surgery. However, ASA is associated with an increased likelihood of AV block and subsequent need for permanent cardiostimulation, as well as greater residual LV outflow tract gradients [40, 41, 44–46]. The need for of repeat ASA or myectomy surgery has been documented in around 7–20% of individuals who have had ASA, a rate that surpasses the reported frequency after surgical myectomy [45].

Non-ASA techniques (coils, polyvinyl alcohol foam particles, cyanoacrylate) and direct endocavitary and intramuscular ablation (radiofrequency, cryotherapy) are alternative methods for which long-term outcome/safety data are not available.

Dilated Cardiomyopathy

Dilated cardiomyopathy (DCM) is defined as left ventricular or biventricular systolic dysfunction and dilation that are not explained by abnormal loading conditions or coronary artery disease. Left ventricular dilation can be defined by echocardiographic parameters such as LV-end diastolic diameter >58 mm in males and >52 mm in females and an indexed LVEDV of ≥75 mL/m^2 in males and ≥62 mL/m^2 in females. Left ventricular global systolic dysfunction is defined by LVEF <50% [48]. Cardiomyopathies are the leading cause of heart transplantation on a global scale, with DCM constituting the majority of patients. Hence, it is universally acknowledged that DCM is the primary etiology of heart transplantation worldwide.

Heart failure was the most prevalent clinical presentation according to a study which enrolled a large cohort of 881 patients diagnosed with DCM. It is worth emphasizing that there was a significantly higher incidence of HF among female patients in comparison to their male counterparts. Furthermore, a distinctive observation is that females exhibited more advanced forms of HF. This is underscored by a higher prevalence of NYHA functional class III-IV symptoms, and a greater frequency of left bundle branch block (LBBB) at the time of diagnosis [49].

A significant proportion of DCM patients still have an unfavourable prognosis, particularly in the short term, with substantial heart failure and arrhythmic risks. Despite the homogeneous phenotype of ventricular enlargement and dysfunction, DCM is a mask term that describes the final common pathway of different pathogenic processes and gene-environment interactions [50], due to the complex and heterogeneous etiology of this disease [51]. Deciphering this etiological diversity is likely to result in better prognostic stratification and ultimately targeted therapy.

A study conducted on the ESC EORP Cardiomyopathy & Myocarditis Registry compared familial and sporadic dilated cardiomyopathy. The findings revealed that patients with familial dilated cardiomyopathy (FDCM) tend to develop symptoms at a younger age and generally have a less severe clinical presentation. This is characterized by a lower NYHA class, decreased levels of B-type natriuretic peptide (BNP) and N-terminal pro B-type natriuretic peptide (NT-proBNP), smaller left ventricular dimensions, and a higher left ventricular ejection fraction. Furthermore, individuals with FDCM tend to exhibit fewer cardiovascular risk factors. Nevertheless, despite these distinctions, FDCM still demonstrates a similar short-term prognosis when compared to the sporadic forms of dilated cardiomyopathy [52]. FDCM is associated with pathogenic variants in more than 60 genes with typical autosomal dominant inheritance, with an estimated prevalence between 1/250 and 1/400 of the population, which is higher than previously reported [53].

For better risk stratification and optimal management of patients, genotype-phenotype correlations have been established among DCM-causing genetic variants associated with progression to advanced heart failure and ventricular arrhythmia. The incidence of heart transplantation (HTx) was found to be greatest among individuals carrying LMNA mutations, with a prevalence of 27%. On the other hand, those carrying RBM20 mutations were transplanted at a much younger age, with a mean age of 28.5 years [54].

Causative genetic variants have the potential to significantly alter the current paradigm of risk estimation for dilated DCM and therefore impact patient care strategies, especially the indications for ICD implantation in primary prevention of sudden cardiac death irrespective of EF and according to high-risk genotypes and their associated risk scores or predictors of SCD. This is the case for genetic variants in LMNA, FLNC, TMEM43, PLN, DSP and RBM20 [3].

Although in many cases of DCM in the young a pathogenic genetic variant is the main trigger, there is remarkable variance between individuals, with differences in age-dependent penetrance, and it is believed that ancillary (genetic, environmental) triggers are needed to provoke a full-blown phenotype (second hit hypothesis). Causative genetic variants are present in around 40% of individuals diagnosed with DCM [55–57]. In specific subgroups such as chemotherapy-induced, alcoholic, or peripartum DCM, the prevalence of the gene variants ranges between 10% and 15% [3, 58–60].

Not only have genetic counselling and testing become a much higher priority in everyday practice according to clinical judgement, but they are also supported by explicit and strong recommendations in patients fulfilling the diagnostic criteria for cardiomyopathy, for whom it could expand the diagnosis, prognostication, therapeutic and reproductive management options [3, 61]. Moreover, it enables genetic counselling and cascade genetic testing in family members [62].

Cardiac magnetic resonance imaging (CMR) is an advanced, precise, and versatile cardiovascular imaging technique [63]. It is widely regarded as the standard for assessing cardiac structure and function in clinical setting [64, 65]. CMR is a commonly employed technique for evaluating myocardial scar and fibrosis through the incorporation of late gadolinium enhancement (LGE) [66]. Recent advancements in mapping techniques have significantly enhanced its quantitative characteristics. These techniques include T1, T2, or T2* mapping, which provide absolute measurements in milliseconds, as well as extracellular volume (ECV) quantification [67, 68]. In a comprehensive examination, cardiovascular magnetic resonance (CMR) has the potential to provide a wide range of valuable information pertaining to cardiac structure, function, tissue characterization, and flow. This detailed understanding of cardiac structure greatly contributes to the accuracy of clinical diagnosis and the enhancement of prognostic discrimination.

The presence of mid-wall fibrosis, as identified by late gadolinium enhancement (LGE), provides strong predictive value in DCM. Fibrosis presence and extent was independently associated with cardiovascular mortality or cardiac transplantation, SCD or aborted SCD, and the composite of HF death, HF hospitalization, or cardiac transplantation [69]. Several extensive studies involving large cohorts and meta-analyses have unequivocally demonstrated that the presence of myocardial scar, as identified through late gadolinium enhancement (LGE), serves as an independent predictor for significant outcomes such as all-cause mortality, future hospitalization, and SCD. Moreover, this prognostic indicator offers supplementary value to conventional risk factors, including LVEF [70–72].

Longitudinal strain assessed by feature tracking CMR analysis also seems to be a valuable emerging tool in describing myocardial deformation patterns and predicting the risk (composite of cardiac death, HTx, and aborted SCD) of DCM patients [73].

Although there have been advancements in understanding the precise mechanisms underlying DCM, the current approach to treatment remains primarily uniform, according to international guidelines. The prevailing HF treatment strategy involves the use of non-specific medications, such as beta-blockers, neurohormonal therapies, and SGLT2 inhibitors, as well as resynchronization therapy when indicated. In the era of precision medicine, specific therapies, that may address the underlying genetic defect or the progression of the disease phenotype, are promisingly starting to evolve (e.g. NCT04572893 phase 2a trial of Danicamtiv in patients with primary DCM due to MYH7 or TTN genetic variants) [74]. They shed light on the importance of identifying the causative etiology, and hence to the development of more individualized therapies [75]. For example, currently, a large number of pre-clinical studies are conducted, with compounds that aim to repair the genetic defect (e.g. antisense and gene therapy), but also that target protein aggregation and integrity, which appear crucial to PLN cardiomyopathy [76, 77]. Preliminary studies on the repair of the TTNtv by CRISPR/Cas9 gene editing in engineered heart muscle fully rescued contractility [78].

Non-dilated Left Ventricular Cardiomyopathy

The definitions of cardiomyopathies have evolved to encompass a much broader spectrum in recent years, given the growing understanding of subclinical phenotypic variations that are increasingly challenging to classify within well-defined categories and clinicians have coined various descriptors. These include "non-dilated hypokinetic cardiomyopathy" or "arrhythmogenic cardiomyopathy without dilation or hypokinesis". Presently, these forms are included in the recent concept of "non-dilated left ventricular cardiomyopathy", aligning with the recommendations outlined in the ESC guideline for cardiomyopathies [3].

Indeed, the recognition of a non-dilated left ventricular cardiomyopathy (NDLVC) phenotype should instigate a multiparametric approach aimed at delineating the underlying etiological substrate, which bears significant clinical implications for therapeutic intervention. The subclinical phase of myocardial dysfunction in its earliest stages can be identified, however, using advanced imaging techniques [79, 80].

Global Longitudinal Strain (GLS) measured by 2D speckle tracking echocardiography stands as the most extensively researched parameter for identifying preclinical cardiac disease, and it exhibits a high level of reproducibility when conducted by skilled operators. The presence of abnormal GLS was linked to the worsening of LVEF, as well as cardiac hospitalization and mortality [81].

Cardiac magnetic resonance is of utmost importance in this scenario, by describing the presence of non-ischaemic LGE distribution or fatty replacement in the absence of LV dilatation, with or without global or regional wall motion abnormalities, or isolated global LV systolic dysfunction (LVEF < 50%) without scarring [3].

The genetic variants associated most frequently with a phenotype of non-dilated left ventricular cardiomyopathy include DSP, FLNC (truncating variants), DES, LMNA, and PLN. However, it is important to note that there is significant overlap in the genetic basis of both dilated cardiomyopathy (DCM) and arrhythmogenic right ventricular cardiomyopathy (ARVC) [3].

The majority of patients diagnosed with NDLVC exhibit no symptoms. However, a subset of patients may present a clinical picture associated with arrhythmia or conduction abnormalities, such as syncope or palpitations, suggesting specific aetiologies, including laminopathies [82], neuromuscular disease, PLN [83], DSP [84] and FLNC [85]—truncating variants).

Additionally, some patients may present with symptoms indicative of diastolic heart failure, such as dyspnea. The treatment of heart failure symptoms should me managed according to the latest guidelines on diagnosis and treatment of heart failure, including SGLT2i in the presence of HFpEF [4, 86].

Arrhythmogenic Right Ventricular Cardiomyopathy

Arrhythmogenic right ventricular cardiomyopathy is predominantly caused by mutations in desmosomal genes and was first classified as the impairment of the right ventricle (RV) either regionally or globally. This impairment is characterized by the gradual loss of cardiac mass, which is subsequently replaced by fibrofatty tissue. Progressive RV systolic dysfunction, malignant ventricular arrhythmias, and even sudden cardiac death can be seen in its progression from subclinical, silent forms to electrical forms with subtle changes on the electrocardiographic tracing, featuring negative T-waves in V1–V2 and minimal structural alterations [87–89].

The term "arrhythmogenic right ventricular cardiomyopathy/ dysplasia" was used prior to the advent of genetic testing and cardiac magnetic resonance imaging (CMR) to characterize the primary myocardial involvement of the right ventricle (RV). Following histopathological analysis, genotype-phenotype correlation studies, and the growing utilization of contrast-enhanced CMR, it has been discovered that the replacement of fibro-fatty tissue in the myocardium is the characteristic phenotypic manifestation of the disease, affecting not only the right ventricle but also the left ventricle. Further classifications have subdivided ARVC into the classic form with right-dominance, the form with biventricular involvement, and the left-dominant form [90], encompassing the more general term of arrhythmogenic cardiomyopathy.

The approach to ARVC diagnosis is based on a multiparametric algorithm, since the first proposed diagnostic criteria were released in 1994 by an International Task Force [91]. Subsequently, in 2010, the major and minor diagnostic criteria for the phenotypic diagnosis were refined by including cutoff values for defining dysfunction and dilation of the right ventricle (RV), along with quantitative histopathological aspects regarding the replacement of fibro-fatty tissue in the myocardium. This criteria upgrade also included a detailed assessment of electrocardiographic anomalies related to depolarization/repolarization and, for the first time, incorporated genotypic diagnosis for the evaluated patient [88]. However, in 2020, improved diagnostic criteria for ACM (the "Padua Criteria") were published as the result of an international expert consensus agreement [90], with the intention of a comprehensive approach for including the phenotypic features characteristic of biventricular/left-dominant involvement, with further refinement in 2023 by the same group [92].

The prevalence of heart failure in ARVC patients is not well-characterized [93, 94], but it may develop in approximately 50% of patients [95]. In addition, the prevalence of heart transplantation (HTx) or mortality resulting from heart failure (HF) in individuals with arrhythmogenic right ventricular cardiomyopathy (ARVC) probands ranges from around 5% to 20% in different cohorts and across diverse racial groups [96–102].

RV dysfunction and biventricular dysfunction are associated with an incremental risk of mortality and HTx [97]. Moreover, studies have shown a negative impact of left ventricular systolic dysfunction [103], atrial arrhythmias [104], and moderate-to-severe tricuspid regurgitation [105] on the progression of heart failure.

The likelihood of developing clinical heart failure seems to be linked to female sex and the presence of T-wave inversion (TWI) in the lateral precordial leads (specifically V4–V6) [95].

Imaging modalities for ARVC diagnosis may also assume a role in forecasting the progression towards heart failure. The presence of a higher extent of late gadolinium enhancement (LGE) within the left ventricle (LV) subepicardial layers of the myocardial wall on CMR demonstrated an inverse relationship with left ventricular ejection fraction (LVEF) [106].

Indeed, it is imperative to acknowledge that genotype exerts a substantial influence on the clinical phenotype of heart failure. Notably, biventricular and left ventricular dysfunction have been closely associated with specific genetic variants within DSP [107] and PLN [100, 108].

Moreover, another noteworthy aspect with potential ramifications for the development of heart failure pertains to the refined characterization of DSP-induced cardiomyopathy. This comprehensive characterization has recognized its correlation with recurrent episodes of myocardial inflammation and injury, resulting in fibrosis, myocardial dysfunction, and an elevated susceptibility to arrhythmias [107]. It is important to note that the available data results from case reports and case series, some of which originated during the pandemic period. During that time, cases initially construed as myocarditis associated with SARS-CoV-2 infection ultimately emerged in relation to pathogenic mutations within the DSP gene [109].

Although the management of individuals with ARVC is predominantly centered around the primary and secondary prevention of life-threatening arrhythmias and mitigating the risk of sudden cardiac death, in accordance with well-established pharmacological and interventional guideline recommendations for arrhythmia management, it is imperative to recognize that the existence of right ventricular systolic dysfunction (RVEF $< 40\%$) and left ventricular systolic dysfunction (LVEF $< 45\%$) represent notable risk factors that may bear considerable weight in the deliberation of ICD (implantable cardioverter-defibrillator) implantation [3, 110, 111]. In addition, progressive HF may not be identified as often as it should be. It is possible that typical signs and symptoms of LV HF, such as dyspnea and orthopnea, may be absent. Instead, the symptoms of RV HF such as abdominal bloating, jugular venous distention, and exhaustion may be more prominent, but often underrecognized [95].

Regarding the management of heart failure, adherence to the recommendations provided by international treatment guidelines on a case-by-case basis should aid the clinician in improving symptoms and functional capacity of patients, with medical treatments adjusted to the phenotype of heart failure (reduced/mildly reduced/preserved EF). In one experimental study, dapagliflozin attenuated ACM-associated cardiac fibrosis and inflammation in the case of a DSG2 mutation [112].

Restrictive Cardiomyopathy

The spectrum of RCM encompasses a wide array of classical etiologies, varying from intrinsic myocyte dysfunction associated with genetic variants, endomyocardial disorders or myocardial extracellular matrix disorders, as well as myocardial diseases with occasional restrictive physiology, often in the context of LVH (e.g. Anderson–Fabry, Danon, glycogenoses, iron overload/storage disorders, carcinoid, endocardial fibroelastosis, chemotherapy, amyloidosis, sarcoidosis, systemic sclerosis etc.) [3, 113] (Fig. 22.2).

Primary RCM is mostly inherited in an autosomal dominant pattern. Sarcomeric structural and regulatory proteins, as well as cytoskeletal intermediate filaments, are associated with RCM phenotype [114].

The classical presentation of RCM is with HFpEF signs and symptoms, with increased jugular venous pressure, tachycardia as a response to reduced cardiac output in advanced stages, as well as hepatomegaly, ascites, and peripheral oedema in decompensated patients.

Diastolic dysfunction with restrictive physiology is generally associated with more advanced stages and milder degrees of diastolic dysfunction are depicted at early diagnosis, echocardiography being the gold standard for diagnosis. In situations of diagnostic uncertainty and to help in the evaluation of cardiac transplant candidacy and timing, cardiac catheterization should be done [115].

The management of RCM involves addressing the root cause of the condition as well as managing any subsequent heart failure symptoms that may manifest as a result of the disease. The symptoms of RCM may be managed with a few different medications. Diuretics are the primary therapeutic approach for managing symptoms associated with heart failure. Their main objective is to alleviate volume overload. However, it is crucial to properly control diuretic administration in order to avoid excessive diuresis. This is particularly important for patients with RCM, as they depend on elevated filling pressures to sustain adequate cardiac output. To lengthen the filling period, beta-blockers or calcium channel blockers are sometimes used [42, 116].

Timely cardiac transplantation planning relies on accurate diagnosis (phenotype and etiology) that rules out all possible inherited and acquired phenocopies [3].

GENETIC	NON-GENETIC
Primary RCM	Amyloidosis (AL)
Variants in sarcomeric, cytoskeletal, nuclear envelope, filamin, titin gene	Endomyocardial fibrosis
Amyloidosis (ATTR)	Hypereosinophilia
Desminopathy	Carcinoid
Anderson-Fabry disease	Endocardial neoplasms
Glycogenoses	Radiotherapy
Danon	Chemotherapy
PRKAG2 variants	Sarcoidosis
Hemochromatosis	Systemic sclerosis
Pseudoxanthoma elasticum	Inflammatory/granulomatous
Primary hyperoxaluria	Drug toxicity
Endocardial fibroelastosis	Diabetic heart disease

Fig. 22.2 Restrictive phenotypes. (Adapted from [3])

Syndromic and Metabolic Cardiomyopathies

Beyond sarcomeric HCM, the "cardiomyopathy mindset" should always keep a high index of suspicion for the presence of inborn errors of metabolism or metabolic storage disorders that can mimic HCM, the so called "HCM phenocopies" in the presence of specific red flags. These inherited rare disorders (e.g. Anderson–Fabry, Danon, Pompe or mitochondrial disease) are usually characterized by multisystemic involvement, but the most prevailing clinical presentation is related to HF symptoms and conduction abnormalities [11, 117].

In Anderson-Fabry disease, accumulation of Gb3 affects all cardiac cell types and tissues, encompassing myocytes, endothelial and smooth muscle cells within intramyocardial vessels, endocardium, valvular fibroblasts, and conduction tissue [118]. Myocardial accumulation of Gb3 leads to progressive LVH and diastolic dysfunction. Fibrosis and involvement of conduction tissue are the underlying causes of ventricular arrhythmias and conduction abnormalities [119].

The 2023 ACC Expert Consensus Decision Pathway on Management of Heart Failure with Preserved Ejection Fraction [120] highlights the importance of discerning between various etiologies of "HFpEF mimics". Classifying individuals with signs of congestion and preserved EF in the HFpEF phenotype should not be considered the ultimate diagnostic approach, but rather a preliminary stage before more investigation into the underlying causes, bearing in mind the fact that certain etiologies can benefit from specific therapies. This is the case of Anderson-Fabry disease, for which treatment strategies include enzyme replacement therapy with agalsidase-α and agalsidase-β [121, 122], or with pharmacological chaperone, migalastat [123, 124], which should be started as soon as possible, before irreversible organ damage has taken place. Enzyme replacement therapy is recommended in all male patients as well as in all symptomatic FD women at the earliest signs of organ involvement [125].

A considerable percentage of individuals have a late-onset phenotype, with dominant cardiac involvement and slow progression due to remaining agalsidase-α enzyme activity. Heart failure in the so-called "cardiac variant" was reported in 21.9% of patients and mean survival free from HF was more frequent in females [125, 126]. Among the untreated population, 19.7% of females and 19.4% of males were reported to have dyspnea and heart failure [127].

Cardiac Amyloidosis

Amyloidosis cardiomyopathy represents a distinct subset which can have features from both restrictive and hypertrophic cardiomyopathy. Despite the fact that over 100 proteins histologically characterized by Congo red staining are known to have the ability to aggregate into amyloid [128, 129], only a dozen produced cardiac amyloidosis and more than 95% of amyloid cardiomyopathies are due to either AL (light-chain amyloidosis) or to ATTR (transthyretin amyloidosis) [130].

The diagnosis of cardiac amyloidosis (CA) relies on a multifaceted algorithm that incorporates both cardiac and extracardiac clues to raise suspicion for the diagnosis. Confirmation of CA can be achieved through the identification of amyloid deposits in cardiac tissue samples obtained via endomyocardial biopsy. Alternatively, a non-invasive approach can be employed, which involves the identification of amyloid deposits in extracardiac tissues through tissue biopsies combined with typical cardiac imaging findings or in the case of ATTR by the combination of diphosphonate scintigraphy coupled with serum and urine tests to rule-out the presence of a monoclonal paraprotein [131].

Ventricular wall thickening, increased ventricular rigidity, and consequently elevated ventricular filling pressure are all consequences of extracellular amyloid infiltration. Additionally, atrial wall infiltration is involved, leading to both functional and electrical changes (e.g., atrial fibrillation (AF) and atrial paralysis), in addition to an elevated risk of developing an atrial thrombosis [132].

In addition to interstitial infiltration, direct amyloid fibril toxicity and non-inflammatory oedema may contribute to cardiac dysfunction in AL and, to a lower degree, in ATTR [133].

Specifically, there is a discrepancy between the extent of the symptoms and the supranormal ejection fraction, which is correlated with significantly elevated levels of NTproBNP and persistent myocardial injury, as indicated by plateau troponin values.

Heart failure in cardiac amyloidosis (CA) is hitherto explained by the hallmarks of the restrictive phenotype and the association of systemic congestion and decreased cardiac output.

AL cardiac amyloidosis is characterized by a more expedited development of heart failure and a worse prognosis compared to ATTR. The prognosis in ATTR is contingent upon many factors, including the specific genetic variant and the extent of cardiac involvement, as well as the neurologic manifestations [134–137].

The management of systemic amyloidosis has seen significant advancements in recent years, benefiting patients with both AL and ATTR forms and leading to enhanced prognoses. Furthermore, recent research has shown that prompt medical intervention may result in a positive change in the patient's medical condition and a reduction in the presence of amyloid infiltration in the heart, as seen using imaging techniques such as cardiac magnetic resonance. The management of AL is overseen by the haematologist in collaboration with the cardiologist especially when there is notable cardiac expression. Therapeutic interventions targeting CA in the context of transthyretin (TTR) substrate include a range of approaches that address different stages of the disease pathophysiology. These strategies include interventions aimed at stabilizing TTR tetramers and inhibiting the aggregation of TTR oligomers (stabilizers), therapies to suppress TTR synthesis (either genetic silencers or gene editors) and antibodies directed against TTR (removers) [138]. Tafamidis was the first stabilizer approved by the FDA and European Medicines Agency (EMA) for treating patients with ATTR-CM, with a proven dose benefit of 80 mg of tafamidis meglumine/day (bioequivalent to 61 mg tafamidis free acid). In the ATTR-ACT randomized trial, including both ATTRv, as well as ATTRwt patients, treatment with tafamidis was associated with lower all-cause mortality (29.5% vs. 42.9%) and lower rate of cardiovascular-related hospitalizations. Furthermore, after 30 months, tafamidis demonstrated efficacy in mitigating symptoms, as evidenced by reduced rates of decline in distance evaluated by the 6-minute walk test and quality of life as measured by the Kansas City Cardiomyopathy Questionnaire score [139]. Recent positive results have been communicated with another stabilizer, acoramidis and results of large Phase 3 trials of genetic silencers (vutrisiran and eplontersen) will be available soon.

CA warrants particular attention in the context of heart failure. Central are fluid balance and euvolemia maintenance. Loop diuretics should be administered in the presence of symptoms of heart failure, even though orthostatic hypotension may lead to intolerance and excessive fluid loss may exacerbate symptoms due to restriction. The potential therapeutic efficacy of ARNIs, betablockers, ACE-Is, or ARBs in managing these patients remains uncertain, and their tolerability may be compromised due to hypotension. Additionally, withdrawal of classical HF medication often results in symptomatic relief and should be taken into account [3, 138, 140].

The introduction of dapagliflozin in individuals with ATTR who were already on tafamidis demonstrated favorable tolerability. However, further investigation is required via randomized controlled studies to assess the effectiveness of SGLT2i treatment in individuals diagnosed with ATTR-CA [141].

Advanced Heart Failure in Genetic Cardiomyopathies

Orthotopic cardiac transplantation represents the final therapeutic option for eligible cardiomyopathy patients [4] with advanced heart failure (NYHA class III-IV) or intractable ventricular arrhythmias. The majority of HCM patients undergoing transplantation exhibit significant impairment in left ventricular systolic function, often referred to as the 'burned-out' phase. It is worth noting that a minority of individuals with HCM may necessitate heart transplantation due to advanced heart failure, even in cases where the left ventricular ejection fraction (LVEF) remains preserved [142]. Advanced HF in DCM patients is encountered in more than 40% of recipients of long-term MCS, whether it's intended as a bridge to heart transplantation or as a destination therapy [143, 144].

In the largest series of HTx in ARVC patients, the use of ventricular assist devices was substantially reduced in ARVC patients, and 1- and 5-year post-HTx survival was greater in ARVC versus non-ARVC HTX recipients. Patients with ARVC also had lower risk of death or graft failure than non-ARVC patients [145]. ARVC poses distinct challenges in pre-transplant management, as RV morphology dysfunction and considerable ventricular arrhythmias restrict the use of inotropes and mechanical support options, respectively [146].

Prior to considering transplantation, a comprehensive evaluation is conducted, and exhaustion of all therapeutic options, including pharmacotherapy, VT endocardial/epicardial ablation and cardiac sympathetic denervation for electrical storm or polymorphic VT is performed [3].

Mechanical circulatory support therapy with left ventricular/biventricular assist devices should be considered for reducing symptoms and the risk of HF hospitalizations in selected cardiomyopathy patients with advanced heart failure (NYHA class III-IV) despite optimal medical therapy, as a bridge to heart transplant for those eligible and awaiting a transplant [147, 148]. However, in the case of patients not suitable for cardiac transplantation, mechanical circulatory support can be an option as bridge to destination, as long as severe right ventricular dysfunction is absent [3, 149]. The 2-year survival rates for patients receiving the latest types of continuous-flow left ventricular assist devices (LVAD) are comparable to those following heart transplantation, although adverse events have a detrimental impact on the quality of life (QOL). In the case of patients with continuous-flow LVADs, survival rates were 80% at 1 year and 70% at 2 years [144, 150].

Conclusions

In embracing the complexities of cardiomyopathy and heart failure, a profound shift in mindset is imperative. The journey from diagnosis to management requires a resilient approach that fosters the recognition of structural, functional, and clinical implications of the disease. A cardiomyopathy mindset entails understanding the intricacies of one's cardiac phenotype, adapting lifestyle choices, and embracing a sense of personalized treatment approach. In addition, the heart failure mindset involves acknowledging the challenges of the standard treatment pillars that may not invariably prove universally suitable for individuals with cardiomyopathies, and such maintaining a vigilant commitment to follow-up. In conclusion, navigating the landscape of cardiomyopathy and heart failure demands a dual commitment to medical approach and a nuanced mindset, the welfare of the patient being the principal objective.

References

1. Elliott P, et al. Classification of the cardiomyopathies: a position statement from the European Society of Cardiology Working Group on Myocardial and Pericardial Diseases. Eur Heart J. 2008;29:270–6.
2. Maron BJ, et al. Contemporary definitions and classification of the cardiomyopathies: an American Heart Association scientific statement from the council on clinical cardiology, heart failure and transplantation committee; quality of care and outcomes research and functional genomics and translational biology interdisciplinary working groups; and council on epidemiology and prevention. Circulation. 2006;113:1807–16.
3. Arbelo E, et al. 2023 ESC Guidelines for the management of cardiomyopathies: developed by the task force on the management of cardiomyopathies of the European Society of Cardiology (ESC). Eur Heart J. 2023;44:3503–626. https://doi.org/10.1093/eurheartj/ehad194.
4. McDonagh TA, et al. 2021 ESC Guidelines for the diagnosis and treatment of acute and chronic heart failure: developed by the Task Force for the diagnosis and treatment of acute

and chronic heart failure of the European Society of Cardiology (ESC) with the special contribution of the Heart Failure Association (HFA) of the ESC. Eur Heart J. 2021;42:3599–726. https://doi.org/10.1093/eurheartj/ehab368.
5. Marian AJ, Braunwald E. Hypertrophic cardiomyopathy: genetics, pathogenesis, clinical manifestations, diagnosis, and therapy. Circ Res. 2017;121:749–70. https://doi.org/10.1161/circresaha.117.311059.
6. Maron MS, et al. Hypertrophic cardiomyopathy is predominantly a disease of left ventricular outflow tract obstruction. Circulation. 2006;114:2232–9.
7. Members ATF, et al. 2014 ESC Guidelines on diagnosis and management of hypertrophic cardiomyopathy: the Task Force for the Diagnosis and Management of Hypertrophic Cardiomyopathy of the European Society of Cardiology (ESC). Eur Heart J. 2014;35:2733–79. https://doi.org/10.1093/eurheartj/ehu284.
8. Olivotto I, et al. The many faces of hypertrophic cardiomyopathy: from developmental biology to clinical practice. J Cardiovasc Transl Res. 2009;2:349–67.
9. Ho CY, et al. Genotype and lifetime burden of disease in hypertrophic cardiomyopathy: insights from the Sarcomeric Human Cardiomyopathy Registry (SHaRe). Circulation. 2018;138:1387–98.
10. Maron BJ, Rowin EJ, Udelson JE, Maron MS. Clinical spectrum and management of heart failure in hypertrophic cardiomyopathy. JACC Heart Fail. 2018;6:353–63.
11. Seferović PM, et al. Heart failure in cardiomyopathies: a position paper from the Heart Failure Association of the European Society of Cardiology. Eur J Heart Fail. 2019;21:553–76.
12. Rowin EJ, et al. Outcomes in patients with hypertrophic cardiomyopathy and left ventricular systolic dysfunction. J Am Coll Cardiol. 2020;75:3033–43. https://doi.org/10.1016/j.jacc.2020.04.045.
13. Zampieri M, et al. Clinical scenarios of hypertrophic cardiomyopathy-related mortality: relevance of age and stage of disease at presentation. Int J Cardiol. 2023;374:65–72.
14. Ishihara K, et al. Predictive factors for decreasing left ventricular ejection fraction and progression to the dilated phase of hypertrophic cardiomyopathy. J Clin Med. 2023;12:5137.
15. Dybro AM, et al. Effects of metoprolol on exercise hemodynamics in patients with obstructive hypertrophic cardiomyopathy. J Am Coll Cardiol. 2022;79:1565–75. https://doi.org/10.1016/j.jacc.2022.02.024.
16. Olivotto I, et al. Mavacamten for treatment of symptomatic obstructive hypertrophic cardiomyopathy (EXPLORER-HCM): a randomised, double-blind, placebo-controlled, phase 3 trial. Lancet. 2020;396:759–69. https://doi.org/10.1016/S0140-6736(20)31792-X.
17. Spoladore R, Maron MS, D'Amato R, Camici PG, Olivotto I. Pharmacological treatment options for hypertrophic cardiomyopathy: high time for evidence. Eur Heart J. 2012;33:1724–33. https://doi.org/10.1093/eurheartj/ehs150.
18. Olivotto I, et al. Impact of atrial fibrillation on the clinical course of hypertrophic cardiomyopathy. Circulation. 2001;104:2517–24.
19. Ha HS, et al. Catheter ablation for atrial fibrillation in hypertrophic cardiomyopathy patients: a systematic review. J Interv Card Electrophysiol. 2015;44:161–70.
20. Providencia R, et al. Catheter ablation for atrial fibrillation in hypertrophic cardiomyopathy: a systematic review and meta-analysis. Heart. 2016;102:1533–43.
21. Zhao D-S, et al. Outcomes of catheter ablation of atrial fibrillation in patients with hypertrophic cardiomyopathy: a systematic review and meta-analysis. Europace. 2016;18:508–20.
22. Gaita F, et al. Usefulness and safety of transcatheter ablation of atrial fibrillation in patients with hypertrophic cardiomyopathy. Am J Cardiol. 2007;99:1575–81.
23. Bassiouny M, et al. Outcomes of nonpharmacologic treatment of atrial fibrillation in patients with hypertrophic cardiomyopathy. Heart Rhythm. 2015;12:1438–47.
24. Bunch TJ, et al. Substrate and procedural predictors of outcomes after catheter ablation for atrial fibrillation in patients with hypertrophic cardiomyopathy. J Cardiovasc Electrophysiol. 2008;19:1009–14.

25. Santangeli P, et al. Catheter ablation of atrial fibrillation in hypertrophic cardiomyopathy: long-term outcomes and mechanisms of arrhythmia recurrence. Circ Arrhythm Electrophysiol. 2013;6:1089–94.
26. Camm AJ, et al. Guidelines for the management of atrial fibrillation: the Task Force for the Management of Atrial Fibrillation of the European Society of Cardiology (ESC). Eur Heart J. 2010;31:2369–429. https://doi.org/10.1093/eurheartj/ehq278.
27. Camm AJ, et al. 2012 focused update of the ESC Guidelines for the management of atrial fibrillation: an update of the 2010 ESC Guidelines for the management of atrial fibrillation. Developed with the special contribution of the European Heart Rhythm Association. Eur Heart J. 2012;33:2719–47. https://doi.org/10.1093/eurheartj/ehs253.
28. Sherrid MV, et al. Treatment of obstructive hypertrophic cardiomyopathy symptoms and gradient resistant to first-line therapy with β-blockade or verapamil. Circ Heart Fail. 2013;6:694–702. https://doi.org/10.1161/circheartfailure.112.000122.
29. Sherrid MV, et al. Multicenter study of the efficacy and safety of disopyramide in obstructive hypertrophic cardiomyopathy. J Am Coll Cardiol. 2005;45:1251–8. https://doi.org/10.1016/j.jacc.2005.01.012.
30. Dybro AM, et al. Randomized trial of metoprolol in patients with obstructive hypertrophic cardiomyopathy. J Am Coll Cardiol. 2021;78:2505–17. https://doi.org/10.1016/j.jacc.2021.07.065.
31. Adelman AG, Shah PM, Gramiak R, Wigle ED. Long-term propranolol therapy in muscular subaortic stenosis. Br Heart J. 1970;32:804–11. https://doi.org/10.1136/hrt.32.6.804.
32. Flamm MD, Harrison DC, Hancock EW. Muscular subaortic stenosis. Prevention of outflow obstruction with propranolol. Circulation. 1968;38:846–58. https://doi.org/10.1161/01.cir.38.5.846.
33. Monda E, et al. Bisoprolol for treatment of symptomatic patients with obstructive hypertrophic cardiomyopathy. The BASIC (bisoprolol AS therapy in hypertrophic cardiomyopathy) study. Int J Cardiol. 2022;354:22–8. https://doi.org/10.1016/j.ijcard.2022.03.013.
34. Stauffer JC, Ruiz V, Morard JD. Subaortic obstruction after sildenafil in a patient with hypertrophic cardiomyopathy. N Engl J Med. 1999;341:700–1. https://doi.org/10.1056/nejm199908263410916.
35. O'Connor MJ, et al. Disopyramide use in infants and children with hypertrophic cardiomyopathy. Cardiol Young. 2018;28:530–5. https://doi.org/10.1017/s1047951117002384.
36. Adler A, et al. Safety of outpatient initiation of disopyramide for obstructive hypertrophic cardiomyopathy patients. J Am Heart Assoc. 2017;6 https://doi.org/10.1161/jaha.116.005152.
37. Desai MY, et al. Dose-blinded myosin inhibition in patients with obstructive hypertrophic cardiomyopathy referred for septal reduction therapy: outcomes through 32 weeks. Circulation. 2023;147:850–63. https://doi.org/10.1161/circulationaha.122.062534.
38. Desai MY, et al. Myosin inhibition in patients with obstructive hypertrophic cardiomyopathy referred for septal reduction therapy. J Am Coll Cardiol. 2022;80:95–108. https://doi.org/10.1016/j.jacc.2022.04.048.
39. Maron BJ, Towbin JA, Thiene G, Antzelevitch C, Corrado D, Arnett D, Moss AJ, Seidman CE, Young JB; American Heart Association; Council on Clinical Cardiology, Heart Failure and Transplantation Committee; Quality of Care and Outcomes Research and Functional Genomics and Translational Biology Interdisciplinary Working Groups; Council on Epidemiology and Prevention. Contemporary definitions and classification of the cardiomyopathies: an American Heart Association Scientific Statement from the Council on Clinical Cardiology, Heart Failure and Transplantation Committee; Quality of Care and Outcomes Research and Functional Genomics and Translational Biology Interdisciplinary Working Groups; and Council on Epidemiology and Prevention. Circulation. 2006;113(14):1807–16. https://doi.org/10.1161/CIRCULATIONAHA.106.174287. Epub 2006 Mar 27. PMID: 16567565.
40. Agarwal S, et al. Updated meta-analysis of septal alcohol ablation versus myectomy for hypertrophic cardiomyopathy. J Am Coll Cardiol. 2010;55:823–34.

41. Alam M, Dokainish H, Lakkis NM. Hypertrophic obstructive cardiomyopathy-alcohol septal ablation vs. myectomy: a meta-analysis. Eur Heart J. 2009;30:1080–7.
42. Brown KN, Pendela VS, Ahmed I, Diaz RR. Restrictive cardiomyopathy. In: StatPearls [Internet]. Treasure Island: StatPearls Publishing; 2019.
43. Bytyçi I, Nistri S, Mörner S, Henein MY. Alcohol septal ablation versus septal myectomy treatment of obstructive hypertrophic cardiomyopathy: a systematic review and meta-analysis. J Clin Med. 2020;9:3062.
44. Leonardi RA, Kransdorf EP, Simel DL, Wang A. Meta-analyses of septal reduction therapies for obstructive hypertrophic cardiomyopathy: comparative rates of overall mortality and sudden cardiac death after treatment. Circ Cardiovasc Interv. 2010;3:97–104.
45. Nguyen A, et al. Surgical myectomy versus alcohol septal ablation for obstructive hypertrophic cardiomyopathy: a propensity score–matched cohort. J Thorac Cardiovasc Surg. 2019;157:306–315.e303.
46. Zeng Z, Wang F, Dou X, Zhang S, Pu J. Comparison of percutaneous transluminal septal myocardial ablation versus septal myectomy for the treatment of patients with hypertrophic obstructive cardiomyopathy—a meta analysis. Int J Cardiol. 2006;112:80–4.
47. Mentias A, et al. Survival after septal reduction in patients> 65 years old with obstructive hypertrophic cardiomyopathy. J Am Coll Cardiol. 2023;81:105–15.
48. Pinto YM, et al. Proposal for a revised definition of dilated cardiomyopathy, hypokinetic non-dilated cardiomyopathy, and its implications for clinical practice: a position statement of the ESC working group on myocardial and pericardial diseases. Eur Heart J. 2016;37:1850–8. https://doi.org/10.1093/eurheartj/ehv727.
49. Halliday BP, et al. Sex- and age-based differences in the natural history and outcome of dilated cardiomyopathy. Eur J Heart Fail. 2018;20:1392–400. https://doi.org/10.1002/ejhf.1216.
50. Sinagra G, Elliott PM, Merlo M. Dilated cardiomyopathy: so many cardiomyopathies! Eur Heart J. 2020;41:3784–6.
51. Merlo M, et al. Evolving concepts in dilated cardiomyopathy. Eur J Heart Fail. 2018;20:228–39.
52. Asselbergs FW, et al. Differences between familial and sporadic dilated cardiomyopathy: ESC EORP Cardiomyopathy & Myocarditis registry. ESC Heart Fail. 2021;8:95–105.
53. McKenna WJ, Judge DP. Epidemiology of the inherited cardiomyopathies. Nat Rev Cardiol. 2021;18:22–36.
54. Kayvanpour E, et al. Genotype-phenotype associations in dilated cardiomyopathy: meta-analysis on more than 8000 individuals. Clin Res Cardiol. 2017;106:127–39.
55. Escobar-Lopez L, et al. Association of genetic variants with outcomes in patients with non-ischemic dilated cardiomyopathy. J Am Coll Cardiol. 2021;78:1682–99.
56. Gigli M, et al. Genetic risk of arrhythmic phenotypes in patients with dilated cardiomyopathy. J Am Coll Cardiol. 2019;74:1480–90.
57. Hey TM, et al. Clinical and genetic investigations of 109 index patients with dilated cardiomyopathy and 445 of their relatives. Circ Heart Fail. 2020;13:e006701.
58. Garcia-Pavia P, et al. Genetic variants associated with cancer therapy–induced cardiomyopathy. Circulation. 2019;140:31–41.
59. Ware JS, et al. Genetic etiology for alcohol-induced cardiac toxicity. J Am Coll Cardiol. 2018;71:2293–302.
60. Ware JS, et al. Shared genetic predisposition in peripartum and dilated cardiomyopathies. N Engl J Med. 2016;374:233–41.
61. Catchpool M, et al. A cost-effectiveness model of genetic testing and periodical clinical screening for the evaluation of families with dilated cardiomyopathy. Genet Med. 2019;21:2815–22.
62. Bordet C, et al. Psychosocial impact of predictive genetic testing in hereditary heart diseases: the PREDICT study. J Clin Med. 2020;9:1365.

63. Patel AR, Kramer CM. Role of cardiac magnetic resonance in the diagnosis and prognosis of nonischemic cardiomyopathy. JACC Cardiovasc Imaging. 2017;10:1180–93.
64. La Gerche A, et al. Cardiac MRI: a new gold standard for ventricular volume quantification during high-intensity exercise. Circ Cardiovasc Imaging. 2012;6:329–38.
65. Seraphim A, et al. Quantitative cardiac MRI. J Magn Reson Imaging. 2020;51:693–711.
66. Kim RJ, et al. The use of contrast-enhanced magnetic resonance imaging to identify reversible myocardial dysfunction. N Engl J Med. 2000;343:1445–53.
67. Messroghli DR, et al. Clinical recommendations for cardiovascular magnetic resonance mapping of T1, T2, T2* and extracellular volume: a consensus statement by the Society for Cardiovascular Magnetic Resonance (SCMR) endorsed by the European Association for Cardiovascular Imaging (EACVI). J Cardiovasc Magn Reson. 2017;19:1–24.
68. Moon JC, et al. Myocardial T1 mapping and extracellular volume quantification: a Society for Cardiovascular Magnetic Resonance (SCMR) and CMR Working Group of the European Society of Cardiology consensus statement. J Cardiovasc Magn Reson. 2013;15:1–12.
69. Gulati A, et al. Association of fibrosis with mortality and sudden cardiac death in patients with nonischemic dilated cardiomyopathy. JAMA. 2013;309:896–908.
70. Assomull RG, et al. Cardiovascular magnetic resonance, fibrosis, and prognosis in dilated cardiomyopathy. J Am Coll Cardiol. 2006;48:1977–85.
71. Becker MA, et al. The prognostic value of late gadolinium-enhanced cardiac magnetic resonance imaging in nonischemic dilated cardiomyopathy: a review and meta-analysis. JACC Cardiovasc Imaging. 2018;11:1274–84.
72. Kuruvilla S, et al. Late gadolinium enhancement on cardiac magnetic resonance predicts adverse cardiovascular outcomes in nonischemic cardiomyopathy: a systematic review and meta-analysis. Circ Cardiovasc Imaging. 2014;7:250–8.
73. Buss SJ, et al. Assessment of myocardial deformation with cardiac magnetic resonance strain imaging improves risk stratification in patients with dilated cardiomyopathy. Eur Heart J Cardiovasc Imaging. 2015;16:307–15.
74. ClinicalTrials.gov. Exploratory study of danicamtiv in patients with primary dilated cardiomyopathy (DCM) Due to genetic variants or other causalities, 2023, March 7. https://classic.clinicaltrials.gov/ct2/show/NCT04572893
75. de Boer RA, et al. Targeted therapies in genetic dilated and hypertrophic cardiomyopathies: from molecular mechanisms to therapeutic targets. A position paper from the Heart Failure Association (HFA) and the Working Group on Myocardial Function of the European Society of Cardiology (ESC). Eur J Heart Fail. 2022;24:406–20.
76. Doevendans PA, Glijnis PC, Kranias EG. Leducq transatlantic network of excellence to CURE phospholamban-induced car-diomyopathy (CURE-PLaN). Circ Res. 2019;125:720–4. https://doi.org/10.1161/CIRCRESAHA.119.315077.
77. Beverborg N, et al. Phospholamban antisense oligonucleotides improve cardiac function in murine cardiomyopathy. Nat Commun. 2021;12:5180.
78. Fomin A, et al. Truncated titin proteins and titin haploinsufficiency are targets for functional recovery in human cardiomyopathy due to TTN mutations. Sci Transl Med. 2021;13:eabd3079.
79. Ponikowski P, et al. 2016 ESC Guidelines for the diagnosis and treatment of acute and chronic heart failure. Eur Heart J. 2016;74:1037–147.
80. Verdonschot JAJ, et al. Value of speckle tracking–based deformation analysis in screening relatives of patients with asymptomatic dilated cardiomyopathy. JACC Cardiovasc Imaging. 2020;13:549–58.
81. Donal E, et al. Multimodality imaging in the diagnosis, risk stratification, and management of patients with dilated cardiomyopathies: an expert consensus document from the European Association of Cardiovascular Imaging. Eur Heart J Cardiovasc Imaging. 2019;20:1075–93. https://doi.org/10.1093/ehjci/jez178.
82. Hasselberg NE, et al. Risk prediction of ventricular arrhythmias and myocardial function in Lamin A/C mutation positive subjects. Europace. 2014;16:563–71.
83. Verstraelen TE, et al. Prediction of ventricular arrhythmia in phospholamban p. Arg14del mutation carriers–reaching the frontiers of individual risk prediction. Eur Heart J. 2021;42:2842–50.

84. Wang W, et al. Clinical characteristics and risk stratification of desmoplakin cardiomyopathy. Europace. 2022;24:268–77.
85. Ortiz-Genga MF, et al. Truncating FLNC mutations are associated with high-risk dilated and arrhythmogenic cardiomyopathies. J Am Coll Cardiol. 2016;68:2440–51.
86. McDonagh TA, et al. 2023 Focused Update of the 2021 ESC Guidelines for the diagnosis and treatment of acute and chronic heart failure: developed by the task force for the diagnosis and treatment of acute and chronic heart failure of the European Society of Cardiology (ESC) with the special contribution of the Heart Failure Association (HFA) of the ESC. Eur Heart J. 2023;44:3627–39. https://doi.org/10.1093/eurheartj/ehad195.
87. Towbin JA, et al. 2019 HRS expert consensus statement on evaluation, risk stratification, and management of arrhythmogenic cardiomyopathy. Heart Rhythm. 2019;16:e301–72.
88. Marcus FI, et al. Diagnosis of arrhythmogenic right ventricular cardiomyopathy/dysplasia: proposed modification of the task force criteria. Circulation. 2010;121:1533–41.
89. Corrado D, Link MS, Calkins H. Arrhythmogenic right ventricular cardiomyopathy. N Engl J Med. 2017;376:61–72.
90. Corrado D, et al. Diagnosis of arrhythmogenic cardiomyopathy: the Padua criteria. Int J Cardiol. 2020;319:106–14.
91. McKenna WJ, et al. Diagnosis of arrhythmogenic right ventricular dysplasia/cardiomyopathy. Task Force of the Working Group Myocardial and Pericardial Disease of the European Society of Cardiology and of the Scientific Council on Cardiomyopathies of the International Society and Federation of Cardiology. Br Heart J. 1994;71:215–8. https://doi.org/10.1136/hrt.71.3.215.
92. Corrado D, et al. Proposed diagnostic criteria for arrhythmogenic cardiomyopathy. European Task Force consensus report. Int J Cardiol. 2023;395:131447.
93. Protonotarios N, et al. Arrhythmogenic right ventricular cardiomyopathy/dysplasia on the basis of the revised diagnostic criteria in affected families with desmosomal mutations. Eur Heart J. 2011;32:1097–104.
94. Bhonsale A, et al. Impact of genotype on clinical course in arrhythmogenic right ventricular dysplasia/cardiomyopathy-associated mutation carriers. Eur Heart J. 2015;36:847–55.
95. Gilotra NA, et al. Heart failure is common and under-recognized in patients with arrhythmogenic right ventricular cardiomyopathy/dysplasia. Circ Heart Fail. 2017;10:e003819.
96. Watkins DA, et al. Clinical features, survival experience, and profile of plakophylin-2 gene mutations in participants of the arrhythmogenic right ventricular cardiomyopathy registry of South Africa. Heart Rhythm. 2009;6:S10–7.
97. Pinamonti B, et al. Prognostic predictors in arrhythmogenic right ventricular cardiomyopathy: results from a 10-year registry. Eur Heart J. 2011;32:1105–13.
98. Kimura Y, et al. Heart failure in patients with arrhythmogenic right ventricular cardiomyopathy: what are the risk factors? Int J Cardiol. 2017;241:288–94.
99. Groeneweg JA, et al. Clinical presentation, long-term follow-up, and outcomes of 1001 arrhythmogenic right ventricular dysplasia/cardiomyopathy patients and family members. Circ Cardiovasc Genet. 2015;8:437–46.
100. Chen S, Chen L, Duru F, Hu SJJOCM. Heart failure in patients with arrhythmogenic cardiomyopathy. J Clin Med. 2021;10:4782.
101. Gilljam T, et al. Heart transplantation in arrhythmogenic right ventricular cardiomyopathy—experience from the Nordic ARVC Registry. Int J Cardiol. 2018;250:201–6.
102. Chen S, et al. Novel risk prediction model to determine adverse heart failure outcomes in arrhythmogenic right ventricular cardiomyopathy. J Am Heart Assoc. 2022;11:e024634.
103. Hulot J-S, Jouven X, Empana J-P, Frank R, Fontaine GJC. Natural history and risk stratification of arrhythmogenic right ventricular dysplasia/cardiomyopathy. Circulation. 2004;110:1879–84.
104. Baturova MA, et al. Atrial fibrillation as a clinical characteristic of arrhythmogenic right ventricular cardiomyopathy: experience from the Nordic ARVC Registry. Circulation. 2020;298:39–43.
105. Jeong H, et al. Characteristics and prognostic implications of tricuspid regurgitation in patients with arrhythmogenic cardiomyopathy. ESC Heart Fail. 2020;7:2933–40.

106. Cipriani A, et al. Arrhythmogenic right ventricular cardiomyopathy: characterization of left ventricular phenotype and differential diagnosis with dilated cardiomyopathy. J Am Heart Assoc. 2020;9:e014628.
107. Smith ED, et al. Desmoplakin cardiomyopathy, a fibrotic and inflammatory form of cardiomyopathy distinct from typical dilated or arrhythmogenic right ventricular cardiomyopathy. Circulation. 2020;141:1872–84.
108. van der Zwaag PA, et al. Phospholamban R14del mutation in patients diagnosed with dilated cardiomyopathy or arrhythmogenic right ventricular cardiomyopathy: evidence supporting the concept of arrhythmogenic cardiomyopathy. Eur J Heart Fail. 2012;14:1199–207.
109. Bookani KR, et al. A case series of desmoplakin cardiomyopathy: a mimic of viral myocarditis. Eur Heart J Case Rep. 2022;6:ytac341.
110. Bosman LP, et al. Predicting arrhythmic risk in arrhythmogenic right ventricular cardiomyopathy: a systematic review and meta-analysis. Heart Rhythm. 2018;15:1097–107.
111. Bosman LP, et al. Comparing clinical performance of current implantable cardioverter-defibrillator implantation recommendations in arrhythmogenic right ventricular cardiomyopathy. Europace. 2022;24:296–305.
112. Yang Z, et al. SGLT2 inhibitor dapagliflozin attenuates cardiac fibrosis and inflammation by reverting the HIF-2α signaling pathway in arrhythmogenic cardiomyopathy. FASEB J. 2022;36:e22410.
113. Rapezzi C, et al. Restrictive cardiomyopathy: definition and diagnosis. Eur Heart J. 2022;43:4679–93.
114. Gallego-Delgado M, et al. Idiopathic restrictive cardiomyopathy is primarily a genetic disease. J Am Coll Cardiol. 2016;67:3021–3.
115. Fenton MJ, et al. Heart and heart–lung transplantation for idiopathic restrictive cardiomyopathy in children. Heart. 2006;92:85–9.
116. Rammos A, Meladinis V, Vovas G, Patsouras D. Restrictive cardiomyopathies: the importance of noninvasive cardiac imaging modalities in diagnosis and treatment—a systematic review. Radiol Res Pract. 2017;2017:2874902.
117. Mehta A, et al. Fabry disease defined: baseline clinical manifestations of 366 patients in the Fabry Outcome Survey. Eur J Clin Investig. 2004;34:236–42.
118. Nair V, Belanger EC, Veinot JP. Lysosomal storage disorders affecting the heart: a review. Cardiovasc Pathol. 2019;39:12–24.
119. Pieroni M, et al. Cardiac involvement in Fabry disease: JACC review topic of the week. J Am Coll Cardiol. 2021;77:922–36.
120. Kittleson MM, et al. 2023 ACC expert consensus decision pathway on management of heart failure with preserved ejection fraction. J Am Coll Cardiol. 2023;81:1835–78. https://doi.org/10.1016/j.jacc.2023.03.393.
121. Banikazemi M, et al. Agalsidase-beta therapy for advanced Fabry disease: a randomized trial. Ann Intern Med. 2007;146:77–86.
122. Mehta A, et al. Enzyme replacement therapy with agalsidase alfa in patients with Fabry's disease: an analysis of registry data. Lancet. 2009;374:1986–96.
123. Hughes DA, et al. Oral pharmacological chaperone migalastat compared with enzyme replacement therapy in Fabry disease: 18-month results from the randomised phase III ATTRACT study. J Med Genet. 2017;54:288–96.
124. Müntze J, Salinger T, Gensler D, Wanner C, Nordbeck P. Treatment of hypertrophic cardiomyopathy caused by cardiospecific variants of Fabry disease with chaperone therapy. Eur Heart J. 2018;39:1861–2.
125. Linhart A, et al. An expert consensus document on the management of cardiovascular manifestations of Fabry disease. Eur J Heart Fail. 2020;22:1076–96.
126. Azevedo O, et al. Natural history of the late-onset phenotype of Fabry disease due to the p. F113L mutation. Mol Genet Metab Rep. 2020;22:100565.
127. Linhart A, et al. Cardiac manifestations of Anderson–Fabry disease: results from the international Fabry outcome survey. Eur Heart J. 2007;28:1228–35.

128. Benson MD, et al. Amyloid nomenclature 2018: recommendations by the International Society of Amyloidosis (ISA) nomenclature committee. Amyloid. 2018;25:215–9.
129. Sipe JD, Cohen AS. History of the amyloid fibril. J Struct Biol. 2000;130:88–98.
130. Garcia-Pavia P, et al. Diagnosis and treatment of cardiac amyloidosis: a position statement of the ESC Working Group on Myocardial and Pericardial Diseases. Eur Heart J. 2021;42:1554–68.
131. Jurcuţ R, et al. Multimodality imaging in cardiac amyloidosis: a primer for cardiologists. Eur Heart J Cardiovasc Imaging. 2020;21:833–44.
132. Nochioka K, et al. Left atrial structure and function in cardiac amyloidosis. Eur Heart J Cardiovasc Imaging. 2017;18:1128–37.
133. Siddiqi OK, Ruberg FL. Cardiac amyloidosis: an update on pathophysiology, diagnosis, and treatment. Trends Cardiovasc Med. 2018;28:10–21.
134. Damy T, et al. Prevalence and clinical phenotype of hereditary transthyretin amyloid cardiomyopathy in patients with increased left ventricular wall thickness. Eur Heart J. 2016;37:1826–34.
135. Rapezzi C, et al. Systemic cardiac amyloidoses: disease profiles and clinical courses of the 3 main types. Circulation. 2009;120:1203–12.
136. Ruberg FL, et al. Prospective evaluation of the morbidity and mortality of wild-type and V122I mutant transthyretin amyloid cardiomyopathy: the Transthyretin Amyloidosis Cardiac Study (TRACS). Am Heart J. 2012;164:222–228.e221.
137. Grogan M, et al. Natural history of wild-type transthyretin cardiac amyloidosis and risk stratification using a novel staging system. J Am Coll Cardiol. 2016;68:1014–20.
138. Adam RD, et al. Progress and challenges in the treatment of cardiac amyloidosis: a review of the literature. ESC Heart Fail. 2021;8:2380–96.
139. Maurer MS, et al. Tafamidis treatment for patients with transthyretin amyloid cardiomyopathy. N Engl J Med. 2018;379:1007–16.
140. Oghina S, et al. The impact of patients with cardiac amyloidosis in HFpEF trials. JACC Heart Fail. 2021;9:169–78.
141. Dobner S, et al. SGLT2 inhibitor therapy for transthyretin amyloid cardiomyopathy: early tolerance and clinical response to dapagliflozin. ESC Heart Fail. 2023;10:397–404.
142. Rowin EJ, et al. Advanced heart failure with preserved systolic function in nonobstructive hypertrophic cardiomyopathy: under-recognized subset of candidates for heart transplant. Circ Heart Fail. 2014;7:967–75.
143. Yoshioka D, et al. Outcome of heart transplantation after bridge-to-transplant strategy using various mechanical circulatory support devices. Interact Cardiovasc Thorac Surg. 2017;25:918–24.
144. Rose EA, et al. Long-term use of a left ventricular assist device for end-stage heart failure. N Engl J Med. 2001;345:1435–43.
145. Giuliano K, et al. Heart transplantation outcomes in arrhythmogenic right ventricular cardiomyopathy: a contemporary national analysis. ESC Heart Fail. 2022;9:988–97.
146. Scheel PJ 3rd, et al. Heart transplantation strategies in arrhythmogenic right ventricular cardiomyopathy: a tertiary ARVC centre experience. ESC Heart Fail. 2022;9:1008–17.
147. Zimpfer D, et al. Two-year outcome after implantation of a full magnetically levitated left ventricular assist device: results from the ELEVATE Registry. Eur Heart J. 2020;41:3801–9.
148. Kirklin JK, et al. Seventh INTERMACS annual report: 15,000 patients and counting. J Heart Lung Transplant. 2015;34:1495–504.
149. Goldstein DJ, et al. Association of clinical outcomes with left ventricular assist device use by bridge to transplant or destination therapy intent: the multicenter study of MagLev technology in patients undergoing mechanical circulatory support therapy with HeartMate 3 (MOMENTUM 3) randomized clinical trial. JAMA Cardiol. 2020;5:411–9.
150. Theochari CA, et al. Heart transplantation versus left ventricular assist devices as destination therapy or bridge to transplantation for 1-year mortality: a systematic review and meta-analysis. Ann Cardiothorac Surg. 2018;7:3.

Chapter 23
Acute Heart Failure: Epidemiology, Treatment, and Outcomes

Laura Antohi, Ovidiu Chioncel, and Marianna Adamo

Abstract Acute heart failure (AHF) represents rapid or gradual onset or worsening of symptoms and/or signs of HF, reflecting diverse abnormalities of congestion and/or hypoperfusion status, leading to either unplanned hospital admission, emergency department (ED) visit or outpatient visit. In patients with history of HF, escalation of therapies, irrespective of venue of care, identifies worsening HF episodes.

Diagnosis must start at the time of the first medical contact and should be based on clinical judgment to integrate patient history with physical examination. Since the sensitivity and specificity of symptoms and signs are only modest, diagnosis of AHF should be further confirmed by appropriate additional investigations such as biomarkers, ECG, chest X-ray, lung ultrasound, laboratory assessment and echocardiography. Coexisting life-threatening clinical conditions that require urgent correction need to be immediately identified and managed, before any other therapeutic measures. The diagnostic workup should continue with the identification of clinical phenotypes, Acutely Decompensated HF (ADHF), Acute Pulmonary Oedema (APO), Acute Right Failure (ARF) and Cardiogenic Shock (CS), that would support the initiation of the early individualized treatments.

Management of AHF represents a continuum of evaluation, initiating therapies, assessing response to implemented therapies and creating a plan for the immediate, short and medium term care.

Keywords Diagnosis · Clinical profiles · Risk stratification · Management

L. Antohi · O. Chioncel (✉)
Intensive Cardiac Care Unit, Emergency Hospital for Cardiovascular Diseases, University for Medicine and Pharmacy, Bucharest, Romania

M. Adamo
Institute of Cardiology and Cardiac Catheterization Laboratory, ASST Spedali Civili di Brescia, Department of Medical and Surgical Specialties, Radiological Sciences, and Public Health, University of Brescia, Brescia, Italy

M. Dorobanţu et al. (eds.), *Current Approach to Heart Failure*,
https://doi.org/10.1007/978-3-031-96562-3_23

Definition

Acute heart failure (AHF) remains a major cause of hospitalization [1] and mortality [1, 2]. Despite several reviews, guidelines and consensus documents, the definition of AHF remains controversial [3–7]. This is partly related to the fact that AHF is a clinical diagnosis and no single biological or hemodynamic parameter is ideally suited to ascertain the diagnosis.

There is a large spectrum of AHF presentations resulting from the interaction between an acute precipitant and a patient's underlying cardiac and overall medical condition, including previous comorbidities [1]. The heterogeneity of the pathophysiology and clinical presentations of this syndrome as well as the variable relationship between the chronic condition and the episodes of acute decompensation remain major factors hindering a simple and thorough definition of this condition.

AHF refers to rapid or gradual onset or worsening of symptoms and/or signs of HF, reflecting diverse abnormalities of congestion and/or hypoperfusion status, leading to either unplanned hospital admission, ED visit or outpatient visit. It is a medical condition, very often life-threatening requiring urgent evaluation with subsequent initiation/intensification of the treatment, including IV therapies or intervention [1].

AHF is a "multi-event disease", and any clinical event associated to worsening signs/symptoms should be acknowledged. These episodes of worsening HF (WHF) are followed by an increased risk of hospitalizations and death and are a major burden on the health care system [8, 9].

Worsening HF can be defined as worsening symptoms and signs of HF in patients with pre-existing HF, requiring intensification of treatment, most often diuretic therapy. It requires a prior diagnosis of HF, excluding episodes of new-onset HF [8, 9]. Including only hospitalizations for AHF, the burden of AHF is largely underestimated, since many patients do present in ED or ambulatory office for worsening signs/symptoms of AHF. Secondly, performance bar measures aimed to decrease hospitalizations may convert into increasing number of emergency department (ED) visits. AHF patients may have comparable risk irrespective of the decision to hospitalize versus administer outpatient intravenous diuretics [2]. In all the cases, the presentation is by definition, unplanned [1, 4, 5].

AHF is the leading cause of hospitalizations, especially in individuals aged 65 years or older, and represents, depending on the type of hospital, 2–10% of all hospitalizations [4–6]. Patients with AHF have a variety of underlying heart diseases, risk factors, comorbidities, and precipitants leading to acute decompensation [6].

AHF is associated with high mortality and re-hospitalization rates. Overall, in-hospital mortality ranges from 2.4% to 10% [3, 6, 7, 10]. The highest in-hospital mortality rate was seen in patients with CS, and 50% of deaths occurred on the first day of admission suggesting that early identification of hypoperfusion signs, as well as appropriateness of initial therapies, is crucial in this setting [11].

For post-discharge mortality, the UK-National Heart Failure Audit reported a 1-year mortality of 30% [12]. In ESC-HF-LT registry, 27% of AHF patients have died at 1-year, 26% have been readmitted due to HF and 44% of patients have died or have been readmitted within 1 year following discharge [11].

AHF may be the first manifestation of HF (new onset) or, more frequently (70% of AHF), related to an acute decompensation of chronic HF [1, 4, 5] and regardless of clinical presentation, either *new onset* or decompensation of chronic HF, these patients are evaluated and treated in different clinical settings, outpatient clinic, ED and in-hospital (HF patient trajectory with multiple AHF episodes is shown in Fig. 23.1). Mortality at discharge may be similar for both clinical presentations, but 1-year mortality and re-hospitalization rates are higher in patients with acutely decompensated chronic HF [13, 14]. AHF episodes may occur in patients with or without previous cardiac dysfunction. Acute loss of myocardial tissue (e.g. AMI, myocarditis) or mechanical cause (spontaneous rupture of MV chordae) lead to AHF especially in patients with previously normal cardiac structure. Usually, these patients have a clear aetiological factor that resolved contributes to HF remission. Of patients with known cardiac dysfunction, some patients have history of HF while others may evolve asymptomatically for variable period of time. In these patients, interaction between acute precipitants and cardiac substrate leads to destabilization.

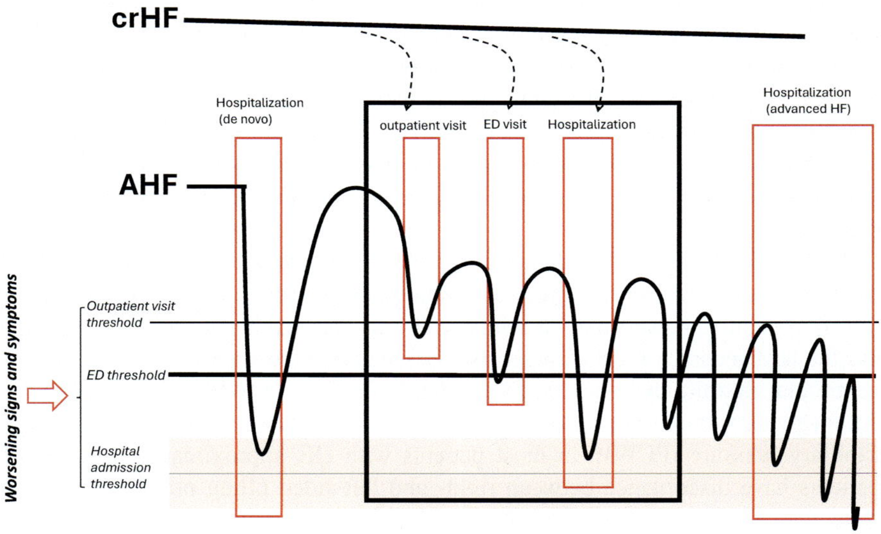

Fig. 23.1 The HF patient trajectory. Following an initial hospitalization for de novo HF, the evolution is marked by a plateau; later on worsening events may occur; worsening HF can be managed in ambulatory setting, or due to the severity of the disease and markers of risk may require hospitalisation; worsening episodes portend different prognosis if patients are managed as outpatients or are hospitalised. True 'worsening' HF (occurring while on adequate GDMT) will represent a new more severe phase—that of advanced HF. *Abbreviations*: *HF* heart failure, *AHF* acute heart failure, *ED* emergency department, *GDMT* guideline directed medical therapy

Diagnosis

The diagnostic must start at the time of the first medical contact and continue in parallel with the initial management [1]. If first contact occurs in pre-hospital phase, pre-hospital assessment and management should not delay the rapid transfer of AHF patients to the most appropriate medical environment [15, 16].

The initial clinical evaluation of patients suspected of AHF should confirm the diagnosis of AHF, assess severity of AHF and identify precipitating factors [17]. Initial diagnosis of AHF should be based on clinical judgment to integrate patient history, assessing the symptoms and assessment of signs/symptoms of congestion and/or hypoperfusion by physical examination.

A history of HF is the most useful parameter. Previously documented cardiac dysfunction (MI, valvular disease, CAD) increase probability of heart failure, and its absence decreases the likelihood [17].

Dyspnea is the most common symptom of AHF. However, the characteristics of dyspnea should be objectively assessed by evaluating the respiratory rate, intolerance of the supine position, and degree of hypoxia. The presence of paroxysmal nocturnal dyspnoea increases the likelihood of the diagnosis of acute heart failure [18].

Symptoms and signs of AHF reflect fluid overload (pulmonary congestion and/or peripheral oedema) or, less often, reduced cardiac output with peripheral hypoperfusion [1, 5]. Congestion is a typical feature of AHF, and physical examination should primarily focus on the presence of congestion which would support the diagnosis of AHF. Left-sided congestion may cause dyspnoea, orthopnoea, paroxysmal nocturnal dyspnoea, cough, tachypnoea, pathological lung auscultation (rales, crackles, wheezing) and hypoxaemia [18]. The absence of rales and a normal chest radiography do not exclude the presence of left-sided congestion. Indeed, 20–30% of patients with elevated pulmonary-artery wedge pressure may have a normal chest radiography [19].

Right-sided congestion may cause increased body weight, bilateral peripheral oedema, decreased urine output, abdominal pain, nausea, jugular vein distension (JVD) or positive hepato-jugular reflux (HJR), ascites and hepatomegaly [18]. JVD has the best accuracy for the diagnosis of AHF and in the absence of isolated right ventricular systolic dysfunction, JVD reliably predicts PCWP > 15 mm Hg [19]. Although, elevation in right atrial pressure (RAP) mirrors an elevation in pulmonary capillary pressure (PCWP) in most patients with HF, approximately 25–30% of patients have discordance between right- and left-sided filling pressures, with an isolated elevation on either side [19–21] (Fig. 23.2).

Symptoms and signs of hypoperfusion indicate severity [13, 22] and may include hypotension, tachycardia, weak pulse, mental confusion, anxiety, fatigue, cold sweated extremities, and decreased urine output. To note, no single element from physical examination can accurately diagnose HF and diagnosis involves integration of multiple physical findings, and diagnosis decisions should be based on comprehensive clinical examination [23, 24].

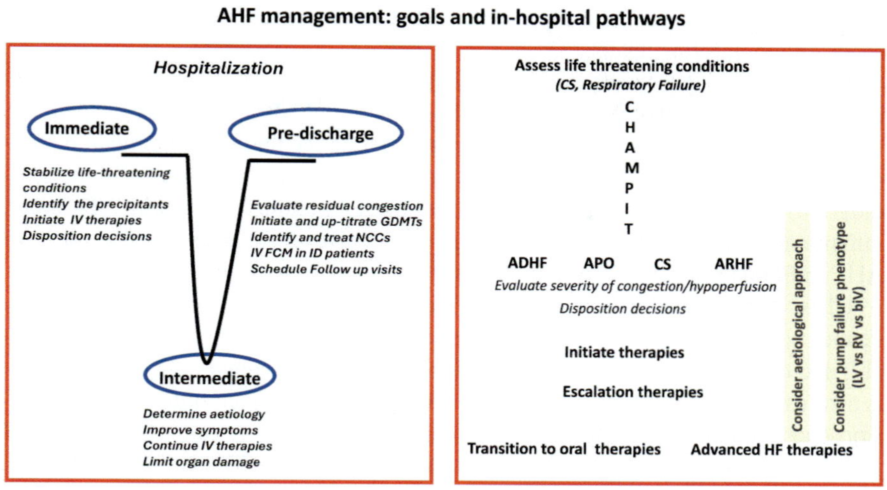

Fig. 23.2 Framework for acute HF management. Left: the timeline for hospitalization may be split in 3 phases, each having different priorities. Right: Acute HF requires for the systematic search and evaluation of life threatening conditions, identifying potential precipitant or specific ethiologies with particular/specific treatment, establishing the clinical phenotype and identifying the optimal timing for escalation of therapies or transition to oral and GDMT before discharge. (Modified after McDonagh et al. [1]). *Abbreviations*: *AHF* acute heart failure, *iv* intravenous, *GDMT* guideline directed medical therapies, *NCC* non cardiac comorbidities, *ID* iron deficit, *CS* cardiogenic shock, *ADHF* acute decompensated heart failure, *APO* acute pulmonary oedema, *ARHF* acute right heart failure, *LV* left ventricle, *RV* right ventricle, *biV* ventricular, *CHAMPIT* acute coronary syndrome, hypertensive emergency, arrhythmias, acute mechanical cause, pulmonary embolism, infection, tamponade

Since the sensitivity and specificity of symptoms and signs, are modest, diagnosis of AHF should be further confirmed by appropriate additional investigations such as ECG, chest X-ray, lung ultrasound, laboratory assessment (with specific biomarkers, mostly natriuretic peptides) and echocardiography [1, 5].

Natriuretic peptides such as B-type natriuretic peptide (BNP) and N-terminal pro-B-type natriuretic peptide (NT-proBNP) are an integral component of HF diagnosis workup in many clinical settings, especially when the diagnosis is uncertain, based on their high negative predictive value [1, 5]. Upon presentation to the ED or CCU/ICU, a plasma NP level (BNP, NT-proBNP or MR-proANP) should be measured in all patients with acute dyspnoea and suspected AHF to help in the differentiation of AHF from non-cardiac causes of acute dyspnoea [1, 5]. The use of these biomarkers has the highest class of recommendation to support exclusion of HF, due to the very high negative predictive value (94–97%). However, natriuretic peptides (NPs) are largely unspecific for HF diagnosis and several clinical conditions other than HF, can result in an increase in NP levels, while other conditions are associated with NPs level lower than expected [25]. An individualized interpretation of biomarker levels, particularly in the setting of competing diagnoses and comorbidities is recommended [26, 27]. Furthermore, patient-level changes need to be interpreted according to baseline levels.

When plasma NP levels are not available or are above the cut-offs, additional investigations (i.e. chest X-ray, echocardiography, lung ultrasound) are needed.

Cardiac imaging is the key step in order to define the underlying cardiac pathology [1]. Along with the initial routine assessment (clinical examination, electrocardiogram) and laboratory parameters (natriuretic peptides, troponins, D-dimer, inflammation markers), imaging modalities are pivotal for accurate diagnosis of AHF in ED and help to guide initial therapeutic and disposition decisions [18].

Chest-X-ray is helpful in identification of pulmonary congestion (pulmonary venous congestion, pleural effusion, interstitial or alveolar oedema and cardiomegaly) and to detect the presence and position of intracardiac devices [1]. Chest X-ray is also useful to identify alternative pathology, especially pneumonia, pleural effusion and pneumothorax. However, clinicians should not rule out AHF in patients with no radiographic signs of congestion, since in about 20–30% patients with AHF, chest X-ray is nearly normal [28]. Also, there is a large interobserver variability in the interpretation of the radiological signs of pulmonary congestion [29, 30].

ECG can provide useful information about underlying cardiac disease or potential precipitants (e.g. myocardial ischemia, arrhythmias, PE), targets for specific therapies (e.g. rate control and anticoagulation for atrial fibrillation, pacing for bradycardia) and may help to select possible candidates for device therapies (cardiac resynchronization therapy, if the patient has left bundle branch block) [1, 5, 31]. To note, ECG may direct further imaging modalities (i.e. coronary angiography for ST elevation MI, CT scan for RV strain, Echocardiography for low QRS voltage).

Echocardiography enables to promptly detect essential structural abnormalities and objectively confirm pulmonary and systemic congestion [30]. Immediate echocardiography is mandatory only in patients with haemodynamic instability (particularly in cardiogenic shock) and in patients suspected of acute life-threatening structural or functional cardiac abnormalities (mechanical complications, acute valvular regurgitation, aortic dissection). Early echocardiography should be considered in all patients with de novo AHF and in those patients with unknown cardiac structure and function or when structure or function have substantially changed since previous studies [5, 18].

The diagnostic value of bedside focused cardiac ultrasound (FoCUS) and lung ultrasound (LUS), provides the shortest path to AHF diagnosis and life-saving therapies during first 2 h after admission [18, 30]. FoCUS examination allows to quickly differentiate the pathophysiology of the hemodynamic instability, through the identification of cardiac tamponade, right or left ventricular (LV) dysfunction, detection of pulmonary (lung B-lines) and right-side congestion (inferior vena cava diameter and respiratory variation) and associated severe valvular dysfunction [30].

Lung ultrasonography has emerged as a valuable modality to detect pulmonary congestion in patients with AHF [30, 32]. This bedside technique enables the detection of interstitial fluid in the pulmonary parenchyma (visualization of B-lines) in a rapid manner, and its ability to rule in and rule out significant interstitial syndrome is superior compared to chest X-ray [33].

Also, the number and extent of B-lines increases with the severity of congestion [33, 34]. However, any condition that causes fluid build-up in the lymphatic interlobular septae at the pleural surface may produce B-lines, thus limiting the ability of pulmonary ultrasound alone to discriminate between AHF from other causes of pulmonary oedema [32]. Other pathological conditions, such as pleural effusion, pneumonia and pneumothorax can be also reliably detected with LUS.

Additional laboratory tests are helpful in the evaluation of patients with AHF. Cardiac troponin may be helpful to exclude myocardial ischaemia as precipitating factor of AHF [35]. However, cardiac troponin, in particular when measured with high-sensitive assays, is elevated in 80–90% of patients with AHF, often without obvious myocardial ischaemia or an acute coronary event [35].

The initial laboratory evaluation should also include a basic assessment of the function of other organ systems (for example, kidney, liver and blood). Blood urea nitrogen (BUN) or urea, creatinine, electrolytes (sodium, potassium), are useful to identify associated non-cardiac comorbidities and may help to guide the treatment [1].

Liver function tests are often impaired in patients with AHF due to haemodynamic derangements, both reduced output and increased venous congestion [36, 37] and identify patients at risk of poor prognosis [36–39].

D-dimer should be measured where acute pulmonary embolism (PE) is suspected [1, 5].

An infection trigger can be evaluated by measurement of inflammatory markers (for example, C-reactive protein and procalcitonin) [40].

Arterial blood gas analysis may be useful when a precise measurement of pH and O_2 and CO_2 partial pressure is needed (i.e. patients with respiratory distress) [1]. Arterial lactate is a prognostic marker in patients presenting with hypoperfusion or hemodynamic instability and its variations, in addition to overall clinical status, markers of end-organ dysfunction and echocardiographic parameters, may guide escalation or weaning of pharmacological or mechanical circulatory support. When arterial blood sample is not available, measurement of the venous lactate offers similar decisional information, since there is no arterio-venous gradient of blood lactate and there are no prognostic differences between venous and arterial lactate [1].

Additional imaging modalities (for example, MRI) are rarely needed during the initial work-up but may be helpful during further investigations.

During the work-up of the diagnostic process, careful evaluation of the potential cause or trigger of acute decompensation should be performed and coexisting life-threatening clinical conditions and/or precipitants that require urgent treatment/correction need to be immediately identified and managed [1].

As stated in the 2021 ESC guidelines, known and treatable causes of AHF must be addressed during initial work-up of AHF diagnosis [1]. Numerous factors may trigger AHF episodes but several of these conditions are considered “life-threatening” causes/aetiologies, follow specific management pathways and triage dispositions and must be identified and treated before initiation of any other standard HF management algorithm process. They included acute coronary syndrome,

hypertension, **a**rrhythmia, acute **m**echanical cause and **p**ulmonary embolism, **i**nfections and **t**amponade (**CHAMPIT**) [1]. In parallel, alternative causes for the patient's symptoms and signs (i.e. worsening COPD, asthma, pulmonary infection, severe anaemia, acute renal failure) [1], should be identified.

The diagnostic workup should continue with the identification of clinical phenotypes (Acutely Decompensated HF, Acute Pulmonary Oedema, Acute Right Failure and Cardiogenic Shock) supporting the initiation of the early individualized treatments.

Acutely decompensated HF (**ADHF**) is the most common form, representing 60–70% of AHF presentations in observational studies [11]. These patients have history of chronic HF and very often previous HF hospitalizations. Typically, they present with symptoms and signs of systemic congestion that worsen gradually. Since the main pathophysiological alteration is progressive fluid retention, signs and symptoms reflect increasing left and right filling pressures, and less often with signs of hypoperfusion. Chest X- ray shows increased cardiothoracic index with pulmonary venous congestion (redistribution and perihilar haze). A large IVC diameter with diminished respiratory variations is a common echo finding [30].

Acute right failure (**ARF**) can be defined as a rapidly progressive syndrome with systemic congestion resulting from impaired RV filling and/or reduced RV output [39]. RV failure is observed in 3–9% of AHF admissions, and the in-hospital mortality of patients with acute RV failure ranges from 5% to 17% [11, 41]. The clinical presentation of acute right ventricular failure may vary depending on the underlying cause and presence of comorbidities [41, 42]. In general, the predominant clinical features of acute right ventricular failure include (1) elevated right atrial and central venous pressure displayed as jugular venous distension; (2) signs of systemic venous congestion due to fluid retention manifesting as peripheral oedema, ascites, pleural effusions, congestive hepatomegaly and hepatojugular reflux, and anasarca; (3) low cardiac output leading to peripheral and organ hypoperfusion; and (4) atrial or ventricular arrhythmias [41, 42]. The initial triage is based on clinical assessment of vital signs and congestion and clinical history (e.g., knowledge of congenital or acquired heart disease, pre-existing pulmonary hypertension, recurrent episodes of pulmonary embolism). The diagnosis or exclusion of aetiologies requiring specific treatment (such as pulmonary embolism, pulmonary hypertension, or acute right myocardial infarction) should be prioritized.

ECG may reveal arrhythmias, signs suggesting right atrial and/or ventricular overload, or ischaemia. Chest X-ray shows an enlarged right contour and the absence of pulmonary venous congestion. Focused echocardiography provides bedside information on right ventricular size and function, as well as data about right filling pressure (IVC diameter and respiratory variations). Arterial blood gases and blood lactate should be assessed in presence of hypoxemia [41, 42].

Acute pulmonary oedema (**APO**) is the second most common clinical presentation of AHF (14–38%), though its reported prevalence and in-hospital mortality may vary considerably by geographic region [43]. Methodological differences among the registries, that are representative for distinct AHF populations from different clinical settings (ED, in-hospital, CCU) and variability of the time-point of classification at different phase of acuity may contribute to the wide differences in the prevalence of APO. Also, overlapping features among AHF clinical profiles and/or the confounding presence of noncardiac comorbidities may lead to incomplete or inaccurate classification. Pathogenesis of this clinical profile is a rapid increase in pulmonary capillary hydrostatic pressure and trans-vascular fluid filtration that exceeds the lymphatic interstitial drainage capacity [43–46]. APO is a high-acuity presentation and the clinical picture is characterized by pulmonary congestion in the face of an acutely increased afterload [43]. Although clinical signs of pulmonary congestion were also reported in other clinical profiles, such as ADHF, the distinctive feature of APO patients is the severity of pulmonary congestion accompanied by respiratory distress (higher respiratory rate > 25/min or use of accessory muscles) and hypoxemia, both contributing to progressive respiratory failure that may lead to cardiorespiratory collapse in hours, or minutes, unless therapeutic action is taken [46].

Since there are variable definitions and due to poor reliability based on clinical diagnosis, several clinical criteria are necessary for diagnosis that require further confirmation through additional tests [45]. Beside symptoms, key clinical findings are respiratory distress and respiratory failure. Diagnostic confirmation requires at least two of the following additional criteria, more specific for AHF: clear signs of pulmonary congestion on chest X ray or CT scan, >3 B-lines in two chest zones on each hemithorax on LUS, signs of elevated filling pressures on echo (E/E' > 15), BNP > 400 pg/ml or N-ProBNP > 900 pg/ml (or 1800 pg/ml in >75 years), elevated pulmonary capillary pressure on catheterization, increased total lung water on pulse contour and thermodilution analysis system [45]. This diagnosis algorithm highlights the importance of respiratory distress and respiratory failure, which should be treated with oxygen and non-invasive ventilation. In some instances, hypoxemia may be too severe or may not be promptly improved by decongestive therapies. The decision to initiate invasive mechanical ventilation must be anticipated and should be based on clinical judgment, considering the overall clinical picture, but should not be delayed until the patient is in extremis or has an altered level of consciousness [43, 44, 46].

Patients with APO often present hypertension on admission, either as precipitant or as reactive stress response. Low SBP at presentation or clinical signs of hypoperfusion, even subtle, portend a poor prognosis [43].

A search for the precipitant and underlying aetiology must be conducted early in the course of hospitalisation. It is important to identify those aetiologies that will not respond to conventional intravenous (IV) therapies, such as mechanical complications of AMI, valvular endocarditis, and prosthetic valve dysfunction [44].

Cardiogenic shock (CS) represents the most severe form of AHF. The prevalence of CS varies according to the definition of CS, clinical setting care and era of data collection. CS accounts for 2–5% of AHF presentations, with a prevalence in intensive care unit (ICU)/ICCU datasets of 14–16% [37, 47]. In-hospital mortality varied between 30% and 60% [37, 47], with nearly half of in-hospital deaths occurring within the first 24 h of presentation [11].

CS is a syndrome caused by a primary cardiovascular disorder in which inadequate CO results in a life-threatening state of tissue hypoperfusion associated with impairment of tissue oxygen metabolism and hyperlactatemia. Depending on its severity, CS may result in multi-organ dysfunction and death [37]. CS may arise in advanced chronic HF when acute precipitants trigger decompensation or may manifest as an acute onset, *de novo* presentation, most often caused by an acute coronary syndrome (ACS) [37].

Based on clinical criteria, diagnosis of CS mandates the presence of clinical signs of hypoperfusion, such as cold sweated extremities, oliguria, mental confusion, dizziness, narrow pulse pressure. Of note, hypoperfusion is not always accompanied by hypotension, as blood pressure may be preserved by compensatory vasoconstriction (with/without pressor agents), albeit at the cost of impaired tissue perfusion and oxygenation. In addition, biochemical manifestations of hypoperfusion, elevated creatinine, metabolic acidosis and elevated serum lactate, are present. The presence of clinical signs of peripheral hypoperfusion even with preserved SBP, is referred as 'pre-shock' and precedes overt CS. Pre-shock may occur in severe AHF presenting with diverse clinical phenotypes and can also be associated with clinical signs of tissue hypoperfusion but without compromising cellular metabolism and having normal lactate [37]. At the end of spectrum of severity, refractory CS' has been defined as CS with ongoing evidence of tissue hypoperfusion despite administration of adequate doses of two vasoactive medications and treatment of the underlying aetiology [37]. The classification proposed by Society for Cardiovascular Angiography and Interventions (SCAI) [48], describes five evolutive stages of CS, from A (at risk of CS) to E (extremis) including a modifier for cardiac arrest (CA). This classification can be applied rapidly bedside upon patient presentation, across all clinical settings. Recently, the SCAI classification has been validated in a large cohort of unselected intensive cardiac care unit (ICCU) patients [49] providing robust mortality risk stratification regardless of CS aetiology, in a manner that was amplified by the presence of CA [50].

A 12-lead ECG should be performed immediately, and in several instances helps to identify underlying causes (ACS, PE, tamponade) [37].

Echocardiography has a central role to identify potential underlying causes and associated pathophysiology, because without identification and treatment of the underlying cause, the outcome is usually fatal. Standard echocardiographic evaluation or FoCUS when available in ED should provide rapidly sufficient information to confirm/exclude tamponade, mechanical complications of AMI, LV outflow tract obstruction, severe valvular lesions. Concomitant assessment of LV and RV function, and estimation of left and right filling pressures should also be included in echo protocols [37, 47].

Since acute respiratory failure is present in almost all CS patients, ABG analysis with determination of blood gases and lactate is recommended in all patients and is highly indicative for the further need of invasive mechanical ventilation [37].

Prognosis

At initial presentation in ED, risk stratification may guide the appropriateness of disposition decisions and of initial therapeutic interventions, during hospitalization risk-stratification may identify the candidates for device therapy or surgical interventions, and at discharge may help to identify high risk patients who require more intense follow-up or to plan elective interventions for selected patients [51, 52].

Once an AHF diagnosis is made and after initial stabilization and management in ED, accurate prognostic information may enhance physician's ability to predict outcomes, thus informing disposition decisions for patients with AHF [53]. Several disposition options regarding the ultimate placement of the patient should be considered, including intensive care unit (ICU), a cardiology ward, or discharge at home. Because the response to AHF treatment is not immediate, an observation period after initial therapy is useful to define the correct disposition [54, 55].

Patient's disposition after complete ED management is one of the most important decisions to be made by emergency physicians [53]. This would allow high-risk patients to receive prompt and aggressive in-hospital therapy, whereas low-risk patients could be safely discharged to home without exposure to potential risk associated to hospitalization and to reduce costly inpatient admissions [53, 56].

AHF hospitalisation represents an important opportunity to assess patient prognosis. [57].

A comprehensive assessment in these patients is necessary to identify multiple prognostic characteristics that may become possible therapeutic targets. Candidate predictors can be obtained from patient demographics, clinical history, physical examination, disease characteristics, laboratory tests, and previous treatment [52, 58].

In general, prognostic studies use a multivariable approach in their design and analysis to determine the important predictors of the studied outcomes and to provide outcome probabilities for different combinations of predictors. The aim is to determine whether an outcome can reliably be attributed to a particular risk factor, with adjustment for other causal factors (confounders) using a multivariable approach. In clinical trials and registries, the predictive factors for post-discharge mortality included age, history of previous hospitalisation, congestion, systolic blood pressure (SBP), heart rate (HR), QRS duration, renal function, markers of organ injury, and non-cardiac comorbidities (such as diabetes, cerebrovascular disease, chronic obstructive pulmonary disease, liver cirrhosis).

Post-hoc analyses derived from observational studies and clinical trials [59–62] have combined various risk markers from multivariable models in risk scores.

AHF Management

AHF management represents a continuum of evaluation, administering therapies, assessing response to implemented therapies and creating a plan for the immediate, short and medium term care.

Treatment itself can be time-split into the following phases (as depicted in Fig. 23.2):

- admission phase—immediate management as per clinical presentation;
- evaluation of response to initial therapies and reassessing for alternate/escalating therapies; continuation/initiation of disease modifying therapies is key (e.g. angiotensin-converting enzyme inhibitors (ACEI), beta-blockers (BB), mineralocorticoid antagonists (MRA));
- pre-discharge phase—evaluation of GDMT prescriptions, discharge and post-discharge planning.

The management during the initial phase—whether pre-hospital or in the emergency room—is the least evidence-based (except for STEMI setting). The initial main goals are to identify:

- potential precipitants or specific etiologies that would require specific therapies (i.e. emergent revascularization for acute STEMI, cardioversion for fast rate atrial fibrillation, antibiotic for infection, anticoagulation/fibrinolysis for pulmonary embolism) (Fig. 23.2);
- respiratory distress—to initiate O_2 therapy and if needed ventilation; respiratory distress is defined by low O_2 saturation (<90%) and polypnea (>25 respirations/minute) or increased breathing work, orthopnea;
- tissue hipoperfusion—to initiate vasoactive medical therapies, evaluate for and initiate mechanical circulatory support; the SCAI classification for cardiogenic shock (CS) should be used to assess clinical, hemodynamic status and guide escalation of therapies, as this has been correlated with survival; the definition of CS has been a matter of debate: the definition in clinical trials requires hemodynamic indices (low cardiac index, increased filling pressures), while in real world setting, the immediate clinical evaluation should identify prolonged capillary filling time, cold clammy skin, altered neurological status, systolic hypotension;
- rapidly initiate decongestion; although, this issue is still debated, there is evidence showing that shorter door-to-diuretic time may be associated to improved in-hospital mortality [63].

The current 2021 ESC HF guidelines describe several phenotypic presentations that may clinically/biologically overlap, but allow for a more systematic approach [1].

Clinical evaluation of hemodynamic status should never rely on one single sign. Although some clinical signs are very specific for identifying HF (e.g. jugular distension, LV 3rd sound), it has been shown that even a proficient clinical will only seldom be able to characterize HF hemodynamics; the clinical ability is much improved when most relevant clinical signs are using in a structured manner [64–66].

The most common presentation profile is that of acute decompensated HF (at least 60% of all hospitalized HF patients) [11]. De novo HF patients will have a far better prognosis as compared with worsening chronic HF, as they can benefit from the initiation of all the medical resources and respond quicker to decongestive therapies [67]. On the other hand, true worsening HF that occurs while patients are already optimally treated are closer to advanced HF and by this become candidates for advanced HF therapies (e.g. percutaneous valve repair (TVR), left ventricular assist devices, heart transplantation) [8, 9].

Disposition Decisions

One key issue is the decision to admit or discharge from the emergency room (ER). Triage may be difficult. This is relevant, as it has been shown that the biology (including the proteonomics) of decompensated AHF patients is different when they require hospitalisation versus that of patients that can be managed in ambulatory setting, having a different (worse) prognosis [68]. As with other algorithms in medicine, one solution is identifying patients at lowest risk—but there is poor evidence for this, as only recently some prospective studies have been designed for this very purpose; also, clinical judgement alone outside using systematic scores is not accurate enough [69]. Among the available models that were derived from the ER setting, some scales appear to provide good to very good discriminative capacity (i.e. Emergency Heart Failure Mortality Risk Grade (EHMRG): c-statistic between 0.74 and 0.81 to predict 7-day mortality; Multiple Estimation of risk based on Emergency department Spanish Score In patients with Acute Heart Failure (MEESSI-AHF): c-statistic 0.80 and 0.84 to predict 30-day mortality) [69–72]. The EHMRG score was prospectively validated for 7 day and 30 day mortality to identify low risk patients in the ACUTE study and the positive COACH intervention trial, and included the following demographic, clinical and biological parameters:

- age
- arrival by ambulance
- active cancer
- metolazone use prior to ER arrival
- systolic blood pressure (SBP) (triage)
- heart rate (HR) (triage)
- oxygen saturation (triage)
- potassium concentration
- creatinine concentration
- troponin level
- ST-depression on 12-lead ECG (30-day model only) [69, 70, 73].

Troponin levels are a significant marker of prognosis and severity of disease and should be included in all risk stratification [68].

Respiratory Support

The initial measure for patients with hypoxemia (defined as peripheral oxygen saturation < 90% or partial arterial oxygen pressure < 60 mm Hg) is supplemental O_2 therapy [74]. This is largely accepted by the medical community. Stepping further, the issue becomes controversial.

Evidence suggest that O_2 supplemental therapy as compared to room air is of no benefit or may even be deleterious in normoxemic patients with coronary artery disease, with decreasing cardiac index, increasing infarct size, both in 'old' and contemporary studies [74–78]. Evidence from AMI trials has been extrapolated to AHF setting as well, and O_2 is currently considered harmful in the setting of normal respiratory parameters [1].

Also, the pivotal 3CPO randomised controlled trial (RCT), published in 2008, has failed to show any survival benefit from non-invasive ventilation using continuous positive airway pressure (CPAP) or noninvasive intermittent positive-pressure ventilation (NIPPV) in acute pulmonary edema, but was associated with a more rapid improvement in respiratory distress versus standard O_2 therapy [79]. According to current consensus, immediate initiation of CPAP is recommended in patients with respiratory distress, with frequent (60–90 min) reassessment of clinical and biological (pH, arterial gas) parameters [18]. Increasing care should be used for predominant right heart failure, as non-invasive ventilation may increase right ventricular afterload and thus, cardiac output.

Cardiogenic Shock (CS)

In the last years, the epidemiology of CS is changing. Firstly, non-AMI CS is becoming more frequent [80] and there is an increased prevalence of the mixed pattern of circulatory shock with both cardiogenic and septic component. Secondly, mortality has been shown that it can be improved by a structured approach in diagnosis and hemodynamic characterization [81]. Hemodynamics is specially important, as the classic initial pattern of interaction between high cardiac filling pressures and high systemic vascular resistances evolves to more complex intertwined patterns during long hospitalisations (e.g. in the SHOCK trial, close to 1/5 of patients developed systemic inflammatory response syndrome with 'warm' low vascular resistances, and if that was related to positive blood cultures, the mortality doubled) [82, 83]. Recently, there has been a surge in the use of pulmonary artery catheter (PAC), which is becoming essential, particularly in CS with right ventricular or bi-ventricular dysfunction, and in those who fail to respond adequately to initial therapies [1, 37].

The current SCAI classification into 5 stages, brings awareness to the fact that CS is a continuum of severity and initiation and escalation of therapies should be done early [37, 48]. After its development it has been further validated and shown to correlate with prognosis [50].

The use of inotropes remains inadvertently high (and increases) in most registry data: 15–30% of AHF will receive an inotrope during hospital stay even though CS incidence is generally reported as less than 5% [3]. Most CS patients will receive at least 1 vasoactive medication, even though the use of vasoactive medications is consistently associated with higher mortality [84, 85]. The most deleterious is probably adrenaline, which has been convincingly shown to increase mortality in the landmark trial from Levy et.al. and several registry analysis in CS patients [86–88]. Best evidence exists for norepinephrine and dobutamine, while clinical RCTs have failed to shown any benefit for the pathophisiologicaly promising drugs levosimendan and milrinone (e.g., SURIVE, RUSSLAN, LIDO for levosimendan and the recent DOREMI for milrinone) [89–92]. One promising inotropic drug, in the pre-CS stages is istaroxime. In the Phase 2a SEISMIC RCT, intravenous infusion istaroxime improved blood pressure and some echocardiography parameters in stage B CS patients (pre-shock) [93].

The current ESC 2021 guidelines recommend the use of dobutamine and/or noradrenaline [1]. Weaning these medications also remains an open question—as this is not always a binary option and continuous modelling strategies may be more appropriate (e.g. using machine learning algorithms [94]). While there is consensus for mean arterial pressure (MAP) target in septic shock, this a matter of debate for CS patients. MAP > 65 mmHg as a reasonable hemodynamic target for CS, is only supported by scarce indirect evidence, such as the association between the mean of all MAP values during the first 24 h of intensive care and mortality in one retrospective study [95]. Given the particular hemodynamic profile of HF patients, with elevated systemic vascular resistance and afterload as an important driver of low cardiac output, this target should be further evaluated and used with precaution.

Short-term mechanical circulatory support (MCS) has only recently gained a positive supporting RCT—the DANGER-SHOCK trial [96]. 179 AMI (with ST elevation MI) related CS patients received either a microaxial flow pump (Impella CP) plus standard care versus 176 patients that received standard care alone. Death from any cause occurred 45.8% in the Impella group vs. 58.5% in the standard of care group (hazard ratio, 0.74; 95% confidence interval [CI], 0.55 to 0.99; P = 0.04). The trial is under scrutiny, if only considering the exceptionally high rates of mortality in both groups (unlike the contemporary real-world cohorts). Until the DANGER-SHOCK trial, there have been a long series of negative RCTs that examined the use of MCS (intraaortic ballon pump (IABP), other Impella trials—IABP-SHOCK II, ISAR-SHOCK, the recent VA-ECMO EURO-SHCOK and ECMO-CS RCTs) and no survival benefit was found in any prior MCS study [97–100]. Even so, there is reported widespread use of MCS use in AMI related CS patients, with more than 30% receiving an IABP—probably due to many years of experience, low complication rates and low price [101].

Decongestion

AHF is governed by congestion (which represents the elevation of cardiac filling pressures) accompanied or not by hypervolemia. Insights form COMPASS-HF trial, showed that HF decompensation is governed by the abrupt increase of filling pressures; at the same time the mean daily weight change in the days preceding the decompensation is in the range of only 1–2 kg (suggesting only a minor role for hypervolemia) [102, 103]. The redistribution of volume from the capacitance veins to the circulatory component due to sympathetic activation, that can occur in a matter of minutes, is significantly related to increased congestion and HF decompensation [104]. The inadequate interrelation heart-kidney and these organs inability to deal with circulatory increased volumes may also be a contributor, as decrease in estimated glomerular filtration rate has been observed to precede by almost 6 month AHF decompensation [105].

Increase in central venous pressure is associated with organ dysfunction, while residual congestion at discharge is associated to poor outcomes [106, 107]. These are compelling arguments to focus on efficiently decongesting patients during hospitalization.

The main class of medication indicated, with a class I, for the treatment of congestion is represented by loop diuretics [1]. Best evidence exists for furosemide—which has been investigated in the DOSE trial [108]. Lessons learned from this trial, are that higher doses (2.5-fold the previous ambulatory at home dose) can increase diuresis with more fluid loss and weight change, while having no impact on the 60-day composite end-point of death/rehospitalization. Current consensus documents are based on these results [1, 109]; the contemporary accepted decongestion strategy is depicted in Fig. 23.3.

Several facts are relevant for the in-hospital use of loop-diuretics that are worth being reappraised:

- loop diuretics increase neuro-hormonal activation, as shown in both animal and human HF models; studies dating back to the 1980's have shown a profound increase in plasma renin activity, plasma norepinephrine and plasmatic aldosterone ([110];
- most neuro-hormonal activation occurs with furosemide administration during orthostatic posture [111, 112]; this is associated with less diuretic response as compared to supine position [111, 112];
- in chronic HF patients receiving loop diuretics, there are short-term deleterious hemodynamic effects with vasoconstriction and transient increase in filling pressures (before the diuretic effect occurs) [110];

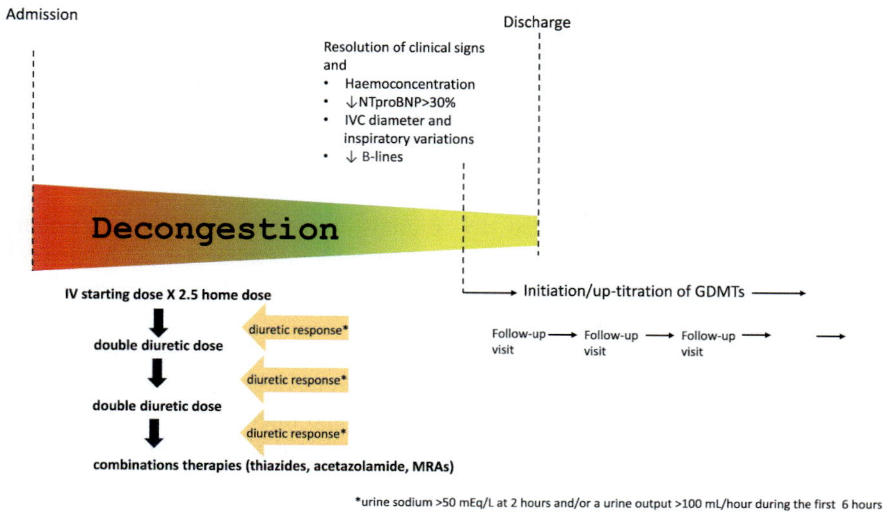

Fig. 23.3 Decongestion management for patients with hypervolemia using the loop diuretic and, if inadequate diuretic response, combinations diuretic therapies; combination therapies can also be used upfront and may help reduce diuretic doses. Evaluation of clinical, biological and echocardiographic response is also important. *Abbreviations*: *iv* intravenous, *GDMT* guideline directed medical therapies, *IVC* inferior vena cava

- to block the neuro-hormonal activation, loop diuretics administration should always be accompanied by neuro-hormonal medications (mainly ACEi and MRAs) [111, 112];
- due to the braking effect and the post-diuretic NaCl retention that occur after each bolus administration, boluses should be administered often [108, 113].

Improving decongestion has been a two decade long focus of clinical trials—all negative in regard to effect on hard-endpoints such as mortality and hospitalization; this occurs as indirect evidence suggests that adequate decongestion at discharge is associated with prognosis and that it improves tolerability of GDMT [114, 115].

Decongestion strategies that can overcome diuretic resistance and/or potentially shorten hospital length of stay (efficient by removal of excess fluid but, again, with no effect on prognosis) include:

- ultrafiltration (in the UNLOAD trial, 48 h net fluid loss was significantly higher than with diuretics 4.6 vs. 3.3 l; p 0.001 [116]),
- using a combination of diuretics:

adding acetazolamide to furosemide in the ADVOR trial improved the percentage of patients discharged without clinical congestion [117]; some patients (e.g. alkalosis) may benefit more from acetazolamide [118];

adding 25–100 mg hydrochlorothiazide to loop diuretics in the CLOROTIC trial also improved diuretic response [119]; Initiation of sacubitril/valsartan in haemodynamically stabilised heart failure patients in hospital or early after discharge: primary results of the randomised TRANSITION study

guiding bumetanide decongestion according to the urinary sodium and diuresis-based protocol, improved cumulative diuresis in the PUSH-AHF trial [120];

no benefit from adding high diuretic dose spironolactone (100 mg) in the ATHENA trial [121].

Decongestion should be guided by diuretic response defined as, urinary sodium > 50 mEq/L at 2 h and/or a urine output >100 mL/hour during the first 6 h [109]. This strategy was associated to better decongestion and greater body weight decrease in PUSH-AHF trial [120].

Decongestion may be less intense in de novo AHF patients, who will benefit from the decongestive effects of the newly initiated medications—ACEI or ARNI, MRAs, SGLT2i; the reduction in plasma volume and interstitial excess water can continue after discharge, during the first weeks after initiation. In true 'worsening' HF, occurring under optimal GDMT, adequate (complete = clinical and echocardiographic) decongestion is more relevant and remains the main objective. On the other hand, this may be difficult to achieve or even deleterious in special HF populations that are preload dependent (as in cardiac amyloidosis and aortic stenosis), or in severe tricuspid regurgitation [22].

Guideline-Directed Medical Therapies (GDMT)

The continuation/initiation/up-titration of GDMT has been perceived as important for HF patients [122].

Hospitalization should be considered as an opportunity to initiate or up-titrate GDMTs—the only effective medical strategy known to improve prognosis in HF patients. The feasibility and effectiveness of a high intensity strategy of up-titration of GDMT have been proven in the STRONG-HF multicenter open-label, randomized clinical trial [123]. Accelerated implementation (within 2 weeks post-discharge) significantly decreased the rate of readmissions for HF; the adjusted risk ratio for the combined primary endpoint of all cause death or HF readmission by day 180 was reduced by 34% (CI 0.50–0.86, p = 0.0021).

The early initiation of ACEI has long been shown to provide an immediate hemodynamic benefit. In severe (NYHA class IV) HF patients, with severely decreased left ventricular ejection fraction, small enalapril doses (as small as 2.5 mg) will shortly (within 1 h) decrease systemic vascular resistance, pulmonary capillary wedge pressure and increase cardiac output [124]. This would eventually translate in sustained prognostic benefit (as shown in the CONSENSUS trial—to only name one of the major ACEI trials [125]).

ARNI has been tested in AHF hospitalised setting, in the PIONEER trial [126]. In stable patients, it decreased NT-proBNP more that Enalapril did and was safe. In the TRANSITION trial this translated in a higher percentage achieving target dose at 10 weeks [127]; it must be said that less than 10% of patients were NYHA class IV at the time of initiation of the medication.

SGLT2i are becoming very relevant for the management of AHF patients. EMPULSE-HF is arguably the only AHF positive trial in the past three decades [128]. Empagliflozin was well tolerated and demonstrated a clinical benefit assessed by a win-ratio analysis (clinical benefit was defined as a hierarchical composite of death from any cause, number of HF events and time to first HFevent, or a 5 point or greater difference in change from baseline in the Kansas City Cardiomyopathy Questionnaire Total Symptom Score at 90 days)—stratified win ratio, 1.36; 95% confidence interval, 1.09–1.68; P = 0.0054. Another interesting advantage of SGLT2i arises from their ability to improve decongestion, with better management of interstitial free water, as shown in the DAPA-RESIST trial [129], and in the EMPA-RESPONSE-AHF trial [130]).

Other Strategies Used for the Management of AHF

There have been several medications investigated in RCTs—most having vasodilatory effects with diuretic effect or not. All RCTs were negative, no significant benefit was proven, with the potential exception of IV isosorbide-dinitrate (ISDN) when compared to the alternate therapy with diuretics and non-invasive ventilation, in the setting of hypertensive pulmonary oedema [131, 132]. Compounds from the natriuretic peptide family (e.g. nesiritide, ularitide), iv nitrates in the ELISABETH trial, hidralazine-isosorbide dinitrate in the GALACTIC trial—all failed to provide any hard-endpoint benefit in AHF patients [133–137].

Non Cardiac Comorbidities

In a recent analysis of ESC-HFA EORP-HF-LT registry, In-hospital and post-discharge mortality gradually increased with number of NCCs [138]. Also, despite of longer hospital stay and a more intense use of i.v. therapies, AHF patients with higher number of NCCs are discharged with suboptimal HF therapies (number and doses) and more severe residual congestion.

While severe comorbidities may impact eligibility for HF therapies, it is important to optimize medical therapy as tolerated and reduce clinical risk and to use admission as a trigger to initiate HF therapies with proven clinical benefit.

In addition to optimization of HF therapies, specific management of NCC during HF hospitalization may improve outcomes. In AFFIRM-AHF trial, enrolling patients with iron deficiency and LVEF < 50% , and who were stabilised after an episode of acute heart failure, treatment with ferric carboxymaltose was safe and reduced the risk of heart failure hospitalisations [139].

Although physicians managing HF patients cite comorbidity burden as a 'reason' for not initiating or uptitrating standard therapies during AHF hospitalization, in the STRONG-HF trial the effects of high intensity care were beneficial irrespective of the number of NCCs or each individual NCC, and application of the rapid up-titration strategy coupled with high-intensity follow-up reduced 180-day mortality and HF readmissions [140].

Post-discharge Management

All patients should be assessed for the indication of device therapies and if judged eligible, regular FU for implementation should already by scheduled.

Short term follow up (FU) is considered essential for the safety of patients and also as a second step to continue the up titration of medications, to improve adherence, according to the evidence provided by the effective STRONG-HF strategy [123]. Two-week FU should include the evaluation of clinical signs and symptoms and routine biology parameters (systolic blood pressure, weight, clinical signs of congestion, creatinine, Na, K and NTpro-BNP).

Along the index hospitalization, true worsening AHF patients may step into an increased risk category and fulfil the criteria for the definition of advanced HF. In this case, they should be referred and evaluated for advanced treatment options including, left ventricular assist devices and heart transplantation (Fig. 23.1).

References

1. Authors/Task Force M, McDonagh TA, Metra M, Adamo M, Gardner RS, Baumbach A, et al. 2021 ESC Guidelines for the diagnosis and treatment of acute and chronic heart failure: developed by the Task Force for the diagnosis and treatment of acute and chronic heart failure of the European Society of Cardiology (ESC). With the special contribution of the Heart Failure Association (HFA) of the ESC. Eur J Heart Fail. 2022;24(1):4–131.
2. Ferreira JP, Metra M, Mordi I, Gregson J, Ter Maaten JM, Tromp J, et al. Heart failure in the outpatient versus inpatient setting: findings from the BIOSTAT-CHF study. Eur J Heart Fail. 2019;21(1):112–20.
3. Chioncel O, Vinereanu D, Datcu M, Ionescu DD, Capalneanu R, Brukner I, et al. The Romanian acute heart failure syndromes (RO-AHFS) registry. Am Heart J. 2011;162(1):142–53 e1.
4. Farmakis D, Parissis J, Lekakis J, Filippatos G. Acute heart failure: epidemiology, risk factors, and prevention. Rev Esp Cardiol (Engl Ed). 2015;68(3):245–8.
5. Ponikowski P, Voors AA, Anker SD, Bueno H, Cleland JGF, Coats AJS, et al. 2016 ESC Guidelines for the diagnosis and treatment of acute and chronic heart failure: the Task Force for the diagnosis and treatment of acute and chronic heart failure of the European Society of Cardiology (ESC) Developed with the special contribution of the Heart Failure Association (HFA) of the ESC. Eur Heart J. 2016;37(27):2129–200.
6. Filippatos G, Angermann CE, Cleland JGF, Lam CSP, Dahlstrom U, Dickstein K, et al. Global differences in characteristics, precipitants, and initial management of patients presenting with acute heart failure. JAMA Cardiol. 2020;5(4):401–10.

7. Kaplon-Cieslicka A, Benson L, Chioncel O, Crespo-Leiro MG, Coats AJS, Anker SD, et al. A comprehensive characterization of acute heart failure with preserved versus mildly reduced versus reduced ejection fraction—insights from the ESC-HFA EORP Heart Failure Long-Term Registry. Eur J Heart Fail. 2022;24(2):335–50.
8. Greene SJ, Bauersachs J, Brugts JJ, Ezekowitz JA, Lam CSP, Lund LH, et al. Worsening heart failure: nomenclature, epidemiology, and future directions: JACC review topic of the week. J Am Coll Cardiol. 2023;81(4):413–24.
9. Metra M, Tomasoni D, Adamo M, Bayes-Genis A, Filippatos G, Abdelhamid M, et al. Worsening of chronic heart failure: definition, epidemiology, management and prevention. A clinical consensus statement by the Heart Failure Association of the European Society of Cardiology. Eur J Heart Fail. 2023;25(6):776–91.
10. Crespo-Leiro MG, Anker SD, Maggioni AP, Coats AJ, Filippatos G, Ruschitzka F, et al. European Society of Cardiology Heart Failure Long-Term Registry (ESC-HF-LT): 1-year follow-up outcomes and differences across regions. Eur J Heart Fail. 2016;18(6):613–25.
11. Chioncel O, Mebazaa A, Harjola VP, Coats AJ, Piepoli MF, Crespo-Leiro MG, et al. Clinical phenotypes and outcome of patients hospitalized for acute heart failure: the ESC Heart Failure Long-Term Registry. Eur J Heart Fail. 2017;19(10):1242–54.
12. Donkor A, Cleland J, McDonagh T, Hardman S. National heart failure audit 2016, July 7.
13. Javaloyes P, Miro O, Gil V, Martin-Sanchez FJ, Jacob J, Herrero P, et al. Clinical phenotypes of acute heart failure based on signs and symptoms of perfusion and congestion at emergency department presentation and their relationship with patient management and outcomes. Eur J Heart Fail. 2019;21(11):1353–65.
14. Butt JH, Fosbol EL, Gerds TA, Andersson C, McMurray JJV, Petrie MC, et al. Readmission and death in patients admitted with new-onset versus worsening of chronic heart failure: insights from a nationwide cohort. Eur J Heart Fail. 2020;22(10):1777–85.
15. Takahashi M, Kohsaka S, Miyata H, Yoshikawa T, Takagi A, Harada K, et al. Association between prehospital time interval and short-term outcome in acute heart failure patients. J Card Fail. 2011;17(9):742–7.
16. Harjola P, Miro O, Martin-Sanchez FJ, Escalada X, Freund Y, Penaloza A, et al. Pre-hospital management protocols and perceived difficulty in diagnosing acute heart failure. ESC Heart Fail. 2020;7(1):289–96.
17. Arrigo M, Parissis JT, Akiyama E, Mebazaa A. Understanding acute heart failure: pathophysiology and diagnosis. Eur Heart J Suppl. 2016;18(Suppl G):G11–8.
18. Mebazaa A, Yilmaz MB, Levy P, Ponikowski P, Peacock WF, Laribi S, et al. Recommendations on pre-hospital and early hospital management of acute heart failure: a consensus paper from the Heart Failure Association of the European Society of Cardiology, the European Society of Emergency Medicine and the Society of Academic Emergency Medicine—short version. Eur Heart J. 2015;36(30):1958–66.
19. Drazner MH, Hellkamp AS, Leier CV, Shah MR, Miller LW, Russell SD, et al. Value of clinician assessment of hemodynamics in advanced heart failure: the ESCAPE trial. Circ Heart Fail. 2008;1(3):170–7.
20. Campbell P, Drazner MH, Kato M, Lakdawala N, Palardy M, Nohria A, et al. Mismatch of right- and left-sided filling pressures in chronic heart failure. J Card Fail. 2011;17(7):561–8.
21. Drazner MH, Brown RN, Kaiser PA, Cabuay B, Lewis NP, Semigran MJ, et al. Relationship of right- and left-sided filling pressures in patients with advanced heart failure: a 14-year multi-institutional analysis. J Heart Lung Transplant. 2012;31(1):67–72.
22. Chioncel O, Mebazaa A, Maggioni AP, Harjola VP, Rosano G, Laroche C, et al. Acute heart failure congestion and perfusion status—impact of the clinical classification on in-hospital and long-term outcomes; insights from the ESC-EORP-HFA Heart Failure Long-Term Registry. Eur J Heart Fail. 2019;21(11):1338–52.
23. Girerd N, Seronde MF, Coiro S, Chouihed T, Bilbault P, Braun F, et al. Integrative assessment of congestion in heart failure throughout the patient journey. JACC Heart Fail. 2018;6(4):273–85.

24. Thibodeau JT, Drazner MH. Reply: the role of the clinical examination in patients with heart failure. JACC Heart Fail. 2018;6(11):971.
25. Baibars M, Ibrahim A, Fang JC, Sipahi I. Natriuretic peptide-guided management of patients with heart failure: a decade of progress but still a controversy. Futur Cardiol. 2010;6(6):743–7.
26. Yancy CW, Jessup M, Bozkurt B, Butler J, Casey DE Jr, Colvin MM, et al. 2017 ACC/AHA/HFSA Focused Update of the 2013 ACCF/AHA Guideline for the management of heart failure: a report of the American College of Cardiology/American Heart Association Task Force on Clinical Practice Guidelines and the Heart Failure Society of America. J Card Fail. 2017;23(8):628–51.
27. Bozkurt B, Coats AJS, Tsutsui H, Abdelhamid CM, Adamopoulos S, Albert N, et al. Universal definition and classification of heart failure: a report of the Heart Failure Society of America, Heart Failure Association of the European Society of Cardiology, Japanese Heart Failure Society and Writing Committee of the Universal Definition of Heart Failure: Endorsed by the Canadian Heart Failure Society, Heart Failure Association of India, Cardiac Society of Australia and New Zealand, and Chinese Heart Failure Association. Eur J Heart Fail. 2021;23(3):352–80.
28. Collins SP, Lindsell CJ, Storrow AB, Abraham WT, Adhere Scientific Advisory Committee I, Study G. Prevalence of negative chest radiography results in the emergency department patient with decompensated heart failure. Ann Emerg Med. 2006;47(1):13–8.
29. Al aseri Z. Accuracy of chest radiograph interpretation by emergency physicians. Emerg Radiol. 2009;16(2):111–4.
30. Celutkiene J, Lainscak M, Anderson L, Gayat E, Grapsa J, Harjola VP, et al. Imaging in patients with suspected acute heart failure: timeline approach position statement on behalf of the Heart Failure Association of the European Society of Cardiology. Eur J Heart Fail. 2020;22(2):181–95.
31. Voors AA, Ponikowski P. Acute heart failure: diagnosis. In: Camm AJ, Lüscher TF, Maurer G, Serruys PW, editors. ESC CardioMed. 3rd ed. Oxford University Press; 2019.
32. Ferre RM, Chioncel O, Pang PS, Lang RM, Gheorghiade M, Collins SP. Acute heart failure: the role of focused emergency cardiopulmonary ultrasound in identification and early management. Eur J Heart Fail. 2015;17(12):1223–7.
33. Volpicelli G, Elbarbary M, Blaivas M, Lichtenstein DA, Mathis G, Kirkpatrick AW, et al. International evidence-based recommendations for point-of-care lung ultrasound. Intensive Care Med. 2012;38(4):577–91.
34. Al Deeb M, Barbic S, Featherstone R, Dankoff J, Barbic D. Point-of-care ultrasonography for the diagnosis of acute cardiogenic pulmonary edema in patients presenting with acute dyspnea: a systematic review and meta-analysis. Acad Emerg Med. 2014;21(8):843–52.
35. Harjola VP, Parissis J, Bauersachs J, Brunner-La Rocca HP, Bueno H, Celutkiene J, et al. Acute coronary syndromes and acute heart failure: a diagnostic dilemma and high-risk combination. A statement from the Acute Heart Failure Committee of the Heart Failure Association of the European Society of Cardiology. Eur J Heart Fail. 2020;22(8):1298–314.
36. Ambrosy AP, Gheorghiade M, Bubenek S, Vinereanu D, Vaduganathan M, Macarie C, et al. The predictive value of transaminases at admission in patients hospitalized for heart failure: findings from the RO-AHFS registry. Eur Heart J Acute Cardiovasc Care. 2013;2(2):99–108.
37. Chioncel O, Parissis J, Mebazaa A, Thiele H, Desch S, Bauersachs J, et al. Epidemiology, pathophysiology and contemporary management of cardiogenic shock—a position statement from the Heart Failure Association of the European Society of Cardiology. Eur J Heart Fail. 2020;22(8):1315–41.
38. Nikolaou M, Parissis J, Yilmaz MB, Seronde MF, Kivikko M, Laribi S, et al. Liver function abnormalities, clinical profile, and outcome in acute decompensated heart failure. Eur Heart J. 2013;34(10):742–9.
39. Biegus J, Hillege HL, Postmus D, Valente MA, Bloomfield DM, Cleland JG, et al. Abnormal liver function tests in acute heart failure: relationship with clinical characteristics and outcome in the PROTECT study. Eur J Heart Fail. 2016;18(7):830–9.

40. Mockel M, de Boer RA, Slagman AC, von Haehling S, Schou M, Vollert JO, et al. Improve Management of acute heart failure with ProcAlCiTonin in EUrope: results of the randomized clinical trial IMPACT EU Biomarkers in Cardiology (BIC) 18. Eur J Heart Fail. 2020;22(2):267–75.
41. Harjola VP, Mebazaa A, Celutkiene J, Bettex D, Bueno H, Chioncel O, et al. Contemporary management of acute right ventricular failure: a statement from the Heart Failure Association and the Working Group on Pulmonary Circulation and Right Ventricular Function of the European Society of Cardiology. Eur J Heart Fail. 2016;18(3):226–41.
42. Konstantinides SV, Meyer G, Becattini C, Bueno H, Geersing GJ, Harjola VP, et al. ESC Guidelines for the diagnosis and management of acute pulmonary embolism developed in collaboration with the European Respiratory Society (ERS): the Task Force for the diagnosis and management of acute pulmonary embolism of the European Society of Cardiology (ESC). Eur Respir J. 2019;2019:54(3).
43. Chioncel O, Ambrosy AP, Bubenek S, Filipescu D, Vinereanu D, Petris A, et al. Epidemiology, pathophysiology, and in-hospital management of pulmonary edema: data from the Romanian Acute Heart Failure Syndromes registry. J Cardiovasc Med (Hagerstown). 2016;17(2):92–104.
44. Chioncel O, Collins SP, Ambrosy AP, Gheorghiade M, Filippatos G. Pulmonary oedema-therapeutic targets. Card Fail Rev. 2015;1(1):38–45.
45. Masip J, Peacock WF, Price S, Cullen L, Martin-Sanchez FJ, Seferovic P, et al. Indications and practical approach to non-invasive ventilation in acute heart failure. Eur Heart J. 2018;39(1):17–25.
46. Masip J. Noninvasive ventilation in acute heart failure. Curr Heart Fail Rep. 2019;16(4):89–97.
47. Chioncel O, Collins SP, Ambrosy AP, Pang PS, Radu RI, Antohi EL, et al. Therapeutic advances in the management of cardiogenic shock. Am J Ther. 2019;26(2):e234–e47.
48. Baran DA, Grines CL, Bailey S, Burkhoff D, Hall SA, Henry TD, et al. SCAI clinical expert consensus statement on the classification of cardiogenic shock: this document was endorsed by the American College of Cardiology (ACC), the American Heart Association (AHA), the Society of Critical Care Medicine (SCCM), and the Society of Thoracic Surgeons (STS) in April 2019. Catheter Cardiovasc Interv. 2019;94(1):29–37.
49. Jentzer JC, van Diepen S, Barsness GW, Henry TD, Menon V, Rihal CS, et al. Cardiogenic shock classification to predict mortality in the cardiac intensive care unit. J Am Coll Cardiol. 2019;74(17):2117–28.
50. Naidu SS, Baran DA, Jentzer JC, Hollenberg SM, van Diepen S, Basir MB, et al. SCAI SHOCK Stage Classification Expert Consensus Update: a review and incorporation of validation studies: this statement was endorsed by the American College of Cardiology (ACC), American College of Emergency Physicians (ACEP), American Heart Association (AHA), European Society of Cardiology (ESC) Association for Acute Cardiovascular Care (ACVC), International Society for Heart and Lung Transplantation (ISHLT), Society of Critical Care Medicine (SCCM), and Society of Thoracic Surgeons (STS) in December 2021. J Am Coll Cardiol. 2022;79(9):933–46.
51. Awad HH, Anderson FA Jr, Gore JM, Goodman SG, Goldberg RJ. Cardiogenic shock complicating acute coronary syndromes: insights from the Global Registry of Acute Coronary Events. Am Heart J. 2012;163(6):963–71.
52. Chioncel O, Collins SP, Greene SJ, Pang PS, Ambrosy AP, Antohi EL, et al. Predictors of post-discharge mortality among patients hospitalized for acute heart failure. Card Fail Rev. 2017;3(2):122–9.
53. Miro O, Levy PD, Mockel M, Pang PS, Lambrinou E, Bueno H, et al. Disposition of emergency department patients diagnosed with acute heart failure: an international emergency medicine perspective. Eur J Emerg Med. 2017;24(1):2–12.
54. Collins SP, Pang PS, Fonarow GC, Yancy CW, Bonow RO, Gheorghiade M. Is hospital admission for heart failure really necessary?: the role of the emergency department and observation unit in preventing hospitalization and rehospitalization. J Am Coll Cardiol. 2013;61(2):121–6.

55. Masri A, Althouse AD, McKibben J, Thoma F, Mathier M, Ramani R, et al. Outcomes of heart failure admissions under observation versus short inpatient stay. J Am Heart Assoc. 2018;7(3):e007944.
56. Michaud AM, Parker SIA, Ganshorn H, Ezekowitz JA, McRae AD. Prediction of early adverse events in emergency department patients with acute heart failure: a systematic review. Can J Cardiol. 2018;34(2):168–79.
57. Cohen-Solal A, Laribi S, Ishihara S, Vergaro G, Baudet M, Logeart D, et al. Prognostic markers of acute decompensated heart failure: the emerging roles of cardiac biomarkers and prognostic scores. Arch Cardiovasc Dis. 2015;108(1):64–74.
58. Passantino A, Monitillo F, Iacoviello M, Scrutinio D. Predicting mortality in patients with acute heart failure: role of risk scores. World J Cardiol. 2015;7(12):902–11.
59. Felker GM, Leimberger JD, Califf RM, Cuffe MS, Massie BM, Adams KF Jr, et al. Risk stratification after hospitalization for decompensated heart failure. J Card Fail. 2004;10(6):460–6.
60. O'Connor CM, Hasselblad V, Mehta RH, Tasissa G, Califf RM, Fiuzat M, et al. Triage after hospitalization with advanced heart failure: the ESCAPE (evaluation study of congestive heart failure and pulmonary artery catheterization effectiveness) risk model and discharge score. J Am Coll Cardiol. 2010;55(9):872–8.
61. Lassus J, Gayat E, Mueller C, Peacock WF, Spinar J, Harjola VP, et al. Incremental value of biomarkers to clinical variables for mortality prediction in acutely decompensated heart failure: the multinational observational cohort on acute heart failure (MOCA) study. Int J Cardiol. 2013;168(3):2186–94.
62. Khazanie P, Heizer GM, Hasselblad V, Armstrong PW, Califf RM, Ezekowitz J, et al. Predictors of clinical outcomes in acute decompensated heart failure: acute study of clinical effectiveness of nesiritide in decompensated heart failure outcome models. Am Heart J. 2015;170(2):290–7.
63. Matsue Y, Damman K, Voors AA, Kagiyama N, Yamaguchi T, Kuroda S, et al. Time-to-furosemide treatment and mortality in patients hospitalized with acute heart failure. J Am Coll Cardiol. 2017;69(25):3042–51.
64. Nohria A, Tsang SW, Fang JC, Lewis EF, Jarcho JA, Mudge GH, et al. Clinical assessment identifies hemodynamic profiles that predict outcomes in patients admitted with heart failure. J Am Coll Cardiol. 2003;41(10):1797–804.
65. Gheorghiade M, Follath F, Ponikowski P, Barsuk JH, Blair JE, Cleland JG, et al. Assessing and grading congestion in acute heart failure: a scientific statement from the acute heart failure committee of the heart failure association of the European Society of Cardiology and endorsed by the European Society of Intensive Care Medicine. Eur J Heart Fail. 2010;12(5):423–33.
66. Hiemstra B, Eck RJ, Keus F, van der Horst ICC. Clinical examination for diagnosing circulatory shock. Curr Opin Crit Care. 2017;23(4):293–301.
67. Greene SJ, Triana TS, Ionescu-Ittu R, Shi S, Guerin A, DeSouza MM, et al. Patients hospitalized for de novo versus worsening chronic heart failure in the united states. J Am Coll Cardiol. 2021;77(7):1023–5.
68. Davison BA, Senger S, Sama IE, Koch GG, Mebazaa A, Dickstein K, et al. Is acute heart failure a distinctive disorder? An analysis from BIOSTAT-CHF. Eur J Heart Fail. 2021;23(1):43–57.
69. Lee DS, Lee JS, Schull MJ, Borgundvaag B, Edmonds ML, Ivankovic M, et al. Prospective validation of the emergency heart failure mortality risk grade for acute heart failure. Circulation. 2019;139(9):1146–56.
70. Collins SP, Pang PS. ACUTE heart failure risk stratification. Circulation. 2019;139(9):1157–61.
71. Wussler D, Kozhuharov N, Sabti Z, Walter J, Strebel I, Scholl L, et al. External validation of the MEESSI acute heart failure risk score: a cohort study. Ann Intern Med. 2019;170(4):248–56.
72. Miro O, Rossello X, Platz E, Masip J, Gualandro DM, Peacock WF, et al. Risk stratification scores for patients with acute heart failure in the emergency department: a systematic review. Eur Heart J Acute Cardiovasc Care. 2020;9(5):375–98.

73. Lee DS, Ross HJ, Investigators CT. Trial of an intervention to improve acute heart failure outcomes. Reply N Engl J Med. 2023;388(13):e46.
74. Sepehrvand N, Ezekowitz JA. Oxygen therapy in patients with acute heart failure: friend or foe? JACC Heart Fail. 2016;4(10):783–90.
75. Bourassa MG, Campeau L, Bois MA, Rico O. The effects of inhalation of 100 percent oxygen on myocardial lactate metabolism in coronary heart disease. Am J Cardiol. 1969;24(2):172–7.
76. Ganz W, Donoso R, Marcus H, Swan HJ. Coronary hemodynamics and myocardial oxygen metabolism during oxygen breathing in patients with and without coronary artery disease. Circulation. 1972;45(4):763–8.
77. Rawles JM, Kenmure AC. Controlled trial of oxygen in uncomplicated myocardial infarction. Br Med J. 1976;1(6018):1121–3.
78. Khoshnood A, Carlsson M, Akbarzadeh M, Bhiladvala P, Roijer A, Bodetoft S, et al. The effects of oxygen therapy on myocardial salvage in ST elevation myocardial infarction treated with acute percutaneous coronary intervention: the supplemental oxygen in catheterized coronary emergency reperfusion (SOCCER) study. Cardiology. 2015;132(1):16–21.
79. Bernard SA, Gray TW, Buist MD, Jones BM, Silvester W, Gutteridge G, et al. Treatment of comatose survivors of out-of-hospital cardiac arrest with induced hypothermia. N Engl J Med. 2002;346(8):557–63.
80. Berg DD, Bohula EA, van Diepen S, Katz JN, Alviar CL, Baird-Zars VM, et al. Epidemiology of shock in contemporary cardiac intensive care units. Circ Cardiovasc Qual Outcomes. 2019;12(3):e005618.
81. Tehrani BN, Truesdell AG, Sherwood MW, Desai S, Tran HA, Epps KC, et al. Standardized team-based care for cardiogenic shock. J Am Coll Cardiol. 2019;73(13):1659–69.
82. Kohsaka S, Menon V, Lowe AM, Lange M, Dzavik V, Sleeper LA, et al. Systemic inflammatory response syndrome after acute myocardial infarction complicated by cardiogenic shock. Arch Intern Med. 2005;165(14):1643–50.
83. Furer A, Wessler J, Burkhoff D. Hemodynamics of cardiogenic shock. Interv Cardiol Clin. 2017;6(3):359–71.
84. Mebazaa A, Parissis J, Porcher R, Gayat E, Nikolaou M, Boas FV, et al. Short-term survival by treatment among patients hospitalized with acute heart failure: the global ALARM-HF registry using propensity scoring methods. Intensive Care Med. 2011;37(2):290–301.
85. Jentzer JC, Wiley B, Bennett C, Murphree DH, Keegan MT, Kashani KB, et al. Temporal trends and clinical outcomes associated with vasopressor and inotrope use in the cardiac intensive care unit. Shock. 2020;53(4):452–9.
86. Tarvasmaki T, Lassus J, Varpula M, Sionis A, Sund R, Kober L, et al. Current real-life use of vasopressors and inotropes in cardiogenic shock—adrenaline use is associated with excess organ injury and mortality. Crit Care. 2016;20(1):208.
87. Leopold V, Gayat E, Pirracchio R, Spinar J, Parenica J, Tarvasmaki T, et al. Epinephrine and short-term survival in cardiogenic shock: an individual data meta-analysis of 2583 patients. Intensive Care Med. 2018;44(6):847–56.
88. Levy B, Clere-Jehl R, Legras A, Morichau-Beauchant T, Leone M, Frederique G, et al. Epinephrine versus norepinephrine for cardiogenic shock after acute myocardial infarction. J Am Coll Cardiol. 2018;72(2):173–82.
89. Follath F, Cleland JG, Just H, Papp JG, Scholz H, Peuhkurinen K, et al. Efficacy and safety of intravenous levosimendan compared with dobutamine in severe low-output heart failure (the LIDO study): a randomised double-blind trial. Lancet. 2002;360(9328):196–202.
90. Moiseyev VS, Poder P, Andrejevs N, Ruda MY, Golikov AP, Lazebnik LB, et al. Safety and efficacy of a novel calcium sensitizer, levosimendan, in patients with left ventricular failure due to an acute myocardial infarction. A randomized, placebo-controlled, double-blind study (RUSSLAN). Eur Heart J. 2002;23(18):1422–32.
91. Mebazaa A, Nieminen MS, Packer M, Cohen-Solal A, Kleber FX, Pocock SJ, et al. Levosimendan vs dobutamine for patients with acute decompensated heart failure: the SURVIVE randomized trial. JAMA. 2007;297(17):1883–91.

92. Mathew R, Visintini SM, Ramirez FD, DiSanto P, Simard T, Labinaz M, et al. Efficacy of milrinone and dobutamine in low cardiac output states: systematic review and meta-analysis. Clin Invest Med. 2019;42(2):E26–32.
93. Metra M, Chioncel O, Cotter G, Davison B, Filippatos G, Mebazaa A, et al. Safety and efficacy of istaroxime in patients with acute heart failure-related pre-cardiogenic shock—a multicentre, randomized, double-blind, placebo-controlled, parallel group study (SEISMiC). Eur J Heart Fail. 2022;24(10):1967–77.
94. Merouani M, Guignard B, Vincent F, Borron SW, Karoubi P, Fosse JP, et al. Norepinephrine weaning in septic shock patients by closed loop control based on fuzzy logic. Crit Care. 2008;12(6):R155.
95. Burstein B, Tabi M, Barsness GW, Bell MR, Kashani K, Jentzer JC. Association between mean arterial pressure during the first 24 hours and hospital mortality in patients with cardiogenic shock. Crit Care. 2020;24(1):513.
96. Moller JE, Engstrom T, Jensen LO, Eiskjaer H, Mangner N, Polzin A, et al. Microaxial flow pump or standard care in infarct-related cardiogenic shock. N Engl J Med. 2024;390(15):1382–93.
97. Seyfarth M, Sibbing D, Bauer I, Frohlich G, Bott-Flugel L, Byrne R, et al. A randomized clinical trial to evaluate the safety and efficacy of a percutaneous left ventricular assist device versus intra-aortic balloon pumping for treatment of cardiogenic shock caused by myocardial infarction. J Am Coll Cardiol. 2008;52(19):1584–8.
98. Thiele H, Zeymer U, Neumann FJ, Ferenc M, Olbrich HG, Hausleiter J, et al. Intraaortic balloon support for myocardial infarction with cardiogenic shock. N Engl J Med. 2012;367(14):1287–96.
99. Banning AS, Sabate M, Orban M, Gracey J, Lopez-Sobrino T, Massberg S, et al. Venoarterial extracorporeal membrane oxygenation or standard care in patients with cardiogenic shock complicating acute myocardial infarction: the multicentre, randomised EURO SHOCK trial. EuroIntervention. 2023;19(6):482–92.
100. Ostadal P, Rokyta R, Karasek J, Kruger A, Vondrakova D, Janotka M, et al. Extracorporeal membrane oxygenation in the therapy of cardiogenic shock: results of the ECMO-CS randomized clinical trial. Circulation. 2023;147(6):454–64.
101. Dhruva SS, Ross JS, Mortazavi BJ, Hurley NC, Krumholz HM, Curtis JP, et al. Use of mechanical circulatory support devices among patients with acute myocardial infarction complicated by cardiogenic shock. JAMA Netw Open. 2021;4(2):e2037748.
102. Chaudhry SI, Wang Y, Concato J, Gill TM, Krumholz HM. Patterns of weight change preceding hospitalization for heart failure. Circulation. 2007;116(14):1549–54.
103. Zile MR, Bennett TD, St John Sutton M, Cho YK, Adamson PB, Aaron MF, et al. Transition from chronic compensated to acute decompensated heart failure: pathophysiological insights obtained from continuous monitoring of intracardiac pressures. Circulation. 2008;118(14):1433–41.
104. Verbrugge FH, Dupont M, Steels P, Grieten L, Malbrain M, Tang WH, et al. Abdominal contributions to cardiorenal dysfunction in congestive heart failure. J Am Coll Cardiol. 2013;62(6):485–95.
105. Chatur S, Vaduganathan M, Peikert A, Claggett BL, McCausland FR, Skali H, et al. Longitudinal trajectories in renal function before and after heart failure hospitalization among patients with heart failure with preserved ejection fraction in the PARAGON-HF trial. Eur J Heart Fail. 2022;24(10):1906–14.
106. Nohria A, Hasselblad V, Stebbins A, Pauly DF, Fonarow GC, Shah M, et al. Cardiorenal interactions: insights from the ESCAPE trial. J Am Coll Cardiol. 2008;51(13):1268–74.
107. Ambrosy AP, Pang PS, Khan S, Konstam MA, Fonarow GC, Traver B, et al. Clinical course and predictive value of congestion during hospitalization in patients admitted for worsening signs and symptoms of heart failure with reduced ejection fraction: findings from the EVEREST trial. Eur Heart J. 2013;34(11):835–43.

108. Felker GM, Lee KL, Bull DA, Redfield MM, Stevenson LW, Goldsmith SR, et al. Diuretic strategies in patients with acute decompensated heart failure. N Engl J Med. 2011;364(9):797–805.
109. Mullens W, Damman K, Harjola VP, Mebazaa A, Brunner-La Rocca HP, Martens P, et al. The use of diuretics in heart failure with congestion—a position statement from the Heart Failure Association of the European Society of Cardiology. Eur J Heart Fail. 2019;21(2):137–55.
110. Francis GS, Siegel RM, Goldsmith SR, Olivari MT, Levine TB, Cohn JN. Acute vasoconstrictor response to intravenous furosemide in patients with chronic congestive heart failure. Activation of the neurohumoral axis. Ann Intern Med. 1985;103(1):1–6.
111. Ring-Larsen H, Henriksen JH, Wilken C, Clausen J, Pals H, Christensen NJ. Diuretic treatment in decompensated cirrhosis and congestive heart failure: effect of posture. Br Med J (Clin Res Ed). 1986;292(6532):1351–3.
112. Okaniwa T, Echizen H, Ishizaki T, Kasao M, Iizuka T. Pharmacodynamic characterization of posture-related diuretic and saluretic responses to furosemide in humans. J Pharmacol Exp Ther. 1990;255(2):716–23.
113. Ellison DH, Felker GM. Diuretic treatment in heart failure. N Engl J Med. 2017;377(20):1964–75.
114. Lucas C, Johnson W, Hamilton MA, Fonarow GC, Woo MA, Flavell CM, et al. Freedom from congestion predicts good survival despite previous class IV symptoms of heart failure. Am Heart J. 2000;140(6):840–7.
115. Lala A, McNulty SE, Mentz RJ, Dunlay SM, Vader JM, AbouEzzeddine OF, et al. Relief and recurrence of congestion during and after hospitalization for acute heart failure: insights from diuretic optimization strategy evaluation in acute decompensated heart failure (DOSE-AHF) and cardiorenal rescue study in acute decompensated heart failure (CARESS-HF). Circ Heart Fail. 2015;8(4):741–8.
116. Costanzo MR, Guglin ME, Saltzberg MT, Jessup ML, Bart BA, Teerlink JR, et al. Ultrafiltration versus intravenous diuretics for patients hospitalized for acute decompensated heart failure. J Am Coll Cardiol. 2007;49(6):675–83.
117. Mullens W, Dauw J, Martens P, Verbrugge FH, Nijst P, Meekers E, et al. Acetazolamide in acute decompensated heart failure with volume overload. N Engl J Med. 2022;387(13):1185–95.
118. Martens P, Verbrugge FH, Dauw J, Nijst P, Meekers E, Augusto SN, et al. Pre-treatment bicarbonate levels and decongestion by acetazolamide: the ADVOR trial. Eur Heart J. 2023;44(22):1995–2005.
119. Trullas JC, Morales-Rull JL, Casado J, Carrera-Izquierdo M, Sanchez-Marteles M, Conde-Martel A, et al. Combining loop with thiazide diuretics for decompensated heart failure: the CLOROTIC trial. Eur Heart J. 2023;44(5):411–21.
120. Ter Maaten JM, Beldhuis IE, van der Meer P, Krikken JA, Postmus D, Coster JE, et al. Natriuresis-guided diuretic therapy in acute heart failure: a pragmatic randomized trial. Nat Med. 2023;29(10):2625–32.
121. Butler J, Anstrom KJ, Felker GM, Givertz MM, Kalogeropoulos AP, Konstam MA, et al. Efficacy and safety of spironolactone in acute heart failure: the ATHENA-HF randomized clinical trial. JAMA Cardiol. 2017;2(9):950–8.
122. Antohi EL, Ambrosy AP, Collins SP, Ahmed A, Iliescu VA, Cotter G, et al. Therapeutic advances in the management of acute decompensated heart failure. Am J Ther. 2019;26(2):e222–e33.
123. Mebazaa A, Davison B, Chioncel O, Cohen-Solal A, Diaz R, Filippatos G, et al. Safety, tolerability and efficacy of up-titration of guideline-directed medical therapies for acute heart failure (STRONG-HF): a multinational, open-label, randomised, trial. Lancet. 2022;400(10367):1938–52.
124. DiCarlo L, Chatterjee K, Parmley WW, Swedberg K, Atherton B, Curran D, et al. Enalapril: a new angiotensin-converting enzyme inhibitor in chronic heart failure: acute and chronic hemodynamic evaluations. J Am Coll Cardiol. 1983;2(5):865–71.

125. Group CTS. Effects of enalapril on mortality in severe congestive heart failure. Results of the Cooperative North Scandinavian Enalapril Survival Study (CONSENSUS). N Engl J Med. 1987;316(23):1429–35.
126. Velazquez EJ, Morrow DA, DeVore AD, Duffy CI, Ambrosy AP, McCague K, et al. Angiotensin-neprilysin inhibition in acute decompensated heart failure. N Engl J Med. 2019;380(6):539–48.
127. Wachter R, Senni M, Belohlavek J, Straburzynska-Migaj E, Witte KK, Kobalava Z, et al. Initiation of sacubitril/valsartan in haemodynamically stabilised heart failure patients in hospital or early after discharge: primary results of the randomised TRANSITION study. Eur J Heart Fail. 2019;21(8):998–1007.
128. Voors AA, Angermann CE, Teerlink JR, Collins SP, Kosiborod M, Biegus J, et al. The SGLT2 inhibitor empagliflozin in patients hospitalized for acute heart failure: a multinational randomized trial. Nat Med. 2022;28(3):568–74.
129. Yeoh SE, Osmanska J, Petrie MC, Brooksbank KJM, Clark AL, Docherty KF, et al. Dapagliflozin vs. metolazone in heart failure resistant to loop diuretics. Eur Heart J. 2023;44(31):2966–77.
130. Boorsma EM, Beusekamp JC, Ter Maaten JM, Figarska SM, Danser AHJ, van Veldhuisen DJ, et al. Effects of empagliflozin on renal sodium and glucose handling in patients with acute heart failure. Eur J Heart Fail. 2021;23(1):68–78.
131. Cotter G, Metzkor E, Kaluski E, Faigenberg Z, Miller R, Simovitz A, et al. Randomised trial of high-dose isosorbide dinitrate plus low-dose furosemide versus high-dose furosemide plus low-dose isosorbide dinitrate in severe pulmonary oedema. Lancet. 1998;351(9100):389–93.
132. Sharon A, Shpirer I, Kaluski E, Moshkovitz Y, Milovanov O, Polak R, et al. High-dose intravenous isosorbide-dinitrate is safer and better than Bi-PAP ventilation combined with conventional treatment for severe pulmonary edema. J Am Coll Cardiol. 2000;36(3):832–7.
133. Mitrovic V, Seferovic PM, Simeunovic D, Ristic AD, Miric M, Moiseyev VS, et al. Haemodynamic and clinical effects of ularitide in decompensated heart failure. Eur Heart J. 2006;27(23):2823–32.
134. Anker SD, Ponikowski P, Mitrovic V, Peacock WF, Filippatos G. Ularitide for the treatment of acute decompensated heart failure: from preclinical to clinical studies. Eur Heart J. 2015;36(12):715–23.
135. Mitrovic V, Forssmann WG, Schnitker J, Felix SB. Randomized double-blind clinical studies of ularitide and other vasoactive substances in acute decompensated heart failure: a systematic review and meta-analysis. ESC Heart Fail. 2018;5(6):1023–34.
136. Freund Y, Cachanado M, Delannoy Q, Laribi S, Yordanov Y, Gorlicki J, et al. Effect of an emergency department care bundle on 30-day hospital discharge and survival among elderly patients with acute heart failure: the ELISABETH randomized clinical trial. JAMA. 2020;324(19):1948–56.
137. Kozhuharov N, Goudev A, Flores D, Maeder MT, Walter J, Shrestha S, et al. Effect of a strategy of comprehensive vasodilation vs usual care on mortality and heart failure rehospitalization among patients with acute heart failure: the GALACTIC randomized clinical trial. JAMA. 2019;322(23):2292–302.
138. Chioncel O, Benson L, Crespo-Leiro MG, Anker SD, Coats AJS, Filippatos G, McDonagh T, Margineanu C, Mebazaa A, Metra M, Piepoli MF, Adamo M, Rosano GMC, Ruschitzka F, Savarese G, Seferovic P, Volterrani M, Ferrari R, Maggioni AP, Lund LH. Comprehensive characterization of non-cardiac comorbidities in acute heart failure: an analysis of ESC-HFA EURObservational Research Programme Heart Failure Long-Term Registry. Eur J Prev Cardiol. 2023;30(13):1346–58.

139. Ponikowski P, Kirwan BA, Anker SD, McDonagh T, Dorobantu M, Drozdz J, et al. Ferric carboxymaltose for iron deficiency at discharge after acute heart failure: a multicentre, double-blind, randomised, controlled trial. Lancet. 2020;396(10266):1895–904.
140. Chioncel O, Davison B, Adamo M, Antohi LE, Arrigo M, Barros M, et al. Non-cardiac comorbidities and intensive up-titration of oral treatment in patients recently hospitalized for heart failure: insights from the STRONG-HF trial. Eur J Heart Fail. 2023;25(11):1994–2006.

Part V
Heart Failure in Special Populations

Chapter 24
Chronic Heart Failure in Frail and Elderly Patients

Maria Dorobanţu and Oana Ioniţă

Abstract With continuous aging of the population and improved medical care, an increased proportion of frail patients is expected. In chronic heart failure, frailty is a major contributor to poor functional status and adverse clinical outcomes.

Frailty and heart failure are frequently interlinked and share common mechanisms. Frailty is associated with a worse prognosis in heart failure and several concerns regarding the risk-benefit balance of intervention in this population group exist. However, most of the heart failure clinical trials suggest that therapeutical benefits are maintained, independent of age and frailty status.

Frailty assessment and early implementation of specific measures are recommended, to reduce its negative impact on heart failure outcomes. Routine evaluation for frailty should be incorporated in daily clinical management and early intervention targeting modifiable components should be instituted.

Keywords Frailty · Elderly · Chronic heart failure · Sarcopenia · Geriatric syndromes

Frailty is an emerging health problem with significant healthcare impact [1]. It is most often defined as a state of aging-related physiological decline, associated with increased vulnerability to stressors and adverse health outcomes [2]. Several definitions have been proposed over the years, defining frailty as disability [3, 4], comorbidity [5], or advanced old age. However, there is significant variability in the rate of age-related functional decline, and frailty can also occur in younger people or in people without comorbidities. Nowadays frailty is recognized as a biological syndrome that underlines this heterogeneity and reflects a state of decreased physiological reserve and vulnerability to stressors [6].

M. Dorobanţu (✉)
University of Medicine and Pharmacy "Carol Davila", Bucharest, Romania

Romanian Academy, Bucharest, Romania

O. Ioniţă
Nord Hospital—Grupul Medical Provita, Bucharest, Romania

M. Dorobanţu et al. (eds.), *Current Approach to Heart Failure*,
https://doi.org/10.1007/978-3-031-96562-3_24

Frailty has become increasingly important in cardiovascular medicine due to the aging of the population and the complexity of these patients [7]. Chronological age is not considered a contraindication for treatment and interventions, and nowadays several patients who were classically considered ineligible for certain procedures benefit from a wide array of interventions and devices [8]. These patients with a complex phenotype and multiple medical comorbidities should be optimally evaluated in order to perform meaningful medical interventions that will improve quality of life and prevent functional decline while avoiding futility.

In Europe and in the United States, cardiovascular disease is the leading cause of mortality in older individuals [9, 10]. Advanced age is the most significant risk factor for the development of cardiovascular disease (CVD) and CVD mortality. Older individuals are living longer as a result of advances in medicine, public health, and technology, with a higher prevalence of clinical and subclinical CVD [11]. The majority of cardiac procedures in the United States are performed in patients older than 65 years [9].

Aging and Frailty

Aging is a complex multifactorial biological process that encompasses some key aging hallmarks: genomic instability, telomere attrition, loss of proteostasis, disabled macroautophagy, mitochondrial dysfunction, chronic inflammation, deregulated nutrient-sensing, cellular senescence, stem cell exhaustion, altered intercellular communication and dysbiosis [12]. While chronological aging (Table 24.1) [14] is not synonymous with frailty, all these hallmarks contribute to each person's aging phenotype and to the decline in the ability to cope with stressors. They are enhanced by the traditional CVD risk factors leading to the appearance of geriatric syndromes (frailty, sarcopenia, cognitive impairment, functional impairment).

Frailty appears as a result of accelerated age-related decline in multiple physiological systems [13] associated with a failure of homeostatic mechanisms to cope. In time the organism's homeostatic reserve is depleted and apparently minor insults

Table 24.1 Definition of older adult

Chronological age	
Most frequently used cut-offs	
Elderly ≥65 years of age	"Young old" 65–74 years of age
	"Middle old" 75–84 years of age
	"Oldest old" ≥85 years of age
Japanese Gerontological Society [13]	"Pre-old age" 65–74 years of age
	"Old age" ≥75 years of age
	"Oldest old" ≥85 years of age

There are variable definitions and no consensus regarding the chronological definition of "older adult". There is a contemporary tendency in the Western societies to continuously increase the age cut-offs

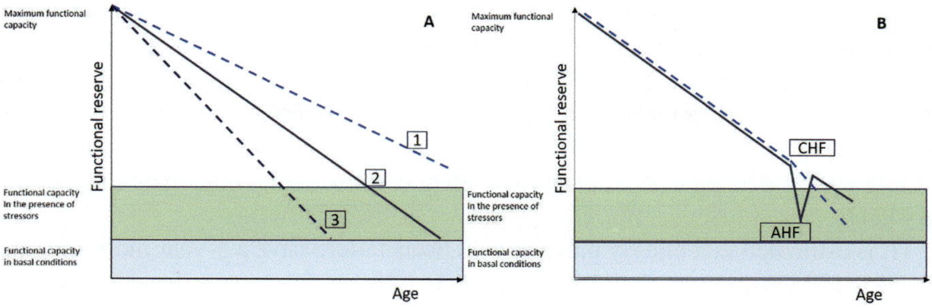

Fig. 24.1 Frailty definition. With aging, both the functional reserve and maximum functional capacity decrease. In non-frail individuals the functional capacity will suffice under normal conditions or under stressors (line 1). However, with frailty, at a certain moment the maximum capacity drops below the threshold required in the presence of stressors (2). The rate of decline is not uniform, with steeper curves in more frail individuals (3). Under the influence of a stressor, three possible transitions can occur: to a physiologically vulnerable status, to a clinically apparent phenotype or to disability and death. In heart failure patients (B) functional reserve can be impaired. Moreover, during episodes of acute heart failure, the level of frailty can be temporarily reached. After an acute decompensation, in some cases reversal to a non-frail status can be achieved. However, any hospitalization in HF is a major progression factor for frailty. *CHF* chronic heart failure, *AHF* acute heart failure. (Modified from Ref. [15] with permission)

(e.g. acute illnesses, minor medical or surgical interventions) can lead to a major and disproportionate change in the health status: from mobile to immobile, from independent to dependent [13, 15] (Fig. 24.1). This increased vulnerability to stressors leads to increased risk for periprocedural complications, disability, hospitalization, and mortality [2].

Frailty and Heart Failure

Frailty assessment is particularly relevant in heart failure (HF) and these two distinct conditions are frequently interlinked. Heart failure is strongly associated with age and older individuals have a higher incidence of heart failure, with worse clinical outcomes [10, 16]. The prognosis and quality of life of elderly patients with HF is still poor despite evidence-based therapies. In elderly people, HF with preserved ejection fraction (HFpEF) is more frequent [16].

In the general population, several studies from the United States report a frailty prevalence of 4–16% in community-dwelling persons over 65 years old [2, 17, 18], while in Europe, the SHAPE study (the Survey of Health, Ageing, and Retirement in Europe) using eight frailty scales reported a frailty prevalence from 6% to 44% in a database of 27,527 individuals aged 50–104 years [19].

In the heart failure population, frailty is more frequent than in the general population, with almost half of heart failure patients being considered frail according to a recent meta-analysis [20]. However, the prevalence of frailty in HF in this work was not age-related. Chronic heart failure alters the skeletal muscle and body composition [7] and might therefore explain the occurrence of a frail phenotype even in younger patients. In the TOPCAT (Treatment of Preserved Cardiac Function Heart Failure with an Aldosterone Antagonist) trial, in a population of HFpEF with a mean age of 71.5 years, up to 94% of the subjects were considered frail, and greater frailty was associated with an increased risk of cardiovascular outcomes and mortality [21].

It is estimated that elderly patients with heart failure have a 5-year mortality rate of 54% [22], with more than half of it due to non-cardiac causes. In older patients comorbidities, frailty, cognitive dysfunction as well as the social environment lead to poorer health outcomes, irrespectively of ejection fraction [15]. The prevalence of frailty seems to be higher in HF patients with HFpEF, most likely due to advanced age and comorbidities. However, the risk of adverse events is increased in frail patients with HF with either preserved or reduced ejection fraction. Frailty in heart failure patients is associated with worse outcomes, reduced access to medical therapy, and an increased rate of adverse events [23]. In a recent meta-analysis of studies reporting the link between frailty and all-cause mortality (29 studies, 18,757 patients) and frailty and hospitalization in patients with chronic heart failure (11 studies, 13,525 patients), frailty was associated with a 48% increase in all-cause mortality and 40% increase in hospitalization [24]. Recent data suggest that frailty has incremental prognostic value independent of the classical cardiovascular risk factors and might be an even more powerful predictor of cardiovascular outcome [25].

Heart Failure and Frailty—Pathophysiology

Frailty and HF share common physio-pathological pathways. Frailty results from cumulative cellular and molecular damage over lifetime [13, 26] which leads in the end to dysregulation in multiple systems and in their interaction. Many organs exhibit cellular redundancy and a physiological reserve, thus making it unclear at which level of cumulative decline frailty becomes evident. Aging has been associated with structural and physiological changes in the brain, endocrine, immune systems, skeletal muscle, respiratory, cardiovascular, renal, and hematopoietic systems [13]. All the associated aging molecular changes, combined with genetic factors, environmental exposure, and specific diseases form the basis of loss of homeostasis and dysregulation of stress response systems. The most important systems affected are the metabolic, musculoskeletal, and stress-response systems. For example, sarcopenia, the age-related loss of skeletal muscle, is a key element in frailty.

Chronic exposure to inflammatory mediators can also lead to pathophysiological changes associated with frailty [26] and changes consistent with low-grade inflammation are frequently seen in frail individuals [27]. The dysregulation of the autonomic nervous system is linked to decreased heart rate variability, cardiac and orthostatic control [27, 28].

Heart failure, through neurohumoral and adrenergic overstimulation, induces a proinflammatory state which leads to changes in muscle composition, muscular mass, and strength and contributes to physical frailty [29]. In chronic heart failure, the sarcopenia is accelerated, and different changes in the composition of the muscle (with reduced capillary-to-fiber ratio, reduced oxidative capacity and mitochondrial content) [30, 31] leading to impaired mitochondrial function and exercise capacity have been described. One link between frailty and chronic HF can also be the upregulated proinflammatory state which leads to insulin resistance, metabolic imbalance, and atherosclerosis progression [32, 33]. In heart failure hemodynamic abnormalities, congestion and hypoperfusion lead to upregulation of the proinflammatory pathways, as well as structural and functional changes in other systems, leading to an increased vulnerability to stressors [6].

In both heart failure and aging, muscle loss occurs. Nutritional deficiency due to malabsorption related to intestinal edema or decreased intake due to depression and cognitive impairment are frequent in heart failure patients and contribute to physical frailty. Recent data show that a lower protein intake in HF patients is associated with lower body mass index, but also with increased signs of congestion [34]. Lower protein intake was strongly associated with higher mortality in this population [35].

Cognitive frailty is defined as the coexistence of physical frailty and cognitive impairment without neurodegenerative diseases [36]. Almost 45% of HF patients present signs of cognitive impairment [37], while cognitive frailty was found in almost 25% of the elderly with HF [38]. Patients with HF and cognitive frailty have an approximately 1.5-fold increased risk for adverse events compared with those without.

Social frailty, defined as a reduction of involvement in social activities is highly prevalent in HF patients and is further associated with worse prognosis [39].

Frailty and heart failure share a bidirectional relationship. Heart failure can accentuate frailty due to hospitalization, associated immobilization, decrease in muscle strength, exercise intolerance, or cognitive impairment. Further, frailty leads to a decreased capacity to respond to stressors like infections or HF decompensations and is associated with worse physical status, comorbidities, cognitive dysfunction, or decreased quality of life. Frailty can also influence the safety-benefit profile of several cardiovascular interventions.

Frailty Assessment

No unified method for the objective measurement of frailty exists and several approaches of assessing frailty that take into consideration the main affected functional domains: physical, cognitive, psychosocial, and nutritional [40] have been described. However, two main conceptual models are the most frequently used. Based on them, several frailty measurement tools have been further developed.

The first approach was proposed by Fried and colleagues in 2001 [2] in the Cardiovascular Health Study and was further validated in the Women's Health and

Table 24.2 Physical Frailty Phenotype assessment [2]

Measure	Definition
Weight loss	Lost 4.5 kg or more than 5% weight unintentionally over the last year
Exhaustion	Self-report of either 'felt that everything I did was an effort' and/or 'could not get going' in the last week
Low physical activity	Self-report, equivalent to $<$270 kCal/week (about 2 h walk) in women and $<$383 kCal/week (about 2.5 h walk) in men
Slow walking	Walking time for 4.57 m (15 feet) at usual pace: slowest 20% ≥7 s for height ≤159 cm in women and ≤173 cm in men or ≥6 s for height $>$159 cm in women and $>$173 cm in men
Weakness	Grip strength measured using a dynamometer ≤(lowest 20% by gender, body mass index) Women: ≤17 kg for BMI ≤23 kg/m^2; ≤17.3 kg for BMI 23.1–26 kg/m^2; ≤18 kg for BMI 26.1–29 kg/m^2; and ≤21 kg for BMI $>$29 kg/m^2 Men: ≤29 kg for BMI ≤24 kg/m^2; ≤30 kg for BMI 24.1–26 kg/m^2; ≤30 kg for BMI 26.1–28 kg/m^2; and ≤32 kg for BMI $>$28 kg/m^2

Score ≥ 3—frailty
Score 2—prefrailty

Aging Study [41]. In their study a specific phenotype of physical frailty has been described, characterized by a decline in the physiological reserve in three or more of the five domains: unintentional weight loss, self-reported exhaustion, weak handgrip strength, slow walking speed, and low physical activity [41]. In the presence of one or two of these criteria, a pre-frailty status is indicated (Table 24.2). Physical frailty as assessed by Fried phenotype has been associated with worse clinical outcomes and poorer quality of life in older community members and also in chronic heart failure patients [6, 42]. Data from a meta-analysis suggest that in the presence of frailty, the risk of death or hospitalization in chronic HF patients is increased by approximately 1.5-fold [42]. Fried phenotype identifies the subjects in an initial stage of reduced functional reserve, with a 2-year mortality of approximately 10% [15]. However, some caveats must be acknowledged when using this assessment, originally derived in a general population cohort, in heart failure patients. There is a significant overlap between the physical frailty and clinical manifestations of HF, making it sometimes difficult to assess if the phenotype is dependent or not on the heart failure status. Furthermore, the measurement cutoffs were derived in the general population and they might not perform as well in HF patients. In clinical practice, the assessment of Fried phenotype might be time-consuming and not feasible in all patients. Moreover, other domains like cognitive impairment, which is frequently met in heart failure patients, are not taken into consideration.

The second most used approach for frailty assessment is the frailty index (FI) or deficit index, developed by Rockwood [3]. It has been proposed and validated in a community of older adults in the Canadian Study of Health and Aging. This model characterizes frailty as a sum of health deficits across multiple domains

Table 24.3 FRAIL score [45]

Domains	Clinical question	Score
Fatigue	Have you felt tired for most or all the time in the last month?	Yes 1; No 0
Resistance	In the last month could you climb a flight of stairs without difficulties?	Yes 1; No 0
Ambulation	In the last month did you have any difficulty walking one block or 300 metres?	Yes 1; No 0
Illnesses	Do you suffer of any of the following illnesses: hypertension, diabetes, cancer, chronic lung disease, congestive heart failure, heart attack, angina, asthma, arthritis, stroke, kidney disease?	≥5 = 1, <5 = 0
Loss of weight	Have you lost more than 5% of your weight in the last year?	Yes 1; No 0

Scale score 0–5
3–5 frail
1–2 pre-frail
0 robust health status

(comorbidity burden, cognitive status, signs, symptoms, abnormal laboratory results, daily living activities, deficits of social support, etc.). FI is expressed as the proportion of the number of deficits present to the number of deficits assessed [3]. It is a more comprehensive approach compared with the frailty phenotype. Some advantages are the ability to apply it to any health dataset, provided enough variables have been collected (as opposed to Fried phenotype where patient presence is needed), the comprehensive assessment of health with a continuous score from fitness to frailty, and the lack of a ceiling effect.

Both frailty frameworks identify well the most vulnerable patients, however, substantial discordance can be found in the more intermediate categories [43], suggesting that in some contexts these two approaches cannot be used interchangeably.

Moreover, in some specific settings, like heart failure patients with diuretic treatment, it is difficult to assess some key parameters, like unintentional weight loss.

Based on these two conceptual models, several modified screening instruments have been developed over time [44–48]. Some simpler scales, suitable for rapid clinical evaluation are presented in Tables 24.3, 24.4 and 24.5. While no perfect frailty measurement exists, there is a common agreement that frailty should be recognized in clinical practice and frailty assessment should be a part of daily care in older patients.

In recent years there has been increased interest in developing new scores for frailty specifically tailored for HF patients. The Heart Failure Association of the ESC proposed a new score, HFA Frailty Score, considering four main domains as main determinants of frailty in HF patients—the clinical, psycho-cognitive, functional, and social domain [23].

Table 24.4 The Study of Osteoporotic Fractures frailty tool (SOF) [46] for assessment of frailty

Clinical question	Score
Weight loss of 5% in the last year	Yes 1; No 0
Inability to stand up from a chair five times without the use of arms	Yes 1; No 0
Do you feel full of energy?	Yes 0; No 1

Score ≥ 2—frail

Table 24.5 Four-item essential frailty toolset (EFT) evaluated in older patients undergoing aortic valve replacement [48]

Clinical question	Score
Five chair rises in less than 15 s	0 points
Five chair rises in more than 15 s	1 point
Unable to complete	2 points
No cognitive impairment	0 points
Cognitive impairment	1 point
Hemoglobin	
Men ≥ 13 g/dl, women ≥ 12 g/l	0 points
Men < 13 g/dl, women < 12 g/l	1 point
Serum albumin	
≥3.5 g/dl	0 points
<3.5 g/dl	1 point

Higher scores are associated with increased mortality and morbidity after aortic valve replacement

Clinical Characteristics, Outcomes, and HF Medication in Frail HF Patients

HF patients with frailty form a special high-risk population, that is older, has more associated comorbidities and worse cardiovascular prognosis. Women tend to be more affected than men [49], with a 25% relative risk compared with men and a worse symptoms profile. As women live longer, they have a greater chance of suffering from frailty than men. Reduced muscular mass can also contribute to physical frailty. In heart failure, women are older at the moment of diagnosis, have more frequent non-ischemic etiologies [50] and a higher burden of comorbidities. Different cardiac geometry with smaller, more hypertrophied hearts can be linked with a higher likelihood than men to develop HF with preserved ejection fraction [51].

Cardiology guidelines recommend evidence-based therapy for all patients with heart failure, independent of age. However, frail elderly patients are typically underrepresented in most of the HF randomized controlled clinical trials. In an older cross-sectional study of HF patients aged more than 64 years discharged from the hospital [52], less than a quarter met the enrolment criteria for the then-contemporary heart failure trials (SOLVD, MERIT-HF, RALES), suggesting a significant discrepancy between trial population and frail patients in the community.

Moreover, in clinical practice, frail patients tend to receive less guideline-directed medication, as their risk-benefit profile is frequently perceived as less favourable. Reasons for undertreatment are clinical concerns regarding polypharmacy, medical interactions, adverse effects, and treatment discontinuation. However, taking into consideration the accentuation of frailty with any hospitalization, the clinical benefit of HF medication might even be bigger in this population [1].

In recent years several studies and registries tried to evaluate frailty and its impact on outcomes in different heart failure settings.

In HF with reduced ejection fraction, a frailty analysis [53] was conducted on combined data from two HFrEF trials: PARADIGM-HF (Prospective comparison of ARNI (Angiotensin Receptor–Neprilysin Inhibitor) with ACEI (Angiotensin-Converting Enzyme Inhibitor) to Determine Impact on Global Mortality and morbidity in Heart Failure) and ATMOSHERE (Aliskiren Trial to Minimize OutcomeS in Patients with HEart failuRE trial) [54, 55], using the Rockwood cumulative deficit approach. In concordance with previous studies, patients with a frailty index higher than 0.21 were defined as frail. The outcomes assessed were the primary endpoints for both trials (composite of HF hospitalization or cardiovascular death), its components, and cardiovascular, non-cardiovascular, and overall hospitalizations. The overall FI was 0.25 ± 0.1, with more than 60% of the 13,625 patients being frail. The frailest patients were older, had a higher burden of HF symptoms and signs, a longer duration of HF, and a higher rate of HF hospitalization. Significantly higher N-terminal proBNP levels were noted in the frailest patients. Congestion and fatigue were twice as prevalent in frail patients. Women were frailer than men and the frailest patients also associated significant levels of anxiety/depression. All outcomes were worse in frail patients, with high rates of all-cause death and hospitalization. The risk of falls and fractures, even though small numbers were registered, paralleled the increase in the frailty index. In the combined population, study drug discontinuation was more common in frail patients (20% versus 14%). However, in PARADIGM-HF, no interaction between treatment and frailty was noticed, showing a consistent sacubitril-valsartan effect in both frail and non-frail patients.

In HF with preserved ejection fraction, TOPCAT investigators [21] reported an even higher mean FI (0.37 ± 0.11), in a population approximately 5 years older, with 94% of patients with a FI ≥ 0.21. These data are in line with results from other studies that show that HFrEF patients tend to younger and be less frail than HFpEF [56]. However, as a comparison, the mean FI in the UK general population (UK Biobank) was 0.139 in those aged more than 65 years [57].

Several post hoc analysis of various trials and registries, focusing on chronic HF patients older than 65 years, have been performed. Besides the analysis of PARADIGM-HF data, angiotensin receptor–neprilysin Inhibitor effectiveness in older patients with HFrEF was assessed in the Get With The Guidelines—Heart Failure registry [58]. The outcome of patients more than 65 years old (mean age 78 years) discharged from the hospital with ARNI has been evaluated. In this registry, 62% of patients older than 65 years were prescribed angiotensin-converting enzyme inhibitor/angiotensin II receptor blocker at discharge, and only 10.9% ARNI. Compared with patients receiving angiotensin-converting enzyme inhibitor/angiotensin II receptor blocker, prescription of sacubitril/valsartan in elderly patients was associated with better post-discharge outcomes, including lower all-cause mortality, suggesting that the benefits of ARNI extend also to older patients.

In HFpEF, a post hoc analysis of the PARAGON-HF (Prospective Comparison of ARNI With ARB Global Outcomes in Heart Failure With Preserved Ejection Fraction) trial [1], evaluated the effects of sacubitril-valsartan according to the frailty status. In the frailest patients, a greater reduction in the primary composite endpoint and total HF hospitalizations with sacubitril/valsartan compared with valsartan was noted when FI was analyzed as a continuous variable. Adverse events, drug discontinuation, falls and fractures were more common in frailer patients, but not different between sacubitril/valsartan and valsartan groups, underlining the safety and tolerance of ARNI independent of frailty class.

The influence of age and frailty on the effects of dapagliflozin has been evaluated in post hoc analysis of DAPA-HF (Dapagliflozin and Prevention of Adverse Outcomes in Heart Failure) [59] and DELIVER (Dapagliflozin Evaluation to Improve the Lives of Patients With Preserved Ejection Fraction Heart Failure) [60] trials. In both analyses, the benefit of dapagliflozin treatment was consistent across the spectrum of frailty, irrespective of frailty class. The absolute reductions in outcomes were even larger in DAPA-HF in more frail patients. While treatment discontinuation and adverse reactions were more common in frail individuals, no difference between study patients and placebo was noted.

Beta-blocker therapy was evaluated in older patients. SENIORS study (Study of the Effects of Nebivolol Intervention on Outcomes and Rehospitalisation in Seniors with Heart Failure) [61] enrolled chronic heart failure patients older than 70 years, and showed that nebivolol was an efficient, well-tolerated medication in this population group.

A retrospective analysis of the OPTIMIZE (Organized Program to Initiate Lifesaving Treatment in Hospitalized Patients With Heart Failure) [62] registry evaluated the clinical effectiveness of initiation of beta-blockers in patients older than 65 years. In a population with a median age of 80 years (versus beta-blockers in HF landmark trials, in which the median age is around 65 years) [62], beta-blocker initiation in HFrEF patients was associated with a significant reduction in all-cause mortality and hospitalizations, although no effect was observed in HFpEF cohort.

Mineralocorticoid receptor antagonists (MRA) in elderly patients were evaluated in a propensity-matched analysis based on a Japanese HF registry [63] in individuals after HF hospitalization, with a median age of 80 years. MRA use was associated with a significant reduction in HF hospitalizations.

One caveat is that the post hoc analysis incorporating frailty or advanced age are effectuated on patients already included in studies, which frequently exclude very high-risk patients. However, all these data suggest that clinical reluctance to use modern HF therapies in frail, elderly patients is not founded on evidence and risk-benefit balance in frail patients might be even more favourable than thought.

Frail patients are not only less likely to have complete HF therapy, but they also tend to receive suboptimal dosage. There is an inverse relationship between frailty status and the probability of receiving optimal chronical HF therapy [64].

While heart failure guideline-directed medical therapy is frequently underused in elderly frail patients, polypharmacy and inappropriate prescription in older people is another significant clinical problem, raising not only concerns about adherence but also about drug-related adverse effects and interactions. Several clinical tools that address the issue of the appropriateness of drug prescription in the elderly have been developed. Two examples are STOPP (screening tool of older people's prescription) START (screening tool to alert to right treatment) criteria [65] or the use of Beers criteria, recently updated by the American Geriatrics Society [66]. As most elderly people have multiple comorbidities and need to take six or even more essential medications, care should be taken in order to keep the essential medication, limit drug interactions, and prioritize treatment for serious conditions over conditions with less impact on life quality [67]. As every prevention of hospitalization will significantly impact on frailty acceleration, clinical efforts should be oriented towards the introduction, up-titration, and maintenance of HF medication.

Device Therapy in Frail HF Patients

Older patients with heart failure have a higher prevalence of cardiac resynchronization therapy (CRT) and implantable cardioverter defibrillator (ICD) [29], most likely due to the higher prevalence of heart failure, longer duration, and more advanced HF. Guidelines do not include an upper age limit for CRT and ICD, but do not recommend ICD in frail patients with a good functional life expectancy lower than 1 year [16, 68, 69]. Most of the device trials included patients with a median age of less than 70 years [69], while in real life a significant proportion of older patients undergo device implantation [70]. The results of Multicenter Automatic Defibrillator Implantation Trial- Cardiac Resynchronization Therapy (MADIT-CRT) have shown a significant reduction of the composite end-point of death and heart failure with CRT and ICD (CRT-D) in patients aged 60–74 years and in patients older than 75 years, with no significant difference observed in people younger than 60 years old [71]. In the elderly patients enrolled in the Multicenter InSync Randomized Clinical Evaluation (MIRACLE) and Multicenter InSync ICD Randomized Clinical Evaluation (MIRACLE-ICD), CRT resulted in significant improvements in NYHA class and left ventricular ejection fraction, irrespective of age [72]. The same results were noticed in a population of octogenarians undergoing CRT implantation [73], with similar clinical benefits as younger patients and similar observed complication rates. These data suggest that all age range patients with appropriate indications according to the current guidelines might benefit from CRT. Data for ICD implantation in elderly patients is more scarce, especially as with advanced age, comorbidities, and geriatric syndromes, tachyarrhythmic death becomes less prevalent [74]. However, in well-selected patients with a high risk of arrhythmic death and few comorbidities other than age, ICD intervention may reduce mortality [74].

Sarcopenia and Frailty

Sarcopenia is characterized as low muscular mass together with low muscular function, strength, and low exercise capacity and it is a significant contributor to frailty. Both share similar risk factors like advanced age, malnutrition, low physical activity, or humoral changes. It is defined as an age-related loss of skeletal muscle more than 2 standard deviations below the mean of a healthy reference group aged 18–40 [16, 75]. It leads to difficulties in performing simple daily tasks like standing from a chair or walking, progressing to functional decline and physical disability. In chronic heart failure, it can be found in 20–50% of the patients with HFrEF [75] and it is a major determinant of outcomes. Several muscular abnormalities, including impaired skeletal muscle energy metabolism, mitochondrial dysfunction, fiber-type transition from type I to type II, and atrophy have been described in HF [76].

Evaluation of sarcopenia is recommended when patients start reporting symptoms such as weakness, falls, difficulty standing from a chair, and a standardized approach has been proposed by the European Working Group on Sarcopenia in Older People [77].

While several treatments, mostly anabolic, have been tested in small studies, the only meaningful therapeutic strategy is exercise training [16]. Exercise is the most effective therapy for muscle wasting in HF, targeting multiple mechanisms like inflammation and hormonal changes [78] and it should combine general physical activity with resistance training. Exercise training and more specific supervised exercise-based cardiac rehabilitation are recommended for frail HF patients in the Guidelines of the European Society of Cardiology for the diagnosis and treatment of acute and chronic HF [16]. In a post-hoc analysis of HF-ACTION trial [79], that evaluated the effects of aerobic supervised training in HFrEF, baseline frailty level modified the treatment effect of aerobic exercise training. In frail patients, a greater benefit was observed, driven by a reduction in all-cause hospitalization. In both frail and non-frail patients, aerobic exercise training was associated with an improvement of quality of life.

Exercise interventions for frailty include aerobic, resistance, and balance exercises, ideally done 2–3 times/week. These exercises should start in a supervised manner and can continue with individualized exercise prescriptions at home. During the supervised time period, the time allocated for each domain should be tailored according to the patient's specific physical impairment and needs. A gradual small increase in exercise from session to session should be promoted, in an individualized manner.

Aerobic exercise can influence the frailty phenotype by improving the maximum oxygen uptake and increasing muscular mass, while resistance training mainly targets the increase in muscle mass and strength. Muscle mass change with exercise is attenuated in older individuals, however, a positive effect on muscular strength has been reported even in the ninth decade [80]. Resistance training can also improve motor performance, gait speed and six-minute walk test. It usually includes functional strengthening exercises and general resistance training for major muscles in the upper and lower extremities. The ideal program combines both aerobic, resistance, and balance training, targeting distinct features of frailty. Moreover, combined regimens of training decreased the fall risk in the frail population [81].

Cardiac rehabilitation interventions have been associated with positive results in HF patients. In EHAB-HF trial (Rehabilitation and Exercise Training after Hospitalization) [82] physical rehabilitation started during hospitalization for acute heart failure and continued after discharge (60 min supervised sessions 3 times per week for 3 months combined with low-intensity home exercise on the nonprogram days) was associated with greater improvement in physical function, 6-minute walk distance, quality of life, reduction in frailty and depression than the usual care. In this study, the outpatient supervised phase was then continued with an independent maintenance phase with individualized exercise prescription.

Screening for Frailty

Due to its high prevalence in HF patients, screening for frailty should be systematically performed. In clinical practice, an HF patient aged 75 or older would be a target for screening [15]. If cardiac surgery, structural interventions or device treatments are contemplated, screening should be considered in patients older than 65 years or sometimes even younger . On the other hand, it is considered futile to screen for frailty in patients completely dependent, approaching the end of life, where palliative care is instituted [15].

Screening should be done either in an outpatient patient with chronic HF or in the inpatient setting, using some of the available tools. For example, in France, The French Health Authority proposed the Triage Risk Screening Tool (TRST), a simple tool that has been validated in two emergency departments in Cleveland [83]. A positive screening result should trigger a battery of cardio-geriatric measures (Table 24.6), pharmacological and non-pharmacological, in order to reduce mortality, hospitalizations, and readmissions for HF and to improve the quality of life and functional status. The non-pharmacological measures include exercise training programs, covering aerobic, strength, and balance exercises and nutritional advice, and eventually fortified diet or protein-energy supplementation. If geriatric syndromes are identified, treatment of malnutrition, sarcopenia, depression, and cognitive impairment should be instituted [15]. This integrated approach to frailty could reduce its negative impact on heart failure outcomes.

Table 24.6 Pharmacological and non-pharmacological interventions for frail patients with chronic heart failure

Domains	Prevention	Treatment
HFrEF	Treatment of risk factors and chronic cardiological diseases	Optimal medical therapy (four pillars: ARNI or ACEi/ARB, beta-blockers, MRA, SGLT2 inhibitors) CRT referral if indicated Optimal diuretic treatment tailored for comorbidities Supervised exercise training programme
HFpEF	Treatment of risk factors and chronic cardiological diseases	Optimal medical therapy (SGLT2 inhibitors) Optimal diuretic treatment Supervised exercise training program
Co-morbidities and polypharmacy	Treatment according to renal function Using a STOPP, START approach, de-escalation of unneeded medication	Periodical check for co-morbidities Medication review Propriety setting if multiple comorbidities present
Sarcopenia	Regular physical exercise	Exercise training program (aerobic, strength, balance exercises) Nutrition plan
Manutrition	Weight monitoring Protein intake (1–1.2 g/kg/day) Regular physical exercise	Exercise training program (aerobic, strength, balance exercises) Protein intake (1.2–1.5 g/kg/day) +/− oral nutritional supplements
Falls	Assess hydration Screening for orthostatic hypotension Regular physical exercise	Identify possible medication or diseases Search for potential precipitating factors Exercise training programme (aerobic, strength, balance exercises) Vitamin D supplementation
Depression	Combatting social isolation	Psychotherapy Medication if needed
Cognitive impairment	Treatment of chronic diseases (Arterial hypertension, atrial fibrillation) Social engagement	Cognitive stimulation Specific treatment and social support Drug adherence
Vaccination	Influenza, pneumococcal	
Social measures	Compliance screening	Social support Nurses

Modified after [15] with permission

ARNI angiotensin receptor neprilysin inhibitors, *ACEi* angiotensin-converting enzyme inhibitors (ACE-I), *ARBs* angiotensin receptor blockers (ARBs), *MRA* mineralocorticoid receptor antagonists, *SGLT2i* sodium-glucose co-transporter 2 inhibitors

Conclusions

Frailty in heart failure patients is a major contributor to poor functional status and adverse clinical outcomes. With continuous aging of the population and improved medical care, an increased proportion of frail patients is expected. Frailty assessment should be a part of routine clinical management of heart failure patients, allowing the initiation of early intervention targeting modifiable components, in order to reduce the impact of frailty and improve heart failure outcomes in this specific population.

References

1. Butt JH, Dewan P, Jhund PS, et al. Sacubitril/valsartan and frailty in patients with heart failure and preserved ejection fraction. J Am Coll Cardiol. 2022;80(12):1130–43.
2. Fried LP, Tangen CM, Walston J, et al. Frailty in older adults: evidence for a phenotype. J Gerontol A Biol Sci Med Sci. 2001;56:M146–56.
3. Rockwood K, Song X, MacKnight C, et al. A global clinical measure of fitness and frailty in elderly people. CMAJ. 2005;173:489–95.
4. Campbell AJ, Buchner DM. Unstable disability and the fluctuations of frailty. Age Ageing. 1997;26:315–8.
5. Winograd CH, Gerety MB, Chung M, et al. Screening for frailty: criteria and predictors of outcomes. J Am Geriatr Soc. 1991;39:778–84.
6. Pandey A, Kitzman D, Reeves G. Frailty is intertwined with heart failure. Mechanisms, prevalence, prognosis, assessment and management. JACC: Heart Fail. 2019;7:1001–11.
7. Afilalo J, Alexander KP, Mack MJ, et al. Frailty assessment in the cardiovascular care of older adults. J Am Coll Cardiol. 2014;63(8):747–62.
8. Dodson JA, Maurer MS. Changing nature of cardiac interventions in older adults. Aging Health. 2011;7(2):283–95.
9. Tsao CW, Aday AW, Almarzooq ZI, American Heart Association Council on Epidemiology and Prevention Statistics Committee and Stroke Statistics Subcommittee, et al. Heart disease and stroke statistics-2023 update: a report from the American Heart Association. Circulation. 2023;147(8):e93–e621.
10. Timmis A, Vardas P, Townsend N, et al. European Society of Cardiology: cardiovascular disease statistics 2021: executive summary. Eur Heart J Qual Care Clin Outcomes. 2022;8(4):377–82.
11. Kumar M, Orkaby A, Tighe C, et al. Life's essential 8: optimizing health in older adults. JACC Adv. 2023;2(7):100560. https://doi.org/10.1016/j.jacadv.2023.100560.
12. López-Otín C, Blasco MA, Partridge L, Serrano M, Kroemer G. Hallmarks of aging: an expanding universe. Cell. 2023;186(2):243–78.
13. Clegg A, Young J, Iliffe S, et al. Frailty in elderly people. Lancet. 2013;381:752–62.
14. Ouchi Y, Rakugi H, Arai H, et al. Joint Committee of Japan Gerontological Society (JGLS) and Japan Geriatrics Society (JGS) on the definition and classification of the elderly. Redefining the elderly as aged 75 years and older: proposal from the Joint Committee of Japan Gerontological Society and the Japan Geriatrics Society. Geriatr Gerontol Int. 2017;17(7):1045–7.
15. Boureau AS, Annweiler C, Belmin J, et al. Practical management of frailty in older patients with heart failure: statement from a panel of multidisciplinary experts on behalf the Heart Failure Working Group of the French Society of Cardiology and on behalf French Society of Geriatrics and Gerontology. ESC Heart Fail. 2022;9(6):4053–63.

16. McDonagh TA, Metra M, Adamo M, ESC Scientific Document Group, et al. 2021 ESC Guidelines for the diagnosis and treatment of acute and chronic heart failure: developed by the Task Force for the diagnosis and treatment of acute and chronic heart failure of the European Society of Cardiology (ESC). With the special contribution of the Heart Failure Association (HFA) of the ESC. Eur J Heart Fail. 2022;24(1):4–131.
17. Woods NF, LaCroix AZ, Gray SL, Women's Health Initiative, et al. Frailty: emergence and consequences in women aged 65 and older in the Women's Health Initiative Observational Study. J Am Geriatr Soc. 2005;53(8):1321.
18. Kiely DK, Cupples LA, Lipsitz LA. Validation and comparison of two frailty indexes: the MOBILIZE Boston Study. J Am Geriatr Soc. 2009;57(9):1532. Epub 2009 Jul 21
19. Theou O, Brothers TD, Mitnitski A, et al. Operationalization of frailty using eight commonly used scales and comparison of their ability to predict all-cause mortality. J Am Geriatr Soc. 2013;61(9):1537.
20. Denfeld QE, Winters-Stone K, Mudd JO, et al. The prevalence of frailty in heart failure: a systematic review and meta-analysis. Int J Cardiol. 2017;236:283289.
21. Sanders NA, Supiano MA, Lewis EF, et al. The frailty syndrome and outcomes in the TOPCAT trial. Eur J Heart Fail. 2018;20(11):1570–7.
22. Virani SS, Alonso A, Aparicio HJ, et al. Heart disease and stroke statistics-2021 update: a report from the American Heart Association. Circulation. 2021;143:e254–743.
23. Vitale C, Jankowska E, Hill L, et al. Heart Failure Association/European Society of Cardiology position paper on frailty in patients with heart failure. Eur J Heart Fail. 2019;21(11):1299–305.
24. Uchmanowicz I, Lee CS, Vitale C, et al. Frailty and the risk of all-cause mortality and hospitalization in chronic heart failure: a meta-analysis. ESC Heart Fail. 2020;7(6):3427–37.
25. Farooqi MAM, Gerstein H, Yusuf S, et al. Accumulation of deficits as a key risk factor for cardiovascular morbidity and mortality: a pooled analysis of 154 000 individuals. J Am Heart Assoc. 2020;9(3):e014686.
26. Dent E, Kowal P, Hoogendijk EO. Frailty measurement in research and clinical practice: a review. Eur J Intern Med. 2016;31:3–10.
27. Fried LP, Cohen AA, Xue QL, et al. The physical frailty syndrome as a transition from homeostatic symphony to cacophony. Nat Aging. 2021;1(1):36–46.
28. Varadhan R, Chaves PH, Lipsitz LA, et al. Frailty and impaired cardiac autonomic control: new insights from principal components aggregation of traditional heart rate variability indices. J Gerontol A Biol Sci Med Sci. 2009;64(6):682–7.
29. Talha KM, Pandey A, Fudim M, et al. Frailty and heart failure: state-of-the-art review. J Cachexia Sarcopenia Muscle. 2023; https://doi.org/10.1002/jcsm.13306. Epub ahead of print.
30. Kitzman DW, Nicklas B, Kraus WE, et al. Skeletal muscle abnormalities and exercise intolerance in older patients with heart failure and preserved ejection fraction. Am J Physiol Heart Circ Physiol. 2014;306(9):H1364–70.
31. Molina AJ, Bharadwaj MS, Van Horn C, et al. Skeletal muscle mitochondrial content, oxidative capacity, and Mfn2 expression are reduced in older patients with heart failure and preserved ejection fraction and are related to exercise intolerance. JACC Heart Fail. 2016;4(8):636–45.
32. Al Zadjali MA, Godfrey V, Khan F, et al. Insulin resistance is highly prevalent and is associated with reduced exercise tolerance in nondiabetic patients with heart failure. J Am Coll Cardiol. 2009;53:747–53.
33. Doehner W, Frenneaux M, Anker SD. Metabolic impairment in heart failure: the myocardial and systemic perspective. J Am Coll Cardiol. 2014;64:1388–400.
34. Sato R, Vatic M, da Fonseca GWP, et al. Sarcopenia and frailty in heart failure: is there a biomarker signature? Curr Heart Fail Rep. 2022;19(6):400–11.
35. Streng KW, Hillege HL, Ter Maaten JM, et al. Clinical implications of low estimated protein intake in patients with heart failure. J Cachexia Sarcopenia Muscle. 2022;13(3):1762–70.
36. Matsue Y, Kamiya K, Saito H, et al. Prevalence and prognostic impact of the coexistence of multiple frailty domains in elderly patients with heart failure: the FRAGILE-HF cohort study. Eur J Heart Fail. 2020;22:2112–9.

37. Cannon JA, Moffitt P, Perez-Moreno AC, et al. Cognitive impairment and heart failure: systematic review and meta-analysis. J Card Fail. 2017;23(6):464–75.
38. Yamamoto S, Yamasaki S, Higuchi S, et al. Prevalence and prognostic impact of cognitive frailty in elderly patients with heart failure: sub-analysis of FRAGILE-HF. ESC Heart Fail. 2022;9(3):1574–83.
39. Jujo K, Kagiyama N, Saito K, et al. Impact of social frailty in hospitalized elderly patients with heart failure: a FRAGILE-HF registry subanalysis. J Am Heart Assoc. 2021;10(17):e019954.
40. Ijaz N, Buta B, Xue QL, et al. Interventions for frailty among older adults with cardiovascular disease: JACC state-of-the-art review. J Am Coll Cardiol. 2022;79(5):482–503.
41. Bandeen-Roche K, Xue QL, Ferrucci L, et al. Phenotype of frailty: characterization in the women's health and aging studies. J Gerontol A Biol Sci Med Sci. 2006;61:262–6.
42. Yang X, Lupon J, Vidan MT, et al. Impact of frailty on mortality and hospitalization in chronic heart failure: a systematic review and meta-analysis. J Am Heart Assoc. 2018;7:e008251.
43. Xue QL, Tian J, Walston JD, et al. Discrepancy in frailty identification: move beyond predictive validity. J Gerontol A Biol Sci Med Sci. 2020;75(2):387–93.
44. Rolfson DB, Majumdar SR, Tsuyuki RT, et al. Validity and reliability of the Edmonton Frail Scale. Age Ageing. 2006;35(5):526–9.
45. Abellan van Kan G, Rolland Y, Bergman H, et al. The I.A.N.A Task Force on frailty assessment of older people in clinical practice. J Nutr Health Aging. 2008;12(1):29–37.
46. Ensrud KE, Ewing SK, Taylor BC, et al. Frailty and risk of falls, fracture and mortality in older women: the study of osteoporotic fractures. J Gerontol A Biol Sci Med Sci. 2007;62:744–51.
47. Jones DM, Song X, Rockwood K. Operationalizing a frailty index from a standardized comprehensive geriatric assessment. J Am Geriatr Soc. 2004;52:1929–33.
48. Afilalo J, Lauck S, Kim DH, et al. Frailty in older adults undergoing aortic valve replacement: the FRAILTY-AVR study. J Am Coll Cardiol. 2017;70(6):689–700.
49. Denfeld QE, Habecker BA, Camacho SA, et al. Characterizing sex differences in physical frailty phenotypes in heart failure. Circ Heart Fail. 2021;14(9):e008076.
50. Azad N, Kathiravelu A, Minoosepeher S, et al. Gender differences in the etiology of heart failure: a systematic review. J Geriatr Cardiol. 2011;8:15–23.
51. Beale AL, Meyer P, Marwick TH, et al. Sex differences in cardiovascular pathophysiology: why women are overrepresented in heart failure with preserved ejection fraction. Circulation. 2018;138:198–205.
52. Masoudi FA, Havranek EP, Wolfe P, et al. Most hospitalized older persons do not meet the enrollment criteria for clinical trials in heart failure. Am Heart J. 2003;146(2):250–7.
53. Dewan P, Jackson A, Jhund PS, et al. The prevalence and importance of frailty in heart failure with reduced ejection fraction—an analysis of PARADIGM-HF and ATMOSPHERE. Eur J Heart Fail. 2020;22(11):2123–33.
54. McMurray JJV, Packer M, Desai AS, et al. Angiotensin–neprilysin inhibition versus enalapril in heart failure. N Engl J Med. 2014;371:993–1004.
55. McMurray JJV, Krum H, Abraham WT, et al. Aliskiren, enalapril, or aliskiren and enalapril in heart failure. N Engl J Med. 2016;374:1521–32.
56. Sze S, Pellicori P, Zhang J, et al. Identification of frailty in chronic heart failure. JACC Heart Fail. 2019;7(4):291–302.
57. Williams DM, Jylhävä J, Pedersen NL, et al. A frailty index for UK Biobank participants. J Gerontol A Biol Sci Med Sci. 2019;74:582–7.
58. Greene SJ, Choi S, Lippmann SJ, et al. Clinical effectiveness of sacubitril/valsartan among patients hospitalized for heart failure with reduced ejection fraction. J Am Heart Assoc. 2021;10(16):e021459.
59. Butt JH, Dewan P, Merkely B, et al. Efficacy and safety of dapagliflozin according to frailty in heart failure with reduced ejection fraction: a post hoc analysis of the DAPA-HF trial. Ann Intern Med. 2022;175(6):820–30.

60. Butt JH, Jhund PS, Belohlávek J, et al. Efficacy and safety of dapagliflozin according to frailty in patients with heart failure: a prespecified analysis of the DELIVER trial. Circulation. 2022;146(16):1210–24.
61. Flather MD, Shibata MC, Coats AJ, SENIORS Investigators, et al. Randomized trial to determine the effect of nebivolol on mortality and cardiovascular hospital admission in elderly patients with heart failure (SENIORS). Eur Heart J. 2005;26(3):215–25.
62. Hernandez AF, Hammill BG, O'Connor CM, et al. Clinical effectiveness of beta-blockers in heart failure: findings from the OPTIMIZE-HF (organized program to initiate lifesaving treatment in hospitalized patients with heart failure) registry. J Am Coll Cardiol. 2009;53(2):184–92.
63. Yaku H, Kato T, Morimoto T, KCHF Study Investigators, et al. Association of Mineralocorticoid Receptor Antagonist Use with All-Cause Mortality and Hospital Readmission in older adults with acute decompensated heart failure. JAMA Netw Open. 2019;2(6):e195892.
64. Sze S, Pellicori P, Zhang J, et al. Effect of frailty on treatment, hospitalisation and death in patients with chronic heart failure. Clin Res Cardiol. 2021;110(8):1249–58.
65. O'Mahony D, Cherubini A, Guiteras ARD, et al. STOPP/START criteria for potentially inappropriate prescribing in older people: version 3. Eur Geriatr Med. 2023;14(4):625.
66. By the 2023 American Geriatrics Society Beers Criteria® Update Expert Panel. American Geriatrics Society 2023 updated AGS Beers Criteria® for potentially inappropriate medication use in older adults. J Am Geriatr Soc. 2023;71(7):2052–81.
67. Tinetti ME, Bogardus ST Jr, Agostini JV. Potential pitfalls of disease-specific guidelines for patients with multiple conditions. N Engl J Med. 2004;351(27):2870–4.
68. Glikson M, Nielsen JC, Kronborg MB, ESC Scientific Document Group, et al. 2021 ESC Guidelines on cardiac pacing and cardiac resynchronization therapy. Eur Heart J. 2021;42(35):3427–520.
69. Heidenreich PA, Bozkurt B, Aguilar D, et al. 2022 AHA/ACC/HFSA Guideline for the Management of Heart Failure: a report of the American College of Cardiology/American Heart Association Joint Committee on Clinical Practice Guidelines. Circulation. 2022;145(18):e895–e1032.
70. Betz JK, Katz DF, Peterson PN, et al. Outcomes among older patients receiving implantable cardioverter-defibrillators for secondary prevention: from the NCDR ICD registry. J Am Coll Cardiol. 2017;69(3):265–74.
71. Penn J, Goldenberg I, Moss AJ, MADIT-CRT Trial investigators, et al. Improved outcome with preventive cardiac resynchronization therapy in the elderly: a MADIT-CRT substudy. J Cardiovasc Electrophysiol. 2011;22(8):892–7.
72. Kron J, Aranda JM Jr, Miles WM, et al. Benefit of cardiac resynchronization in elderly patients: results from the Multicenter InSync Randomized Clinical Evaluation (MIRACLE) and Multicenter InSync ICD Randomized Clinical Evaluation (MIRACLE-ICD) trials. J Interv Card Electrophysiol. 2009;25(2):91–6.
73. Killu AM, Wu JH, Friedman PA, et al. Outcomes of cardiac resynchronization therapy in the elderly. Pacing Clin Electrophysiol. 2013;36(6):664–72.
74. Savelieva I, Fumagalli S, Kenny RA, et al. EHRA expert consensus document on the management of arrhythmias in frailty syndrome, endorsed by the Heart Rhythm Society (HRS), Asia Pacific Heart Rhythm Society (APHRS), Latin America Heart Rhythm Society (LAHRS), and Cardiac Arrhythmia Society of Southern Africa (CASSA). Europace. 2023;25(4):1249–76.
75. Mirzai S, Eck BL, Chen PH, et al. Current approach to the diagnosis of sarcopenia in heart failure: a narrative review on the role of clinical and imaging assessments. Circ Heart Fail. 2022;15(10):e009322.
76. Fulster S, Tacke M, Sandek A, et al. Muscle wasting in patients with chronic heart failure: results from the studies investigating co-morbidities aggravating heart failure (SICA-HF). Eur Heart J. 2013;34:512–9.
77. Cruz-Jentoft AJ, Bahat G, Bauer J, Writing Group for the European Working Group on Sarcopenia in Older People 2 (EWGSOP2), and the Extended Group for EWGSOP2,

et al. Sarcopenia: revised European consensus on definition and diagnosis. Age Ageing. 2019;48:16–31. https://doi.org/10.1093/ageing/afy169.

78. von Haehling S, Steinbeck L, Doehner W, et al. Muscle wasting in heart failure: an overview. Int J Biochem Cell Biol. 2013;45(10):2257–65.
79. Pandey A, Segar MW, Singh SR, et al. Frailty status modifies the efficacy of exercise training among patients with chronic heart failure and reduced ejection fraction: an analysis from the HF-ACTION trial. Circulation. 2022;146(2):80–90.
80. Liu CK, Fielding RA. Exercise as an intervention for frailty. Clin Geriatr Med. 2011;27(1):101–10. https://doi.org/10.1016/j.cger.2010.08.001.
81. Delmonico MJ, Beck DT. The current understanding of sarcopenia: emerging tools and interventional possibilities. Am J Lifestyle Med. 2017;11:167–81.
82. Kitzman DW, Whellan DJ, Duncan P, et al. Physical rehabilitation for older patients hospitalized for heart failure. N Engl J Med. 2021;385(3):203–16.
83. Meldon SW, Mion LC, Palmer RM, et al. A brief risk-stratification tool to predict repeat emergency department visits and hospitalizations in older patients discharged from the emergency department. Acad Emerg Med. 2003;10(3):224–32.

Chapter 25
Heart Failure in Pregnancy

Larysa Strilchuk and Renata Cífková

Abstract Cardiovascular disease (CVD) is the most common cause of non-obstetric complications of pregnancy. The number of pregnant women with CVD is steadily increasing, so heart failure (HF) rates may increase proportionally. HF may complicate pregnancy-specific CVD (peripartum cardiomyopathy, hypertensive disorders of pregnancy, and amniotic fluid embolism) and nonspecific ones (myocarditis, valvular heart disease, arrhythmias, congenital heart defects, coronary heart disease, various cardiomyopathies, etc.).

Pregnant women with acute HF must be immediately referred to an intensive care unit in a tertiary care center, where hemodynamically unstable patients with severe HF must undergo an urgent cesarean section, irrespective of gestation time. Urgent delivery is also advocated if the fetus is unviable. If the fetus is viable and it is possible to stabilize the mother's condition, delivery can be postponed.

Assessment of cardiovascular risk is a cornerstone of HF prevention. Women with a history of CVD or preeclampsia need thorough counseling including symptom assessment, maternal/fetal risk evaluation, adjustment of medications, general health evaluation, and appropriate education.

In general, HF in pregnancy is a life-threatening complication comprising a broad spectrum of medical conditions. Management of HF in pregnancy generally resembles management in nonpregnant patients, however, avoiding potentially teratogenic drugs must be kept in mind.

Keywords Heart failure · Pregnancy · Peripartum cardiomyopathy

---

L. Strilchuk
Department of Therapy No. 1, Medical Diagnostics, Hematology and Transfusiology, Lviv Danylo Halytsky National Medical University, Lviv, Ukraine

R. Cífková (✉)
Center for Cardiovascular Prevention, Charles University in Prague, First Faculty of Medicine and Thomayer University Hospital, Prague, Czech Republic

Department of Medicine II, Charles University in Prague, First Faculty of Medicine, Prague, Czech Republic
e-mail: renata.cifkova@ftn.cz

M. Dorobanţu et al. (eds.), *Current Approach to Heart Failure*,
https://doi.org/10.1007/978-3-031-96562-3_25

Table 25.1 Risk factors of maternal HF [9, 34]

Demographic risk factors	Obstetric risk factors	Other risk factors
Black race Age > 40 years Tobacco use Alcohol use Drug abuse	Multiple gestation Gestational or chronic hypertension Preeclampsia/eclampsia Preterm delivery Postpartum hemorrhage Placenta accreta/abruption/previa Gestational diabetes mellitus	Prior HF Family history of HF Hyperlipidemia Pre-existing diabetes mellitus Obesity Obstructive sleep apnea Chronic kidney disease Anticoagulant use History of chemotherapy

Introduction

Pregnancy renders high-level physiological stress on the woman's organism, unveiling latent disorders and triggering new unfavorable conditions [12], including cardiovascular disease (CVD) and their main complication—heart failure (HF). The prevalence of HF in pregnant women with CVD varies from 13% in ones with pre-existing cardiac disease (Registry of Pregnancy and Cardiac Disease, ROPAC) [58] to ≈33% in women with pre-existing cardiomyopathy [31]. Risk factors of maternal HF may be divided into several categories (Table 25.1).

Epidemiology of Heart Failure in Pregnancy

In pregnant women of the developed world, CVDs are the most common cause of non-obstetric deaths and complications. For instance, in the USA CVDs account for more than 1/4 of all maternal deaths [11], and HF—for over 9% of in-hospital maternal deaths. An analysis of the U.S. Nationwide Inpatient Sample (2001–2011), which included >50 million pregnancy-related hospitalizations, showed that the overall rate of HF was 112 cases per 100,000 hospitalizations of pregnant women. About 60% of HF cases occurred postpartum, 27.3%—by delivery, and 13.2%—antepartum [42]. It is worth noticing that most cases of CV death occur within the first 4 weeks postpartum due to previously undiagnosed cardiomyopathies. Despite this fact, many women have insurance only for the pregnancy period, and most US practices provide a single follow-up visit ≈6 weeks after delivery [66].

An analysis of CVD trends showed that the number of pregnant women with CVD from 2003 to 2012 increased by 24.7% [32], so HF rates in pregnancy may increase proportionally. Stergiopoulos et al. [66] explain the increasing trend of pregnancies complicated by CVD by the lack of preconception risk stratification, lack of knowledge by patients and healthcare providers, poor transitions of care, and lack of proper counseling regarding pregnancy risks. They also notice that, even with all necessary counseling and warnings about the risks, some women with CVD opt for pregnancy regardless. According to systematic reviews and meta-analyses, the common categories of CVD contributing to HF in pregnancy are valvular heart disease (58.4%; 95% confidence interval [CI]: 35.0–78.5), congenital heart disease (23%; 95% CI; 7.8–51.5), and cardiomyopathies (7.0%; 95% CI: 4.0–12.1) [24, 25].

Risk of Heart Failure in Pregnancy

Heart failure in pregnancy places both women and fetuses/infants at high risk of different complications, the most frequent maternal ones being pulmonary edema, renal failure, respiratory distress syndrome, preterm delivery, admission to an intensive care unit, respiratory failure, arrhythmias, and death [9, 42, 46]. The most frequent infant risks include prematurity, small-for-gestational-age status, low Apgar scores, infant respiratory distress syndrome, prolonged intensive care unit stay, and death. HF increases the probability of infant death by 7.7 times [46]. In ROPAC, maternal mortality in women with HF was almost tenfold higher than in women without it (4.8% vs. 0.5%) [58].

HF and maternal and fetal deaths may be preventable, given that the susceptible women have close peripartum multidisciplinary counseling and follow-up. According to Keepanasseril et al. [30], up to 68% of maternal mortality may be prevented. It means that the relevant healthcare providers must be prepared to provide necessary medical care for pregnant women with HF and to prevent HF development in this population.

Definitions and Guidelines

According to the American Heart Association (AHA), American College of Cardiology, and Heart Failure Society of America guidelines (2022), HF is a complex clinical syndrome with symptoms and signs that result from any structural or functional impairment of ventricular filling or ejection of blood (of note, the authors recognized that this definition does not cover asymptomatic stages). In a subchapter dedicated to HF and pregnancy, the AHA provides three recommendations:

1. In women with a history of HF or cardiomyopathy, including previous peripartum cardiomyopathy (PPCM), patient-centered counseling regarding contraception and the risks of CV deterioration during pregnancy should be provided.
2. In women with acute HF caused by PPCM and left ventricle ejection fraction (LVEF) <30%, anticoagulation may be reasonable at diagnosis, until 6–8 weeks postpartum, although the efficacy and safety are uncertain.
3. In women with HF or cardiomyopathy who are pregnant or currently planning for pregnancy, angiotensin-converting enzyme inhibitors (ACEi), angiotensin receptor blockers (ARB), angiotensin receptor-neprilysin inhibitors (ARNi), mineralocorticoid receptor antagonists (MRA), sodium-glucose cotransporter inhibitors (SGLT2 inhibitors), ivabradine, and vericiguat should not be administered because of significant risks of fetal harm [22].

The definition of HF by the European Society of Cardiology (ESC) guidelines (2021) states that HF is a condition due to a structural and/or functional abnormality of the heart that results in elevated intracardiac pressures and/or inadequate cardiac output at rest and/or during exercise. These guidelines also include a detailed description of its cardinal symptoms (breathlessness, ankle swelling, and fatigue) and signs (elevated jugular venous pressure, pulmonary rales, and peripheral edema). ESC guidelines classify HF in pregnancy into pre-existing before conception and new, presenting during gestation, and pay special attention to the diagnosis and pharmacotherapy of these two HF subtypes [38].

Hemodynamic Changes in Pregnancy

The Clinical Management Guidelines for Obstetrician–Gynecologists (ACOG) call pregnancy a natural stress test, as it is a physiological condition associated with altered hemodynamics (Table 25.2) and increased demands on a woman's cardiovascular system [1], so women of suboptimal baseline CV status can easily decompensate during pregnancy [66].

Table 25.2 Physiologic hemodynamic changes in pregnancy and the early postpartum period [2, 9, 12, 29, 66]

Parameter	Expected change	Timeline
Plasma volume	Gradual increase by 30–50% (physiologic anemia)	Late second trimester (28–32 weeks of gestation), then plateau
	Further increase	Delivery (systemic circulation gets 200–400 mL of uteroplacental blood per each uterine contraction)
	Normalization	3–6 weeks postpartum, or even longer
Stroke volume	Gradual increase by 30–50%, decrease, and increase	Increase up to the late second trimester (28–32 weeks of gestation), then plateau and decrease due to uterine compression of the inferior vena cava, then increase during labor and early postpartum period
Cardiac output	Gradual increase by 30–50% (twin pregnancies portend a more prominent increase)	From early pregnancy till late second trimester (28–32 weeks of gestation), then plateau until delivery
	Further increase	Delivery: within an hour after delivery returns to pre-labor levels, but stays elevated compared to the nonpregnant value
Heart rate	Increase by 10–15 bpm	Parallel to cardiac output increase in pregnancy and further increase during delivery (due to pain and anxiety); within an hour after delivery returns to pre-labor levels, but stays elevated compared to the nonpregnant value

(continued)

Table 25.2 (continued)

Parameter	Expected change	Timeline
Blood pressure	Decrease by ~10 mm Hg from baseline	Parallel to cardiac output increase
	Increase by 15–25% (SBP) and 10–15% (DBP)	Delivery (due to pain and anxiety)
Systemic vascular resistance	Decrease	Parallel to cardiac output increase

SBP systolic blood pressure, *DBP* diastolic blood pressure

Hemodynamic changes in physiologic pregnancy include a marked increase in the circulating blood volume, stroke volume, and cardiac output by 30–50% [66]. Other changes in circulatory dynamics include tachycardia, decreased vascular resistance, hypercoagulability, and increased vascular wall vulnerability [29].

Causes of Heart Failure in Pregnancy

In pregnant women, HF may complicate a wide range of CVDs including pregnancy-specific ones (PPCM, hypertensive disorders of pregnancy (HDP), and amniotic fluid embolism) and nonspecific ones for this group of cardiac diseases (myocarditis, valvular heart disease, arrhythmias, arrhythmogenic right ventricular dysplasia, left ventricular noncompaction, congenital heart defects, coronary heart disease, pulmonary embolism, pulmonary hypertension, spontaneous coronary artery dissection, and various cardiomyopathies [hypertrophic, familial, Takotsubo, chemotherapy-related, related to other systemic illness, Chagas, tachycardiomyopathy]) [9, 15, 18].

Non-pregnancy-specific causes of HF might be further classified according to the primary causative mechanism:

(a) diseases increasing vascular resistance (hypertensive cardiomyopathy, pulmonary congestion, and right heart failure),
(b) aortic root pathologies (Marfan syndrome, Takayasu's arteritis, and atherosclerotic disease), and
(c) heart disease itself due to obstruction or ventricular failure/congenital cardiac abnormalities and proximal vasculature (cardiomyopathies and ischemic heart disease) [2, 18].

Peripartum Cardiomyopathy

PPCM is a significant cause of increased fetomaternal morbidity and mortality. The multifaceted presentation and varied course of PPCM make it hard to diagnose and investigate. According to the definition, PPCM is a new-onset HF with no

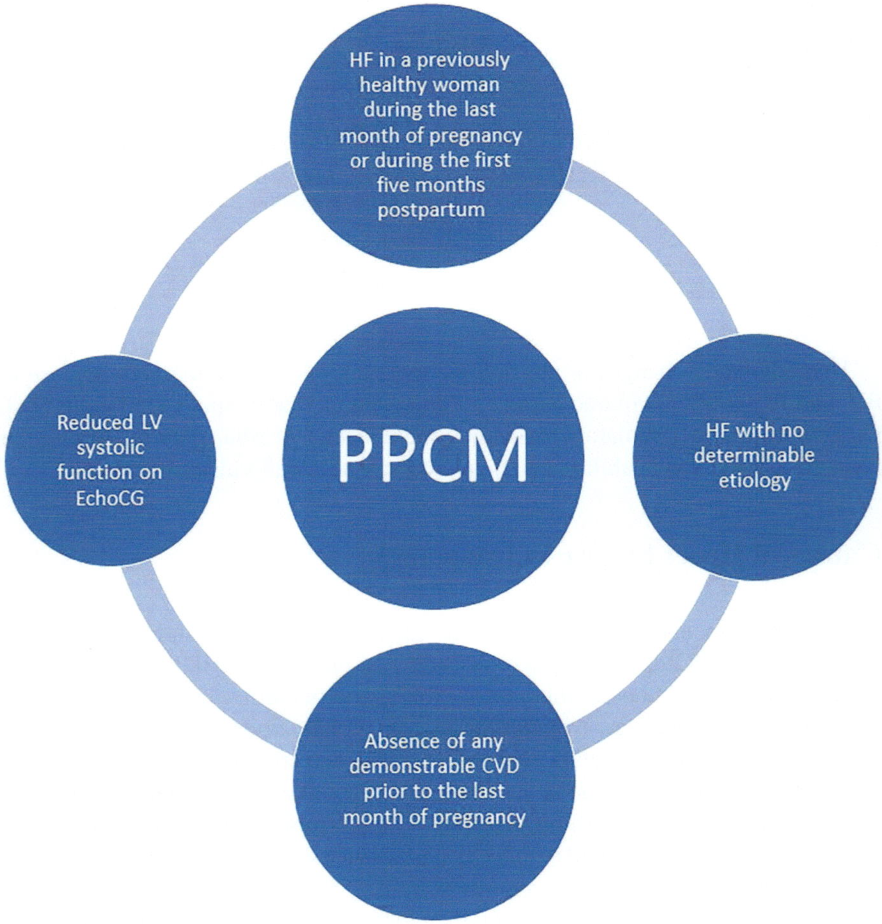

Fig. 25.1 Diagnostic criteria of PPCM

determinable cause, which occurs in the peripartum period (from the last month of pregnancy to the first 5 months postpartum) [45]. Current diagnostic criteria for PPCM are presented in the Fig. 25.1.

The pathophysiologic background of PPCM is not established yet. Different authors propose different hypotheses (genetic susceptibility, viral or antigen-induced myocarditis, pathological immune response to fetal antigens, or pathological CV response to hemodynamic changes of pregnancy, hormonal abnormalities, angiogenic imbalance, the influence of stress-activated cytokines, and nutritional deficiencies (e.g., selenium)) [26]. In general, we agree with a so-called two-hit paradigm, which states that PPCM results from the vascular humoral insult during pregnancy in genetically predisposed women [23]. Risk factors of PPCM include

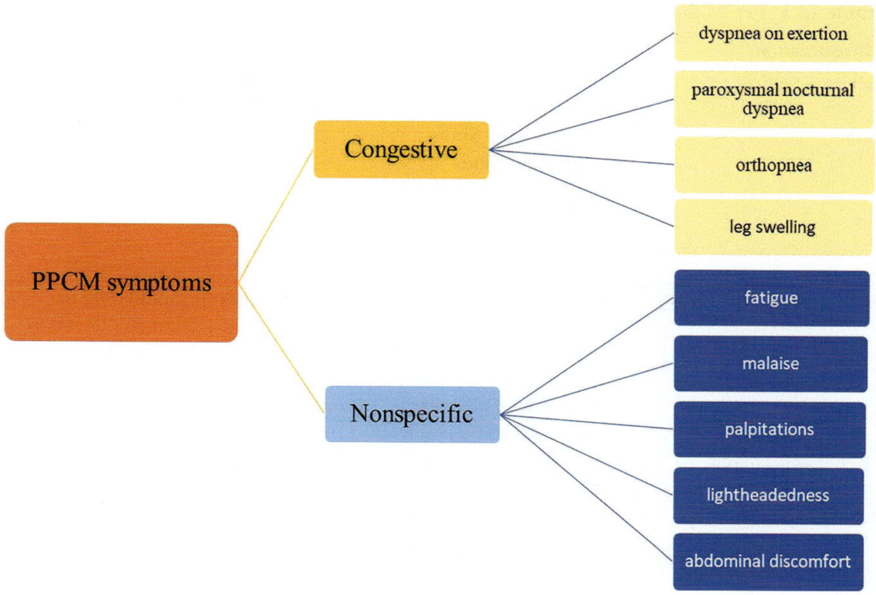

Fig. 25.2 Symptoms of PPCM

multiparity, African-American race, age > 30 years, HDP, history of eclampsia/pre-eclampsia, in vitro fertilization, use of tocolytic agents, smoking, and malnutrition [7, 8, 15, 56].

The clinical manifestation of PPCM, in general, resembles any other systolic HF and includes dyspnea, orthopnea, cough (especially in the horizontal position), palpitations, leg swelling, chest tightness, fatigue, and dizziness (Fig. 25.2). On physical examination, sinus tachycardia, an increased jugular venous pressure, and bilateral crepitations in the lungs may be present. Some features of PPCM may resemble the physiological symptoms of late pregnancy, so this medical condition may be overlooked and, therefore, not treated [12, 26]. Also, similar presentation may be conditioned by extracardiac causes like anemia, thyroid dysfunction, or infection [9].

The timeline of decompensation or new-onset HF may provide a hint for diagnosis: women with pre-existing cardiomyopathy or valvular heart disease tend to become symptomatic in the late second trimester, when the hemodynamic changes are maximal, whereas women with PPCM usually develop overt clinical manifestation later in pregnancy (third trimester) or even up to 6 months postpartum [12, 19, 35, 53, 58].

Diagnosis of PPCM is usually a diagnosis of exclusion, as most instrumental and laboratory findings are nonspecific (Table 25.3). Echocardiography is at the central point of diagnosis, as it also helps to reveal the other causes of HF, assess complications of PPCM, and predict outcomes [6, 26].

Table 25.3 PPCM diagnosis [12, 15, 26]

Investigation	Typical findings	Comments
Electrocardiography	Nonspecific ST-segment changes and T wave abnormalities. Sinus tachycardia, sinus arrhythmia, atrial fibrillation, atrial flutter, and ventricular tachycardia were also reported.	Normal ECG does not rule out the possibility of PPCM.
Chest X-ray	May show cardiomegaly with pulmonary edema, signs of pulmonary venous congestion, or pleural effusion with alveolar shadowing and septal lines.	In pregnancy, it should only be performed if other methods fail to clarify symptoms (the fetal dose is < 0.01 mGy).
Echocardiography	LV ejection fraction of <45%; often (but not always)—LV dilatation; right ventricular enlargement and/or dysfunction. Four-chamber enlargement, mitral or tricuspid regurgitation, and elevated pulmonary artery pressure may also be found.	Is considered the most effective imaging technique; is useful for outcome prediction.
Exercise testing (semi-recumbent cycle ergometry, treadmill walking. Or upright cycle ergometry)	Decreased functional capacity of the heart, blood pressure response, and exercise-induced arrhythmias.	Is used for follow-up in women with CVD or asymptomatic valvular heart diseases. The ESC guidelines recommend exercise testing in women with known heart disease before pregnancy for risk assessment.
Cardiac magnetic resonance	Can reveal left ventricle systolic dysfunction, intracardiac thrombi, and signs of tissue injury (fibrosis, necrosis, leakage of capillaries, hyperemia, etc.)	Disadvantages: use of gadolinium contrast, which enters the placenta and may be teratogenic; high cost; low availability in a limited resource setting.
Endomyocardial biopsy	Non-diagnostic histological findings.	Is rarely performed. May bring advantages if an alternative diagnosis, which would require a different treatment strategy, is suspected.

(continued)

Table 25.3 (continued)

Investigation	Typical findings	Comments
Laboratory markers	C-reactive protein and leucocyte count—↑; hemoglobin level—↓. BNP or NT-proBNP—↑; troponin T—normal.	These findings are nonspecific. NT-proBNP may be slightly elevated in normal pregnancy (19–20 pg/mL compared to 10 pg/mL in nonpregnant women), but women with preeclampsia usually have higher values. Serial BNP levels can aid in detecting the adverse CV events during pregnancy.

BNP Brain natriuretic peptide, *NT-proBNP* N-terminal pro-brain natriuretic peptide

Outcomes of PPCM vary from complete recovery to heart transplantation or even death. Baseline LVEF <30% predicts a lower likelihood of recovery [39]. Subsequent pregnancies may also be complicated by the relapse of PPCM [26].

Management of PPCM is based on the guidelines for other forms of HF with reduced ejection fraction and expert opinions, paying particular attention to avoiding teratogenic agents or drugs that are excreted into breast milk.

The pharmacotherapy of PPCM includes volume management with a loop diuretic (together with sodium restriction), afterload reduction (hydralazine, nitrates), and rhythm control (selective beta1-blockers: metoprolol, bisoprolol, carvedilol; digoxin). Hemodynamically unstable patients with PPCM are treated with intravenous diuretics, nitrates, and, if needed, non-invasive ventilation and continuous positive airway pressure. In case of cardiac shock, vasopressors and inotropes are administered, and if they fail, mechanical circulatory support is indicated [12, 40]. Wearable cardiac defibrillators may be used in severe cases until intracardiac device implantation or till recovery of ejection fraction for a period of 3–6 months [23]. Severe refractory cases may require heart transplantation. In the postpartum period, ACEIs, ARBs, MRA, ARNI, SGLT2 inhibitors, ivabradine, and vericiguat can be initiated [12].

Recent advances and perspective trends in PPCM management include prolactin inhibition with bromocriptine (for patients with LVEF <25% or with cardiogenic shock at a dose of 2.5 mg twice daily for 2 weeks followed by 2.5 mg once daily for 6 weeks along with anticoagulation), antisense therapy against microRNA-146a, vascular endothelial growth factor agonism and apheresis of anti-angiogenic proteins, serelaxin, perhexiline, and pentoxifylline [21, 55].

As thromboembolism is the most frequent severe complication of PPCM [23], in case of LVEF ≤35% (according to ESC) or ≤30% (according to the AHA) anticoagulation is recommended [22, 38]. As warfarin is teratogenic and new direct-acting oral anticoagulants have not been studied in the population of pregnant women, low molecular weight heparin and unfractionated heparin should be used for this purpose [8].

In the postpartum period, women with PPCM who are not breastfeeding may receive standard HF therapy according to current guidelines. Clinically stable women who are breastfeeding may be treated with beta-blockers, enalapril, and spironolactone. In contrast, ARBs, ARNi, and ivabradine should be avoided during lactation due to the lack of information about their compatibility with breastfeeding [26].

Other Causes of Heart Failure in Pregnancy

Hypertensive Disorders in Pregnancy

Women with HDP are at risk of developing HF, with preeclampsia in particular (fourfold increased risk of HF compared with their normal pregnancy counterparts) [73].

Preferred first-line antihypertensive agents for pregnant women are:

- labetalol (100–200 mg orally twice daily),
- extended-release nifedipine (30–60 mg orally once a day),
- and α-methyldopa (250 mg orally 2–3 times daily).

Second-third-line agents include:

- hydralazine (10 mg orally 4 times daily),
- thiazide diuretics (12.5 mg orally once a day),
- and clonidine (0.1–0.3 mg orally twice a day or 0.1 mg in a transdermal patch every day).

Urgent treatment in cases of systolic blood pressure $\geq$ 160 mm Hg or diastolic blood pressure $\geq$ 110 mm Hg for >15 min can be provided with intravenous labetalol and hydralazine or oral immediate release nifedipine if intravenous access is not available [52].

Cardiomyopathies Other Than Peripartum Cardiomyopathy

Patients with cardiomyopathies usually experience the onset of HF some weeks before delivery and postpartum [58]. According to the ROPAC, most women with hypertrophic cardiomyopathy tolerate pregnancy well. However, about 23% of them experience HF or arrhythmias, particularly ventricular ones [20]. Women with left ventricle outflow obstruction may be treated with beta.blockers, and women with volume overload—with diuretics [49]. Once per trimester, clinical check-ups and echocardiography are recommended. Regarding the delivery mode, vaginal delivery (possibly, with an assisted second stage) is a safe option in most cases [4].

Valvular Heart Disease

Among pregnant women with various valvular diseases, 23% of mothers with mitral regurgitation, 31.8% with moderate mitral stenosis, and 48.1% with severe mitral stenosis develop HF [57, 58, 70].

As for asymptomatic patients with severe mitral stenosis or symptomatic patients with moderate mitral stenosis, the ESC guidelines on CVD in pregnancy advise percutaneous mitral valvuloplasty before pregnancy [55]. If left untreated, mitral stenosis can lead to HF with pulmonary edema, atrial arrhythmias, cerebrovascular events, and death [60, 69, 70]. Beta1-selective beta-blockers and activity restriction are the mainstream treatment for such patients who are symptomatic or have significant pulmonary hypertension. In cases of substantial pulmonary hypertension despite optimal pharmacotherapy, pregnant women may be subject to percutaneous transvenous mitral commissurotomy (preferably after 20 weeks of gestation) [55, 71].

Regurgitant lesions are generally better tolerated in pregnant women compared to stenotic lesions. However, in case of the presence or progression of symptoms despite optimal pharmacotherapy before pregnancy, the medical team should consider valvular repair or replacement in the preconception stage [47], as women with regurgitant lesions may develop pulmonary edema after delivery [48].

Asymptomatic aortic stenosis may be tolerated, whereas women with symptomatic aortic stenosis need an intervention before pregnancy. Intervention before pregnancy is also recommended in case of severe systolic dysfunction or if symptoms develop during an exercise stress test. In severely symptomatic women, balloon valvuloplasty can be done during pregnancy [63].

Aortic regurgitation is usually well tolerated in the absence of left ventricular dysfunction. Operated congenital defects (ventricular or atrial septum defect, patent ductus arteriosus) also carry a low risk of HF [37].

Arrhythmias

Arrhythmia-related complications of pregnancy may range from isolated premature ventricular contractions to life-threatening arrhythmias like atrial fibrillation or sustained ventricular tachycardia. Atrial fibrillation in pregnant women is associated with a high risk for preeclampsia and congestive HF [13].

According to the Heart Rhythm Society Consensus (2023), the majority of arrhythmias in pregnant women are benign, the most prevalent being sinus arrhythmia, supraventricular tachycardia, and premature beats (the latter are seen in 50–60% of pregnant patients). Arrhythmias in pregnancy may affect both the mother and the fetus, so all possible risks must be discussed, and a multidisciplinary team is needed. In cases of hemodynamically significant maternal arrhythmias, the most effective available therapy (cardioversion, antiarrhythmic drug infusion, or catheter ablation) must be used. Antiarrhythmic drug use during pregnancy and the postpartum period is, in general, similar to the nonpregnant patients; however, fetal safety must be considered [28].

Amniotic Fluid Embolism

This rare labor complication may lead to cardiovascular collapse, pulmonary edema, seizure activity, and bleeding diathesis. It is thought that in cases of amniotic fluid embolism, large amounts of amniotic fluid and fetal squames get into the maternal circulation and trigger acute pulmonary hypertension followed by left ventricle failure that needs inotropic support [44].

Coronary Heart Disease

In the ROPAC, CHD was relatively rare (<2% of maternal cardiovascular conditions) [57], but as maternal age gradually advances globally, the likelihood of CHD in pregnant women may also increase [52]. Coronary heart disease in pregnancy usually presents as acute coronary syndrome. The latter must be suspected in cases of a typical clinical picture similar to those in nonpregnant patients. High-sensitivity troponin may be used to support the diagnosis. The management of acute coronary syndrome in pregnancy, including indications for acute revascularization, also meets general guidelines, but fetal monitoring needs to be provided [4]. Myocardial infarction is usually caused by spontaneous coronary artery dissection, or the coronary arteries are not obstructed. The third trimester and postpartum are the highest-risk periods. In patients with STEMI, timely coronary reperfusion by percutaneous coronary intervention (PCI) is recommended. Fetal radiation protection with lead shielding and radiation reduction measures should be implemented. If PCI is not readily available, thrombolysis is very rarely used because of the risk of maternal hemorrhage. An invasive approach is also recommended in unstable patients with non-STEMI or in case of high atherosclerotic burden. Stable patients at low risk can be managed conservatively. Post-PCI low-dose aspirin is considered safe throughout pregnancy, and clopidogrel may be used with caution for the shortest duration possible. Other antiplatelet agents should be avoided.

Management of Heart Failure in Pregnancy

Multidisciplinary Team

Women with HF in pregnancy must be managed by a multidisciplinary team (cardio-obstetric team, pregnancy heart team) including core specialists (cardiologist and obstetrician) who are responsible for key clinical decisions and various additional experts who provide care and support when it is needed (Table 25.4).

Table 25.4 Multidisciplinary team for management of HF in pregnancy [3, 6, 12]

Doctor	Tasks
General practitioner	Close monitoring of pregnancy in mild cases
Obstetrician	Decision on the preferred timing and mode of delivery (in case of advanced PPCM lower segment cesarean section could be considered)
Cardiologist	Decision on treatment of underlying CVD and their complications
Anesthesiologist (intensivist)	Choice of optimal anesthesia (dense epidural anesthesia can minimize the hemodynamic instability)
Pediatrician (neonatologist)	Control the neonate condition, especially in case of preterm birth
Nurses, midwives, doulas	Provide relevant care
Pharmacist	Provide relevant care if needed
Cardiac surgeon	
Social worker	

This team should provide:

- a preconception cardiovascular risk assessment,
- obstetric and fetal risk assessment during pregnancy,
- and outcomes prediction.

In the postpartum period, the multidisciplinary team provides counseling on medication safety during lactation, medication weaning, and planning of subsequent pregnancies [40].

The inclusion of a wide spectrum of medical and non-medical professionals in the multidisciplinary team ensures uninterrupted care throughout the entire maternal health continuum from preconception to postpartum. The set of involved professionals may be tailored according to the patient's needs and institutional resources. As these resources may be limited, the pregnancy heart team may work through co-located clinics, case conferences, or independent service lines. Regular meetings of the team help to create and implement a detailed, individualized, and regularly updated management plan, which must include delivery management and postpartum aspects [33, 68, 72].

Cardio-obstetrics needs to evolve further, as this multidisciplinary field of medicine may help to prevent maternal morbidity and mortality. Primary care clinicians must also have a general knowledge of the fundamental aspects of HF in pregnancy [40].

Management of Acute Heart Failure in Pregnancy

Acute HF during pregnancy can be secondary to pre-existing cardiomyopathy, coronary heart disease, PPCM, stress/toxic cardiomyopathy, severe valvular heart disease, or myocardial ischemia due to coronary artery dissection or atherosclerosis

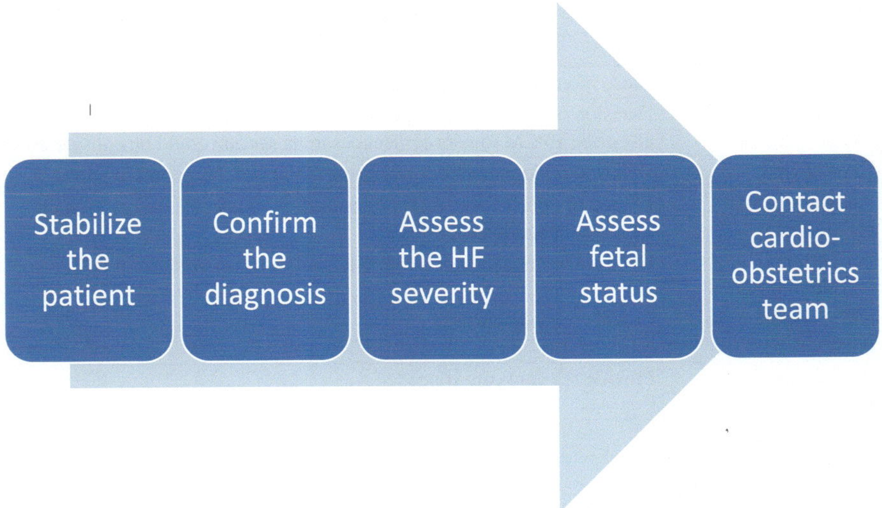

Fig. 25.3 Initial management algorithm for pregnant/postpartum women with acute HF [9]

[43]. Hypertensive disorders in pregnancy, preeclampsia, in particular, may induce the development of HF.

The Guidelines of the Heart Failure Association of the ESC Study Group on PPCM state that pregnant women with acute HF must be immediately referred to an intensive care unit in a tertiary care center, where a multidisciplinary team is responsible for rapid diagnosis and appropriate therapy. Stabilization of a mother is of utmost importance (Fig. 25.3). Hemodynamically unstable women with severe HF must undergo an urgent cesarean section, irrespective of gestation time [65]. Urgent delivery is also advocated if the fetus is unviable. If the fetus is viable and it is possible to stabilize the mother's condition, delivery can be postponed, and dexamethasone can be administered for fetal lung maturation [37].

Women with acute decompensated HF with SBP > 110 mm Hg may require vasodilators and, in case of shock, inotropes and mechanical circulatory support [37].

In an ante-, intra- or postpartum period, acute pulmonary edema may develop, usually as a complication of preeclampsia or eclampsia [54]. Patients with acute pulmonary edema typically present with dyspnea, orthopnea, chest discomfort, cough, and wheezing. Progressive dyspnea with nocturnal dyspnoic paroxysms in case of acute pulmonary edema should not be confused with physiologic late pregnancy dyspnea caused by an enlarged uterus and abdominal muscle distension [14].

Stabilized or subacute pulmonary edema in pregnancy is treated similarly to those of nonpregnant patients. Treatment includes:

- oxygen therapy,
- fluid restriction,
- intravenous loop diuretics,

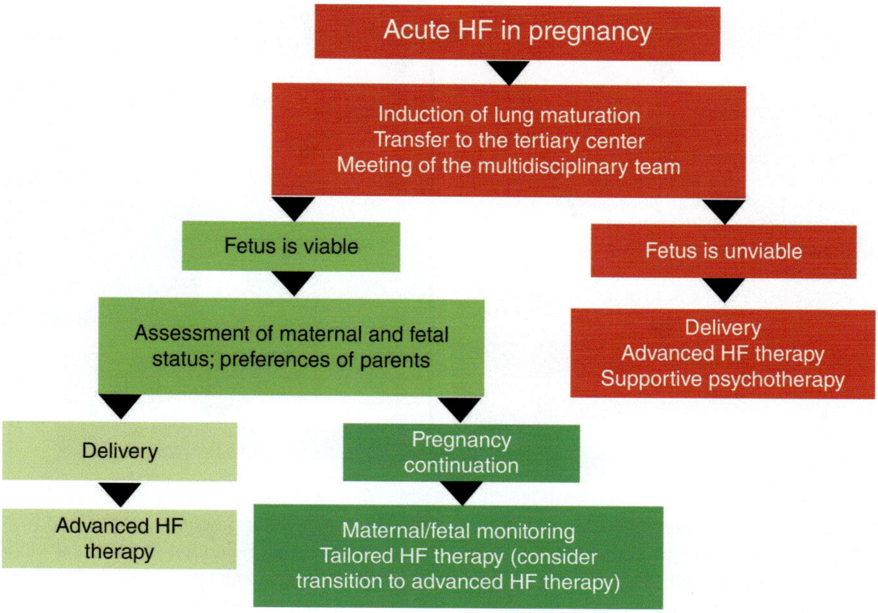

Fig. 25.4 Management of acute HF in pregnancy: workup and decision making. (Modified from [55])

- central hemodynamic monitoring,
- and vasodilators, preferably nitroglycerin [55, 65].

Pregnant women with acute HF must be immediately referred to an intensive care unit, where further management strategy depends on fetus viability and the possibility of stabilizing the mother's condition (Figs. 25.4 and 25.5). If stabilization is possible, the delivery may be delayed. In contrast, if the woman is hemodynamically unstable, she must undergo urgent delivery by cesarean section irrespective of the gestation period [65].

Prevention of acute pulmonary edema in pregnant women can be provided by thorough clinical monitoring, restricted fluid intake, and administration of 100–150 mg of aspirin for women with moderate/high risk of preeclampsia, administered from week 12 to weeks 36–37 [51, 55].

Timing and Mode of Delivery

According to the modern point of view, spontaneous labor and vaginal birth are preferred for most pregnant women with CVD [10, 17, 55]. During vaginal delivery, instrumentation may be used to shorten the second stage of labor [27].

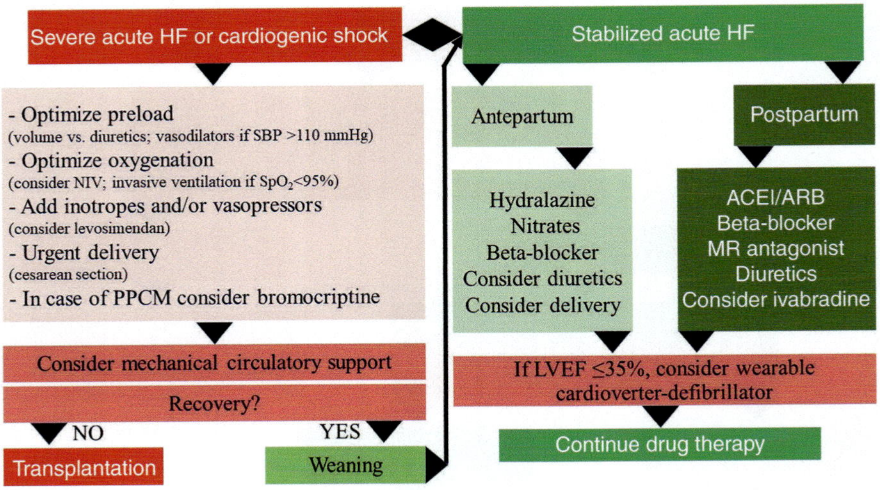

Fig. 25.5 Management of severe and stabilized acute HF during/after pregnancy. (Modified from [55]). Note: Diuretics should be used with caution due to potential reduction in placental blood flow. *ACEI* angiotensin-converting enzyme inhibitor, *ARB* angiotensin receptor blocker, *LVEF* left ventricular ejection fraction, *MR* mineralocorticoid receptor, *NIV* non-invasive ventilation, *PPCM* peripartum cardiomyopathy, *SpO_2* peripheral oxygen saturation

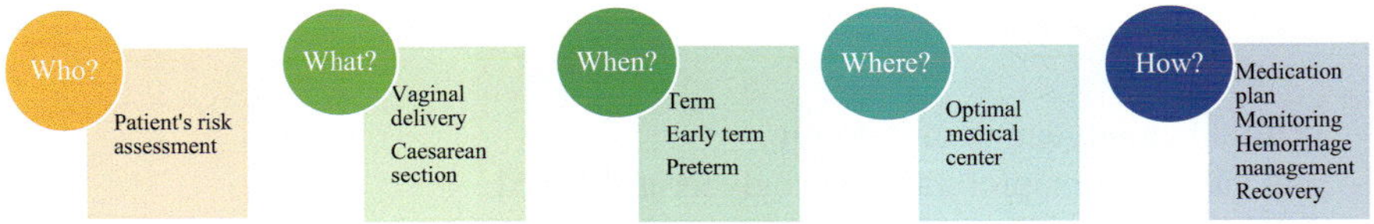

Fig. 25.6 The delivery framework plan

The timing of delivery is decided by the cardio-obstetric team depending upon maternal, obstetric, and fetal risks balance. Cesarean delivery is usually reserved for the most decompensated cases, like women with advanced HF requiring inotropic therapy or mechanical circulatory support [26, 40]. In hemodynamically unstable women with severe HF, urgent cesarean section should be considered irrespective of gestational duration [5, 55].

The ACOG recommends elective induction of labor for pregnant women with CVD between 39 and 40 weeks of gestation if the patient does not have a spontaneous onset of labor or clinical indications for preterm delivery [1].

According to the scientific statement of the American Heart Association (2023), the delivery framework plan must answer the questions “who” (patient’s risk assessment), “what” (vaginal/caesarian delivery), “when” (term, early term or preterm), “where” (type of medical center), and “how” (medication plan, monitoring, hemorrhage management, and recovery) (Fig. 25.6; [41]).

Prevention: Preconception Counseling and Postpartum Follow-Up

Maternal HF needs the vigilance of healthcare providers and comprehensive counseling of high-risk women before, during, and after pregnancy. Preconception counseling must include individual risk estimation, shared decision-making, and explaining potential adverse events during pregnancy and labor to the woman [40].

Assessment of cardiovascular risk is a cornerstone of preconception counseling. The most frequently used pregnancy risk indices are CARPREG II (Cardiac Disease in Pregnancy) and ZAHARA (Zwangerschap bij Aangeboren HARtAfwijkingen [pregnancy with coronary heart disease]) (Table 25.5) [2]. The CARPREG risk index is based on prior cardiac events, NYHA functional class, left heart obstruction, and systemic/sub-aortic ventricular systolic dysfunction [62], whereas the ZAHARA score enlists eight items to consider: prior arrhythmias, NYHA class ≥II,

Table 25.5 Assessment of cardiovascular risk in pregnancy [36, 61]

Parameter	CARPREG II	ZAHARA	mWHO
Risk predictors	Prior cardiac events or arrhythmias; baseline NYHA III-IV functional class or cyanosis; mechanical valve; ventricular dysfunction; high-risk left-sided valve disease or left ventricular outflow tract obstruction; pulmonary hypertension; coronary artery disease; high-risk aortopathy; no prior cardiac intervention; late pregnancy assessment	History of arrhythmia; cardiac medications before pregnancy; NYHA functional class ≥II; severe left heart obstruction; severe systemic atrioventricular (AV) valve regurgitation; severe pulmonary AV valve regurgitation; mechanical valve prosthesis and cyanotic heart disease	Four risk classes (WHO I, II, III and IV) are defined according to the conditions of specific heart lesions and the clinical cardiac risk status such as mechanical valve, systemic right ventricle, Fontan circulation or pulmonary hypertension
Calculation system	Each predictor is assigned a weighted point score; the sum of points represents the risk score. Increasing number of predictors corresponds to increasing risk of maternal CV complications	Weighted risk score; the sum of the points corresponds to an estimated risk of adverse events	A range of risk estimates from class I (no increase in maternal mortality and no/low increase in maternal morbidity) to class IV (extremely high risk of maternal mortality or severe morbidity)
Population	Both congenital and acquired heart conditions	Exclusively for women with coronary heart disease	Both congenital and acquired heart conditions

left heart obstruction, cardiac medication before pregnancy, systemic atrioventricular valve regurgitation, pulmonary atrioventricular valve regurgitation, mechanical valve prosthesis, and cyanotic heart disease [16]. The modified World Health Organization (mWHO) classification of cardiac lesions is also widely used for risk prediction in pregnant women with HF [55]. This classification has been validated with the help of the ROPAC prospective data [4].

Women with a history of CVD or preeclampsia need special, thorough counseling including symptom assessment, maternal/fetal risk evaluation, adjustment of medications, general health evaluation, cardiovascular risk screening with the mWHO scoring system, and appropriate education of the patient [9, 68]. If the woman presents already pregnant, the cardio-obstetric team needs to create a roadmap for her safe pregnancy, delivery, and the postpartum period [9].

Women at high risk of complication require a detailed plan of delivery including an ideal location (preferably a high-intensity cardiac environment where cardiac surgery, mechanical heart support, or even heart transplantation may be rapidly implemented). Despite the cesarean section usually being associated with an increased risk of infection and bleeding, it offers benefits concerning timing, care coordination, and anticoagulation management [4].

According to the American College of Obstetricians and Gynecologists guidelines, women with CVD need an early postpartum follow-up visit to either the primary care provider or cardiologist within 7–14 days of delivery, and women with hypertensive disorders—within 7–10 days of delivery [1].

In the case of PPCM, the relevant working group of the Heart Failure Association advises providing a regular 6-month follow-up with echocardiography until LVEF recovers to >50% [64].

During postpartum counseling future pregnancies (after evaluation by a multidisciplinary team), contraception, follow-up schedule, and future cardiovascular risk should be discussed. Counseling needs to be disease-specific [26, 40]. Future pregnancies should be avoided in very high-risk conditions including Eisenmenger's syndrome, severe pulmonary hypertension, and severe residual left ventricular dysfunction in PPCM [37].

Summary of General Rules for Heart Failure Management in Pregnant Women

Usually, diuretics are the first line of treatment, especially loop diuretics, which provide decongestion. Amiloride can be used because aldosterone antagonists (spironolactone) are teratogenic and should be avoided [2, 37]. ACEIs and ARBs, which are widely used in nonpregnant patients, are also contraindicated in pregnancy [59].

Beta-blockers improve symptoms and increase survival in patients with systolic dysfunction [50]. They are generally considered safe in pregnancy, but they may be associated with an increased risk of fetal growth retardation and hypoglycemia.

Nevertheless, beta-blockers may be used if the mother's life is at risk [67]. Cardioselective agents (metoprolol, bisoprolol) should be used, especially in mitral stenosis, dilatation cardiomyopathy, PPCM, or atrial fibrillation [37], as they are less likely to interfere with uterine contraction and have lower rates of fetal growth retardation. Unselective beta-blockers such as atenolol are no longer recommended in pregnancy.

As pregnant women have an increased intravascular blood volume, they may require higher dosages of drugs to achieve therapeutic plasma concentrations. Apart from that, increased renal perfusion and hepatic metabolism make drug clearance faster, so pregnant women require dose monitoring and timely adjustment [55].

Conclusion

HF in pregnancy is a life-threatening complication of a broad spectrum of medical conditions. Pregnant women are a unique population of patients, so the management of HF in pregnancy must include interdisciplinary collaboration of cardiologists, gynecologists, and other specialists. Management of HF in pregnancy generally resembles management in nonpregnant patients, however, avoiding potentially teratogenic drugs must be kept in mind. Bromocriptine efficacy and safety remain unclear, and further randomized clinical trials are warranted to elucidate the benefits of this drug. Important gaps in knowledge should also be addressed including optimal anticoagulation strategy, risk stratification, prognostic evaluation, management during a subsequent pregnancy, and long-term treatment.

Management of pregnant women with HF requires the collaboration of all levels of medical care and non-medical professionals (pharmacists, social workers, etc.). Considering the broad spectrum of medical, social, religious, moral, and personal issues involved in getting children, the decision-making needs to be shared. Population-level education, further scientific investigations, and individual counseling may improve the healthcare for pregnant women with HF including outcomes both for mothers and children.

References

1. ACOG Practice Bulletin No. 212: pregnancy and heart disease. Obstet Gynecol. 2019;133:e320–56.
2. Albakri A. Heart failure in pregnancy: a review of clinical status and meta-analysis of diagnosis and medication safety. Med Clin Arch. 2018;3:e1000144. https://doi.org/10.15761/MCA.1000144.
3. Arany Z, Elkayam U. Peripartum cardiomyopathy. Circulation. 2016;133(14):1397–409. https://doi.org/10.1161/CIRCULATIONAHA.115.020491.
4. Assenza GE, Dimopoulos K, Budts W, Donti A, Economy KE, Gargiulo GD, Gatzoulis M, Landzberg MJ, Valente AM, Roos-Hesselink J. Management of acute cardiovascular com-

plications in pregnancy. Eur Heart J. 2021;42(41):4224–40. https://doi.org/10.1093/eurheartj/ehab546.

5. Bauersachs J, Arrigo M, Hilfiker-Kleiner D, Veltmann C, Coats AJS, Crespo-Leiro MG, De Boer RA, van der Meer P, Maack C, Mouquet F, et al. Current management of patients with severe acute peripartum cardiomyopathy: practical guidance from the Heart Failure Association of the European Society of Cardiology Study Group on Peripartum Cardiomyopathy. Eur J Heart Fail. 2016;18:1096–105. https://doi.org/10.1002/ejhf.586.
6. Bauersachs J, König T, van der Meer P, et al. Pathophysiology, diagnosis and management of peripartum cardiomyopathy: a position statement from the Heart Failure Association of the European Society of Cardiology Study Group on Peripartum Cardiomyopathy. Eur J Heart Fail. 2019;21(7):827–43. https://doi.org/10.1002/ejhf.1493.
7. Bello N, Rendon ISH, Arany Z. The relationship between preeclampsia and peripartum cardiomyopathy: a systematic review and meta-analysis. J Am Coll Cardiol. 2013;62(18):1715–23. https://doi.org/10.1016/j.jacc.2013.08.717.
8. Bhattacharyya A, Basra SS, Sen P, Kar B. Peripartum cardiomyopathy: a review. Tex Heart Inst J. 2012;39(1):8–16.
9. Bright RA, Lima FV, Avila C, Butler J, Stergiopoulos K. Maternal heart failure. J Am Heart Assoc. 2021;10(14):e021019. https://doi.org/10.1161/JAHA.121.021019.
10. Canobbio MM, Warnes CA, Aboulhosn J, Connolly HM, Khanna A, Koos BJ, Mital S, Rose C, Silversides C, Stout K, On behalf of the American Heart Association Council on Cardiovascular and Stroke Nursing; Council on Clinical Cardiology; Council on Cardiovascular Disease in the Young; Council on Functional Genomics and Translational Biology; and Council on Quality of Care and Outcomes Research. Management of pregnancy in patients with complex congenital heart disease: a scientific statement for healthcare professionals from the American Heart Association. Circulation. 2017;135:e50–87. https://doi.org/10.1161/CIR.0000000000000458.
11. Center for Disease Control and Prevention. Pregnancy mortality surveillance system. 2019. Available at: https://www.cdc.gov/reproductivehealth/maternalinfanthealth/pregnancy-mortality-surveillance-system.htm. Accessed 12 June 2023.
12. Chaudhari K, Choudhary M, Chaudhari K, et al. Advancement in current therapeutic modalities in postpartum cardiomyopathy. Cureus. 2022;14(3):e22813. https://doi.org/10.7759/cureus.22813.
13. Chokesuwattanaskul R, Thongprayoon C, Bathini T, O'Corragain OA, Sharma K, Prechawat S, Ungprasert P, Watthanasuntorn K, Pachariyanon P, Cheungpasitporn W. Incidence of atrial fibrillation in pregnancy and clinical significance: a meta-analysis. Adv Med Sci. 2019;64:415–22. https://doi.org/10.1016/j.advms.2019.07.003.
14. Cypher RL. Pulmonary edema in obstetrics: essential facts for critical care nurses. AACN Adv Crit Care. 2018;29(3):327–35. https://doi.org/10.4037/aacnacc2018958.
15. Dash D, Mody R, Malan SR, Ahmed N, Mody B. Peripartum cardiomyopathy: a 2022 update. Iberoam J Med. 2022;4(2):104–12. https://doi.org/10.53986/ibjm.2022.0016.
16. Drenthen W, Boersma E, Balci A, Moons P, Roos-Hesslink JW, et al. Predictors of pregnancy complications in women with congenital heart disease. Eur Heart J. 2010;31:2124–32.
17. Easter SR, Rouse CE, Duarte V, Hynes JS, Singh MN, Landzberg MJ, Valente AM, Economy KE. Planned vaginal delivery and cardiovascular morbidity in pregnant women with heart disease. Am J Obstet Gynecol. 2020;222:77.e1–77.e11. https://doi.org/10.1016/j.ajog.2019.07.019.
18. Elkayam U, Goland S, Pieper PG, Silverside CK. High-risk cardiac disease in pregnancy: part I. J Am Coll Cardiol. 2016;68(4):396–410. https://doi.org/10.1016/j.jacc.2016.05.048.
19. Elkayam U. Clinical characteristics of peripartum cardiomyopathy in the United States: diagnosis, prognosis, and management. J Am Coll Cardiol. 2011;58(7):659–70. https://doi.org/10.1016/j.jacc.2011.03.047.
20. Goland S, van Hagen IM, Elbaz-Greener G, Elkayam U, Shotan A, Merz WM, Enar SC, Gaisin IR, Pieper PG, Johnson MR, et al. Pregnancy in women with hypertrophic cardiomyopathy:

data from the European Society of Cardiology initiated Registry of Pregnancy and Cardiac disease (ROPAC). Eur Heart J. 2017;38:2683–90. https://doi.org/10.1093/eurheartj/ehx189.
21. Halkein J, Tabruyn SP, Ricke-Hoch M, Haghikia A, Nguyen NQ, Scherr M, Castermans K, Malvaux L, Lambert V, Thiry M, Sliwa K, Noel A, Martial JA, Hilfiker-Kleiner D, Struman I. MicroRNA-146a is a therapeutic target and biomarker for peripartum cardiomyopathy. J Clin Invest. 2013;123(5):2143–54. https://doi.org/10.1172/JCI64365.
22. Heidenreich PA, Bozkurt B, Aguilar D, Allen LA, Byun JJ, Colvin MM, Deswal A, et al. 2022 AHA/ACC/HFSA Guideline for the Management of Heart Failure: a report of the American College of Cardiology/American Heart Association Joint Committee on Clinical Practice Guidelines. Circulation. 2022;145(18):e895–e1032. https://doi.org/10.1161/CIR.0000000000001063. Erratum in: Circulation. 2022;145(18):e1033. Erratum in: Circulation. 2022;146(13):e185. Erratum in: Circulation. 2023;147(14):e674.
23. Honigberg MC, Givertz MM. Peripartum cardiomyopathy. BMJ. 2019;364:k5287. https://doi.org/10.1136/bmj.k5287.
24. Hossinzadeh R, Parizad R, Tabrizi MT, Khojasteh ZG, Ainehchi N. Prevalence of heart diseases in pregnant women referred to the heart diseases clinic for obstetrics. Int J Women's Health Reprod Sci. 2018;62:55–8.
25. Indira I, Sunitha K, Jyothi. Study of pregnancy outcome in maternal heart disease. IOSR J Dental Med Sci. 2015;14:6–10.
26. Iorgoveanu C, Zaghloul A, Ashwath M. Peripartum cardiomyopathy: a review. Heart Fail Rev. 2021;26(6):1287–96. https://doi.org/10.1007/s10741-020-10061-x.
27. Jayasooriya G, Silversides C, Raghavan G, Balki M. Anesthetic management of women with heart failure during pregnancy: a retrospective cohort study. Int J Obstet Anesth. 2020;44:40–50. https://doi.org/10.1016/j.ijoa.2020.06.001.
28. Joglar JA, Kapa S, Saarel EV, Dubin AM, Gorenek B, Hameed AB, Lara de Melo S, et al. HRS expert consensus statement on the management of arrhythmias during pregnancy. Heart Rhythm. 2023;2023:S1547-5271(23)022464. https://doi.org/10.1016/j.hrthm.2023.05.017. Epub ahead of print.
29. Kamiya CA, Yoshimatsu J. Pharmacological treatment for cardiovascular disease during pregnancy and lactation. J Cardiol. 2019;73(5):363–9. https://doi.org/10.1016/j.jjcc.2018.12.020.
30. Keepanasseril A, Pfaller B, Metcalfe A, Siu SC, Davis MB, Silversides CK. Cardiovascular deaths in pregnancy: growing concerns and preventive strategies. Can J Cardiol. 2021;37:1969–78. https://doi.org/10.1016/j.cjca.2021.09.022.
31. Lima FV, Parikh PB, Zhu J, Yang J, Stergiopoulos K. Association of cardiomyopathy with adverse cardiac events in pregnant women at the time of delivery. JACC Heart Fail. 2015;3:257–66. https://doi.org/10.1016/j.jchf.2014.10.008.
32. Lima FV, Yang J, Xu J, Stergiopoulos K. National trends and in-hospital outcomes in pregnant women with heart disease in the United States. Am J Cardiol. 2017;119:1694–700.
33. Lindley KJ. Call for action to address increasing maternal cardiovascular mortality in the United States: strategies for improving maternal cardiovascular care. Circulation. 2022;145:502–4. https://doi.org/10.1161/CIRCULATIONAHA.122.058772.
34. Lindley KJ. Heart failure and pregnancy: thinking beyond peripartum cardiomyopathy. J Card Fail. 2021;27(2):153–6. https://doi.org/10.1016/j.cardfail.2020.09.475.
35. Liu LX, Arany Z. Maternal cardiac metabolism in pregnancy. Cardiovasc Res. 2014;101(4):545–53. https://doi.org/10.1093/cvr/cvu009.
36. Lu CW, Shih JC, Chen SY, Chiu HH, Wang JK, Chen CA, Chiu SN, et al. Comparison of 3 risk estimation methods for predicting cardiac outcomes in pregnant women with congenital heart disease. Circ J. 2015;79:1609–17. https://doi.org/10.1253/circj.CJ-14-1368.
37. Mahilmaran A. Heart failure in pregnancy. Indian J Cardiovasc Dis Women-WINCARS. 2018;3:161–6.
38. McDonagh TA, Metra M, Adamo M, Gardner RS, Baumbach A, Böhm M, Burri H, ESC Scientific Document Group, et al. 2021 ESC Guidelines for the diagnosis and treatment of

acute and chronic heart failure. Eur Heart J. 2021;42(36):3599–726. https://doi.org/10.1093/eurheartj/ehab368.
39. McNamara DM, Elkayam U, Alharethi R, Damp J, Hsich E, Ewald G, Modi K, Alexis JD, Ramani GV, Semigran MJ, et al. Clinical outcomes for peripartum cardiomyopathy in North America: results of the IPAC Study (Investigations of Pregnancy-Associated Cardiomyopathy). J Am Coll Cardiol. 2015;66:905–14. https://doi.org/10.1016/j.jacc.2015.06.1309.
40. Mehta LS, Warnes CA, Bradley E, Burton T, Economy K, Mehran R, Safdar B, Sharma G, Wood M, Valente AM, Volgman AS, On behalf of the American Heart Association Council on Clinical Cardiology; Council on Arteriosclerosis, Thrombosis and Vascular Biology; Council on Cardiovascular and Stroke Nursing; and Stroke Council. Cardiovascular considerations in caring for pregnant patients: a scientific statement from the American Heart Association. Circulation. 2020;141:e884–903. https://doi.org/10.1161/CIR.0000000000000772.
41. Meng ML, Arendt KW, Banayan JM, Bradley EA, Vaught AJ, Hameed AB, Harris J, Bryner B, Mehta LS. Anesthetic care of the pregnant patient with cardiovascular disease: a scientific statement from the American Heart Association. Circulation. 2023;147(11):E657–73. https://doi.org/10.1161/CIR.0000000000001121.
42. Mogos MF, Piano MR, McFarlin BL, Salemi JL, Liese KL, Briller JE. Heart failure in pregnant women: a concern across the pregnancy continuum. Circ Heart Fail. 2018;11:e004005.
43. Monsieurs KG, Nolan JP, Bossaert LL, Greif R, Maconochie IK, Nikolaou NI, Perkins GD, Soar J, Truhlář A, Wyllie J, Zideman DA, ERC Guidelines 2015 Writing Group. European resuscitation council guidelines for resuscitation 2015: section 1. Executive summary. Resuscitation. 2015;95:1–80.
44. Moore J, Baldisseri MR. Amniotic fluid embolism. Crit Care Med. 2005;33(10 Suppl):S279–85. https://doi.org/10.1097/01.ccm.0000183158.71311.28.
45. Mubarik A, Chippa V, Iqbal AM. Postpartum cardiomyopathy. Treasure Island: StatPearls Publishing; 2022.
46. Ng AT, Duan L, Win T, Spencer HT, Lee MS. Maternal and fetal outcomes in pregnant women with heart failure. Heart. 2018;104:1949–54.
47. Nishimura RA, Otto CM, Bonow RO, Carabello BA, Erwin JP, Fleisher LA, Jneid H, Mack MJ, McLeod CJ, O'Gara PT, et al. 2017 AHA/ACC focused update of the 2014 AHA/ACC Guideline for the Management of Patients with Valvular Heart Disease: a report of the American College of Cardiology/American Heart Association Task Force on Clinical Practice Guidelines. Circulation. 2017;135:e1159–95. https://doi.org/10.1161/CIR.0000000000000503.
48. Ouzounian JG, Elkayam U. Physiologic changes during normal pregnancy and delivery. Cardiol Clin. 2012;30:317–29. https://doi.org/10.1016/j.ccl.2012.05.004.
49. Owens AT. Pregnancy in hypertrophic cardiomyopathy. Eur Heart J. 2017;38:2691–2. https://doi.org/10.1093/eurheartj/ehx304.
50. Packer M, Bristow MR, Cohn JN, Colucci WS, Fowler MB, Gilbert EM, Shusterman NH. The effect of carvedilol on morbidity and mortality in patients with chronic heart failure. U.S. Carvedilol Heart Failure Study Group. N Engl J Med. 1996;334(21):1349–55. https://doi.org/10.1056/NEJM199605233342101.
51. Parikh P, Blauwet L. Peripartum cardiomyopathy and preeclampsia: overlapping diseases of pregnancy. Curr Hypertens Rep. 2018;20(8):69. https://doi.org/10.1007/s11906-018-0868-9.
52. Park K, Bairey Merz C, Bello N, et al. Management of women with acquired cardiovascular disease from preconception through pregnancy and postpartum. J Am Coll Cardiol. 2021;77(14):1799–812.
53. Patel PA, Roy A, Javid R, Dalton JA. A contemporary review of peripartum cardiomyopathy. Clin Med (Lond). 2017;17(4):316–21. https://doi.org/10.7861/clinmedicine.17-4-316.
54. Pordeus ACB, Katz L, Soares MC, Maia SB, Amorim MMR. Acute pulmonary edema in an obstetric intensive care unit: a case series study. Medicine (Baltimore). 2018;97(28):e11508. https://doi.org/10.1097/MD.0000000000011508.
55. Regitz-Zagrosek V, Roos-Hesselink JW, Bauersachs J, Blomström-Lundqvist C, Cífková R, De Bonis M, Iung B, ESC Scientific Document Group, et al. 2018 ESC Guidelines for the

management of cardiovascular diseases during pregnancy. Eur Heart J. 2018;39(34):3165–241. https://doi.org/10.1093/eurheartj/ehy340.
56. Ricke-Hoch M, Pfeffer TJ, Hilfiker-Kleiner D. Peripartum cardiomyopathy: basic mechanisms and hope for new therapies. Cardiovasc Res. 2020;116(3):520–31. https://doi.org/10.1093/cvr/cvz252.
57. Roos-Hesselink J, Baris L, Johnson M, De Backer J, Otto C, Marelli A, Jondeau G, Budts W, Grewal J, Sliwa K, et al. Pregnancy outcomes in women with cardiovascular disease: evolving trends over 10 years in the ESC registry of pregnancy and cardiac disease (ROPAC). Eur Heart J. 2019;40:3848–55. https://doi.org/10.1093/eurheartj/ehz136.
58. Ruys TPE, Roos-Hesselink JW, Hall R, Subirana-Domènech MT, Grando-Ting J, Estensen M, Crepaz R, Fesslova V, Gurvitz M, De Backer J, et al. Heart failure in pregnant women with cardiac disease: data from the ROPAC. Heart. 2014;100:231–8. https://doi.org/10.1136/heartjnl-2013-304888.
59. Say L, Chou D, Gemmill A, Tunçalp Ö, Moller AB, Daniels J, Gülmezoglu AM, Temmerman M, Alkema L. Global causes of maternal death: a WHO systematic analysis. Lancet Glob Health. 2014;2(6):e323–33. https://doi.org/10.1016/S2214-109X(14)70227-X.
60. Silversides CK, Colman JM, Sermer M, Siu SC. Cardiac risk in pregnant women with rheumatic mitral stenosis. Am J Cardiol. 2003;91:1382–5. https://doi.org/10.1016/s0002-9149(03)00339-4.
61. Silversides CK, Grewal J, Mason J, Sermer M, Kiess M, Rychel V, Wald RM, Colman JM, Siu SC. Pregnancy outcomes in women with heart disease: the CARPREG II study. J Am Coll Cardiol. 2018;71(21):2419–30. https://doi.org/10.1016/j.jacc.2018.02.076.
62. Siu SC, Sermer M, Colman JM, Alvarez AN, Mercier AL, et al. Prospective multicenter study of pregnancy outcomes in women with heart disease. Circulation. 2001;104:515–21.
63. Sliwa K, Azibani F, Baard J, et al. Reducing late maternal death due to cardiovascular disease—a pragmatic pilot study. Int J Cardiol. 2018a;272:70–6.
64. Sliwa K, Petrie MC, Hilfiker-Kleiner D, et al. Long-term prognosis, subsequent pregnancy, contraception and overall management of peripartum cardiomyopathy: practical guidance paper from the Heart Failure Association of the European Society of Cardiology Study Group on Peripartum Cardiomyopathy. Eur J Heart Fail. 2018b;20(6):951–62. https://doi.org/10.1002/ejhf.1178.
65. Sliwa K, van der Meer P, Petrie MC, Frogoudaki A, Johnson MR, Hilfiker-Kleiner D, Hamdan R, et al. Risk stratification and management of women with cardiomyopathy/heart failure planning pregnancy or presenting during/after pregnancy: a position statement from the Heart Failure Association of the European Society of Cardiology Study Group on Peripartum Cardiomyopathy. Eur J Heart Fail. 2021;23:527–40. https://doi.org/10.1002/ejhf.2133.
66. Stergiopoulos K, Lima FV, Butler J. Heart failure in pregnancy: a problem hiding in plain sight. J Am Heart Assoc. 2019;8:e012905. https://doi.org/10.1161/JAHA.119.012905.
67. Swan L, Lupton M, Anthonhy J, Yentis S, Steer P, Gatzoulis M. Controversies in pregnancy and congenital heart disease. Congenit Heart Dis. 2006;1:27–34. https://doi.org/10.1111/j.1747-0803.2006.00005.x.
68. Tamirisa KP, Dye C, Bond RM, Hollier LM, Marinescu K, Vaseghi M, Russo AM, Gulati M, Volgman AS. Arrhythmias and heart failure in pregnancy: a dialogue on multidisciplinary collaboration. J Cardiovasc Dev Dis. 2022;9(7):199. https://doi.org/10.3390/jcdd9070199.
69. Thorne S. Risks of contraception and pregnancy in heart disease. Heart. 2006;92:1520–5.
70. van Hagen IM, Thorne SA, Taha N, Youssef G, Elnagar A, Gabriel H, ElRakshy Y, Iung B, Johnson MR, Hall R, et al. Pregnancy outcomes in women with rheumatic mitral valve disease: results from the registry of pregnancy and cardiac disease. Circulation. 2018;137:806–16. https://doi.org/10.1161/CIRCULATIONAHA.117.032561.
71. Vaughan G, Tune K, Peek MJ, et al. Rheumatic heart disease in pregnancy: strategies and lessons learnt implementing a population-based study in Australia. Int Health. 2018;10(06):480–9.

72. Victor RG, Lynch K, Li N, Blyler C, Muhammad E, Handler J, Brettler J, Rashid M, Hsu B, Foxx-Drew D, et al. A cluster-randomized trial of blood-pressure reduction in black barbershops. N Engl J Med. 2018;378:1291–301. https://doi.org/10.1056/NEJMoa1717250.
73. Wu P, Haththotuwa R, Kwok CS, Babu A, Kotronias RA, Rushton C, Zaman A, Fryer AA, Kadam U, Chew-Graham CA, et al. Preeclampsia and future cardiovascular health: a systematic review and meta-analysis. Circ Cardiovasc Qual Outcomes. 2017;10:e003497. https://doi.org/10.1161/CIRCOUTCOMES.116.003497.

Chapter 26
Cardiac Involvement in Cirrhotic Portal Hypertension—From Diastolic Mild Dysfunction to Right Heart Failure

Teodora Radu, Speranta Iacob, Bogdan Dorobanţu, and Liana Gheorghe

Abstract End stage liver disease (ESLD) is associated with cardiovascular complications that can range from hyperdynamic circulation to up–front heart failure in cirrhotic cardiomyopathy (CCM). Patients with cirrhosis can present with pulmonary involvement and the most common manifestations are porto-pulmonary hypertension (PoPH) and hepatopulmonary syndrome (HPS). Transplant eligibility and medical management are different in the presence of these entities.

The prevalence of CCM is high among cirrhotic patients, but because of the absence of symptoms at rest and the preserved left ventricle systolic function, the diagnosis is frequently missed. Severity of CCM correlates with the severity of the liver disease and is associated with worse outcomes before and after transplant. Introduction of new criteria in 2019 that include new imaging techniques like global longitudinal strain and a more detailed diastolic function assessment aims to improve recognition.

PoPH is a life-threatening complication despite its low prevalence. A mean pulmonary artery pressure above 45 mmHg is an absolute contraindication for liver transplant. Invasive diagnostic confirmation is mandatory and specific medical therapies can improve the hemodynamic profile, allowing listing for transplant. At the opposite end, patients with HPS and high symptom burden, with severe hypoxemia should be listed for transplant early, as no other treatment option exists.

Keywords Cirrhotic cardiomyopathy · Porto-pulmonary hypertension · Hepatopulmonary syndrome · End stage liver disease · Liver transplant

T. Radu (✉)
"Carol Davila" University of Medicine and Pharmacy, Bucharest, Romania

Emergency Institute for Cardiovascular Disease "Prof. Dr. C. C. Iliescu", Bucharest, Romania

S. Iacob · B. Dorobanţu · L. Gheorghe
"Carol Davila" University of Medicine and Pharmacy, Bucharest, Romania

Fundeni Clinical Institute, Bucharest, Romania

M. Dorobanţu et al. (eds.), *Current Approach to Heart Failure*,
https://doi.org/10.1007/978-3-031-96562-3_26

Introduction—The Hyperdynamic Syndrome

Hyperdynamic syndrome (HS) is a hallmark of cirrhosis pathophysiology and is characterized by high cardiac output (CO), low systemic vascular resistances (SVR), tachycardia, low blood pressure, increase in total body fluid, with a paradoxical state of hypovolemia of the systemic circulation due to an increase in blood volume in the splanchnic circulation [1].

In the cirrhotic liver the pressure gradient between vena porta and inferior vena cava causes a redistribution of the blood flow to the splanchnic circulation, which in turn promotes formation of collateral vessels to by-pass the liver (portosystemic shunts). Sheer stress and bacterial translocation caused by portal hypertension favours release of inflammatory cytokines, endothelial dysfunction and nitric oxide synthase activation. The diseased liver suffers a decline in its metabolic and immunologic functions and as a consequence increased levels of splanchnic vasodilators and inflammatory cytokines are not cleared. The portosystemic shunts are responsible for redirecting the blood from the splanchnic circulation to the systemic circulation along with multiple vasodilatory mediators like prostacyclines, nitric oxide (NO), endocannabinoides and carbon monoxide (CO) [2]. There is also a decreased response to vasoconstrictor molecules and a neoangioformation in the mesenteric vessels correlated with the increased levels of vasodilators and inflammation [3].

Reduction in SVR triggers a compensatory increase in CO by increase in heart rate and also total blood volume. The drop in arterial pressure is registered by arterial baroreceptors and causes neurohormonal activation through the renin—angiotensin—aldosterone system (RAAS) and sympathetic nervous system (SNS). This causes renal vasoconstriction and consecutive water and sodium retention. As the disease progresses splanchnic vasodilation can no longer be compensated through the mechanisms of hyperdynamic circulation [4]. Portal hypertension and fluid retention that concentrates in the splanchnic compartment determines formation of ascites. The bacterial translocation favours infections (spontaneous bacterial peritonitis) and the increase in pressure in the portosystemic shunts leads to variceal bleeding. Persistent renal vasoconstriction in the context of central hypovolemia can lead to hepato—renal syndrome [5]. The continuing worsening of the hyperdynamic state affects most organs in the body and represents the primary cause of heart (CCM) and lung (HPS, PoPH) involvement, and also neurological changes (encephalopathy) and kidney function alteration (hepato-renal syndrome).

Cirrhotic Cardiomyopathy (CCM)

Definition and Physiopathology

CCM was defined for the first time in 2005 at the World Congress of Gastroenterology at Montreal. It is defined by the presence of left ventricle (LV) systolic or diastolic dysfunction, sometimes accompanied by electrophysiological changes (the most common is long QT) in patients with end stage liver disease, in the absence of known cardiovascular disease.

In the initial stages it was presumed it was related to alcohol toxic effects on the myocardium, but in the later years it was demonstrated that it can be present in patients with all types of cirrhosis. The cardiac dysfunction severity and progression is correlated with the severity and progression of the liver disease, independent of its cause.

The pathophysiological mechanisms are not completely understood. The main drive for CCM is the hyperdynamic syndrome associated with ESLD. Arterial baroreceptor activation determines RAAS and SNS feedback, probably contributing to the cardiac remodelling and hypertrophy in cirrhosis. The blood that is redirected from the splanchnic circulation through portosystemic shunts carries vasoactive mediators that are not being inactivated by the liver such as adrenaline and noradrenaline, atrial natriuretic peptide, glucagon, renin, substance P, aldosterone, vasopressin etc. Excretion of bile salts is reduced in the diseased liver and causes a high efflux of bile acids and bilirubin entering systemic circulation. Because of the high cholesterol and bile salts concentration, severe and longstanding cholestasis has toxic effects on the myocites and on the sinus node, causing arrhythmia, interfering with signalling pathways and inducing apoptosis (through the Farnesoid X Receptor) [6], affecting the quality of the cells' membrane (cholecardia) and the number and function of beta adrenergic receptors [7]. Another postulated mechanism in CCM is the proinflammatory state accentuated by the low hepatic immunological and metabolic function, allowing for cytokines (Il-6, Il-8 Il-1b, TNFἀ, TGF-β) and negative inotropes vasodilators like NO, CO, endocannabinoids to reach myocardial fibres and induce dysfunction through a shift in myosin heavy chain isoform from the more powerful α-subtype to the weaker β-isoform and also by inducing apoptosis [8]. The most common cannabinoid is anandamide, released from cell membrane phospholipids. It induces impaired contractility in the myocardium by acting on Cannabinoid-1 (CB1) receptor. TNFἀ (elevated in context of infection) is responsible for increased release of anandamide. Together with Il-1b, TNFἀ also stimulates production of NO, thus the role of inflammation in promoting cardiac impairment. Decreased cardiac response to stress/ exercise (chronotropic and inotrope impairment) is a consequence of SNS prolonged and over-activation. Sympathetic excess activity causes direct myocardial damage (noradrenaline exposure) and a desensitization of β-adrenergic receptor that includes down-regulation and also an alteration of the receptor with decreased cAMP production resulting in energetic and metabolic inefficacy [9].

Because of absence of symptoms at rest and because the systemic vasodilation that accompanies ESLD masks the LV systolic dysfunction, the diagnosis is frequently missed. There is no single diagnostic test that can establish or exclude the presence of CCM alone. Unfortunately, during stress like infection, haemorrhage or surgery, the LV function can deteriorate and manifest as up-front heart failure (HF) causing an increase in morbidity and mortality. It is an important cause for cardiovascular events (pulmonary edema, death) in the initial perioperative setting after liver transplant (LT) because of the abrupt increase of SVR as systemic circulation returns to normal, causing the LV dysfunction to be unmasked by the sudden increase in afterload. Another setting that can unmask CCM is transjugular intrahepatic portosystemic shunt (TIPS) insertion. Some patients develop HF after the intervention due to the increased amount of blood that is diverted from the splanchnic to the systemic circulation, causing increased preload. Large volume paracentesis can also determine HF decompensation—by reducing the abdominal pressure and increasing preload [10]. Furthermore, CCM can be a causative/contributing factor in the development of hepato–renal syndrome and cirrhosis decompensation [11].

Diagnosis

The 2005 World Congress of Gastroenterology diagnostic criteria are [12]:

- Systolic Dysfunction (any of the following)
  - Blunted contractile response on stress testing
  - LVEF < 55%
- Diastolic Dysfunction (any of the following)
  - Deceleration time of the E wave > 200 ms
  - Isovolumetric relaxation time > 80 ms
  - E/A < 1
- Supporting criteria
  - Electrophysiological abnormalities
  - Abnormal chronotropic response
  - Electromechanical uncoupling
  - Prolonged QTc interval
  - Enlarged left atrium
  - Increased myocardial mass
  - Increased brain natriuretic peptide (BNP) and/or pro-BNP
  - Increased troponin I

In the context of novel echocardiographic techniques becoming widely available such as Tissue Doppler and strain (GLS) and considering the new guidelines for the evaluation of LV diastolic function published in 2016 by the European Association of Cardiovascular Imaging and American Society of Echocardiography the CCM diagnostic criteria were up-dated in 2019. The new criteria put an emphasis on LV diastolic function and aim to improve LV subclinical systolic dysfunction detection by introducing GLS.

The 2019 Cirrhotic Cardiomyopathy Consortium diagnostic criteria are [11]:

- Systolic Dysfunction (any of the following)
  - GLS < 18 or GLS > 22
  - LVEF <= 50%
- Diastolic Dysfunction (>3 of the following)
  - Septal e' velocity < 7 cm/s
  - E/e' ratio > 15
  - Left atrial volume index > 34 ml/m^2
  - Tricuspid regurgitation velocity > 2.8 m/s
- Areas for future research which require further validation
  - Electrocardiographic changes
  - Abnormal chronotropic or inotropic response
  - Electromechanical uncoupling
  - Myocardial mass change
  - Chamber enlargement
  - Serum biomarkers
  - Cardiac magnetic resonance imaging

Cardiac Evaluation

Ecocardiography

Patients with cirrhosis have non-specific symptoms overlapping with HF symptoms (breathlessness from ascites, low exercise tolerance from peripheral muscle wasting, edema and pleural effusions due to low protein levels and sodium and water retention) making a clinical diagnosis challenging.

Transthoracic echocardiography is the first line investigation in identifying patients with CCM. HF can be classified according to the LV ejection fraction—HF with preserved EF (LVEF > 50%), HF with reduced EF (LVEF < 40%) and mid-range (EF 40–50%) [13].

The prevalence of CCM varies according to the diagnostic criteria used. Using the 2005 criteria the prevalence is estimated at 50–70% and using the 2019 criteria it drops to 29–55.7%. Systolic dysfunction was more prevalent using the new criteria including GLS than by the sole use of conventional LVEF [14]. The majority of the patients with CCM have normal resting LVEF using 2D echocardiography and GLS can detect subclinical dysfunction. A recent meta-analysis [15] showed a variability of diastolic dysfunction prevalence from 61% of patients when applying the 2005 criteria, to 45% when using TDI.

Using the 2005 criteria diastolic dysfunction was overestimated, as the parameters used were preload sensitive (E/A, TDE, isovolumic relaxation time). They increase with volume overload and decrease with diuretic treatment, paracentesis. Also, they have a U shape evolution, and patients with advanced diastolic dysfunction and young, normal subjects have similar patterns, making it difficult to discern normal from pathologic. Introducing to the diastolic function evaluation Tissue Doppler parameters and left atrial enlargement, which are not preload dependent, have made the diagnosis more accurate, but there are still caveats. Myocardial relaxation is impaired in all forms of cardiac disease, thus a reason to use (e') velocity decline in the diagnosis of CCM, as it precedes the decline in ((E/A), yet) but a reduction in (E/A) but not in (e') velocity is more indicative of hypovolemia. Left atrial dilation can be caused in cirrhotic patients also by the hyperdynamic state even if diastolic dysfunction is not yet present. Tricuspid valve regurgitation velocity can also be increased in cirrhotic patients with PoPH, with no relation to diastolic impairment, but these patients are rare.

Recent retrospective studies have failed to prove that the current diagnostic criteria can help in risk stratifying CCM patients. A clinical study showed that patients diagnosed by 2005 criteria had a higher risk of cardiovascular events at 1 year follow-up after LT, but patients diagnosed using the 2019 criteria did not [16]. Another retrospective study showed similar 6 year mortality in patients with or without CCM diagnosed mostly as by the presence of altered GLS [17].

GLS expressed as a percentage of longitudinal shortening, predominantly reflects the function of subendocardial longitudinal fibers, as opposed to conventional LVEF which is based also on the radial LV function. As longitudinal function is the first affected (more prone to ischemic damage and wall stress), it would seem logical that a decline in GLS should be encountered early in CCM patients. Despite that, GLS evidence in cirrhotic patients is not homogenous. A study did not find a difference in GLS between cirrhotic patients and controls, despite demonstrating increased LVEF dependent of liver disease severity in cirrhotic patients [18]. Another study found increased resting GLS associated with advanced liver disease, and also, low and high GLS were correlated with higher mortality [19]. A possible explanation would be the systemic vasodilation that progresses with liver disease, promoting LV contractility.

Although not included in the diagnostic criteria, other cardiac changes have been noted in cirrhotic patients, some of them having an impact on prognosis. One clinical trial has found that increased thickness of the myocardial septum is associated with worse prognosis after LV [44]. Left ventricle hypertrophy can be due to SNS over activation. Increased cardiac mass and dilated cardiac chambers and pulmonary artery that correlate with the severity of the liver disease have also been reported in studies [20, 21]. An autopsy study demonstrated that right ventricle dilation and hypertrophy was more common in cirrhotic patients [22].

Stress testing is challenging in liver cirrhosis patients because, as was mentioned before, patients often have blunted inotrope and chronotropic response during exercise/stress. The ESLD patients also have a low functional capacity. Even when challenged with pharmacological inotrope stressors like dobutamine the cardiac response is still abnormal. Vasodilator (adenosine) response is also impaired because of the already vasodilated state in cirrhosis. An increase in LA filling pressures during exercise/stress is used to unmask HF with preserved ejection fraction (HFpEF) and could be suggestive of CCM in cirrhotic patients. As most of the time LV systolic impairment is silent at rest in early stages CCM, abnormal stress tests could be useful for diagnosis. Limitation comes from a lack in standardized definitions of inotrope and chronotropic impairment and clear cut offs in defining abnormal tests. A study using dobutamine stress echocardiography demonstrated an increase in CCM diagnosis from 7.7% at rest to 61.5%. Systolic dysfunction was defined as a < 10% increase in EF and diastolic dysfunction was defined as an increase in E/e' ratio during dobutamine infusion [23].

Cardiopulmonary Testing (CPET) and ECG Treadmill Testing

Although CPET does not provide information included in the diagnostic criteria for CCM, multiple clinical studies have demonstrated a good correlation between mortality and peak oxygen consumption or anaerobic threshold values in patients on transplant waiting list and post LT. One study showed that a peak VO2 less than 60% of the predicted value was the only other parameter apart from MELD score that predicted mortality in the following year [25]. Another study demonstrated that a lower anaerobic threshold was associated with higher mortality in the first 3 months after LT [26]. CPET can help differentiate between limited exercise capacity causes (cardiovascular performance, pulmonary pathology, peripheral muscle wasting or deconditioning). Chronotropic incompetence can be unmasked during exercise, adding supportive information in CCM diagnosis. In this context, CPET can be considered to better stratify risk in CCM patients.

Another simpler exercise test, is the ECG treadmill test. A recent study [27] has demonstrated a chronotropic incompetence (CI) prevalence of 68.8% in patients with cirrhosis awaiting LT. CI prevalence was higher among patients with more severe liver disease (higher MELD/ Child scores) and among patients with alcohol related liver disease. The test was performed as a part of pre LT evaluation. CI was not associated with worse prognosis after LT in this study and the results did not alter transplant decision.

Modified heart rate reserve (MHRR), a new parameter derived from peak effort heart rate and resting heart rate, was proven to be independent of beta blocker use. Low MHRR was associated with increased risk of HF after LT [28].

ECG

Electrocardiographic changes were considered supporting evidence of CCM according to 2005 diagnostic criteria, but are no longer considered as such in the newer 2019 criteria. QT prolongation is frequent in cirrhotic patients (up to 50%), it is independent of liver disease cause but it is correlated with its severity. It is a hallmark of cell membrane alterations secondary to excess bile salts and vasoactive substances determinated by portosystemic shunts. They determine malfunctions in membrane Ca and K channels, Na/K ATPase and Ca ATPase which are responsible for Ca and K intracellular homeostasis and the repolarization of the cardiomyocytes. SNS over activation and excess noradrenaline also has a role in QT prolongation [29]. Electromechanical uncoupling refers to a lack of synchrony between electrical and mechanical systole and is related to QT interval prolongation. The clinical significance of these changes are not clearly demonstrated. It can be demonstrated using pulsed Doppler (decreased preejection time (PEET), increased LV ejection time (LVET), decreased ratio PEEP/LVET, opposite modifications compared to HFrEF) [30]. The presence of atrial fibrillation (5.4% prevalence) is associated with worse perioperative prognosis after LT [31]. NOACs are not recommended in advanced Child C patients.

Biomarkers

The most commonly used cardiac biomarkers are BNP/ NT pro BNP. BNP is a marker of LV dysfunction and strain, as it is released in the context of high intracardiac pressure. Some studies mentioned BNP as a screening marker for identification of cirrhotic patients at higher risk for complications related to portal hypertension, but it should be interpreted in the context of a comprehensive clinical evaluation [32]. Liver disease decompensation is associated with volume overload, atrial enlargement and increased filling pressures. An increase in BNP/ NT pro BNP compared to healthy controls, with higher values during acute settings like ascites, encephalopathy or bacterial spontaneous peritonitis are expected [33], as well as in other frequent complications associated with liver cirrhosis as sepsis, acute or chronic renal failure, shock of any etiology [32]. A study showed the correlation between NT pro BNP and both the severity of the liver dysfunction and cardiac impairment, but not to the presence of hyperdynamic circulation alone [34]. NT pro BNP values correlate with MELD score and Child classification, and also with poor outcomes on the waiting list and after LT. One study found 37% of patients with NT pro BNP above 2000 pg/ml had cardiac complications after LT compared with 9% in patients with lower NT pro BNP [20].

Troponins are a marker of myocardial ischemia, useful in acute coronary syndromes. Troponin is also increased in the context of myocardial wall stress—for example volume overload and high cardiac output HF in CCM patients. There is data linking increased troponin to adverse outcomes in cirrhotic patients. One study showed that pretransplant elevated troponin levels, diabetes and a history of cardiovascular disease are strongly associated with cardiovascular adverse events after LT [35].

Galectin 3 is a newer biomarker, with an outstanding role in chronic inflammation. Increased levels are associated with more severe liver disease. It is a marker of remodelling and fibrosis in HF [36] but it is also increased in liver fibrotic processes [37], mainly in non-alcoholic steatohepatitis, which limits its use in CCM. Another recent biomarker associated with liver disease is endocan (endothelial cell specific molecule-1) found in endothelial cells, primarily in the liver but also kidney and lung. Various articles have shown correlation with survival and with CCM in cirrhotic patients but further data is necessary to clarify its utility [38].

Cardiac Magnetic Resonance (CMR)

CMR can be used to further characterise cardiac function, especially when other studies have been inconclusive. It is not included in the 2019 diagnostic criteria and more clinical trials are needed to determine its utility in CCM diagnosis but CMR allows for a more accurate LVEF assessment and also provides myocardial structural information. A pharmacological agent (dobutamine) can be used to evaluate inotropic/chronotropic incompetence. Gadolinium enhancement (LGE) and extracellular volume fraction calculation (ECV) can provide more information regarding myocardial fibrosis and possible reversibility. EVf is a mark of pericellular edema, which is reversible, but fibrosis on LGE is a non-reversible change. Fibrosis can be a pathophysiological substrate for diastolic dysfunction. A clinical study showed that an increase in ECV is associated with liver disease progression and also demonstrated a connection between high ECV and post LT worse outcomes [39]. Patients with more advanced liver disease and ascites had more elevated EVf values. ESLD is associated with iron metabolism anomalies that can lead to iron overload and myocardial increased iron levels. T2* imaging is used to quantify iron deposition in the heart or liver. A study showed that lower than 20 ms T* values correlate with advanced liver disease (MELD > 25 and Child C) and values lower than 15 ms were associated with worse outcomes after LT [40].

Risk Scores to Estimate Cardiovascular Pre-transplant Risk

CAR-OLT score was developed to assess cardiovascular risk. The CAR-OLT score is based on variables like age, sex, race, educational and working status, history of heart failure or atrial fibrillation, diabetes, arterial hypertension, association of hepatocarcinoma, pulmonary hypertension or pre-transplant mechanical ventilation. It is based on following patients after transplant and comparing the group who experienced a cardiovascular event to those who did not. Cardiovascular events were defined as cardiovascular death, myocardial infarction, revascularization, HF, atrial fibrillation, cardiac arrest, pulmonary embolism, transient ischemic attack and/or stroke. A score below 23 has a 99% negative predictive value for a cardiac contraindication for transplant listing (about 30% of patients) and can be listed without further testing. 30% of patients had a score above 40 which predicted high cardiac risk [41].

In a recent study authors have demonstrated using the HFA-PEFF score in cirrhotic patients that the score is elevated in more than 50% of cases. HFA-PEFF is a score that was designed to help diagnose HFpEF, composed of echocardiographic and serologic criteria [24]. An elevated score was associated with higher mortality in cirrhotic patients. The main reason for that is the fact that HFpEF diagnosis relies much on the presence of diastolic dysfunction and higher scores imply higher LA filling pressures, thus worse prognosis. HFA-PEFF could be a useful tool in risk stratifying CCM patients, yet the score has not been validated in this population and further studies are necessary [42].

Treatment

There are no clear guidelines in regard to the management of patients with CCM. Regarding HF guideline medical treatment in CCM, some considerations must be noted. Patients with Child C decompensated cirrhosis, with ascites cannot tolerate angiotensin converting enzyme inhibitors (ACEi) or angiotensin receptor blockers (ARBs) because a further decrease in SVR and arterial pressure is associated with worsening renal function. ACEi/ ARBs should not be used in this population, their use being restricted to patients in less advanced stages of liver disease [47]. There are no clinical trials investigating the use of sacubitril/valsartan in cirrhotic patients with CCM.

Patients with reduced ejection fraction should be treated with beta-blockers as recommended by current guidelines. Considering that over activation of SNS and increased exposure to noradrenaline is one of the pathophysiological mechanisms of CCM beta-blocker use in this population is beneficial. Carvedilol has proven benefits in patients with compensated liver disease reducing risk of first variceal bleeding compared to prophylactic endoscopic variceal ligation and the risk of cirrhosis decompensation and ascites, increasing survival compared to Propranolol, thus being the first line choice [43]. One clinical trial found that beta-blockers had protective effect on perioperative cardiac adverse events in LT patients [44]. A positive effect on QT prolongation is also to be expected with beta-blocker treatment, although increased QT has not been associated with increased mortality or malignant arrhythmia and should not represent the sole reason for treatment. Patients with compensated child A and child B cirrhosis usually tolerate beta-blockers. The best way to monitor beta-blocker tolerance is by measuring blood pressure. Maintaining a MAP over 70 mmHg reduces the risk of hepato-renal syndrome. In case of worsening hypotension, ascites and decline in renal function, beta-blockers should be withheld [45].

Another medication that can be added in case of tachycardia and LV diastolic dysfunction (LVDD) is Ivabradine. It does not have the negative inotrope effect of beta-blockers or their effect on blood pressure. Ivabradine acts at the sinoatrial node level, inhibiting the pacemaker current (If). A study demonstrated that, by using carvedilol and adding ivabradine if target heart rate was not met (55–60 beats per minute), patients exhibited a trend towards improvement of LVDD and a lower risk of kidney injury and encephalopathy, a lower NT pro BNP and decreased mortality at 1 year [46].

Clinical trials to investigate the usefulness of sodium glucose transporter 2 inhibitors (SGLT2i) in cirrhotic patients with refractory ascites are ongoing. Up to date there are only case reports of cirrhotic patients associating diabetes in which a SGLT2i was initiated for glucose control. Their effects are dual—diuretic and hypoglycemic. The diuretic effect favours osmotic diuresis and natriuresis, inhibiting the SNS and RAAS, with a trend towards improvement of hyponatremia [48]. The hypoglycemic effects are associated with improvement of nutritional status and hepatic function probably by improving glucose metabolism, important in the context of increasing number of cases of non-alcoholic steatohepatitis (NASH) cirrhosis [60]. Also, studies have shown improvement in liver fibrosis and steatosis (measured by fibroscan) with the use of SGLT2i in type 2 diabetic patients and NASH, but without cirrhosis [61]. Also, SGLT2 inhibitors have proven anti-inflammatory properties, reducing liver inflammation, a key driver of fibrosis progression [62].

In advanced cirrhosis patients with ascites and volume overload the treatment consists of sodium restriction, paracentesis, serum albumin infusions and high dose mineralocorticoid antagonist (MRA) combined with loop diuretics [49].

Implications of CCM Regarding Liver Transplant Patient Selection

As mentioned before, LT surgery is associated with high circulatory stress and frequent cardiac complications. The anhepatic stage of surgery implies clamping of inferior vena cava, vena porta and hepatic artery, switching to total veno-venous by-pass with secondary hypomagnesaemia, increased ischemia and decrease in preload. After graft reperfusion, a high quantity of vasoactive molecules are washed into systemic circulation together with an increase in preload (unclamping of IVC) and afterload (increase in SVR). The graft is exposed to a conservation solution with high potassium concentration that can be a cause of hyperkalemia. To avoid excess vasoactive substances and potassium, the graft is washed via the hepatic artery or portal vein and the fluid is flushed by IVC venting before reperfusion. There are also large quantities of blood products infused during surgery that can have potential negative cardiac effects and also citrate can cause low calcium levels. The reperfusion phase is the most difficult, hemodynamically unstable phase and many patients develop reperfusion syndrome [65]. It is defined as a fall in blood pressures of more the 30% from baseline in the 5 min after graft reperfusion. In the context of subclinical heart suffering that is associated with CCM, the cardiovascular system adapts poorly to the hemodynamic changes [54]. Cardiac arrest during LT appears in 5% of transplants, most of them during reperfusion period, with a mortality of 50% (total intra-operatory and in-hospital). Patients who arrested usually had a higher MELD [55].

Cardiac adverse events occur in 25–40% of recipients with a high mortality (about 30% of patients with HF) during the first year after transplant. The most frequent events are myocardial infarction, HF and arrhythmias [56]. Post-operative systolic dysfunction after LT was observed with an incidence of 3–7% [57]. Pulmonary edema diagnosed by clinical or radiological criteria was reported in up to 50% of patients [59].

Higher MELD score, dilated LA, increased E/e' ratio and sinus tachycardia were associated with increased risk of cardiovascular events [58]. In another study authors found no difference in pulmonary wedge pressure, etiology or severity of liver disease, but HF was more likely to develop in patients who are older and had higher pretransplant pulmonary artery pressures [57]. History of HF and high number of blood infusions during surgery were also linked to the risk for developing HFrEF after LT [56]. One study testing cardiac response to sudden increase in preload, in order to mimic the reperfusion phase, reported that non-responders had higher MELD and were more likely to have alcohol cirrhosis, more dilated LA and a lower SVR. Non-responders had higher rates of cardiovascular events after LT [50].

CCM patients undergoing LT should be monitored using invasive hemodynamic assessment and adding intra-operatory transoesophageal echocardiography can help better understand the preload and afterload changes and the cardiac response. After surgery patients at high risk of developing HF should be followed-up closely by a cardiologist to ensure timely initiation of HF guidelines medical therapies.

There are case reports of acute HF early after LT, in some complete recovery was seen, others evolved with cardiogenic shock unresponsive to medical therapy, requiring LV assist device (intra-aortic balloon pump/ECMO/BIVAD) [51]. In a series of cases of acute HF after LT authors found an incidence of acute HF after LT of 3% (9 out of 298). 6 of the 9 patients were considered Takotsubo cardiomyopathy, made a full recovery and 3 patients (30%) died [53]. Another article reports to cases of Takotsubo after cardiac arrest during LT surgery. The LVEF drops to 30% with ensuing cardiogenic shock needing inotrope and vasopressor support. LVEF normalized in the following days [52]. All patients reported had a normal LV systolic function with mildly impaired diastolic function pretransplant. Although Takotsubo cardiomyopathy can occur after a stressing event like surgery, in this clinical context CCM cannot be ruled out. Another recent study [63] evaluated retrospectively 1760 LT recipients, of whom 601 patients had a post-transplant transthoracic echocardiography. Patients with pre-transplant LVEF < 50% were excluded. They found 69 patients with new LVEF < 40% (11% of patients with post-transplant echo and 4% of the hole cohort). The only risk factors found were pre transplant low normal EF (50–55%) and wall motion abnormalities. Other recipient and donor characteristics were similar, including LA dilation and pulmonary pressure. Half of the patients recovered LV function in 30 days. Over all, patients who required echo post-transplant, irrespective of LVEF had a higher mortality.

Reversal of the hyperdynamic syndrome effects on circulation after LT does not happen instantly, it is a process that can take up to 9 months. The first 3 months after

LT, LV systolic and diastolic function can sometimes deteriorate compared to pre-transplant assessment. This is the time frame in which patients are at the highest risk to develop HF. Cardiac function usually improves 6–12 months after LT. There is also improvement of exercise tolerance and cardiac output [64].

As cardiac function appears to improve after LT, CCM is not a contraindication for transplant. The management of patients before, during and after transplant plays an important role in improving their prognosis and careful cardiology monitoring of these patients is necessary during the process.

All LT candidates should perform a basic cardiac evaluation (ECG, echocardiography, NT pro BNP), followed by more advanced investigations if CCM is suspected in order to better stratify risk. The general agreement is that an LVEF below 40% in the context of optimal HF guideline medical treatment (as tolerated in the context of liver disease) is an absolute contraindication for transplant. A LVEF below 50% is a relative contraindication for transplant and must determine CCM and coronary artery disease (CAD) pretransplant evaluation [65]. It is important to exclude CAD in all patients with systolic LV dysfunction, as CAD has a different treatment entirely. Percutaneous revascularization of proximal hemodynamic significant coronary stenosis (>70%) in asymptomatic patients should be performed only in patients who are LT candidates, who have a high risk of acute coronary event in the first 30 days after LT and revascularization improves prognostic. If ineligible for transplant, revascularization and double antiplatelet therapy in asymptomatic cirrhotic patients is associated with high bleeding risk and no clear benefit. In patients with preserved systolic function and impaired diastolic relaxation, CAD screening should be performed according to local guidelines, related to the presence of symptoms or atherosclerosis risk factors. A recent retrospective study [66] analysed patients who were listed for liver transplant in their institution between 2010 and 2019—a total of 1771 patients that had 1634 stress echocardiography tests and 1266 coronary angiographies as required by the local protocol. The authors found that the most important risk factors for CAD were older age, male sex, diabetes, hypertension, tobacco use (pack years), family history of CAD and personal history of CAD and based on this, they devised CAD—LT risk score that stratifies CAD risk in low (≤2%), intermediate (3–9%) and high (≥10%). If non-invasive testing is performed in intermediate risk patients and invasive coronary angiography in high risk patients, half of the tests could be avoided and 97% of severe CAD patients (requiring surgery or percutaneous intervention) are diagnosed.

To conclude, more information from clinical trials is needed on the impact of the new diagnostic criteria on diagnosing and risk stratifying patients with CCM. It continues to be an underdiagnosed condition despite negative impact on outcomes after LT and TIPS and increased awareness is required. Stress tests, advanced imaging techniques and adapted risk scores from HFpEF can improve the diagnosis and risk assessment in CCM and further trials are expected. On-going studies with new medication from HFrEF guidelines (SGLT2i, ivabradine) will shed more light on their mechanisms of action and utility in CCM. There is no algorithm to predict development of post-transplant HF complications in patients with preserved systolic LV function. The assessment and management of cardiac complications should be tailored to each patient individual clinical presentation and risk factors in a multidisciplinary team. Older patients, with previous history of heart failure, patients with higher MELD and patients with pre-transplant low-normal EF or abnormal wall motion should be monitored more closely.

Porto-Pulmonary Hypertension (PoPH)

Definition

Pulmonary Hypertension Definition

According to the ESC Guidelines for the diagnosis and management of pulmonary hypertension (PH) [67] the definition of PH relies on right heart catheterization (RHC). Although the hemodynamic assessment is mandatory, the final diagnosis and classification must consider the whole clinical setting. PH is defined by a mean pulmonary arterial pressure (mPAP) > 20 mmHg at rest (a threshold that was reduced from a previous value of more than 25 mmHg in the previous guidelines [68] after the 6th World Symposium on Pulmonary Hypertension [69]).

To differentiate pre- and post-capillary PH measurements of pulmonary vascular resistance (PVR) and pulmonary arterial wedge pressure (PAWP) are necessary. The normal value for PVR < 2 WU (160 dyn·s/cm^5)—a threshold that was reduced from a previous value of more than 3 WU (240 dyn·s/cm^5) in the previous guidelines. For PAWP although the threshold for normal is <12 mmHg, all clinical trials and also European Heart Failure Association recommend using >15 mmHg cut-off to define post—capillary PH (classified as group 2 PH associated with left heart disease).

Pre-capillary PH (group 1, pulmonary arterial hypertension—PAH) is defined as a mPAP > 20 mmHg in the context of PVR > 2 UW and PAWP < 15 mmHg.

Post-capillary PH is defined as mPAP > 20 mmHg and PAWP > 15 mmHg. PVR is used to differentiate between patients with post-capillary PH who have a significant pre-capillary component (PVR > 2 WU—combined post- and pre-capillary PH) and those who do not (PVR ≤ 2 WU—isolated post-capillary PH). Another parameter used to characterize post-capillary PH is the trans-pulmonary pressure gradient (TPG) which is the difference between mPAP—PAWP. A TPG > 12 mmHg in patients with combined post and pre-capillary PH is indicative of a disproportionate pre-capillary component.

Another situation, when patients have mPAP > 20 mmHg with normal PAWP < 15 mmHg and normal PVR < 2 WU, is defined as unclassified PH.

Clinical pulmonary hypertension classification [67] is listed below:

GROUP 1 Pulmonary arterial hypertension (PAH)

- 1.1 Idiopathic
  - 1.1.1 Non-responders at vasoreactivity testing
  - 1.1.2 Acute responders at vasoreactivity testing
- 1.2 Heritable
- 1.3 Associated with drugs and toxins
- 1.4 Associated with:
  - 1.4.1 Connective tissue disease
  - 1.4.2 HIV infection
  - 1.4.3 Portal hypertension
  - 1.4.4 Congenital heart disease
  - 1.4.5 Schistosomiasis
- 1.5 PAH with features of venous/capillary (PVOD/PCH) involvement
- 1.6 Persistent PH of the newborn

GROUP 2 PH associated with left heart disease

- 2.1 Heart failure:
  - 2.1.1 with preserved ejection fraction
  - 2.1.2 with reduced or mildly reduced ejection fraction
- 2.2 Valvular heart disease
- 2.3 Congenital/acquired cardiovascular conditions leading to post-capillary PH

GROUP 3 PH associated with lung diseases and/or hypoxia

- 3.1 Obstructive lung disease or emphysema
- 3.2 Restrictive lung disease
- 3.3 Lung disease with mixed restrictive/obstructive pattern
- 3.4 Hypoventilation syndromes
- 3.5 Hypoxia without lung disease (e.g. high altitude)
- 3.6 Developmental lung disorders

GROUP 4 PH associated with pulmonary artery obstructions

- 4.1 Chronic thromboembolic PH
- 4.2 Other pulmonary artery obstructions

GROUP 5 PH with unclear and/or multifactorial mechanisms

- 5.1 Haematological disorders
- 5.2 Systemic disorders
- 5.3 Metabolic disorders
- 5.4 Chronic renal failure with or without haemodialysis
- 5.5 Pulmonary tumour thrombotic microangiopathy
- 5.6 Fibrosing mediastinitis

Portopulmonary Hypertension Definition and Classification

Group 1 PAH (mPAP > 20 mmHg, PVR > 2 WU, PAWP < 15 mmHg) in the context of the presence of portal hypertension, irrespective of the presence of the liver disease, is commonly named porto-pulmonary hypertension (PoPH). It can also be associated with periportal fibrosis, portal vein thrombosis, hepatic vein sclerosis and congenital anomalies of portal circulation, The prevalence is 2–6% in the population with portal hypertension [70, 71] and represent 5–15% of PAH patients in registries [72–74]. In patients with ESLD on waiting list for LT prevalence of PoPH is reported higher in some trials, variating from 2% [75], 5.3% [76] to 10% [77], but in this last study the authors used only echocardiography, no RHC, which might have led to an over-estimation. It must be considered that most existing PoPH studies have used the older version of diagnostic criteria with mPAP ≥ 25 mmHg, PAWP ≤ 15 mmHg, and PVR > 3 WU.

Portal hypertension is present in ESLD patients and is defined by an increase in the pressure gradient between the portal vein and the IVC, which is hemodynamically defined by a hepatic venous pressure gradient up to 5 mm Hg, trans-splenic pressure ≥ 15 mmHg, and a portal vein pressure ≥ 21 mmHg [78].

PoPH is classified according to severity in mild (mPAP ≤ 35 mmHg), moderate (mPAP between 35 and 44 mmH) and severe (mPAP ≥ 45 mmHg). That is important because of a clinical trial that demonstrated that a mPAP > 50 mmHg was associated with a mortality of 100% after LL and patients with moderate PoPH had 50% mortality risk. High PVR (>5 WU) and TPG (> 37 mmHg) were also associated with adverse outcomes. In patients with mild PoPH or TPG < 15 mmHg no cardio-pulmonary death was registered [79]. In this context patients with ESLD and PoPH are considered for LT only if mPAP is below 35 mmHg (with or without vasodilatory medication).

Physiopathology

The mechanisms that cause patients with cirrhosis to develop PoPH are not completely clear. On histologic analysis similar alterations in the pulmonary vasculature with those found in idiopathic and other group 1 PAH patients were found. There was evidence of fibrosis, thrombosis, platelet aggregation, vasoconstriction, vascular remodelling composed of intimal proliferation, medial hypertrophy and smooth muscle proliferation, plexiform lesions.

The most common mechanism that was proposed was that excess of vasoconstrictor mediators from the splanchnic vascular compartment, not neutralised by the liver, such as endothelin-1, estradiol and serotonin, which were found to be in higher quantities in cirrhotic patients' plasma, enter the systemic circulation though the portosystemic shunts and cause proliferation (excess estrogen signaling) along with vasoconstriction. Also, there is a disequilibrium in the vasodilator molecules in the pulmonary endothelium, with prostacyclin and nitric oxide deficit. Endotoxin and bacterial translocation favour inflammation, with release of proinflammatory cytokines (interleukin 6) and proangiogenic factors that could have a role in pulmonary vascular remodelling. Another proposed mechanism is that hyperdynamic circulation determines increased shear stress and promotes endothelial dysfunction and endothelial cell injury, with activation and suppression of specific genes that participate in the vascular remodeling process [105]. As only a small percentage of cirrhotic patients develop PoPH, hereditary influence cannot be ruled out. BMPR2 mutations are found frequently in familial PAH. Lower circulating levels of BMPR2 and higher concentration of estrogen have been described in PoPH patients compared with patients with cirrhosis but without PoPH. Endotoxin and estrogen also have a role in regulating the BMPR2 gene expression. Genetic variants involved in estrogen signaling increased the risk of POPH [80].

Although there is no correlation between severity or cause of liver disease, female sex and autoimmune disease were found to be associated with a higher risk for developing PoPH. Patients with chronic hepatitis C infection had a lower risk of PoPH in clinical studies [81]. Another study [99] found that primary biliary cholangitis was more frequent among patients with cirrhosis and PoPH than in those without PoPH.

Diagnostic

Clinical diagnosis is challenging as liver and heart disease symptoms overlap. The most common symptom of PoPH is effort dyspnea, which is easy to be misinterpreted as usual fatigue caused by the underlying liver disease. Patients can also have other clinical signs of PH—left parasternal systolic murmur, diastolic murmur on the pulmonic site and jugular vein distension. Ascites and lower limb edema can be found but they are also present in decompensated liver cirrhosis. Chest pain, palpitations and syncope can be present in PH patients. Patients with PoPH had more fatigue (31% versus 23%), less exertional dyspnea (81% versus 86%), more edema (33% versus 21%) and more abdominal distension (12% versus 3%) than patients with idiopathic PAH [86]. As the pulmonary hypertension progresses exertional dyspnea worsens.

PoPH must be distinguished from hepato-pulmonary syndrome, which is characterized by platipnea (decreased oxygen saturation in orthostatic position) and is caused by vasodilatation in the pulmonary arterioles.

Portal hypertension can be documented invasively (rarely) and is defined as hepatic vein pressure gradient >10 mmHg. Most often clinical examination, non-invasive imaging (CT, endoscopy) showing oesophageal varices and hepatic elastography are enough.

Transthoracic echocardiography is the first line investigation used to screen patients with portal hypertension for PoPH. Because of the high CO in this population, tricuspid regurgitation velocity of >2.8 m/s (a right ventricle to right atrium pressure gradient—RV/RA > 35 mmHg) can over-estimate the diagnosis and cause an excess of RHCs. In liver transplant echocardiographic screening for PoPH, a cut-off of >50 mmHg estimated systolic arterial pressure (sPAP) is used, as it has a 97% sensitivity and a 77% specificity to identify moderate and severe PoPH patients [82]. Other authors recommend to perform RHC at a lower threshold of 38 mmHg, ensuring a specificity of 82% and a negative predictive value of 100%. In this particular centre, a cut-off of 30 mmHg had resulted in a specificity of 54% with 85% of RHC being negative [83].

Special attention must be paid to several other echo parameters when screening for pulmonary hypertension. They represent indirect signs of PH and by calculating the PH probability, they help diagnosis [67]:

- RV dilation (RV/LV > 1 in 4 chamber view)
- RA dilation (RA area > 18 cm^2)
- Pulmonary artery (PA) diameter > aortic root diameter
- PA diameter > 25 mm
- Flattening of the interventricular septum, D shape LV
- RVOT < 105 ms and/or mid-systolic notching
- IVC diameter > 21 mm with decreased inspiratory collapse
- Pulmonary valve diastolic regurgitation velocity > 2.2 m/s
- Pericardial effusions
- RV systolic dysfunction TAPSE < 18 mm, TDI systolic velocity of tricuspid annulus S < 9.5 cm/s, TAPSE/ PAPs < 0.55, reduced RV fractional area change < 35%

In the presence of these other echo signs of PH, a lower tricuspid regurgitation velocity (2.8–3.4 m/s) is associated with a high probability of PH and should determine further investigations and RHC.

The American Association for the Study of Liver Diseases recommends RHC in patients with sPAP ≥ 45 mm Hg and/or evidence of high mPAP founded on TTE (pulmonary artery dilation, right atrium dilation). The European Respiratory Society and the Mayo Clinic use sPAP ≥ 50 mm Hg.

Optimal follow-up time for patients on LT waiting list is unclear, but current guidelines recommend 1 year echo reevaluation [67].

RHC is necessary to confirm the diagnosis and differentiate it from PH secondary to the unclassified PH characteristic to hyperdynamic circulation (elevated CO, high mPAP, low PVR) or the similar to left heart disease in volume overload (high mPAP and PAWP, low PVR). It is important because only confirmed true PoPH can be treated with PAH vasodilatory medication.

Other investigations can help support the PoPH diagnosis. ECG can show RV hypertrophy, right axis deviation, and right bundle branch block, suggestive of right heart strain. A chest X ray can show enlarged heart and proximal vessels, with pruning of the peripheral pulmonary circulation. Thoracic CT scan can show signs of pulmonary hypertension (enlarged right cardiac chambers and pulmonary artery, dilated IVC, IVC contrast reflux), it can show signs of portal hypertension, and also exclude other common causes of PH like chronic thromboembolic PH or pulmonary parenchymal disease.

Risk stratification and decision to up-grade medical therapy should be done according to PAH guidelines [67] every 3–6 months based on a combination of investigations (clinical evaluation—WHO class, syncope, worsening symptoms and 6MWT; biochemical—BNP/ NT pro BNP; echocardiography—RA area and presence of pericardial effusions; RHC hemodynamic data—CI, mixed venous oxygen saturation and RAP). A score of 1–3 is assigned to each variable according to its value, where low risk is 1 point, intermediate-risk is 2 points and high risk is 3 points. The average score is indicative of the global patient risk. The disadvantage of this 3 strata model is that 70% of patients are included in the intermediate risk group. A simpler, 4 strata model was designed based on registry data, using just 3 variables (WHO class, NT pro BNP, 6 MWD) to better asses risk in the intermediate risk group [84].

Therapy

Presence of PoPH is associated with worse outcomes. In patients who did not receive medical therapy for PoPH and did not undergo LT, one study showed a 5 year survival of 14%, with 54% of deaths occurring in the 1st year. When pulmonary vasodilatory medication was used, survival at 5 years improved to 45% [85].

An study followed 174 PoPH patients from the REVEAL registry for 3 years and compared their evolution to that of idiopathic PAH patients. The authors found that patients with PoPH had a better hemodynamic profile and functional class, but despite of that, they had worse outcomes. Patients with PoPH were less likely to be on medical therapy [86]. Another report, also from the REVEAL registry, encompassing 156 patients followed for 1 year [72], also showed worse outcomes for PoPH patients (83% survival compared to 93% in idiopathic PAH). Data from the Spanish registry for PAH, REPAH, also confirmed better hemodynamic profile of PoPH patients, with worse survival (49.3% versus 68.7% at 5 years) and lower treatment rates compared to idiopathic PAH. Treated PoPH patients also had a better survival [73].

Medical therapy used in PAH patients improves survival in PoPH patients. The pulmonary vasodilatory medication acts on 3 pathways:

- The nitric oxide (NO) pathway—phosphodiesterase 5 inhibitors (PDE5i) Sildenafil, Tadalafil and soluble guanylate cyclase (sGC) stimulator—Riociguat;
- Endothelin pathway—endothelin receptor antagonists (ERAs) Macitentan, Bosentan, Ambrisentan;
- Prostacyclin pathway—prostacyclin (PGI2) Epoprostenol, Treprostinil and prostacyclin receptor agonists Selexipag;

In severe PAH and high risk patients up-front double or triple therapy should be used. In PoPH, because of side effects that can be more severe in ESLD patients due to a longer half time and risk of liver toxicity, treatment should start with monotherapy, up—titrating to double and triple therapy with caution. The aim of treatment is to lower the mPAP below 35 mmHg and make the patient eligible for LT, but also improve his PH risk and survival. In patients who are not at low risk the treatment should up-graded when possible.

Patients with PoPH have been excluded from most PAH trials. Most data is coming from registries.

NO promotes vasodilation by increasing the levels of secondary messenger cGMP which in turn produces smooth muscle relaxation. PDE5i act by preventing the degradation of cGMP, which results in increasing effects of NO. Riociguat's mechanism of action is represented by increased production of cGMP, determining a rise in NO action.

An initial study in 2005 [87] included 14 PoPH patients and demonstrated a positive effect of sildenafil on NT pro BNP and 6 MWT. Another study [88] showed improvement of PVR and mPAP allowing patients to be listed for LT. A more recent study included 25 patients who were treated either with sildenafil or tadalafil. The authors [89] demonstrated improved functional class WHO and hemodynamics, with no effect on 6 MWT.

PATENT 1 and 2 clinical trials with Riociguat were the first clinical trials for PAH that did not exclude PoPH patients. The total number of PoPH patients included in PATENT 1 was 13. It was demonstrated that in this population Riociguat is safe and improves functional capacity (WHO class and 6 MWT), effects that were maintained in the 2 year open label PATENT 2 [92].

ERAs decrease pulmonary hypertension by blocking endothelin-1 receptors, favouring vasodilation. Bosentan was the first in class drug. Multiple studies have demonstrated its efficacy and safety in this population [90, 91].

PORTICO is the only randomised trial ever designed specifically for PoPH patients. It showed Macitentan improves hemodynamic profile (35% reduction in PVR) and the most frequent adverse event was edema, with no hepatic safety concerns. 9% of patients on macitentan had adverse effects that required drug interruption [93].

An open label trial with Ambrisentan showed improved PVR, mPAP, CI and RAP, with improvement in WHO class but no change in 6 MWT. 31 patients were included, only 19 finished the study extension. The most frequent adverse events were edema and headache [94]. Neither PORTICO nor PATENT included Child C patients, only A and B.

Prostacyclin analogues have vasodilator, antithrombotic and antiproliferative effects. The most studied is epoprostenol, which has demonstrated hemodynamic benefits and multiple case series are published with PoPH patients improving and becoming eligible for transplant [96]. The negative part is that epoprostenol is not stable at room temperature and requires continuous i.v. administration through a tunnelled cathether. Lead infections and acute occlusions can complicate long term administration and abrupt stop is associated with severe rebound PH. Treprostinil, which is more easily to administer subcutaneously, is being increasingly used with similar efficacy [97]. It is also associated with administration site pain. Also used in patients with PoPH is inhaled iloprost [98]. Side effects of the class are jaw bone pain, muscle pain, headaches and diarrhoea, making treatment difficult to tolerate.

Data from the French PAH registry was analysed. The authors included 637 PoPH patients evaluated between 2007 and 2017. The majority of patients were initiated on monotherapy (74%, either an ERA or a PDE5i); 15% were initiated on double oral combination therapy and 1% on triple therapy. Patients on double therapy had a better hemodynamic response. The majority of patients were Child A, mean MELD was 11. Baseline sex, age, 6 MWT and MELD/ Child class were independent risk factors. Patients who underwent liver transplant had a better survival, specific PAH medication was stopped or down-titrated after transplant in most cases [95].

A retrospective study in Japan [99] included 386 PoPH patients, the data was obtained from the general medical data base and was based on the diagnosis. In the first 90 days 20.5% of patients received monotherapy and 16.6% received double therapy. Prostacyclin was used in 8.8% of cases. This is low considering that the Japanese PAH registry data [100] has demonstrated that dual therapy had a significant effect on PVR, mPAP and CI, while monotherapy showed improvement without reaching statistical significance. 66% of patients were on dual therapy, the reported survival at 3 and 5 years were better than in other registries (88% and 80.2% respectively).

In conclusion, specific PAH therapy in PoPH is underused although it improves survival and the effect on hemodynamic profile can make a patient eligible for LT.

Supportive therapeutic measures consist of sodium restriction, diuretics to treat congestion and oxygen in order to maintain a $SpO_2 > 90\%$ to prevent further vasoconstriction in the pulmonary circulation. Anticoagulants are not recommended as they increase the risk of bleeding in this population. Calcium channel blockers increase splanchnic vasodilation and are also contraindicated.

Implication for LT Decision

As was discussed, severe PoPH (mPAP > 45 mmHg) is an absolute contraindication for LT as an early trial demonstrated 100% mortality in the perioperative setting in these patients. These patients should be treated with PAH specific medication in order to improve survival and functional capacity. Patients with moderate PoPH should be treated with specific PAH medication with a double end point—lowering mortality but also, if the mPAP is reduced to less than 35 mmHg, LT can be considered. The French PAH registry data showed better outcomes in patients who were eligible for LT [95]. A metanalysis [101] and a retrospective study [102] showed that in selected PoPH cases, when LT is both necessary because of ESLD and also safe because of the improved mPAP with vasodilatory medication, combining LT and specific therapy is associated with improved survival. Half of the patients are able to interrupt medication after transplant. Long time survival after LT in PoPH patients is not as good as in non PoPH transplant candidates (60% at 5 years) and elevated PVR before surgery are associated with worse outcomes. The American Association for the Study of Liver Diseases recommends that LT should be considered in patients with mPAP < 35 mmHg and PVR < 5 WU [104]. The guidelines of the International Society of Liver Transplantation also consider for transplant patients with mPAP > 35 mmHg if they have PVR < 3 WU [103]. That is based on a study [106] that showed 1 year survival of 69% (11 out of 16 patients, with only one death due to cardiovascular causes) and by that time 63% of the patients had been weaned off PAH specific therapy. The hypothesis the authors started from was that the mPAP can be increased also because of concomitant overload and high CO which are common in ESLD. Elevated PVR could help identify patients with more significant pulmonary vascular disease component, at higher risk during LT surgery.

As with LT, considering TIPS in patients with PoPH requires careful selection. Increasing the preload of an already strained right ventricle can lead to heart failure decompensation. Severe PoPH is an absolute contraindication for TIPS [105].

To conclude, patients with ESLD that are candidates for LT should be screened for PoPH with transthoracic echocardiography. It is important that the diagnosis is confirmed by RHC and that the patients are managed in expert centres with experience in both diseases. PoPH patients should receive specific PAH medication and this should be initiated as soon as possible, as it improves survival.

Hepatopulmonary Syndrome

Definition and Classification

The hepatopulmonary syndrome (HPS) is defined by a combination of 3 criteria:

- hypoxemia
- presence of intrapulmonary vascular dilatation (IPVD)
- ESLD

IPVD cause increased alveolar—arterial oxygen gradient $P(A\text{-}a)O_2$ in room air (>15 mmHg, or >20 mmHg in patients >64 years of age). This results in right to left shunting and hypoxemia.

IPVD can be found in up to 40–60% of cirrhotic patients, but only 15–30% of patients have associated hypoxemia and meet the diagnostic criteria for HPS [107]. Patients with HPS have worse outcomes and it is important to be diagnosed early. During LT surgery patients have increased mortality compared to non HPS patients, but less so compared to PoPH patients. As HPS is mostly reversible after LT and there is no other therapeutic option, listing for LT should be considered early, preferably in centres with experience.

HPS is classified based on PaO2 (arterial oxygen tension) in

- mild>80 mmHg
- moderate 60–79 mmHg
- severe 50–59 mmHg
- very severe <50 mmHg

Pathophysiology

The physiology of HPS is not clearly known but it is linked to the hyperdynamic circulation associating liver cirrhosis. In HPS patients there is an imbalance in the vascular tone with the predominance of vasodilation. There are multiple mechanisms responsible for hypoxemia, not only arteriovenous shunting but also ventilation-perfusion mismatch and diffusion alteration. Because of its impaired function there is an inadequate liver clearance of vasoactive substances from the splanchnic circulation such as NO, PGI2, vasoactive intestinal peptide, endothelin-1 etc. In combination with the opening of the portosystemic these molecules reach the pulmonary circulation and determine a functional vasodilatation of the pulmonary arterioles. As was discussed earlier, cirrhosis is associated with increased levels of bile acids in the systemic and pulmonary circulation. Bacterial translocation determines increased levels of endotoxins. This determines activation of pulmonary macrophages, which produce inflammatory cytokines like and TNFα̇ and trigger production of vasodilators (NO, CO) and angiogenetic factors like vascular endothelial growth factor (VEGF) [108]. Reducing gut bacteria with antibiotic treatment can help reduce HPS incidence. Sorafenib, which has anti-VEGF effects, is being studied in HPS. Excess endothelin-1 in liver disease can cause both vasoconstriction and vasodilation. Stimulating the receptor ET-1B activates NOS and production of NO. This causes endothelial dysfunction and lead to IPVD and shunts, blood being redirected to the arterial circulation before reaching the alveoli. Possible therapies using ET-1B blockage or NO inhibition are being studied [109].

Because of the vasodilation there is an increase in blood flow to the alveoli, yet ventilation remains unchanged, creating ventilation—perfusion mismatch. Also due to vasodilation the exchange of oxygen in the alveoli is altered, the molecules having to pass through a thicker layer. The blood cells travel at higher speed because of the hyperdynamic circulation, which makes the time for oxygenation shorter [109].

Diagnostic

Most patients are asymptomatic and HPS must be actively searched. On clinical examination patients can present with cyanosis and digital clubbing. The pathognomonic sign is dyspnea and platypnea due to orthodeoxia (decrease of SpO2 of 5% or more in orthostatic position compared to supine) [110].

In patients with dyspnea, peripheral oxygen saturation should be measured using a pulse-oximetry. Measurements in standing position should also be performed. If below 96%, arterial blood gasses analysis should be performed. If PaO2 is below 80 mmHg and P(A-a)O2 > 15 mmHg a contrast enhanced transthoracic echocardiography (CE-TTE) using agitated saline serum should be performed to confirm the intrapulmonary shunt (presence of bubbles in the left atria after 3–6 cardiac cycles) [111].This is the gold standard in HPS diagnosis as it can differentiate from intracardiac shunts (presence of microbubbles in the first 3 cycles). Transoesophageal echocardiography has more sensitivity for intracardiac shunts but because of the theoretical risk of variceal bleeding it is less used. Also, pulmonary function tests must be performed to exclude a concomitant pulmonary comorbidity. If HPS is confirmed, there is no associated lung disease, and PaO2 is below 60 mmHg (corresponding to a SpO2 < 90%) patients should be listed for transplant with an exception from the MELD score. Patients with PaO2 > 60 mmHg should be followed and listed for LT according to MELD score.

Technetium macroaggregated albumin lung perfusion scan (^{99m}TcMAA) is a less sensitive and more invasive way to screen for HPS. It cannot distinguished from intrapulmonary from intracardiac shunts. The macroaggregates are normally trapped in the pulmonary vessels but in HPS patients or in patients with an intracardiac shunt, they bypass the pulmonary circulation and there is brain and kidneys up-take which can be measured [112].

Contrast thoracic CT scan can also show signs of intrapulmonary shunts [113].

Pulmonary arteriography can be performed in case of suspected large intrapulmonary shunts that might be suitable for embolization.

HPS can coexist with other cardiac and pulmonary comorbidities and increase the severity of hypoxemia they determine. It is important to exclude them as part of the diagnosis process (tuberculosis, asthma, pulmonary idiopathic fibrosis, heart failure etc.).

Prognosis and Liver Transplant Decision

Medical treatment for HPS has not yet proven efficient. Patients with mild and moderate HPS, with PaO2 > 60 mmHg should be followed-up periodically.

In patients with severe HPS, long term oxygen therapy should be recommended. These patients should be listed for LT with priority, as they have a worse outcome than patients with ESLD without HPS.

In patients with very severe disease, PaO2 < 50 mmHg there is a high risk of negative outcomes during transplant surgery and decision to go ahead with LT is centre based.

After LT, the majority of patients improve in the next 6–12 months (1977) [114]. Perioperative management is crucial, as induction of anesthesia can cause severe drop in SpO2. During surgery and in post-operatory setting it is important to avoid both hypovolemia and volume overload. Hypoxemia can worsen after LT and in some cases use of ECMO was necessary [115].

Coexistence of PoPH and HPS within one patient has been reported. Intrapulmonary vasodilatation is common in PoPH and the concomitant diagnoses of PoPH and HPS are increasingly being described and are not mutually exclusive conditions. Patients with cirrhosis and concomitant HPS and PoPH are difficult to manage, usually they are treated with PAH targeted therapy, HPS is managed supportively and afterwards are referred to LT in order to expedite resolution of HPS [106].

In summary, in HPS, hypoxemia is generally progressive and post LT outcomes are worse in very severe cases. As LT cures HPS, the disease is an indication for LT. In PoPH, post liver transplant outcome can be unpredictable and mortality increases with worsening pulmonary hypertension. Vasodilators are key in reducing pulmonary pressure. A standard exception from MELD score can be requested if pulmonary pressure is adequately reduced on specific medication. Diagnosis and management of these pulmonary complications related to liver disease are challenging and require a multidisciplinary approach involving hepatologists, cardiologists and pulmonologists.

References

1. Iwakiri Y, Groszmann RJ. The hyperdynamic circulation of chronic liver diseases: from the patient to the molecule. Hepatology. 2006;43:S121–31. https://doi.org/10.1002/hep.20993.
2. Moreau R, Lebrec D. Molecular mechanisms of systemic vasodilation and hyperdynamic circulatory state of cirrhosis. In: Sanyal AJ, Shah VH, editors. Portal hypertension. Clinical gastroenterology. Humana Press; 2005. p. 51–64. https://doi.org/10.1007/978-1-59259-885-4_4.
3. Licata A, Mazzola A, Ingrassia D, et al. Clinical implications of the hyperdynamic syndrome in cirrhosis. Eur J Intern Med. 2014;25:795–802. https://doi.org/10.1016/j.ejim.2014.09.004.
4. Møller S, Bendtsen F, Henriksen JH. Effect of volume expansion on systemic hemodynamics and central and arterial blood volume in cirrhosis. Gastroenterology. 1995;109:1917–25. https://doi.org/10.1016/0016-5085(95)90759-9.
5. Arroyo V, Terra C, Ginès P. Advances in the pathogenesis and treatment of type-1 and type-2 hepatorenal syndrome. J Hepatol. 2007;46:935–46. https://doi.org/10.1016/j.jhep.2007.02.001.
6. Gao J, Liu X, Wang B, et al. Farnesoid X receptor deletion improves cardiac function, structure and remodeling following myocardial infarction in mice. Mol Med Rep. 2017;16:673–9. https://doi.org/10.3892/mmr.2017.6643.
7. Kaur H, Premkumar M. Diagnosis and management of cirrhotic cardiomyopathy. J Clin Exp Hepatol. 2022;12:186–99. https://doi.org/10.1016/j.jceh.2021.08.016.
8. Møller S, Lee SS. Cirrhotic cardiomyopathy. J Hepatol. 2018;69:958–60. https://doi.org/10.1016/j.jhep.2018.01.006.
9. Chayanupatkul M, Liangpunsakul S. Cirrhotic cardiomyopathy: review of pathophysiology and treatment. Hepatol Int. 2014;8:308–15. https://doi.org/10.1007/s12072-014-9531-y.
10. Sharma A, Fletcher A, Lipscomb GR. Pulmonary oedema after therapeutic ascitic paracentesis: a case report and literature review of the cardiac complications of cirrhosis. Eur J Gastroenterol Hepatol. 2010;22:241–5. https://doi.org/10.1097/meg.0b013e32833110f7.
11. Izzy M, VanWagner LB, Lin G, et al. Redefining cirrhotic cardiomyopathy for the modern era. Hepatology. 2020;71:334–45. https://doi.org/10.1002/hep.30875.
12. Moller S, Henriksen JH. Cardiovascular complications of cirrhosis. Gut. 2008;57:268–78. https://doi.org/10.1136/gut.2006.112177.
13. Meunier-McVey N. 2021 ESC guidelines for the diagnosis and treatment of acute and chronic heart failure. EMJ Cardiol. 2021:22–5. https://doi.org/10.33590/emjcardiol/21f1011.
14. Razpotnik M, Bota S, Wimmer P, et al. Prevalence of cirrhotic cardiomyopathy according to the old and new diagnostic criteria. J Hepatol. 2020;73:S740–1. https://doi.org/10.1016/s0168-8278(20)31930-9.
15. Shahvaran SA, Menyhárt O, Csedrik L, Patai ÁV. Diagnosis and prevalence of cirrhotic cardiomyopathy: a systematic review and meta-analysis. Curr Probl Cardiol. 2021;46:100821. https://doi.org/10.1016/j.cpcardiol.2021.100821.

16. Ali SA, Arman HE, Shamseddeen H, et al. Cirrhotic cardiomyopathy: predictors of major adverse cardiac events and assessment of reversibility after liver transplant. J Cardiol. 2023;82:113–21. https://doi.org/10.1016/j.jjcc.2023.04.007.
17. Cesari M, Chiara Frigo A, Piano S, Angeli P. Prevalence and prognostic value of cirrhotic cardiomyopathy as defined according to the proposed new classification. Clin Exp Hepatol. 2021;7:270–7. https://doi.org/10.5114/ceh.2021.108708.
18. Pagourelias ED, Sotiriou P, Papadopoulos CE, et al. Left ventricular myocardial mechanics in cirrhosis: a speckle tracking echocardiographic study. Echocardiography. 2016;33:223–32. https://doi.org/10.1111/echo.13010.
19. Mechelinck M, Hartmann B, Hamada S, et al. Global longitudinal strain at rest as an independent predictor of mortality in liver transplant candidates: a retrospective clinical study. J Clin Med. 2020;9:2616. https://doi.org/10.3390/jcm9082616.
20. Bernal V, Pascual I, Lanas A, et al. Cardiac function and aminoterminal pro-brain natriuretic peptide levels in liver-transplanted cirrhotic patients. Clin Transpl. 2012;26:111–6. https://doi.org/10.1111/j.1399-0012.2011.01438.x.
21. Silvestre OM, Bacal F, Ramos D de S, et al. Impact of the severity of end-stage liver disease in cardiac structure and function. Ann Hepatol. 2013;12:85–91. https://doi.org/10.1016/s1665-2681(19)31389-4.
22. Wehmeyer MH, Heuer AJ, Benten D, et al. High rate of cardiac abnormalities in a postmortem analysis of patients suffering from liver cirrhosis. J Clin Gastroenterol. 2015;49:866–72. https://doi.org/10.1097/mcg.0000000000000323.
23. Barbosa M. Cirrhotic cardiomyopathy: isn't stress evaluation always required for the diagnosis? WJH. 2016;8:200. https://doi.org/10.4254/wjh.v8.i3.200.
24. Pieske B, Tschöpe C, de Boer RA, et al. How to diagnose heart failure with preserved ejection fraction: the HFA–PEFF diagnostic algorithm: a consensus recommendation from the Heart Failure Association (HFA) of the European Society of Cardiology (ESC). Eur Heart J. 2019;40:3297–317. https://doi.org/10.1093/eurheartj/ehz641.
25. Dharancy S, Lemyze M, Boleslawski E, et al. Impact of impaired aerobic capacity on liver transplant candidates. Transplantation. 2008;86:1077–83. https://doi.org/10.1097/tp.0b013e318187758b.
26. Prentis JM, Manas DMD, Trenell MI, et al. Submaximal cardiopulmonary exercise testing predicts 90-day survival after liver transplantation. Liver Transpl. 2012;18:152–9. https://doi.org/10.1002/lt.22426.
27. Główczyńska R, Borodzicz-Jażdżyk S, Peller M, et al. Chronotropic incompetence in end-stage liver disease. PLoS One. 2022;17:e0270784. https://doi.org/10.1371/journal.pone.0270784.
28. Rudzinski W, Waller AH, Prasad A, et al. New index for assessing the chronotropic response in patients with end-stage liver disease who are undergoing dobutamine stress echocardiography. Liver Transpl. 2012;18:355–60. https://doi.org/10.1002/lt.22476.
29. Karagiannakis DS, Papatheodoridis G, Vlachogiannakos J. Recent advances in cirrhotic cardiomyopathy. Dig Dis Sci. 2015;60:1141–51. https://doi.org/10.1007/s10620-014-3432-8.
30. Scarlatescu E, Marchenko SP, Tomescu DR. Cirrhotic cardiomyopathy—a veiled threat. Cardiol Rev. 2022;30:80–9. https://doi.org/10.1097/crd.0000000000000377.
31. Chokesuwattanaskul R, Thongprayoon C, Bathini T, et al. Liver transplantation and atrial fibrillation: a meta-analysis. World J Hepatol. 2018;10:761–71. https://doi.org/10.4254/wjh.v10.i10.761.
32. Tsai S-H, Lin Y-Y, Chu S-J, et al. Interpretation and use of natriuretic peptides in non-congestive heart failure settings. Yonsei Med J. 2010;51:151. https://doi.org/10.3349/ymj.2010.51.2.151.
33. Yildiz R, Yildirim B, Karinkaoglu M, et al. Brain natriuretic peptide and severity of disease in non-alcoholic cirrhotic patients. J Gastroenterol Hepatol. 2005;20:1115–20. https://doi.org/10.1111/j.1440-1746.2005.03906.x.

34. Henriksen JH, Goetze JP, Fuglsang S, et al. Increased circulating pro-brain natriuretic peptide (PROBNP) and brain natriuretic peptide (BNP) in patients with cirrhosis. Relation to cardiovascular dysfunction and severity of disease. J Hepatol. 2003;38:29. https://doi.org/10.1016/s0168-8278(03)80497-x.
35. Coss E, Watt KDS, Pedersen R, et al. Predictors of cardiovascular events after liver transplantation: a role for pretransplant serum troponin levels. Liver Transpl. 2011;17:23–31. https://doi.org/10.1002/lt.22140.
36. Shah RV, Chen-Tournoux AA, Picard MH, et al. Galectin-3, cardiac structure and function, and long-term mortality in patients with acutely decompensated heart failure. Eur J Heart Fail. 2010;12:826–32. https://doi.org/10.1093/eurjhf/hfq091.
37. Pejnovic N, Jeftic I, Jovicic N, et al. Galectin-3 and IL-33/ST2 axis roles and interplay in diet-induced steatohepatitis. World J Hepatol. 2016;22:9706. https://doi.org/10.3748/wjg.v22.i44.9706.
38. Voiosu AM, Bălănescu P, Daha I, et al. The diagnostic and prognostic value of serum endocan in patients with cirrhotic cardiomyopathy. Rom J Intern Med. 2018;56:182–92. https://doi.org/10.2478/rjim-2018-0007.
39. Wiese S, Hove J, Mo S, et al. Myocardial extracellular volume quantified by magnetic resonance is increased in cirrhosis and related to poor outcome. Liver Int. 2018;38:1614–23. https://doi.org/10.1111/liv.13870.
40. Lewin SM, Kallianos K, Nevah MI, et al. Cardiac MRI T2* in liver transplant candidates: application and performance of a novel imaging technique to identify patients at risk for poor posttransplant cardiac outcomes. Transplant Direct. 2018;4:e363. https://doi.org/10.1097/txd.0000000000000803.
41. VanWagner LB, Ning H, Whitsett M, et al. A point-based prediction model for cardiovascular risk in orthotopic liver transplantation: the CAR-OLT score. Hepatology. 2017;66:1968–79. https://doi.org/10.1002/hep.29329.
42. Dimitroglou Y, Tsartsalis D, Vasilieva L, et al. HFA-PEFF score as an independent predictor of 2-year mortality in liver cirrhosis patients. Eur J Gastroenterol Hepatol. 2023;35:204–11. https://doi.org/10.1097/meg.0000000000002472.
43. Turco L, Reiberger T, Vitale G, La Mura V. Carvedilol as the new non-selective beta-blocker of choice in patients with cirrhosis and portal hypertension. Liver Int. 2023;43:1183–94. https://doi.org/10.1111/liv.15559.
44. Safadi A, Homsi M, Maskoun W, et al. Perioperative risk predictors of cardiac outcomes in patients undergoing liver transplantation surgery. Circulation. 2009;120:1189–94. https://doi.org/10.1161/circulationaha.108.847178.
45. Tergast TL, Kimmann M, Laser H, et al. Systemic arterial blood pressure determines the therapeutic window of non-selective beta blockers in decompensated cirrhosis. Aliment Pharmacol Ther. 2019;50:696–706. https://doi.org/10.1111/apt.15439.
46. Premkumar M, Rangegowda D, Vyas T, et al. Carvedilol combined with ivabradine improves left ventricular diastolic dysfunction, clinical progression, and survival in cirrhosis. J Clin Gastroenterol. 2020;54:561–8. https://doi.org/10.1097/mcg.0000000000001219.
47. Hsu W-F, Yu S-H, Lin J-T, et al. Renal effects of angiotensin-converting enzyme inhibitors and angiotensin receptor blockers in patients with liver cirrhosis: a nationwide cohort study. Gastroenterol Res Pract. 2019;2019:1–8. https://doi.org/10.1155/2019/1743290.
48. Refardt J, Imber C, Nobbenhuis R, et al. Treatment effect of the SGLT2 inhibitor empagliflozin on chronic syndrome of inappropriate antidiuresis: results of a randomized, double-blind, placebo-controlled, crossover trial. J Am Soc Nephrol. 2023;34:322–32. https://doi.org/10.1681/asn.2022050623.
49. Brankovic M, Lee P, Pyrsopoulos N, Klapholz M. Cardiac syndromes in liver disease: a clinical conundrum. J Clin Transl Hepatol. 2023;11(4):975–86. https://doi.org/10.14218/jcth.2022.00294.

50. Escobar B, Taurá P, Martínez-Palli G, et al. Stroke volume response to liver graft reperfusion stress in cirrhotic patients. World J Surg. 2014;38:927–35. https://doi.org/10.1007/s00268-013-2289-x.
51. Sharma S, Prasad A, Karamchandani K. Extracorporeal membrane oxygenation in a patient with cirrhotic cardiomyopathy: a case report. J Cardiothorac Vasc Anesth. 2019;33:173–5. https://doi.org/10.1053/j.jvca.2018.02.017.
52. Sharma S, Karamchandani K, Wilson R, et al. Acute heart failure after orthotopic liver transplantation: a case series from one center. BMC Anesthesiol. 2018;18:102. https://doi.org/10.1186/s12871-018-0560-2.
53. Farr M, Verna E, Takayama H, et al. Acute myocardial failure after liver transplantation: Tako-Tsubo or undiagnosed cirrhotic cardiomyopathy? Transplantation. 2014;98:790–1. https://doi.org/10.1097/00007890-201407151-02708.
54. Aggarwal S, Kang Y, Freeman JA, et al. Postreperfusion syndrome: hypotension after reperfusion of the transplanted liver. J Crit Care. 1993;8:154–60. https://doi.org/10.1016/0883-9441(93)90021-c.
55. Matsusaki T, Hilmi IA, Planinsic RM, et al. Cardiac arrest during adult liver transplantation: a single institution's experience with 1238 deceased donor transplants. Liver Transpl. 2013;19:1262–71. https://doi.org/10.1002/lt.23723.
56. Sakr AE, Fraser GE, Doctorian TP, et al. Predictors of systolic heart failure and mortality following orthotopic liver transplantation: a single-center cohort. Transplant Proc. 2019;51:1950–5. https://doi.org/10.1016/j.transproceed.2019.04.063.
57. Eimer MJ, Wright JM, Wang EC, et al. Frequency and significance of acute heart failure following liver transplantation. Am J Cardiol. 2008;101:242–4. https://doi.org/10.1016/j.amjcard.2007.08.056.
58. Scholte NTB, Lenzen MJ, van der Hoven B, et al. In-hospital cardiovascular events after liver transplantation: predictors and long-term outcome. Neth Hear J. 2018;26:506–11. https://doi.org/10.1007/s12471-018-1144-y.
59. Zardi EM, Abbate A, Zardi DM, et al. Cirrhotic cardiomyopathy. J Am Coll Cardiol. 2010;56:539–49. https://doi.org/10.1016/j.jacc.2009.12.075.
60. Miyamoto Y, Honda A, Yokose S, et al. The effects of SGLT2 inhibitors on liver cirrhosis patients with refractory ascites: a literature review. J Clin Med. 2023;12:2253. https://doi.org/10.3390/jcm12062253.
61. Zhou P, Tan Y, Hao Z, et al. Effects of SGLT2 inhibitors on hepatic fibrosis and steatosis: a systematic review and meta-analysis. Front Endocrinol. 2023;14:1144838. https://doi.org/10.3389/fendo.2023.1144838.
62. Xu Z, Hu W, Wang B, et al. Canagliflozin ameliorates nonalcoholic fatty liver disease by regulating lipid metabolism and inhibiting inflammation through induction of autophagy. Yonsei Med J. 2022;63:619. https://doi.org/10.3349/ymj.2022.63.7.619.
63. Eyvazian VA, Gordin JS, Yang EH, et al. Incidence, predictors, and outcomes of new-onset left ventricular systolic dysfunction after orthotopic liver transplantation. J Card Fail. 2019;25:166–72. https://doi.org/10.1016/j.cardfail.2018.10.013.
64. Torregrosa M, Aguadé S, Dos L, et al. Cardiac alterations in cirrhosis: reversibility after liver transplantation. J Hepatol. 2005;42:68–74. https://doi.org/10.1016/j.jhep.2004.09.008.
65. Barman PM, VanWagner LB. Cardiac risk assessment in liver transplant candidates: current controversies and future directions. Hepatology. 2021;73:2564–76. https://doi.org/10.1002/hep.31647.
66. Rachwan RJ, Kutkut I, Timsina LR, et al. CAD-LT score effectively predicts risk of significant coronary artery disease in liver transplant candidates. J Hepatol. 2021;75:142–9. https://doi.org/10.1016/j.jhep.2021.01.008.
67. Giles R. The 2022 ESC/ERS guidelines for the diagnosis and treatment of pulmonary hypertension. Eur Heart J. 2022;43(38):3618–731. https://doi.org/10.55788/c838601b.
68. Galie N. 2015 ESC/ERS Guidelines for the diagnosis and treatment of pulmonary hypertension. The Joint Task Force for the Diagnosis and Treatment of Pulmonary Hypertension of

the European Society of Cardiology (ESC) and the European Respiratory Society (ERS). Eur Respir J. 2015;46:903–75. Eur Respir J 46:1855–1856. https://doi.org/10.1183/13993003.51032-2015.
69. Galiè N, McLaughlin VV, Rubin LJ, Simonneau G. An overview of the 6th world symposium on pulmonary hypertension. Eur Respir J. 2019;53:1802148. https://doi.org/10.1183/13993003.02148-2018.
70. Castro M, Krowka MJ, Schroeder DR, et al. Frequency and clinical implications of increased pulmonary artery pressures in liver transplant patients. Mayo Clin Proc. 1996;71:543–51. https://doi.org/10.4065/71.6.543.
71. Mandell MS, Groves BM. Pulmonary hypertension in chronic liver disease. Clin Chest Med. 1996;17:17–33. https://doi.org/10.1016/s0272-5231(05)70296-3.
72. McGoon M, Miller D, Barst R. REVEAL registry: one year outcome of patients with portopulmonary hypertension (PoPH). In: American Thoracic Society 2009 international conference; 2009. https://doi.org/10.1164/ajrccm-conference.2009.179.1_meetingabstracts.a4915.
73. Lazaro Salvador M, Quezada Loaiza CA, Rodríguez Padial L, et al. Portopulmonary hypertension: prognosis and management in the current treatment era—results from the REHAP registry. Intern Med J. 2021;51:355–65. https://doi.org/10.1111/imj.14751.
74. Navarro-Vergara DI, Roldan-Valadez E, Cueto-Robledo G, Jurado-Hernandez MY. Portopulmonary hypertension: prevalence, clinical and hemodynamic features. Curr Probl Cardiol. 2021;46:100747. https://doi.org/10.1016/j.cpcardiol.2020.100747.
75. Hadengue A, Benhayoun MK, Lebrec D, Benhamou J-P. Pulmonary hypertension complicating portal hypertension: prevalence and relation to splanchnic hemodynamics. Gastroenterology. 1991;100:520–8. https://doi.org/10.1016/0016-5085(91)90225-a.
76. Krowka MJ, Swanson KL, Frantz RP, et al. Portopulmonary hypertension: results from a 10-year screening algorithm. Hepatology. 2006;44:1502–10. https://doi.org/10.1002/hep.21431.
77. Chen H-S, Xing S-R, Xu W-G, et al. Portopulmonary hypertension in cirrhotic patients: prevalence, clinical features and risk factors. Exp Ther Med. 2013;5:819–24. https://doi.org/10.3892/etm.2013.918.
78. Rodríguez-Almendros N, Toapanta-Yanchapaxi LN, Aguirre Valadez J, et al. Hipertensión portopulmonar: Revisión actualizada. Arch Cardiol Mex. 2018;88:25–38. https://doi.org/10.1016/j.acmx.2016.11.002.
79. Krowka M. Pulmonary hemodynamics and perioperative cardiopulmonary-related mortality in patients with portopulmonary hypertension undergoing liver transplantation. Liver Transpl. 2000;6:443–50. https://doi.org/10.1053/jlts.2000.6356.
80. Jasso-Baltazar EA, Peña-Arellano GA, Aguirre-Valadez J, et al. Portopulmonary hypertension: an updated review. Transplant Direct. 2023;9:e1517. https://doi.org/10.1097/txd.0000000000001517.
81. Kawut SM, Krowka MJ, Trotter JF, et al. Clinical risk factors for portopulmonary hypertension. Hepatology. 2008;48:196–203. https://doi.org/10.1002/hep.22275.
82. Kim W. Accuracy of doppler echocardiography in the assessment of pulmonary hypertension in liver transplant candidates. Liver Transpl. 2000;6:453–8. https://doi.org/10.1053/jlts.2000.7573.
83. Raevens S, Colle I, Reyntjens K, et al. Echocardiography for the detection of portopulmonary hypertension in liver transplant candidates: an analysis of cutoff values. Liver Transpl. 2013;19:602–10. https://doi.org/10.1002/lt.23649.
84. Hoeper MM, Pausch C, Olsson KM, et al. COMPERA 2.0: a refined four-stratum risk assessment model for pulmonary arterial hypertension. Eur Respir J. 2022;60:2102311. https://doi.org/10.1183/13993003.02311-2021.
85. Swanson KL, Wiesner RH, Nyberg SL, et al. Survival in portopulmonary hypertension: mayo clinic experience categorized by treatment subgroups. Am J Transplant. 2008;8:2445–53. https://doi.org/10.1111/j.1600-6143.2008.02384.x.

86. Krowka MJ, Miller DP, Barst RJ et all (2012) Portopulmonary hypertension: a report from the US-based REVEAL registry. Chest. https://doi.org/10.1378/chest.11-0160. Epub 2011 Jul 21. PMID: 21778257.
87. Reichenberger F, Voswinckel R, Steveling E, et al. Sildenafil treatment for portopulmonary hypertension. Eur Respir J. 2006;28:563–7. https://doi.org/10.1183/09031936.06.00030206.
88. Gough MS, White RJ. Sildenafil therapy is associated with improved hemodynamics in liver transplantation candidates with pulmonary arterial hypertension. Liver Transpl. 2009;15:30–6. https://doi.org/10.1002/lt.21533.
89. Fisher JH, Johnson SR, Chau C, et al. Effectiveness of phosphodiesterase-5 inhibitor therapy for portopulmonary hypertension. Can Respir J. 2015;22:42–6. https://doi.org/10.1155/2015/810376.
90. Savale L, Magnier R, Le Pavec J, et al. Efficacy, safety and pharmacokinetics of bosentan in portopulmonary hypertension. Eur Respir J. 2013;41:96–103. https://doi.org/10.1183/09031936.00117511.
91. Halank M, Miehlke S, Hoeffken G, et al. Use of oral endothelin-receptor antagonist bosentan in the treatment of portopulmonary hypertension. Transplantation. 2004;77:1775–6. https://doi.org/10.1097/01.tp.0000122420.86904.89.
92. Cartin-Ceba R, Halank M, Ghofrani H, et al. Riociguat treatment for portopulmonary hypertension: a subgroup analysis from the PATENT-1/-2 studies. Pulm Circ. 2018;8:1–4. https://doi.org/10.1177/2045894018769305.
93. Sitbon O, Bosch J, Cottreel E, et al. Macitentan for the treatment of portopulmonary hypertension (PORTICO): a multicentre, randomised, double-blind, placebo-controlled, phase 4 trial. Lancet Respir Med. 2019;7:594–604. https://doi.org/10.1016/s2213-2600(19)30091-8.
94. Preston IR, Burger CD, Bartolome S, et al. Ambrisentan in portopulmonary hypertension: a multicenter, open-label trial. J Heart Lung Transplant. 2020;39:464–72. https://doi.org/10.1016/j.healun.2019.12.008.
95. Savale L, Guimas M, Ebstein N, et al. Portopulmonary hypertension in the current era of pulmonary hypertension management. J Hepatol. 2020;73(1):130–9. https://doi.org/10.1016/j.jhep.2020.02.021. Epub 2020 Mar 5. Erratum in: J Hepatol. 2020 Nov;73 (5):1293–1294. PMID: 32145258.
96. Sussman N, Kaza V, Barshes N, et al. Successful liver transplantation following medical management of portopulmonary hypertension: a single-center series. Am J Transplant. 2006;6:2177–82. https://doi.org/10.1111/j.1600-6143.2006.01432.x.
97. Hollatz TJ, Musat A, Westphal S, et al. Treatment with sildenafil and treprostinil allows successful liver transplantation of patients with moderate to severe portopulmonary hypertension. Liver Transpl. 2012;18:686–95. https://doi.org/10.1002/lt.23407.
98. Melgosa MT, Ricci GL, García-Pagan JC, et al. Acute and long-term effects of inhaled iloprost in portopulmonary hypertension. Liver Transpl. 2010;16:348–56. https://doi.org/10.1002/lt.21997.
99. Atsukawa M, Takano M, Omura J. Treatment pattern and clinical outcomes in portopulmonary hypertension: a database study in Japan. JGH Open. 2022;6:763–73. https://doi.org/10.1002/jgh3.12820.
100. Tamura Y, Tamura Y, Taniguchi Y, et al. Clinical management and outcomes of patients with portopulmonary hypertension enrolled in the Japanese multicenter registry. Circ Rep. 2022;4:542–9. https://doi.org/10.1253/circrep.cr-22-0098.
101. Deroo R, Trépo E, Holvoet T, et al. Vasomodulators and liver transplantation for portopulmonary hypertension: evidence from a systematic review and meta-analysis. Hepatology. 2020;72:1701–16. https://doi.org/10.1002/hep.31164.
102. Cartin-Ceba R, Swanson KL, Vargas H, et al. Clinical outcomes after liver transplantation in patients with portopulmonary hypertension. Transplantation. 2020;105(10):2283–90. https://doi.org/10.1164/ajrccm-conference.2020.201.1_meetingabstracts.a2916.

103. Sendra C, Carballo-Rubio V, Sousa JM. Hepatopulmonary syndrome and portopulmonary hypertension: management in liver transplantation in the Horizon 2020. Transplant Proc. 2020;52:1503–6. https://doi.org/10.1016/j.transproceed.2020.02.057.
104. Martin P, DiMartini A, Feng S, et al. Evaluation for liver transplantation in adults: 2013 practice guideline by the American Association for the Study of Liver Diseases and the American Society of Transplantation. Hepatology. 2014;59:1144–65. https://doi.org/10.1002/hep.26972.
105. Krowka MJ, Fallon MB, Kawut SM, et al. International liver transplant society practice guidelines. Transplantation. 2016;100:1440–52. https://doi.org/10.1097/tp.0000000000001229.
106. DuBrock HM, Runo JR, Sadd CJ, et al. Outcomes of liver transplantation in treated portopulmonary hypertension patients with a mean pulmonary arterial pressure ≥35 mmHg. Transplant Direct. 2020;6:e630. https://doi.org/10.1097/txd.0000000000001085.
107. Abrams GA, Jaffe CC, Hoffer PB, et al. Diagnostic utility of contrast echocardiography and lung perfusion scan in patients with hepatopulmonary syndrome. Gastroenterology. 1995;109:1283–8. https://doi.org/10.1016/0016-5085(95)90589-8.
108. Varghese J, Ilias-basha H, Dhanasekaran R, et al. Hepatopulmonary syndrome—past to present. Ann Hepatol. 2007;6:135–42. https://doi.org/10.1016/s1665-2681(19)31918-0.
109. Raevens S, Geerts A, Van Steenkiste C, et al. Hepatopulmonary syndrome and portopulmonary hypertension: recent knowledge in pathogenesis and overview of clinical assessment. Liver Int. 2015;35:1646–60. https://doi.org/10.1111/liv.12791.
110. Gómez FP, Martínez-Pallí G, Barberà JA, et al. Gas exchange mechanism of orthodeoxia in hepatopulmonary syndrome. Hepatology. 2004;40:660–6. https://doi.org/10.1002/hep.20358.
111. Bozkurt HS. Portabl pulse oxymetry and contrast echocardiography in hepatopulmonary syndrome diagnosis. mtd. 2022; https://doi.org/10.35514/mtd.2022.62.
112. Wolfe JD, Tashkin DP, Holly FE, et al. Hypoxemia of cirrhosis: detection of abnormal small pulmonary vascular channels by a quantitative radionuclide method. Am J Med. 1977;63(5):746–54. https://doi.org/10.1016/0002-9343(77)90161-9.
113. Herve P, Le Pavec J, Sztrymf B, et al. Pulmonary vascular abnormalities in cirrhosis. Best Pract Res Clin Gastroenterol. 2007;21:141–59. https://doi.org/10.1016/j.bpg.2006.07.011.
114. Swanson KL, Wiesner RH, Krowka MJ. Natural history of hepatopulmonary syndrome: impact of liver transplantation. Hepatology. 2005;41:1122–9. https://doi.org/10.1002/hep.20658.
115. Monsel A, Mal H, Brisson H, et al. Extracorporeal membrane oxygenation as a bridge to liver transplantation for acute respiratory distress syndrome-induced life-threatening hypoxaemia aggravated by hepatopulmonary syndrome. Crit Care. 2011;15:R234. https://doi.org/10.1186/cc10476.

Further Reading

DuBrock HM, Krowka MJ. The myths and realities of portopulmonary hypertension. Hepatology. 2020;72:1455–60. https://doi.org/10.1002/hep.31415.

Correction to: Assessment of Left Ventricular Contractile Reserve in Heart Failure

Serban Mihaileanu and Laura Antohi

Correction to: Chapter 8 in: M. Dorobanţu et al. (eds.), *Current Approach to Heart Failure*, https://doi.org/10.1007/978-3-031-96562-3_8

In the original version of the book, the following belated corrections have been incorporated:

The author name "Şerban Mihailеănu" has been changed to "Serban Mihaileanu" in the Frontmatter, and in Chapter 8.

The updated version of this chapter can be found at
https://doi.org/10.1007/978-3-031-96562-3_8

M. Dorobanţu et al. (eds.), *Current Approach to Heart Failure*,
https://doi.org/10.1007/978-3-031-96562-3_27

Index

M. Dorobanţu et al. (eds.), *Current Approach to Heart Failure*,
https://doi.org/10.1007/978-3-031-96562-3

B

C

N

U

V

MIX
Papier aus verantwortungsvollen Quellen
Paper from responsible sources
FSC® C105338

If you have any concerns about our products,
you can contact us on
ProductSafety@springernature.com

In case Publisher is established outside the EU,
the EU authorized representative is:
Springer Nature Customer Service Center GmbH
Europaplatz 3, 69115 Heidelberg, Germany

Printed by Libri Plureos GmbH
in Hamburg, Germany